591562

Su

THE NURSING PROCESS IN LATER MATURITY

Ruth Beckmann Murray

M. Marilyn Wilson Huelskoetter

Dorothy Lueckerath O'Driscoll

School of Nursing
St. Louis University

Prentice-Hall, Inc., Englewood Cliffs, New Jersey 07632

THE NURSING PROCESS IN LATER MATURITY

Library of Congress Cataloging in Publication Data
MURRAY, RUTH
    The nursing process in later maturity.

    Includes bibliographies and index.
    1. Geriatric nursing.   I. Huelskoetter, M.
Marilyn Wilson, joint author.   II. O'Driscoll,
Dorothy Lueckerath, joint author.   III. Title.
RC954.M87   610.73′65   79-15999
ISBN 0-13-627570-2

*This book is dedicated to the elderly—
who are vulnerable,
who face physical and emotional pain, loneliness, and death,
who have inspired us with their wisdom, integrity, and
forebearance.*

THE NURSING PROCESS IN LATER MATURITY
*Ruth Beckmann Murray, M. Marilyn Wilson Huelskoetter,
and Dorothy Lueckerath O'Driscoll*

Printed in the United States of America

10 9 8 7 6 5

Editorial/production supervision
    and interior design by Ian M. List
Chapter opening design by Virginia M. Soulé
Cover design by Virginia M. Soulé
Manufacturing buyer: Cathie Lenard

PRENTICE-HALL INTERNATIONAL, INC., *London*
PRENTICE-HALL OF AUSTRALIA PTY. LIMITED, *Sydney*
PRENTICE-HALL OF CANADA, LTD., *Toronto*
PRENTICE-HALL OF INDIA PRIVATE LIMITED, *New Delhi*
PRENTICE-HALL OF JAPAN, INC., *Tokyo*
PRENTICE-HALL OF SOUTHEAST ASIA PTE. LTD., *Singapore*
WHITEHALL BOOKS LIMITED, *Wellington, New Zealand*

contents

v

GROUP WORK WITH THE PERSON IN LATER MATURITY   82

4

unit **II**

SOCIETY AND LATER MATURITY:
Implications for Nursing Process
119

COMMUNITY RESOURCES FOR THE PERSON/FAMILY IN LATER MATURITY   160

7

LEGAL ISSUES AFFECTING THE PERSON IN LATER MATURITY   191

8

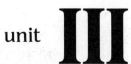

unit **III**

NORMAL AGING CHANGES IN LATER MATURITY:
Implications for Nursing Process
213

PHYSICAL CHANGES IN LATER MATURITY   214

9

COGNITIVE CHARACTERISTICS IN LATER MATURITY   241

EMOTIONAL DEVELOPMENT IN LATER MATURITY   **260**

11

unit **IV**

PHYSICAL ILLNESS IN LATER MATURITY:
Related Nursing Process
379

PROBLEMS OF MOBILITY IN LATER MATURITY   380

15

**PROBLEMS OF NEUROREGULATION
AND SENSORY PERCEPTION
IN LATER MATURITY   415**

**PROBLEMS OF TRANSPORTING
AND EXCHANGING OXYGEN
AND NUTRIENTS
IN LATER MATURITY   455**

PROBLEMS OF CELL PROLIFERATION AND PAIN IN LATER MATURITY   482

18

WITHDRAWAL AND THE SCHIZOPHRENIC SYNDROME IN LATER MATURITY   576

22

SUSPICION AND THE PARANOID PROCESS IN LATER MATURITY   600

to the reader

Major reasons for the lengthening of life span can be quickly categorized: better medical care, better nutrition, better use of preventive measures, a generally higher standard of living and more leisure time, and research in many areas that contributes toward making life more comfortable and healthier for more people.

However, society's attitudes, and thereby the attitudes of each of us, toward those who have lived long enough to become part of the aged statistics cannot be so quickly listed and resolved. The medical and nursing professions have not been quick to plan for or implement health care to meet the unique needs of people in later maturity—the not-so-old and the very old. Too often, the caring professions have reflected society's attitude; the 83-year-old is expected to behave and recuperate the way the 38-year-old does.

Theory about the biopsychosocial influences upon and biopsychosocial processes within the person/family in later maturity, in the era you may call old age, is drawn from several disciplines. The content is planned to help you increase your skill in assessing, diagnosing, planning for, implementing, and evaluating care for the person aged 65 or over who is generally well or ill. We discuss nursing diagnoses and interventions along with medical diagnoses and treatment. Because we have found that both nursing students and staff have difficulty formulating long-term and short-term goals, we have included statements that may help you in developing care plans. Chapter 2 on the nursing process sets the foundation for discussion of the nursing process throughout the book. We have purposefully developed the chapters on the helping relationship (Chapter 3) and on group process (Chapter 4) because their content is sometimes covered superficially in texts. Yet that content is basic to your understanding of and work with the elderly.

We have included both nursing and medical knowledge about physical and psychosocial aspects as well as our insights and experience. We feel that you as a professional will be able to synthesize and use the depth and breadth of scientific knowledge and experimental insight that this combined approach permits. In turn, you should feel more comfortable in collaborating as a member of the multidisciplinary team or in doing research to prevent illness or improve health care.

We hope to stimulate you to look at the person/family in later maturity with a more positive, yet realistic, attitude. We hope to stimulate your sense of empathy and compassion for the person you care for through an understanding of the aging process and all the social attitudes and stressors imposed upon the person.

We use the term *you* throughout the text in order to speak to you and involve you as an active reader. We hope that this will stimulate the integration of this information into your nursing so that your care will be more knowledgeable, compassionate, and practical.

We have looked at the person as a whole. We explain reasons for the elderly person's behavior so that you can better understand *why* he behaves as he does. We have taken a multidisciplinary approach by integrating information on physical, emotional, sociocultural, family, and legal aspects. We feel that as a professional you can take this information and apply insights as you move into care of the aged person/family. Your approach is crucial to maintaining the dignity of the person and the quality of his life.

Lastly, remember how very important you are to the elderly person with whom you work. Through an appraisal of your involvement with the person living through the last developmental stage you will grow in self-knowledge, self-acceptance, and fulfillment. These qualilties, which indicate a personal depth and integrity, may then become the basis for further compassionate, knowledgeable care.

ACKNOWLEDGMENTS

The authors thank their families for their support, patience, and assistance. Without the help of C. Edwin Murray, Frank, Michele, and Matthew Huelskoetter, and Patrick O'Driscoll with extra home responsibilities, this book would not be possible.

We thank Sister Mary Teresa Noth, Dean, School of Nursing, *St. Louis University,* for her encouragement, and Dr. Joseph Callahan, psychiatrist, for his suggestions and inspiration of ideas.

Special thanks goes to Karen Murphy and Sally Lehnert for their conscientious assistance in typing and preparing this manuscript and to Kathy Imbs and Carol Kramer for their help with typing.

Special thanks also to Sister Michele McConville, C.Pp.S., R.N., M.S.N., Assistant Professor of Psychiatric Nursing, for her contributions to Chapter 14.

In addition, the following persons are acknowledged for reviewing the manuscript, partially or in total: Margaret P. Benner, R.N., M.S.N, Assistant Professor, School of Nursing, *University of Delaware;* Marjorie J. Elmore, R.N., Ed.D., Professor Emeritus, Orvis School of Nursing, *University of Nevada;* Bernadene C. Hallinan, R.N., M.S., Director of Nursing, Chairperson of

Health Science Division, *Howard Community College;* Joan Hrubetz, R.N., Ph.D., Assistant Dean of Students, School of Nursing, *St. Louis University;* Sharon L. Roberts, R.N., M.S., Associate Professor, School of Nursing, *California State University at Long Beach;* Sister Marilyn Schwab, O.S.B., R.N., M.S.N., Nursing Consultant; Benedictine Nursing Center, Mt. Angel, Oregon; and Judith Proctor Zentner, R.N., M.A., Assistant Professor, Department of Nursing, Lenoir Rhyne College.

We also thank Prentice-Hall, Inc., especially William Gibson and Fred Henry, College Editors, and Ian List, the Production Editor, who gave valuable guidance during the preparation of the text.

St. Louis, Missouri   RUTH BECKMANN MURRAY, R.N., M.S.N.
M. MARILYN WILSON HUELSKOETTER, R.N., M.S.N.
DOROTHY LUECKERATH O'DRISCOLL, R.N., M.S.N.

AUTHORS

RUTH BECKMANN MURRAY, R.N., M.S.N., Professor of Psychiatric Nursing and Director, Continuing Nursing Education, School of Nursing, *St. Louis University,* St. Louis, Missouri.

M. MARILYN WILSON HUELSKOETTER, R.N., M.S.N., Associate Professor of Psychiatric Nursing and Chairman, Psychiatric Nursing Section, School of Nursing, *St. Louis University,* St. Louis, Missouri.

DOROTHY LUECKERATH O'DRISCOLL, R.N., M.S.N., J.D., Formerly Assistant Professor, School of Nursing, *St. Louis University,* St. Louis, Missouri, and *University of Missouri, Columbia.*

THE PERSON IN LATER MATURITY:
Basic Nursing Practice

unit **I**

introduction to
the person
in later maturity

Study of this chapter will enable you to:

1. Define later maturity, rather than old age, as the last developmental stage.

2. Define biological, psychological, and social aging.

3. Discuss personal definitions of *old* and *age* and factors that influence these definitions.

4. Explore personal values, attitudes, and feelings about aging and later maturity and explore the relationship of these to your behavior with persons in later maturity.

5. Discuss major theories of physiological aging.

6. Discuss major theories of psychosocial aging.

7. Use knowledge about theories of aging to explore the interdependence of physical, psychological, and social aging within the senior.

8. Critique research reports about the elderly, considering factors that influence the findings in research studies on the elderly.

1

WHAT IS LATER MATURITY?

Later maturity refers to the *last developmental stage in life, which begins after retirement, usually 65 to 70 years of age* in the United States. Traditionally, this era has been called old age. However, this stage may cover 30 or 40 years; no other developmental era covers such a time span. Therefore, some people refer to the *young-old, ages 65 or 70 to 75 or 80* years, and the *old-old, ages 75 or 80 years until death.* The end stage of later maturity is marked by dependency on others for assistance in meeting basic needs and may be called old age by some authors.[10]

Chronological age is a poor marker for development, but old age and retirement have been linked in our minds. Since some people are retiring before age 65 and the work years are now legally extended until age 70 or 75 for some groups of people, future age definitions of later maturity may change. Some people still feel middle-aged at 70 or even 75. What was once considered old age—45 to 65 years—is now middle age. As people live longer, it is likely that the period of middle age will be lengthened and that later maturity will begin at age 70 or 75.[2,51]

The definitions of old, aging, and aged are pertinent to later maturity, but they are not necessarily the same in meaning. *Old* is defined as *having existed for a long time or being advanced in years.*[15] *Aged* is defined as *that point in the life span of a person when changes of aging markedly interfere with functioning.*[49] *Aging* is commonly thought of as *those changes associated with declining function after the person reaches maturity.*[9] It has been said that aging begins with the onset of differentiation in utero or at birth. Some biologists believe that aging begins when the ability to reproduce ceases.

The person may be considered as old as he feels. *Biological age* refers to *the person's physiological status and position in time relative to his potential life span.*[23] *Psychological age* refers to *the person's ability to adapt to his environment using sensory functions, perceptual ability, memory, learning, problem-solving skills, motor skills, motivational level, attitudes, and personality characteristics.*[23] *Social age refers to the person's involvement in various roles in the family, at work, and in the community, how well he fulfills the expectations of others, and his interests and activities.*[23] Biological, psychological, and social age are interdependent, each involving certain processes, and the person may not be equally old in all biological, psychological, and social aspects.

Personal Definitions of Old and Age

The words *old* and *age* have different meanings to each of us, depending upon our self-image, personal patterns of adjustment, emotional conflicts, past experiences with elderly people, sociocultural and ethnic background, religion, and personal age. To the 4-year-old, 20 is ancient! To the teen-ager, 30 is old. To the 30-year-old, 50 begins to look younger. To the 75-year-old, old means

3

anyone over 80. To the average white American, old is associated with retirement from the job. To the Mexican-American, 50 years may be considered old.[3] The word *old* has negative connotations to many people in the United States, but in some cultures the old are revered.

The repulsion about growing old that exists is unrealistic when you consider the alternative. But the old are usually revered in cultures in which few people survive for a long number of years. Common fears and other negative feelings relate closely to the cultural attitudes found in the United States, which are learned by each of us. These attitudes and related feelings are hard to dispel.

No other developmental era is so rigidly stereotyped. In no way can all older people be alike any more than all toddlers, adolescents, or young adults can be alike. Their diversity is influenced not only by genetic, biological, environmental, cultural, religious, and familial differences, but also by the many years of unique stresses and experiences. Seniors must be perceived as individuals, each having a wide range of personality characteristics, distinct patterns of coping with life, and unique relationships to others.

SELF-AWARENESS AND LATER MATURITY

In order to perceive the senior as a unique person, you must consider your personal definitions, values, attitudes, and feelings about old age and aging. What does old age mean to you? What do you *value* or *consider important:* beauty, youth, and strength or wisdom, thoughtfulness, experience, and age? What is your *mental set* or *attitude* toward elderly people, which in turn affects your *behavior,* or *overt reactions?* Are the elderly useless or helpful? Irritating or lovable? Stingy or generous? Slow or deliberate? What is your *feeling* or *subjective response* when you are with the elderly? Do you feel pleasure or impatience, respect or repugnance? Do you fear growing old or do you look forward to later maturity? Certainly your behavior and feelings will vary, depending upon who you are and your situation. But your values and attitudes are a basic part of you and are more difficult to change.

After you have tried to be honest in answering the above questions, turn to the exercises in the Appendix of this chapter to gain further self-understanding. The exercises are included to help you assess your feelings and attitudes toward aging and elderly people. Your past experiences with others, fears, conflicts, and personality characteristics become the basis for your present values, attitudes, and feelings which are not necessarily right or wrong. They are a part of you, and as such, affect your behavior, level of compassion, and effectiveness as you nurse people.

When you initially care for elderly people, you may feel afraid, disgusted, or impatient. These feelings are not unusual. It is important that you face these feelings and try to understand your values and attitudes. Try to be open, honest, and accepting of yourself. Look at your strengths as well as your limits in caring for the elderly. Share your feelings with a trusted confidant so that you can gain another view of aging. Observe and listen to the feedback you receive from the elderly. If you remain open, you can learn how they see you, and if necessary, you can try to change in a desired direction. Work through feelings of anxiety, anger, depression, or rejection so that you can care for the person in later maturity more comfortably and effectively. Use every opportunity to learn about yourself as an aging person. Various courses and people may help. A searching attitude is imperative. You can begin to understand the basis for your feelings and express them more effectively. In turn, you can learn to deal with your feelings and perhaps change to positive feelings toward old people and old age.

Certainly, you won't like every old person you care for, but you will be more effective if you are not sad, angry at, or disgusted with him just because he is old and if you appreciate his strengths as well as his limits. If you can respect the person simply because he is a human being like yourself, accept his limits, and perceive him as a unique person, he will respond to your acceptance. As you understand and accept the person, he will share more of himself with you. His sharing is gratifying and will enable you to give even more of yourself. And so a helping relationship develops—one in which both of you mature.

This book will help you to realize that the active, alert, healthy, older people whom you know are not exceptions and that some of the physical characteristics you see are part of the normal aging process rather than characteristics of pathology. Understanding the normal psychological aspects of aging and some of the common deviations from normalcy will help you realize that common stereotypes are destructive to the dignity and worth of the person. Your knowledge will help you more accurately assess, plan, and give individualized care.

NUMBER OF PEOPLE REACHING LATER MATURITY

Feeling interested in and comfortable with the elderly people with whom you work is important. The aged are here to stay, and they will become even more visible. According to the 1976 Census figures, over 10 percent of the United States population—22 million people—are 65 years or older. Fourteen million of these elderly citizens are between 65 and 74 years; over 6 million are between 75 and 84, and almost 2 million are 85 or older. Compare that to the 20 percent who are middle-aged and the 69 percent who are under 45 and who will grow old someday. Life expectancy is increasing faster for females than for males, and while life expectancy for nonwhites is increasing, it still lags behind that of whites.[10] Among the aged Black population there are equal numbers of women and men living, but generally there are two aged women for every aged man.[41]

The increased number of people in the stage of later maturity is partly the result of increased average life expectancy. The primary reason is that more young people are reaching old age than ever before because of improved maternal-child care, communicable disease control, nutritional status, medical care for adults, sanitation, and general standard of living.[8,35] In 1900 the life expectancy in the United States was 43 years. Now the average man lives 78 years; the average woman lives 81 years.[4]

The increasing number of people in later maturity will influence health care delivery as well as our general society. The unique needs of the persons aged 65 to 85 and of those over 85 need to be considered separately and carefully. Well-conducted research can assist nurses to understand the elderly and find specific ways to help them.

THEORIES OF AGING

Research and the Elderly Person

Studies of the person in later maturity can be conducted through observation, interview, and formal research procedures. Although conclusions drawn from observation of and interview with the person are subjective, formal research studies may also yield data with limited or subjective results. Certain problems exist in doing research with elderly persons.

When you conduct your own research or read the results of others' research, be mindful that the following factors often color the research:

1. Young researchers are likely to interpret data negatively because of their own personal biases and because of society's stereotyping of the elderly person.
2. Medical professionals doing research treat normal aging as pathology.
3. Questions asked on tests designed to obtain data match the researcher's mind set and are likely to obtain results that he expects.
4. Normal caution of the elderly is interpreted into a low score; the elderly are less concerned with doing something quickly.
5. Concepts of intelligence are defined in terms of abilities useful in youth rather than in terms of wisdom and adulthood.
6. Some tests on intelligence and attitudes are so frankly childish that the senior recognizes the absurdity of the task and performs accordingly.
7. Norms for test scores are higher now than earlier because of a generally better educated population and are therefore not applicable to seniors.
8. Fatigue during test taking, visual impairment, and lack of reinforcement for their efforts and competence may account for lower scores.
9. Lack of longitudinal studies prevents understanding how a person devel-

ops through the years, since research is frequently cross-sectional. Studying various age groups and piecing together to compare age groups or to
describe a whole person is likely to give different information from that
gained by studying the same person over a period of time.
10. Research is often conducted in the medical, psychiatric, or institutional
    setting. Therefore, the results may not be applicable to elderly people in
    general.[3,6]

In addition, most studies are done on middle-class persons and people who stay
at home because they are easy to interview and involve in research. Results of
studies frequently fail to acknowledge the variables of culture, race, socioeconomic class, occupation, and religion. A realistic understanding of the aging
person requires longitudinal studies that look at a number of variables.[6,31,43]

Biological Theories of Aging

Rapid advances in molecular biology, protein chemistry, and immunology
have resulted in a proliferation of research findings on aging and age-related
changes.

Theories of biological aging are usually divided into two general categories. The *Error Accumulation Theories* state that aging results from environmental insults. The *Genetic Program Theories* suggest that aging is the natural
outcome of a systematic genetic program that regulates the growth and development process.[25]

Most researchers no longer believe that one general overall theory will account for all aspects of the aging process. Aging is a highly complex phenomenon requiring different explanations for different aspects of the process.[47]

Biological aging is thought to basically arise from changes at the molecular or genetic level. Thus, discussion of theories will be limited to those that are
based on molecular changes at the genetic level.[19] The *Autoimmunity and Enzyme Theories* will also be surveyed because of their popularity.

Biologic Clock Theory suggests that an *identifiable clock of aging* exists in
each of us. This is believed to be a genetically determined program that dictates aging and dying and their rate of occurrence. Researchers agree that it
may be possible to discover the location(s) of this "clock of aging" and its
mechanism of operation. Some also feel that it will be possible to interfere with
this mechanism and thus prevent senescence.[42]

Researchers who adhere to the concept of a biological clock present varied
evidence. The lives of rats can be extended from 50 percent to 100 percent by
feeding them a low-caloric but nutritionally adequate diet. The rats fail to
mature in comparison to control animals, but they resume normal growth and
development when placed on a normal diet. These rats live considerably
longer than the controls.[14,30] Gerontologists postulate this as evidence for a
programmed, controlled developmental process of aging.[28] Strehler's *Condon-
Restriction Theory* also postulates a biologic clock. It proposes that vital ge-

netic *"code words"* that control production of cellular elements are systematically repressed. This repression results in biologic manifestations of aging.[50]

Tissue experiments add evidence for a biological clock. Human embryo fibroblasts have the capacity to double on the average of 50 times in vitro before showing signs of deterioration and death. Hayflick proposes that the clock of aging lies within the cell nucleus; just as the cell has a finite life span, so has man. The nucleus and not environmental influences on the cell body cause the deterioration of these fibroblasts around their fiftieth doubling. When the nucleus is removed from older cells and placed in young cell bodies, and vice versa, the nuclei still continue to divide the 50 times. When frozen cells are thawed, they also continue their 50 divisions.[18,20,21,22] Cells taken from persons of various ages show a correlation between age and the remaining numbers of doublings.[21]

Embryogenesis and differentiation are genetically controlled; according to von Hahn, *aging regulator genes* may also exist that are switched on in order to replace the previous regulator genes. This happens at a determined moment in the cell's life span, perhaps after its last mitosis. These aging regulator genes may produce a repressor that cannot be inactivated by normal inducee molecules. The result for the cell, therefore, is a loss of genetic information because of blocking of the transcription step in protein synthesis.[43]

Error Accumulation Theories propose that genetic mutations cause aging. These mutations have been experimentally produced by radiation. Organisms receiving high doses of radiation undergo a process of deterioration similar to that of aging. Perhaps mutations damage nuclear DNA at a rate faster than it can be repaired; this continues until the cell deteriorates and dies.[48] The *Redundant Message Theory* states that aging occurs when the system of genetic redundancy is exhausted, particularly in essential genes. Genetic redundancy refers to a process whereby reserve sequences serve as replacements when errors accumulate in functioning genes.[32] Another variation of this theory is the *Error Catastrophe Hypothesis* which states that the accuracy of protein synthesis is decreased because of the faulty selection of amino acids by enzymes.[35]

There are many other researchers working in this area, far too many for coverage in this book.

Free Radical Theory has been described by Harman. Free radicals are defined as nonionic chemical intermediates that have an odd number of electrons, causing them to react readily with other compounds. They can be generated from chemicals commonly found in food, tobacco smoke, air, and water, as well as from radiation interacting with cellular water. Free radicals are thought to react with unsaturated fatty acids to form nonfunctional peroxide molecules that cause intracellular disruption and eventually death. Experiments with various substances called *antioxidants* inhibit this free radical damage. Some of these substances are 2-mercaptoethylamine (2MER) and butylated hydroxytoluene (BHT).[26] Other researchers have experimented with vitamins C and E and selenium.[16]

Cross Linkage Theory states that molecules covalently link together in the aging process. This linkage results in aggregates or knots that lose the ability to function normally and is observed during growth and development in collagen. Cross linking may lead to progressive failure of biochemical mechanims.[7]

With many of these theories, the question of cause or effect of aging must be raised.

Autoimmunity Theories state that impaired or decreased immune response is crucial in determining cell death or cell changes that lead to the aging process. Perhaps the rate of aging can be slowed by manipulating the immune system through diet, temperature, or other means.[52] Researchers are currently experimenting with thymosin, a hormone of the thymus gland that decreases in amount with age. Since thymosin is vital to the stimulation of lymphocyte production, knowledge of it might hold clues to the immunity factor of aging. Thymosin added to the circulation should increase resistance to infection, cancer, and other deteriorative changes. This hypothesis is being tested with aging cells in tissue culture.[43]

Hormone and Enzyme Theories link aging to a centralized endocrine control in the brain, specifically the hypothalamus and pituitary, although reproductive hormones may be involved. Some researchers see the biological time clock as a pituitary hormone, which Denckla labels DECO (decreasing oxygen consumption). Others have labeled this a death hormone. Denckla theorizes that the thyroid is the critical gland in aging; thyroxine is still released, but it is prevented from being properly used by the cells through the blocking action of the hormone DECO.[42] The effect of age on concentrations of brain monoamine neurotransmitters (serotonin, dopamine, norepinephrine) is also under study.[25,42] Researchers are hopeful that reduced intake of the amino acid trytophan will alter the metabolism and levels of monoamine neurotransmitters and will result in the control of aging.[20] Thus clinical intervention in human aging may be possible through drugs or diet.[25]

With additional technology and continued study, the answer to biological aging will be found. When it is, efforts will be made to prolong human life span. You should be aware of these efforts and the possible repercussions—social, ethical, and biological—and you should try to preserve the quality of life and the dignity of the individual now and whenever human lifespan modification efforts might begin.

Psychosocial Theories of Aging

Little is known about the adult psychosocially. In the past emphasis has been on study of the child and adolescent. There are several theories about certain aspects of psychosocial aging, but inadequate evidence exists to formulate a single theory of psychological or social aging. Some researchers indicate that genetic endowment is not the primary determinant of longevity, that age of parents at death shows little correlation with longevity of offspring, and that life-style, personality, and environmental factors are more important factors. The way a person ages depends to a great degree on previous personality, psychological drives, and ability to satisfy needs.[37,38]

Developmental or Continuity Theory contends that adaptation to aging can proceed in several directions, depending on the aging person's past life. Personality types and ability to adjust to stresses and the social milieu remain stable over the life span. Barring serious illness or social upheaval, patterns of aging are believed to be predictable from knowing the person in his younger years. Factors such as work status, health, financial resources, marital status, and social attitudes and resources all more strongly affect the older person's capacity to lead a satisfying life than does the person's chronological age.[10]

Erikson's *Epigenetic Theory of development states that each stage of life has a psychosexual crisis that must be accomplished and lays the foundation for the new stage.* He states that the elderly person's behavior and feelings depend on how he has lived his earlier life and on whether or not he has mastered earlier developmental crises. His theory will be discussed further in Chapter 12. Havighurst and Duvall state specific developmental tasks for the elderly, which are discussed in Chapter 12.[12,17]

Disengagement Theory was proposed by Cumming and Henry after cross-sectional studies were made on a limited population in the 1950's. They postulated that most old people disengage. The basic concepts of Disengagement Theory are as follows:

1. The process of mutual withdrawal of the aging person and society from each other is typical of most aged people and helps both society and the person prepare for the person's death.
2. The disengagement process is biologically and psychologically intrinsic and inevitable.
3. The process is not only correlated with successful aging, but it is necessary for aging; it is preferable for the person not to resist the forces that shrink his social world.
4. The process benefits both the elderly and society.[9,29]

Activity Theory was formulated by Havighurst, Maddox, and Palmore to refute Disengagement Theory. Activity Theory is currently the more popular theory. The concepts are as follows:

1. The majority of normal aging people maintain a fairly high level of activity and engagement.
2. The amount of engagement or disengagement is more influenced by past life-styles and by social and economic forces than by an intrinsic or inevitable process.
3. The maintenance of physical, mental, and social activity is usually necessary for successful aging, and the person should maintain the interests and activities of middle age as long as possible.[9,17,36]

Since these two theories are on opposite ends of the continuum, it is likely that most people fall somewhere in between. Evidence from longitudinal studies show that during a 10-year-period elderly men had almost no overall reduction in activities or life satisfaction and that women had small reduction in activities and life satisfaction.[23] Although the person in later maturity reduces activities in some areas, such as work, he often increases activities in other areas, depending on past life-style and external factors. Load shedding may occur in old-old age as energy decreases; the senior is less involved with other people, social roles, or physical activity, but the person who is mentally alert continues and may increase the use of cognitive abilities.[5]

Sometimes disengagement is involuntary because of the lack of opportunity for social contacts because of poor health, death of peers, or the lack of transportation or finances, or because a group of primarily younger people do not welcome the older person. The older person also has a better opportunity to use his time as he wants and tends to be less concerned about others' approval. Thus he may select activities that give him pleasure but that are not part of a group, which can be interpreted as disengagement.[6] Mindel found that the older person may not be active in organizations or group roles but is nonetheless engaged in life and reality.[33]

Disengagement may occur in the person who is ill and close to death, but disengagement is *not* inevitable and it is not intrinsic. Birren and Neugarten have redefined disengagement. They say that it may be a part of successful aging.[5,34] Life satisfaction is highly correlated with remaining active for Blacks and whites.[13,23,34] Research indicates that the senior need not engage in the entire range of available activities in order to experience high morale, which Activity Theory originally postulated.[44] Instead, the activity must be meaningful in terms of status, achievement, and recognition for it to contribute significantly to morale. Certain personality types who have always been less active will feel comfortable being less active in later maturity. Activity levels in later maturity are proportionate to levels at about age 40. The more passive person may be annoyed at being prodded into performing a social role in which he is no longer interested or in which he never did have any interest. This person may not volunteer for activity unless he senses the outcome will be attention, approval, or preferential treatment.[24]

We do not know much about the aging of any one person. In this book we will synthesize the insights of numerous researchers and the experiences of the authors with the elderly person.

REFERENCES

1. ADLER, WILLIAM, "An Autoimmune Theory of Aging," in *Theoretical Aspects of Aging*, ed. Morris Rockstein. New York: Academic Press, Inc., 1974, pp. 33–42.

2. BENAIM, S., and I. ALLEN, eds., *The Middle Years*. London: T. V. Publications, Limited, 1967.

3. BENGSTON, V., J. CUELLAR, and P. KAGAN, "Stratum Contrasts and Similarities in Attitudes Toward Death," *Journal of Gerontology*, 23: No. 1 (1977), 76–88.

4. BIRCHENALL, JOAN, and MARY STREIGHT, *Care of the Older Person.* Philadelphia: J. B. Lippincott Company, 1973.

5. BIRREN, JAMES, *The Psychology of Aging.* Englewood Cliffs, N. J.: Prentice-Hall, Inc., 1964.

6. BISCHOF, LEDFORD, *Adult Psychology.* New York: Harper & Row, Publishers, Inc., 1969.

7. BJORKSTEN, J., "The Crosslinking Theory of Aging," *Journal of American Geriatric Society,* 16: No. 4 (1968), 408–27.

8. BROTMAN, H., "Life Expectancy—Comparison of National Levels in 1900 and 1974 and Variations in State Levels, 1969–1971," *The Gerontologist,* 17: No. 1 (1977), 12–22.

9. BUSSE, E., and E. PFEIFFER, eds., *Behavior and Adaptation in Late Life.* Boston: Little, Brown & Company, 1969.

10. CAMERON, MARCIA, *Views of Aging.* Ann Arbor, Mich.: The University of Michigan, Institute of Gerontology, 1976.

11. CUMMING, E., and W. E. HENRY, *Growing Old: The Process of Disengagement.* New York: Basic Books, Inc., 1961.

12. DUVALL, EVELYN, *Family Development,* 4th ed. Philadelphia: J. B. Lippincott Company, 1971.

13. ERIKSON, ERIK, *Childhood and Society,* 2nd ed. New York: W. W. Norton and Co., 1963.

14. GOODRICK, CHARLES, "Body Weight-Increment and Length of Life: The Effect of Genetic Constitution and Dietary Protein," *Journal of Gerontology,* 33: No. 2 (1978), 184–90.

15. GURALNICK, D., ed., *Webster's New World Dictionary,* 2nd college ed. New York: The World Publishing Co., 1972.

16. HARMAN, D., "Free Radical Theory Inhibitors on the Mortality Rate of LAF Mice," *Journal of Gerontology,* 23: No. 4 (1968), 476.

17. HAVIGHURST, R. J., and R. ALBRECHT, *Older People.* New York: Longmans, Green Publishers, 1953.

18. HAYFLICK, LEONARD, "The Longevity of Cultured Human Cells," *Journal of the American Geriatrics Society,* 22: No. 1 (1974), 1–12.

19. ———, "The Strategy of Senescence," *The Gerontologist,* 14: No. 1 (1974), 37–45.

20. ———, "Cell Biology of Aging," *Bio Science,* 25: No. 10 (1975), 629–37.

21. ———, "Current Theories of Biological Aging," *Federation Proceedings,* 34: No. 1 (1975), 9–13.

22. ———, "The Cell Biology of Human Aging," *New England Journal of Medicine,* 295: No. 23 (December 2, 1976), 1302–8.

23. Health Services and Mental Health Administration, *Working with Older People, Biological, Psychological and Sociological Aspects of Aging, Volume II.* Rockville, Md.: U.S. Department of Health, Education and Welfare, May, 1972.

24. KALSON, LEON, "MASH: A Program of Social Interaction Between Institutionalized Aged and Adult Mentally Retarded Persons," *The Gerontologist,* 16: No. 4 (1976), 340–48.

25. KENT, SAUL, "Why Do We Grow Old?" *Geriatrics,* 31: No. 2 (1976), 135–36.

26. ———, "Do Free Radicals and Dietary Antioxidants Wage Intracellular War?" *Geriatrics,* 32: No. 1 (1977), 127–36.

27. KNAPP, M., "The Activity Theory of Aging," *The Gerontologist,* 17: No. 6 (1977), 553–59.

28. KOGAN, NATHAN, "Attitudes Toward Old People: The Development of a Scale and an Examination of Correlates," *Journal of Abnormal and Social Psychology,* 62: (1961), 44–54.

29. MADDOX, G. L., "Disengagement Theory: A Critical Evaluation," *The Gerontologist,* 4: (1974), 80–83.

30. McCAY, C., G. SPEILING, and L. BARNES, "Growth, Aging, Chronic Diseases, and Life Span in Rats," *Archives of Biochemistry and Biophysics,* 2: (August, 1943), 469–70.

31. McNULTY, J. A., and W. CAIRD, "Memory Loss with Age: An Unsolved Problem," *Psychological Reports,* 20: (1967), 283–88.

32. MEDVEDEV, Z., "Repetition of Molecular-Genetic Information as a Possible Factor in Evolutionary Changes of Life Span," *Experimental Gerontology,* 7: No. 4 (1972), 227–38.

33. MINDEL, C., and C. VAUGHN, "A Multi-dimensional Approach to Religiosity and Disengagement," *Journal of Gerontology,* 33: No. 1 (1978), 103–8.

34. NEUGARTEN, BERNICE, and Associates (eds.), *Personality in Middle and Late Life.* New York: Atherton Press, 1964.

35. ORGEL, L., "Aging of Clones of Mammalian Cells," *Nature,* 243: (June 22, 1973), 441–45.

36. PALMORE, E., "The Effects of Aging on Activities and Attitudes," *The Gerontologist,* 8: No. 4 (1968), 259–63.

37. ———, ed., *Normal Aging.* Durham, N.C.: Duke University Press, 1970.

38. ———, and F. JEFFERS, eds. *Predictions of Life Span: Recent Findings.* Lexington, Mass.: D. C. Heath & Company, 1971.

39. PRYOR, W., "Free Radicals in Biological Systems," *Scientific American,* 223: (1970), 70.

40. RAHE, R., J. McKEAN, and A. RANSOM, "A Longitudinal Study of Life Changes and Illness Patterns," *Journal of Psychosomatic Research,* 10: (1967), 355–66.

41. RANDALL, OLLIE, "Aging in America Today—New Aspects of Aging," *The Gerontologist,* 17: No. 1 (1977), 6–11.

42. ROSENFELD, ARTHUR, "Are We Programmed to Die?" *Saturday Review,* October 2, 1976, 12–17.

43. ———, *Prolongevity.* New York: Alfred A. Knopf, Inc., 1976.

44. SAUER, WM., "Morale of the Urban Aged: A Regression Analysis by Race," *Journal of Gerontology,* 32: No. 5 (1977), 600–608.

45. SCHONFELD, D., and W. DONALDSON, "Immediate Memory as a Function of Intraseries Variation," *Canadian Journal of Psychology,* 20: (1966), 218–27.

46. SEGALL, P., C. MILLER, and P. TIMIRAS, "Aging and CNS Monoamines," *Abstracts Tenth International Congress of Gerontology,* 2: No. 87 (1975), n.p.

47. SHOCK, NATHAN, "Physiological Theories of Aging," in *Theoretical Aspects of Aging,* ed. Morris Rockstein. New York: Academic Press, Inc., 1974, pp. 119–36.

48. SINEX, F., "The F' Histone Pool in the Post-Mitotic Tissue," *Abstracts Tenth International Congress of Gerontology,* 2: No. 90 (1975), n.p.

49. "Standards for Geriatric Nursing Practice," *American Journal of Nursing,* 70: No. 9 (1970), 1894–95.

50. STREHLER, B., *et al.,* "Condon Restriction Theory of Aging and Development," *Journal of Theoretical Biology,* 33: (1971), 429.

51. VEDDER, C. B., *Problems of the Middle-Aged.* Springfield, Ill.: Charles C Thomas Publishers, 1965.

52. WALFORD, R., "Immunologic Theory of Aging: Current Status," *Federation Proceedings,* 33: (1974), 3020.

CHAPTER APPENDIX: PERSONAL MEANING OF OLD AGE

What does *old* mean to you? This may be difficult to assess, but look for clues about yourself in the following self-discovery exercises.

In the first exercise complete the sentences as spontaneously as possible. Do not pause to think. There is no right or wrong answer.

1. When I contemplate growing old, I . . .
2. Growing old makes me feel . . .
3. Growing old means getting . . .
4. The older I become, the . . .
5. Old people never . . .
6. When I get old, I will lose . . .
7. Seeing an old person makes me . . .
8. A person can be considered old when . . .
9. When I am old, I . . .
10. As I look back on the preceding statements, I feel aging is . . .

After you have completed your statements, identify how you felt as you wrote. Were you angry, tense, or fearful? Could you think of nothing to write? Consider further some of your feelings if you can. For example, explain your feelings of fear. Fear of what? Fear of loss of power? Fear of the unknown? Fear of dependency? Fear of loss of prestige or beauty?

Look carefully at your answers. Do you see any similarities in them? Are any words or phrases repeated? Can you identify any meaning attached to them? Can you begin to realize what getting old might mean to you?

Try the second exercise. Name as quickly as you can three elderly people whom you feel have had the greatest impact on your life. Then list five traits that you have associated with each person.

Name	*Name*	*Name*
1. _____	1. _____	1. _____
2. _____	2. _____	2. _____
3. _____	3. _____	3. _____
4. _____	4. _____	4. _____
5. _____	5. _____	5. _____

Identify your feelings as you thought of each person. Do your present feelings relate to past experiences with the person? Do your feelings relate to the meaning of *old* to you? Now look at the list of characteristics. Are there similarities between the three persons? Is each person markedly different? What feelings are associated with the traits you have listed? Do the similar characteristics you have listed indicate any values in your life?

Look at the following example for clarification:

Grandmother	*Mother*	*Father*
1. loves to teach	1. tolerant	1. lively
2. inspiring	2. warm	2. funny
3. generous	3. wise	3. hard-working
4. narrow-minded	4. *loving*	4. kind
5. *loving*	5. interesting	5. *loving*

You might say, "I felt pleased and happy when I wrote these traits. *Old* means to be loving and generous, and I feel secure about aging. I certainly value love as an important part of my life."

Another interesting way to identify feelings is through the "draw-a-picture" method. In the following space draw any picture that will depict an old person to you. Do not worry about your artistic skills. Be creative, and have fun.

Now look at your picture. Who does it remind you of? Identify your feelings and ideas about your picture. After you have assessed yourself, look at the following sketches:

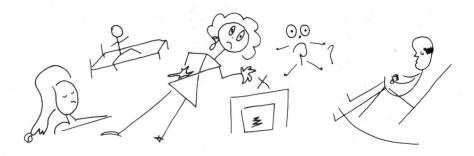

What ideas and feelings do you have as you look at these pictures? Do they remind you of anyone? Sometimes it is easier to identify feelings expressed by others than to express them yourself.

Another way to learn about your feelings about elderly people is to carefully observe your behavior and listen to your words and the tone of your voice. For one week keep a brief diary about your reactions when you meet an older person. Do your eyes meet his? Do you smile at him? Do you stand aside as if you might be contaminated? Do you brusquely shove him aside in a line? Also try to note how you speak to the older person. Is your voice kind and gentle, condescending, sneering, harsh? How do you say the word *old* when you are referring to older people? Look for a consistent pattern in your behavior and verbal response.

The ability to look at your feelings, attitudes, and behavior honestly involves the following process:

Feeling	*Attitude*	*Behavior*
I feel afraid of losing youth and beauty.	I have a disparaging attitude toward old age.	I can't be around old people very long.

Being honest also involves avoiding such self-deceptions as: "I'm never afraid." "I don't have any feelings about old age." "I won't get old."

Search for the basis of your feelings; dare to face your conflicts about growing old. Don't avoid these feelings when you become involved in experiences with others. Have a searching attitude. Continue asking yourself the following questions about aging and the elderly:

1. What are my feelings now?
2. What have I felt in the past?
3. Are my present feelings related to past experiences?
4. What do my feelings mean? How do they effect my behavior?
5. What are my values? What is really important? What would I want to keep at almost any cost?

Use the information gained from these exercises to develop a self-awareness and an objective perspective about the elderly.

nursing practice in later maturity

Study of this chapter will enable you to:

1. Define nursing and the five steps of the nursing process.

2. Describe why and how to assess the elderly person/family.

3. Formulate an assessment tool based on information presented in this chapter.

4. Obtain a nursing history during assessment, using skillful communication methods.

5. Determine a nursing diagnosis that is based on assessment and related to actions that you can take to overcome client problems.

6. Write short-term and long-term patient-care goals and a plan of care for the elderly person/family.

7. Discuss various interventions that are especially useful in individualizing care for the elderly person/family.

8. Implement appropriate interventions for an elderly client.

9. Evaluate the effectiveness of your nursing approach and care measures, using information presented in this chapter.

10. Discuss the importance of standards of practice for nursing the elderly person/family.

11. Discuss your philosophy of nursing.

12. Relate information about the nursing process from this chapter to the content in the remaining chapters.

2

In this chapter five steps in the nursing process will be explored in relation to the elderly. (Most texts discuss only three or four steps.) The five steps are assessment, statement of nursing diagnosis, formulation of patient-care goals and plan of care, intervention, and evaluation. Application of the nursing process to the person/family in later maturity will also be discussed in the following chapters.

DEFINITIONS OF NURSING

Many leaders in nursing have defined nursing. You may want to read various references at the end of this chapter to help you formulate your own definition of nursing.

The authors define *nursing* as *an art and science in which health-related activities, verbal and nonverbal, tangible and intangible, are systematically performed by a specially educated, compassionate person to promote or maintain biopsychosocial health, to comfort, protect, or stabilize during life or in the face of death, or to aid recovery of the person/family/group. These activities, legally defined, involve the use of self and may be performed independently or collaboratively with other health team members, but always with the person/family/group as actively involved as possible in the process.*

THE NURSING PROCESS

As a nurse, you do more than can be overtly seen by others. You use the *nursing process,* a dynamic method through which nursing is practiced.

The *nursing process is an ongoing systematic series of actions, interactions, and transactions with a person(s) in need of health care, using the problem-solving method, so that empathic and intellectual processes and scientific knowledge form the basis for your outward actions observable to others. The problem-solving process in nursing is analogous to the problem-solving process used by other professionals.*[21]

Johnson describes three phases of the problem-solving process: (1) the preparation phase, during which the problem is identified; (2) the production phase, during which the person thinks of and tries a particular solution; and (3) the judgment phase in which the selected solution is evaluated.[18] In nursing the problem-solving method can be divided into the steps of assessment, statement of the nursing diagnosis, identification of patient-care goals and plan of care (all of which are the preparation phase), intervention (the production phase), and evaluation (the judgment phase).

Assessment

In *assessment, data about the person, family, group, or situation are obtained by means of astute observation and examination, purposeful communication, and the use of special skills and techniques, through using scientific knowledge about the person and his behavior along with information from other health team members to gain a broader perspective.* The information about the objective and subjective status of the person(s) is critically analyzed, interrelated, and interpreted through using inferences, knowledge, personal or health team experience, records, and a variety of other sources as indicated. Nursing judgments are made based on this information.[2,3]

First-level assessment is done on initial contact with the elderly person/family to determine the perceived health threat, the ability to adapt to the threat, and immediate necessary actions. Second-level assessment continues throughout the time of contact with the person(s); it adds depth and breadth to the understanding of physical, emotional, mental, spiritual, family, social, and cultural characteristics and needs. This more comprehensive view of the person(s) enables you to plan and give care better suited to the whole individual or situation.[2,3,33,35]

A nursing history form or assessment tool is an organized means of recording the information obtained in the first and second-level assessments. It is distinct from a medical history in that it focuses on the *meaning* of illness and health care to the person instead of primarily on pathology. The form serves as a guide to obtain information that does not repeat data collected by other health team members, although it may include aspects of the medical or social history that is pertinent to nursing care. The nursing assessment or history provides a composite picture of the client; other health team members may use it as an introduction to the client.

Although the form used and the kind of information collected must be adapted to your individual work setting and clientele, Bower states that the *nursing history* should include the following information:

1. Previous experience with illness, hospitalization, health agencies, nurses, and nursing, and the meaning of these experiences for the present situation.
2. Intellectual understanding and interpretation of the health problem, diagnostic and treatment regimen, and specific questions or concerns.
3. Educational level and intellectual capacity.
4. Language usage and communication pattern.
5. Usual patterns of living, health, and religious practices and recreational pursuits.
6. Occupational and social roles and responsibilities.
7. Developmental status and level of behavior.
8. Usual behavior patterns in the presence of stress or crisis.

9. Close relationships with others and their ability to help in the present situation.
10. Expectations, goals, and needs related to health care.[3]

The nursing history should also include daily preferences and idiosyncratic patterns of living. For example, the elderly person may regularly have tea at mid-afternoon. If this pattern is not continued after admission to a hospital or residence, the person may feel a sense of loss and become irritable or depressed. Also, many elderly persons drink prune juice or a glass of water upon arising each morning. Adhering to this pattern promotes their wellness physically and their feelings of being cared for. Such preferences, minor to us, can only be obtained through a careful history.

You may think that obtaining a lengthy assessment or nursing history is too time-consuming and is impractical. But it is a necessary activity for individualizing care. A nurse-patient relationship is begun during assessment. Assessment conveys interest and concern, and it establishes a sense of mutual trust. A nursing diagnosis and realistic care objectives cannot be formulated without the information obtained in a nursing history or without the client's involvement. Nor can the last step, evaluation of the process, be done effectively unless there are baseline data. Every nursing unit should have a guide for assessment, and all of the nurses should be involved in its development, trial usage, and revision so that the tool can be useful in daily practice.

Communication skills will help you obtain assessment and nursing history data. Use open-ended statements. Indicate your observation of the senior's behavior or your understanding of his implied communication. Remaining silent so that the senior can elaborate on his answers and being attentive to the nonverbal behavior that accompanies verbal behavior, and to its meaning, can add considerably to the total amount of information collected. Asking a barrage of direct questions will tend to stifle the senior's expression, resulting in superficial or brief answers. The interviewer who is too active obtains less pertinent data. *An assessment tool is not meant to be used as a probe.* Ask questions related to what the senior is saying to fill in the needed information. In that way you may get information that was not anticipated, but which is important. Information about certain aspects, such as the senior's interpretation of reality or ability to abstract, can best be obtained by observation, attentive listening, or indirect questions. You will probably not be able to fill in all the spaces on the guide the first time you meet the person/family. In fact, you will probably get more accurate information if you use the assessment tool as a guide over a period of several visits to determine patterns of behavior and the usual health-illness status of the senior instead of making conclusions about the person based on one observation or interview. The more skillful you are as a communicator, the better your data will be as the basis for continued care.

Guides to Assessment

If you are working in an agency that has a pertinent, adequate assessment tool, use it to develop a care plan. If such a tool is not available, you may have to develop your own.

One way to begin developing an assessment tool or nursing history is to write all of the factors or characteristics that you observe when you are admitting a patient or elderly resident, opening a case with a client, beginning a series of group sessions, making a home visit, or beginning care for the first time. Next write the questions asked and information sought when you talk with the person/family/group. Recall the theory about characteristics and needs of the elderly person that would be helpful in determining what information to seek. Organize your ideas into logical categories.

Reread the assessment tool you just wrote. If you do not regularly use an assessment tool or do not have one committed to memory, perhaps you found it difficult to think initially of all the points that you now feel are important and added to the tool. Then practice using the tool. Refine it with usage so that it will be applicable to the person/family in later maturity and to your setting.

In the Appendix at the end of this chapter you will find several assessment tools that can help you formulate your own tool or nursing history. These guides are extensive in order to assist you in formulating your own. They demonstrate variety in structure and completeness to convey that at this point in nursing no one best assessment tool or nursing history form exists. Suggested techniques for phrasing the questions are given in two tools. What is useful in one health care setting or with elderly patients may not be useful in a residential setting for the family in later maturity. You will have to formulate a guide to serve you and your clients.

Another tool is the OARS Multidimensional Functional Assessment Questionnaire to assess physical and mental status, socioeconomic resources, and self-care capacity. The manual can be obtained from OARS Program, Box 3003, Duke University Medical Center, Durham, North Carolina 27710.

Regardless of the tool's format, the tool will enable you to assemble information systematically; determine the need for more information; select and organize information; recall knowledge and theory that apply to the person; and locate other sources of information, such as past records, the family, or other health team members. The tool will also enable you to continue to appraise the person/situation over time in order to validate prior information for use in the person's/family's care.

Following are obstacles that must be avoided when you use an assessment tool: (1) having a partial or stereotyped view of the person, (2) perceiving him as an object or thing instead of as a person, (3) viewing the person in terms of his potential to meet *your* needs instead of in terms of how you can better meet his needs, and (4) using the tool as a task in itself instead of as a basis for individualized patient care.

Statement of Nursing Diagnosis

Once a sufficient amount of information has been collected about the senior and his situation, the information can be analyzed and interpreted so that an explicit statement can be made about the presenting problem or unmet needs, related to health, that require nursing care.

The word *diagnosis* means to *state a decision or opinion after careful examination and analysis of facts in a situation or condition;* the word diagnosis is not limited to medical conditions.[13] *Nursing diagnosis is a description of behavior at variance with the desired state of health, a commonly recurring condition or unmet needs that interfere with health and adaptation,* or *the present or anticipated problem or difficulty experienced by the person/family which is amenable to nursing intervention.* The diagnostic statement or label provides a guideline for intervention and indicates prognosis, potential, or desired outcome.[8,30]

Nursing diagnoses do not label medical entities. They refer to conditions that can be helped by nursing action. Diagnoses that may be applicable to the psychological and physical status of the elderly include anxiety; confusion; emotional or social deprivation; disengagement; mourning; impaired adjustment to crisis, stress, or the aging process; maladaptive family process; altered level of consciousness (lethargy, stupor, coma), lack of understanding; noncompliance with treatment; pain; altered ability to perform activities of daily living (or self-care); impaired mobility, impaired nutritional-hydration status; impaired elimination process; impaired oxygen-carbon dioxide exchange; impaired integrity of the skin; impaired sensory processes (blindness, deafness, paresthesias); negative self-concept; impaired verbal communication (aphasic, mute, asocial, poverty of ideation); suspicion; withdrawal; agitation; and insomnia. Certainly this list is not conclusive; various medical problems would also generate nursing diagnoses pertinent to the physical and psychological status that results.

Formulation of Patient-Care Goals and Plan of Care

After assessment and statement of nursing diagnosis, various nursing actions, approaches, or solutions are considered in view of the nature and probable source of the person's unmet needs. At this point *patient-care goals, statements about a predicted or desired client outcome,* can be formulated cooperatively with the person/family. *Short-term goals are individualized to the person, are derived from the diagnosis, and can be accomplished in a short span of time. Long-term goals are future oriented and state the ultimate desired result of nursing intervention.*[12]

Priority of goals is affected by the following criteria:

1. Nursing diagnosis identified in collaboration with the senior/family.
2. Severity of health problem or senior's life situation.
3. Potential for recovery or susceptibility to relapse.

4. Amount of time needed by the senior or nurse.
5. Receptivity to nursing care by the senior.
6. Cost in terms of money or energy to the senior, nurse, agency, and society.
7. Demands of external constraints, such as agency policies or legal factors.[3]

Short-term goals for the elderly *hospitalized* patient might include relief from pain or insomnia; long-term goals might include increased mobility or self-care. Short-term goals for the person admitted to a *nursing home* might include orientation to the agency and its policies; long-term goals might include resolution of the crisis of death of spouse and admission to the home.

When goals are formulated and priorities are set, the details of meeting these goals can be written in the nursing care plan. The **nursing care plan** is a *record summarizing the information obtained from assessment that is required to implement approriate nursing care and to meet specific goals for the elderly person/family at a given time.* The written plan includes the client's need and problems; patient-care goals and priority in reaching them; **nursing orders,** or the *approaches of action that have been selected from the available alternatives;* expected behavioral outcomes; and evaluative criteria to measure actions. Care measures prescribed by the physician and general measures determined by the person's situation or agency policy are also included in the plan.

The care plan is begun when the senior is admitted to the agency, and it must be updated throughout his stay as more information is obtained or as his condition changes. The nurse who first contacts the person is usually responsible for beginning a care plan. Thereafter, all nursing personnel should be encouraged to write observations and care suggestions on the plan. Only then can the following *purposes* of the care plan be realized:

1. To communicate information about the person/family and appropriate nursing actions or approaches.
2. To provide individualized and comprehensive care.
3. To provide coordination and continuity of care.
4. To facilitate ongoing and accurate evaluation of care.[3]

The nursing care plan will be used for a long period of time in the nursing home, residential center for the aged, or extended care facility. Since hospital stays are frequently limited in duration, both the nursing care plan and the nursing history are justified for short-term care intervals and should become a permanent part of the senior's record so that it is available for understanding the person on future admissions and for further care planning. Additionally, a copy of the care plan (and history) should be sent with the senior upon transfer to another agency.

Intervention

Intervention refers to all of the actions that you engage in, as well as the approach you use, to promote the client's well-being.[26] According to the definition of nursing given earlier, intervention includes verbal and nonverbal communication; visible actions; and your approach and reactions to the person as you promote or maintain biopsychosocial health; comfort, protect, or enhance stability; or aid recovery of the client. Intervention occurs when you prevent harm or further dysfunction or assist the senior to function as effectively as possible within the limits imposed by his condition. Many tasks done unwittingly are nursing interventions and should be defined as such to the client. The scientific rationale for doing the nursing activity should also be explained to the client.

Nursing interventions with the elderly person/family include the following:

1. Giving sickness care, including intensive care or daily care procedures, such as feeding, bathing, range of motion exercises, and turning.
2. Enabling the senior to perform his own hygiene and grooming.
3. Implementing medical procedures and treatments ordered by the physician.
4. Encouraging the senior to use energy-saving devices.
5. Adapting procedures or techniques to the home situation.
6. Encouraging a regimen of activity or rehabilitation to reduce disengagement.
7. Maintaining communication with the senior, for example, by listening to him reminisce.
8. Reducing sensory and emotional immobility, for example, by visiting with an elderly couple or bringing the person a bouquet of flowers.
9. Meeting spiritual needs by maintaining the pattern of worship, calling the minister, reading a passage from the Bible, or saying a prayer at the person's request.
10. Maintaining communication with the family or significant others.
11. Teaching and counseling the person/family to help them become more adaptive or independent.
12. Reducing anxiety by being supportive and available to the person and family experiencing death.
13. Referring the elderly person/family to health, social, and welfare agencies as indicated.

The list could go on and on. Through nursing interventions you help the person/family meet the needs that can't be met by the self. To summarize, nursing interventions (actions) include (1) helping the person/family cope with an actual or potential stressor; (2) eliminating a source of stress; (3) helping the senior develop a new behavior, strengthen an existing one, or modify or diminish a present behavior; (4) supporting the senior in his present behavior; (5) preventing further injury or complications; and (6) manipulating the environment to promote adaptation.[3]

The elderly person may have many needs to be met—physical, social, emotional, and spiritual. Often the following basic needs are overlooked, but they can be met with little extra effort on your part if you remember that the elderly person desires to:

1. Be recognized as a person and not regarded as a room number, a disease, a problem, "grandma," or less of a person because of his age.
2. Be listened to.
3. Be comforted, to have distress recognized, and perceive that health care workers are making efforts to make him physically and emotionally comfortable. The aged person can tolerate pain if he is not being neglected.
4. Be remembered; the person fears being overlooked and forgotten.
5. Learn what is causing his health problems or distress in terminology that he can understand.
6. Know what treatment and care is being planned, the possible length of treatment, and what generally can be expected as an end result.
7. Receive quality care.
8. Have some self-determination about what activities he will take part in so long as he does not injure others or himself.

Family members of the patient often have basic needs that are overlooked. Even though the family members may also be aged, they deserve the same consideration as the patient. They should not be treated as infants or as incompetents. Family members also need to be comforted emotionally, and sometimes physically, when they are feeling guilty or worried. They need to be informed as fully as possible about the situation and expected results of the treatment and care. Family members also need encouragement and support as they encounter the stress of illness in the loved one and work to restore and maintain well-being and prevent further complications in the patient.

Thus, intervention includes the *independent functions* of doing all hygiene and comfort measures; planning and creating an environment conducive to wholeness and safety from injury and risk; teaching and counseling, either formally or informally; offering of self to impart strength and courage to another as he copes with problems; socializing in a purposeful manner; or making a referral to another agency when indicated. Intervention includes the *dependent function* of doing all the ministrations or procedures that implement the medical regimen outlined by the physician or other health team members. Intervention also includes *coordinating care* given by other health team members; collaborating with others to provide continuity of care; and directing others, including the family, to give care to the person.

Bower classifies intervention into three nursing actions: supportive, generative, and protective. *Supportive nursing actions provide comfort, treatment, and restoration. These measures augment the person's present adaptive capacity, help him cope more effectively with stress, and prevent further health problems.* In addition, supportive interventions maximize the person's/family's strengths and provide guidance, encouragement, or relief to enable the person to regain health. *Generative nursing actions are innovative and rehabilitative. They help the person/family develop different approaches to coping with stress or crisis and* are especially used when assisting another with struggles involved in role changes or identity crisis. *Protective nursing actions are measures that promote health and prevent disease; improve or correct situations,* such as immunizations, health teaching, or anticipatory guidance; or *prevent complications and disease sequelae.*[3]

Since the nursing process is a problem-solving method, your nursing actions should be considered as hypotheses to be tested in practice. When the actions are demonstrated to be effective and can be validated as the best way to meet needs, they become part of the ongoing individualized nursing care plan.[27]

Evaluation

Evaluation is the purposeful examination and use of measurement data, devices, and methods to determine effectiveness or nursing actions and your approach toward achieving short-range and long-range patient-care goals, as well as to determine the problems that have been resolved, that are still unresolved, and new ones that have arisen. It is the last step of the nursing process, but it cannot be separated from assessment, formulating a nursing diagnosis, determining objectives and planning care, and intervention.

Evaluation includes first predicting outcomes through long-term and short-term goals. These outcomes are expressed as behavioral objectives (patient responses) that you expect to see after nursing intervention and they indicate progress in achievement of stated goals. The current behaviors of the patient act as a baseline for expected change within a certain time limit. Statements of goals help you not only to determine specific interventions to use but also the specific patient behaviors that would indicate that these goals have been achieved.[12] When a behavioral objective (predicted outcome) is reached, a new objective corresponding to progress in status is written.[12]

Behavioral objectives based on priorities of care establish the criteria for evaluation and must be either observable to the client or nurse or measurable in some way so that the cause of unexpected outcomes can be determined and further negative effects can be avoided.

Nursing can be evaluated for effort, effect, and efficiency.[6]

Measuring *effort* involves asking the following questions: What has been done compared to what was desired? What has been done compared to the stated objective of care? Was as much done as could have been done?[6]

Measuring *effect* involves seeking information about change or lack of change in the client's situation. Was the change important? Intended? Expected? Safe? Necessary? Desirable to the client and the nurse?[6]

Measuring *efficiency* involves seeking information on how the actions were performed in terms of energy, time, and materials. If the results of nursing care were satisfactory, how many actions were necessary to accomplish care? Were the actions coordinated? Could fewer actions have produced the same results? If the nursing care outcomes were not those that were expected or desired, what factors may be responsible? Were outcomes unsatisfactory because needs were inadequately identified, because of lack of skill in intervention, or because of other factors over which the nurse or patient had no control? Less than satisfactory outcomes may result from many variables in the senior's life situation.[6]

Evaluation should be continuous so that the insights gained can be used to reassess the person, modify plans, and improve care throughout the nursing process. Evaluation benefits the senior and the nurse because it provides a final statement about patient progress and is a critical examination of nursing practice. Areas to scrutinize include the use of knowledge in practice; accuracy of assessment and diagnosis; effectiveness of intervention; consistency of approach; success of communication; and cooperation of other health team members.[28]

Evaluation of care is directly related to *accountability, the state of being responsible for your actions and being able to explain, define, or measure the results of your decision making.* Accountability involves measuring your effectiveness against a set of criteria—the agency's policies, the unit's general care standards, the Standards of Nursing Practice, or the client's care objectives. Accountability involves validating intangibles, such as attitudes and subtle nuances, as well as overt care measures. You are accountable to the person/family/group, agency, doctor, other health team members, and the community. Your accountability assures optimum health care delivery.[27]

In summary, your responsibility is to:

1. Assess thoroughly the senior's health care needs. *This cannot be delegated.* Tools can be utilized, but it is your responsibility to validate any information on a nursing history form collected by someone other than yourself.
2. Determine nursing diagnosis based on your assessment.
3. Plan with the team, supervise others, and teach care measures needed by the person/family. You must assume responsibility for the patient-care objectives and the level of care rendered; thus, your responsibility will include supervising, teaching, and assigning personnel according to their qualifications and the senior's needs.
4. Give care when indicated, acting as a role model for other staff members.
5. Evaluate care and determine whether or not goals have been met. You must take corrective action as indicated. Through this process you demonstrate accountability.

As you read the steps of the nursing process, you are no doubt keenly aware that the process is continuous and circular and that some of the steps of the process overlap. For example, while you are doing one intervention, such as bathing the person, you are simultaneously assessing him and mentally or verbally making a plan with him on how you will continue with your intervention of giving skin care and ambulating the person. You may think that your mental or verbal care plan is sufficient to help you do your care, but you will find that a written plan of major goals or objectives and specific ways of accomplishing them is essential if you want to provide for consistency in care. Other nursing team members cannot read your mind and you cannot read their minds. If each of you shares what you know and plan, both the nursing team and client benefit.

STANDARDS OF PRACTICE FOR LATER MATURITY

Formulating standards of nursing practice is a necessary prerequisite to evaluating the quality of care given to the client. Factors to consider in developing standards are (1) type of agency, (2) scope of care, (3) units of care, and (4) evaluation approaches.[11]

Type of agency refers to the hospital, public health department, home health care agency, physician's office, extended care agency, industry, or another form of health care setting. *Scope of care* includes whether care is provided by one professional group, a number of professional groups working together in one agency, or all of the health disciplines that might be involved in providing comprehensive community health care. Usually standards of care and evaluation focus on care provided to the individual client by one professional group. *Units of care* encompass either sporadic or long-term care that may be preventive, acute, or restorative. Physiologic, psychologic, and social factors are considered. *Evaluation approaches* vary; usually evaluations are made on the process, structure, and outcome of care. *Process* focuses on clinical decisions and the actions of health practitioners. *Structure* focuses on properties of health care facilities, equipment, manpower, and financing. *Outcome* focuses on the end results of health care, which are specified in terms of client health, welfare, and satisfaction. Client opinions, reactions, and behaviors should also be included.[11]

Various organizations and authors have formulated standards of care. The Standards of Geriatric Nursing prepared by the American Nurses' Association have as their purpose to fulfill the profession's obligation to provide and improve nursing practice. The Standards provide a means for determining the quality of nursing that a client receives, regardless of the level of the worker who provides the service, and apply to nursing practice in any setting. The Standards of Nursing Practice are stated according to the steps of assessment, planning, intervention, and evaluation and can be a useful guide to you and your agency. Copies of the Standards can be obtained from the American Nurses' Association, 2420 Pershing Road, Kansas City, Missouri 64108.

As a nurse, you are in a special position to think about the meaning and sequence of life as you care for the person or family, ill or well. Your philosophy of nursing should be the foundation for your use of knowledge and skill in nursing practice. Often nurses prefer to avoid thinking about philosophy. Now that you have a general perspective on the nursing process as the methods for giving care, consideration of the guiding principles about people and health care is essential. You may want to return to a study of various philosophers or writers in nursing in order to help you clarify your own philosophy of care.

The following paragraphs reflect *the authors'* basic beliefs about nursing and care for the person/family in later maturity.

Life is a movement, a changing and growing process. You, the nurse, as a living being, constantly undergo change. The health care system in which you work is changing, and your roles are affected by these changes. The people you care for are also changing; they are maturing as individuals. They are not just a conglomerate mass isolated by an age bracket. The elderly person, with his potential for change and further development, is intrinsically valuable. He is unique and different; yet he is similar to yourself in basic needs. The senior continues to adapt to his changing self and changing life situation. He maintains a faith in something or someone greater than himself and uses his inner strengths as well as his relationships with others to maximize his potential. His behavior falls on a continuum from wellness to illness to dying, and he attempts to remain responsible to himself, others, and his environment as long as possible.

You, the nurse, functioning as an individual citizen and as a professional health worker, can add much to the dimension of the elderly person's life. You can be significant to the well-being and ongoing development of the elderly person/family by demonstrating a humanistic concern for the whole person; by being compassionate, empathic, courteous, and authentic in your behavior; and by treating the person with dignity when he is ill and approaching death, just as you would treat the person who is young, rich, or beautiful. What you are and do is significant to those in your care. You can enter into a partnership with the person that is based on trust. You can assure the person that his rights will be honored, that appropriate information will be shared with him, and that he can contribute to the care plan. You are responsible for the overall welfare of the person to whom you give service. You are responsible for personalizing his care while you help him adapt to his health-illness status through goal-directed service.

Giving the kind of high-level care just described is possible if you are aware of your own values, biases, and beliefs and if you base your nursing practice on a belief system. Thus, your knowledge of the nursing process, your methods of practice, and your awareness of the philosophy underlying your actions must be combined with a knowledge about the person/family in later maturity.

REFERENCES

1. BATES, BARBARA, *A Guide to Physical Examination.* Philadelphia: J. B. Lippincott Company, 1974.

2. BELAND, IRENE, and JOYCE PASSOS, *Clinical Nursing: Pathophysiological and Psychosocial Approaches,* 3rd ed. New York: Macmillan Publishing Co., Inc., 1975.

3. BOWER, FAY, *The Process of Planning Nursing Care: A Theoretical Model.* St. Louis: The C. V. Mosby Company, 1972.

4. BUCKINGHAM, WILLIAM, MARSHALL SPAIBERG, and MARTIN BRANDFONBRENER, *A Primer of Clinical Diagnosis.* New York: Harper & Row, Publishers, Inc., 1971.

5. CHAMBERS, WILLA, "Nursing Diagnosis," *American Journal of Nursing,* 62: No. 1 (1962), 102–4.

6. CURTIS, JOY, MARILYN ROTHBERT, and BERNICE CHRISTIAN, "A Practical Evaluation of Nursing Care as Part of the Nursing Process," *Nursing Digest,* 3: No. 3 (1975), 20–21.

7. DAUBENMIRE, M. JEAN, and IMOGENE KING, "Nursing Process Models: A Systems Approach," *Nursing Outlook,* 21: No. 8 (1973), 512–17.

8. GEBBIE, KRISTINE, and MARY LAVIN, eds., *Classification of Nursing Diagnosis.* St. Louis: The C. V. Mosby Company, 1975.

9. GEITGEY, DORIS, "Self-Pacing—A Guide to Nursing Care," *Nursing Outlook,* 17: No. 8 (1969), 48–49.

10. GEORGE, MADELON, KAZUYOSHI IDE, and CLARA VAMBERRY, "The Comprehensive Health Team: A Conceptual Model," *Journal of Nursing Administration,* 1: No. 2 (1971), 9–13.

11. GLENNIN, CLAIRE, "Formulation of Standards of Nursing Practice Using a Nursing Model," in *Conceptual Models for Nursing Practice,* eds. Joan Riehl and Callista Roy. New York: Appleton-Century-Crofts, 1974, pp. 234–46.

12. GRUBBS, JUDY, "An Interpretation of the Johnson Behavioral System Model for Nursing Practice," in *Conceptual Models for Nursing Practice,* eds. Joan Riehl and Callista Roy. New York: Appleton-Century-Crofts, 1974, pp. 160–94.

13. GURALNIK, DAVID, ed., *Webster's New World Dictionary of the American Language,* 2nd college ed. New York: The World Publishing Company, 1972.

14. HARMER, B., and V. HENDERSON, *Textbook of the Principles and Practice of Nursing.* New York: Macmillan Publishing Co., Inc., 1955.

15. HENDERSON, VIRGINIA, "The Nature of Nursing," *American Journal of Nursing,* 64: No. 8 (1964), 62–68.

16. ———, *The Nature of Nursing.* New York: Macmillan Publishing Co., Inc., 1966.

17. HOCKSTEIN, ELLIOT, and A. RUBIN, *Physical Diagnosis.* New York: McGraw-Hill Book Company, 1964.

18. JOHNSON, DONALD, *Psychology: A Problem-Solving Approach.* New York: Harper & Row, Publishers, Inc., 1961.

19. JOHNSON, DOROTHY, "The Significance of Nursing Care," *American Journal of Nursing,* 61: No. 11 (1961), 63–66.

20. JUDGE, RICHARD, and GEORGE ZUIDEMA, eds., *Physical Diagnosis: A Physiologic Approach to Clinical Examination,* 2nd ed.   Boston: Little, Brown & Company, 1968.

21. KING, IMOGENE, "A Conceptual Frame of Reference for Nursing," *Nursing Research,* 17: No. 1 (1968), 27–31.

22. LEWIS, LUCILLE, "This I Believe—About the Nursing Process, Key to Care," *Nursing Outlook,* 16: No. 5 (1968), 26–29.

23. MACKINNON, R., and R. MICHELS. *Psychiatric Interview in Clinical Practice.* Philadelphia: W. B. Saunders Company, 1971.

24. MCCAIN, R. FAYE, "Nursing by Assessment—Not Intuition," *American Journal of Nursing,* 65: No. 4 (1965), 82–84.

25. MORGAN, WILLIAM, and GEORGE ENGEL, *The Clinical Approach to the Patient.* Philadelphia: W. B. Saunders Company, 1969.

26. MUNDINGER, MARY, and GRACE JAURON, "Developing a Nursing Diagnosis," *Nursing Outlook,* 23: No. 2 (1975) 94–98.

27. MURRAY, RUTH, and JUDITH ZENTNER, *Nursing Concepts for Health Promotion,* 2nd ed.   Englewood Cliffs, N. J.: Prentice-Hall, Inc., 1979.

28. O'DRISCOLL, DOROTHY, "The Nursing Process and Long-Term Care," *Journal of Gerontological Nursing,* 2: No. 3 (1976), 34–37.

29. ORLANDO, IDA, *The Dynamic Nurse-Patient Relationship.* New York: McGraw-Hill Book Company, 1961.

30. ———, *The Discipline and Teaching of Nursing Process.* New York: G. P. Putnam's Sons, 1972.

31. Patient Assessment: Taking a Patient's History," *American Journal of Nursing,* 74: No. 2 (1974), 293–324.

32. PEPLAU, HILDEGARDE, *Interpersonal Relations in Nursing.* New York: G. P. Putnam's Sons, 1952.

33. RIEHL, JOAN, and SISTER CALLISTA ROY, eds., *Conceptual Models for Nursing Practice.* New York: Appleton-Century-Crofts, 1974.

34. RUBIN, REVA, "Body Image and Self-Esteem," *Nursing Outlook,* 16: No. 6 (1968), 20–23.

35. SAXTON, DOLORES, and PATRICIA HYLAND, *Planning and Implementing Nursing Intervention.* St. Louis: The C. V. Mosby Company, 1975.

36. SHERMAN, JACQUES, and SYLVIA FIELDS, *Guide to Patient Evaluation.* Flushing, New York: Medical Examination Publishing Co., Inc., 1974.

37. SNYDER, JOYCE, and MARGO WILSON, "Elements of a Psychological Assessment," *American Journal of Nursing,* 77: No. 2 (1977), 235–39.

38. YURA, HELEN, and MARY WALSH, *The Nursing Process,* 2nd ed.   New York: Appleton-Century-Crofts, 1973.

CHAPTER APPENDIX: ASSESSMENT GUIDES

SOCIOCULTURAL ASSESSMENT

(For use on admission to the hospital, nursing home, or residence for senior citizens)

I. *Identifying Data*

Name: Sex:

Age: Race/Ethnicity:

Date of Admission/or First Contact: Referral Source:

Previous Occupation, or Present Employment:

II. *Environment*

Describe the neighborhood and geographical area in which you reside (resided). What about it is/was important to you?

Describe your current/previous home and arrangement of space inside. What health hazards are/were present?

What transportation facilities do/did you use?

What leisure activities/recreation do you pursue? Where? With whom?

What was/is the environment at work? What health hazards were/are present?

III. *Socioeconomic Level and Life-Style*

How would you describe your socioeconomic level and life-style? How do you think these have affected your health?

How has your health status affected your life-style?

What changes do you expect to occur in your life-style as a result of growing older/this illness and hospitalization/or admission to this center?

What special practices or foods do you consider essential to your life-style?

IV. *Family Patterns*

Marital Status:

Children:

Other Important Members of Family:

Who resides in the home with you?

What is the usual daily living pattern in your family?

What family events are important?

What rituals are important in your family?

How do the daily living pattern and rituals affect your health?

Family Functions and Interaction:

> What is your role in the family? (What does your family depend on you for?)
>
> How are decisions made in the family?
>
> Who helps provide for the family?
>
> Who has the responsibility for the various family tasks?
>
> What are your special concerns in your family?

V. *Religious Practices*

What church or religious denomination do you belong to as a member?

Are you active?

Are there special beliefs you adhere to? How do these affect your health?

How do you see your relationship to God during this period of time? What effect does God have on your health/illness?

If you do not subscribe to a particular religious creed, what are your basic beliefs and values?

How do these affect your health/illness?

What can the nurse do to assist you in practicing religious rituals/beliefs during your illness or during your stay at this center?

VI. *Memberships*

What groups/organizations in the community do you belong to?

What is your role in these groups? How much satisfaction do you get from group activities?

VIII. *Personal Values (consider expressed ideal vs. real)*

What are your ideas about the following:

Man and the environment relationship?

Privacy vs. group interaction (being with others)?

Possessions (personal vs. shared)?

Time Orientation:

Do you like to have things done promptly?

Do you rely on past experience primarily?

Do you like to plan ahead into the future?

How do you feel if you know that you or someone else is going to be late to an event?

Work/Activity—Leisure Orientation:

How much time do you spend in work tasks daily?

Do you prefer to be busy instead of sitting and thinking, reading, or relaxing?

What do you do to relax?

How much time do you spend in leisure daily?

Attitude toward Change:

How do you feel when you hear the word change?

How often do you make or have you made changes in your life?

What changes would you like to make in yourself? In others? In your environment?

Education:

Level of school achievement?

How important is education to you?

What do you consider necessary for achievement?

Health-Illness Values/Definitions:

When do you consider yourself or members of your family healthy?

When do you consider them ill?

What do you do when you or members of your family become ill?

What customs, special practices, or rituals do you and your family engage in to keep healthy? Do you and your family have any specific beliefs or observe any specific traditions concerning health?

Note: This tool could be adapted by the nurse who is working in the home health care agency.

PHYSICAL ASSESSMENT

(For use on admission to the hospital, nursing home, or residence for senior citizens)

The Health History Includes the Following Data:

I. *Identifying Data*

Name: Sex:

Address: Race/Ethnicity:

Age:

Marital status: If widowed, when?

Occupation: If retired, date of retirement:

Reason for contacting health agency:

II. A concise statement of the *chief complaint* and its duration.

III. Concise chronological description of the *present health status or illness.*

IV. *Past medical history* beginning as far back as the person can remember and continuing up to the time when he considered himself to be in good health.

Childhood:

Medical:

Surgical, including accidents:

Psychiatric:

Obstetrical—number and outcome of pregnancies, abnormalities, or complications:

Hospitalizations—include names of hospitals, dates, attending physicians, and problems:

Previous routine or periodic examinations:

Exposure to known case of illness, travel in foreign country, exposure to toxic substances:

Allergies—to what and reaction:

V. *Personal and social history*

Childhood—birth (when, where), family group, education, environment, problems:

Adulthood—employment history, military service:

Sexual and marital history—marital status, sexual activity, children:

Present life-style—descriptions of home, occupation, family life, affiliations, habits:
  Tobacco:
    Type—cigarettes, cigars, pipe, chewing, snuff:
    Age at which use began:
    Current level of usage:
  Beverages:
    Coffee, tea, cola:
    Type of alcoholic beverage and estimate of average daily or weekly consumption:
  Drugs:
    Drug use, including legal and illegal drugs, prescribed and over-the-counter drugs:
    Present schedule and dosage: (sleeping tablets, aspirin, weight-reducing drugs, antihistamines, folk remedies, laxatives, enemas, vitamins):
  Personal habits:
    Sleep:
    Working hours:
    Travel:
    Vacation:
    Hobby or leisure activities:
    Nutrition and hydration (sample 1 day diet and fluid intake); special diet needs:
    Elimination habits:
  Family history:
    Health status of relatives:
    Presence of specific diseases—diabetes, tuberculosis, cancer, mental illness, illness similar to the patient's present illness:
    Family tree—including grandparents, parents, siblings, children:
  Religious practices:
    Denomination:
    Church location:
    Pastor:
    Usual attendance:

Review of Systems and Physical Examination Includes the Following Data:

I. *Measurement of Vital Signs*

Height:
Weight:
Temperature:
Pulse—rate and character:
Respiration—rate and character:
Blood pressure; note arm and position:

II. *General Appearance*

An opening statement describing muscular development, posture, position of body, body movements, nutritional state, appearance of acute or chronic illness, whether he appears his age, state of personal hygiene.

History of weakness, fatigue, malaise, fever, chills, weight gain or loss.

Skin—color, temperature, turgor, moisture, pigment changes, bruises, pressure areas, decubitus, lesions, rashes and scars (location), dryness, texture, appearance of nails, size and shape of fingers, use of hair dyes or other agents:

Head—history of headache, head injury, dizziness, syncope:

Exam: 1. Skull—deformities:
      2. Scalp and scaling:
      3. Hair—color, pattern of baldness, parasites:
      4. Face—expression, edema, muscle tics, paralysis:

Eyes—history of pain, use of glasses, last change in refraction, diplopia, infection, glaucoma, cataract:

Exam: 1. Vision—near, distant, and peripheral:
      2. Pupils—reaction to light and accommodation, equality of size:
      3. Condition of lids, conjunctiva, and sclera; movements, expression, presence of discharge:

Ears—history of earaches, hearing loss, use of hearing aid, tinnitus, vertigo, discharge, pain, infection, mastoiditis:

Exam: 1. External—auditory meatus, tympanic membrane, general appearance:
      2. Hearing—distance whispered word heard:

Nose—history of sinus pain, epistaxis, obstruction, discharge, postnasal drip, colds, sneezing:

Exam: 1. External—size, shape, sense of smell, difficulty in breathing, discharge:
   2. Internal—patency, polyps, septal deviation, others:

Mouth—history of toothache, recent extractions, soreness or bleeding of lips, gums, mouth, tongue, or throat; disturbance of taste; thirst; hoarseness; tonsillectomy:

Exam: 1. Lips—pallor, cyanosis, lesions, dryness:
   2. Teeth—natural, state of repair, dentures:
   3. Gums—bleeding, retracted, color, hypertrophic:
   4. Tongue—color, size, deviation, hydration, lesions, tremors, paralysis:
   5. Pharynx—motion of palate, uvula, tonsils, gag reflex; posterior pharynx—hoarseness, difficulty speaking or swallowing, ulcerations, inflammation:

Neck—history of pain, limitation of motion, thyroid enlargement:

Exam: 1. General—stiffness, range of motion, tenderness, veins, pulses, bruits:
   2. Thyroid—enlargement, nodules, tenderness:
   3. Lymph glands—size, consistency, tenderness:

Cranial Nerves (See Chapter 16 for description of examination)

Thorax—history of pain, breast lumps, discharge, or operations:

Exam: 1. Chest—size, shape, and movements:
   2. Breasts—nipple discharge, areola, contour, symmetry, masses (size, location, shape, consistency, fixation), skin ulceration, axillary nodes:

Heart—history of pain or distress, palpitation, dyspnea (relate to effort), orthopnea, paroxysmal nocturnal dyspnea, edema, nocturia, cyanosis, heart murmur, rheumatic fever, hypertension, coronary artery disease, anemia; last EKG:

Exam: 1. Inspection
    (a) Apex beat, relation to midclavicular or midsternal line, intercostal space:
    (b) Other pulsations:
   2. Palpation
    (a) Size, vigor of apex beat:
    (b) Left sternal lift, epigastric palpation, thrills:

3. Percussion
   (a) Distance of dullness from midsternal line in left second to sixth or seventh interspace:
4. Auscultation
   (a) Quality and intensity of S1 and S2 in each value area:
   (b) Splitting:
   (c) Extra sounds—S3 and S4
   (d) Murmur—location, radiation, systolic or diastolic, intensity, frequency, character—crescendo, decrescendo, holosystolic:

Lungs—history of pain, cough, sputum (character and amount), hemoptysis, wheezing, asthma, shortness of breath, bronchitis, pneumonia, tuberculosis or contact therewith, date of last X-ray or skin test:

Exam: 1. Inspection
   (a) Breathing pattern:
   (b) Symmetry:
   (c) Venous pattern:
2. Palpation
   (a) Vocal fremitus:
   (b) Use of accessory muscles:
3. Percussion—locate by interspace dullness, flatness, hyperresonance, or tympany:
4. Auscultation
   (a) Type of breath sounds—vesicular, bronchial, or bronchovesicular:
   (b) Adventitial sounds—rales, cavernous breathing, asthmatic breathing, pleural friction rub:
   (c) Vocal resonance—bronchophony:

Abdomen—history of appetite, food intolerance, dysphagia, heartburn, pain or distress after eating, colic, jaundice, belching, nausea, vomiting, hematemesis, flatulence; character and color of stools, change in bowel habits; rectal conditions, ulcer, gallbladder disease, hepatitis, appendicitis, colitis, parasites, hernia.

Exam: 1. Inspection
   (a) Distention:
   (b) Masses:
   (c) Peristalsis (visible):
2. Palpation
   (a) Tenderness on light or deep palpation:
   (b) Masses (exact location, consistency, mobility, nodularity, pulsation):

   (c) Rigidity:
   (d) Organ outlines (liver, spleen):
3. Percussion
   (a) Abdominal distention (air or ascites):
   (b) Bladder distention:
4. Auscultation
   (a) Bowel sounds:
   (b) Bruits:

Extremities and Back—history of intermittent claudication, varicose veins, thrombophlebitis, joint pain, stiffness, swelling, arthritis, gout, bursitis, flat feet, infection, fracture, muscle pain, cramps; assistance devices utilized (prostheses, cane, crutches, walker, wheelchair):

Exam: 1. Blood vessels—pulse, veins:
      2. Joints—tenderness, deformities, crepitation, range of motion of each:
      3. Edema—location, pitting, discoloration:
      4. Reflexes:
      5. Sensation—pain and temperature, vibration, position:
      6. Muscular function—standing on toes, strength of movement:
      7. Gait and stance—walking, standing with eyes closed:
      8. Back—pain (location and radiation, especially to the extremities), stiffness, limitation of motion:

Genitourinary—history of urinary tract—renal colic, frequency, nocturia, polyuria, oliguria, hesitancy, urgency, dysuria, narrowing of stream, dribbling, incontinence, hematuria, albuminuria, pyuria, kidney disease, facial edema, renal stone, cystoscopy; genital (male)—testicular pain, scrotal change; nodules in scrotum; (female)—menstrual history, vaginal bleeding or discharge, menopause and associated symptoms, date of last Pap smear; venereal disease—gonorrhea or syphilis (note date, treatment, complications); sexual—drive, activity, pleasure, discomfort, impotence:

Examination of the Male Genitalia and Urinary Tract:
      1. Penis:
      2. Scrotum—size, symmetry, consistency, tenderness, masses, atrophy:
      3. Inguinal region—pulses, lymph glands, hernia, parasites:
      4. Character of urine; presence of indwelling catheter, date of last change:

Examination of the Female Reproductive System:
      1. External genitalia
         (a) Vulva—ulceration:

(b) Urethra—discharge:

(c) Pelvic relaxation—cystocele, rectocele, prolapse uterus (degree):

2. Internal genitalia

(a) Speculum exam of vagina (discharge, ulcerations, irregularities):

(b) Cervix (ulceration, irregularity), Pap smear:

Examination of the Rectum:

1. External inspection for external hemorrhoids, perianal skin, pilonidal sinus:

2. Internal palpation—sphincter tonicity, abscess; prostate enlargement; rectal masses, impaction:

Central Nervous System—general history—syncope, loss of consciousness, convulsions, meningitis, encephalitis, stroke; mentative—aphasia (describe), emotional status, mood, orientation, memory, change in sleep pattern, psychiatric illness; motor—tremor, weakness, paralysis (describe involvement), clumsiness of movement; sensory—neurologic pain, reduced sensation, paresthesia:

Hematopoietic—history of bleeding tendencies of skin or mucous membrane, anemia and treatment, blood type, transfusion and reaction, blood dyscrasia, exposure to toxic agents or radiation:

Endocrine—history of nutrition and growth, thyroid function (tolerance to heat and cold, change in skin, relationship between appetite and weight, nervousness, tremors, thyroid medication); diabetes or its symptoms (polyuria, polydipsia, polyphagia); hirsutism, secondary sex characteristics, hormone therapy:

Activities of Daily Living Survey

	Independent	Needs Assistance (Describe type needed)	Dependent
Bathing			
Dressing			
Toileting*			
Feeding			
Transferring			
Ambulating			
Turning in bed			

* Describe whether the person can ask to be taken to the bathroom or is totally incontinent.

Note: This tool could be adapted by the nurse who is working in the home health care agency.

PSYCHOLOGICAL ASSESSMENT

(For use on admission to the hospital, nursing home, or residence for senior citizens)

I. *Identifying data*

    Name: Sex:

    Age: Race/Ethnicity:

    Marital Status:

    Children:

    Other members of household:

    Occupation (Past or Present):

    Where employed: How long?

    Ever active in different occupation?

    If yes, why did you change?   When?

    Date of admission/first contact?   Referral source:

II. *Health History*

Have you had previous admissions to a hospital? To another nursing home or residence?

Describe significant aspects of your health history.

What does it mean for you to be in the hospital/nursing home/residence?

What is your usual source of health care?

How accessible are health services? Is transportation easily available? Do you have some form of health insurance?

What medication do you currently use?

Describe any drug allergies:

What do you consider your major present problem or area of concern?

When did the problem begin? Was the onset sudden or gradual?

What does this problem/illness mean to you?

What do you consider as the stressful event that triggered your problem?

Have you ever experienced a similar problem? If you have, what was the problem and how did you handle it? Were your coping patterns successful?

III. *Life-Style Patterns*

What is your usual pattern of living? Are you able to care for own activities of daily living? What time of the day do you feel most alert?

What is your present living situation and environment? Are there any hazards to health or development?

How do your present circumstances differ from your usual pattern of living? Have things changed with your aging/illness/disability? If so, how?

IV. *Perceptual Ability*

Describe your sensory ability or any impairment related to:

Sight:

Hearing:

Smell:

Taste:

Touch:

Balance:

Pain or unusual body perceptions:

Do bright lights or loud noises bother you?

If you are more sensitive to light or noise now, is it related to your illness or to conditions existing in the hospital/residence?

Do you have special visions? If so, describe them and when and where they occur?

Do you hear voices? If so, what do they say and are you able to converse with them?

What are your food preferences? What foods are not tasteful or enjoyable to you?

What kinds of feelings do you have in various body parts? Are you especially aware of any body part or function?

What situations require assistance for you to maintain balance/mobility? What kind of assistance do you need?

V. *Emotional Status*

Self-concept:

How would you describe yourself?

How do you feel you handle yourself and your life?

What would you describe as your attitude toward life?

What are the most important values to you?

What do you like best about yourself?

If it were possible, what is the primary aspect of yourself that you would like to change?

Do you prefer doing things alone or with others?

Ego ideal:

What goals or aspirations do you presently have?

Do you feel you have managed to achieve your goals in life?

Super ego:

Which of the following comes first for you? Pleasure, your goals, or essential tasks?

How do you respond to situations that require you to do something you are reluctant to do:
    Do you ignore the task?
    Do you plunge in and complete it as soon as possible?
    Do you delay the task as long as possible?
What rules or customs are difficult for you to follow?

What do you consider the most important teachings that were given to you by your parents or family? That you have lived by?

What causes you to feel guilty?

Relations to others:

Do you share your feelings with another with ease or with difficulty? With whom do you share your feelings?

Who can you trust to help you in time of need?

Who or what do you care about most in your life?

Who do you think cares most about you?

How do you see your life fitting into the lives of others?

How dependent on/independent of your family/friends are you?

Sense of autonomy:

What does the term "fate" mean to you?

What do you feel has control over what is happening to you?

How much control do you exert over others?

How has aging/illness/hospitalization/admission to nursing home or residence affected your feelings of control or lack of control?

Reaction and coping with situations:

What situations or persons make you feel calm, secure, happy?

What situations or persons cause you to feel upset, embarrassed, anxious, or angry?

How do you handle persons or situations that cause you to feel discomfort, anxiety, or anger?

What usually results from your behavior?

Adaptive pattern:

What is your usual pattern of relating to those close to you? To strangers? To a group situation?

How much does another's reaction or behavior influence how you will act?

How important is another person's behavior or feelings to you?

What is your reaction to frustration? To success?

Which of the following are you likely to do?

Go along with the person or situation to keep peace?

Blame others if something goes wrong for you?

Consider yourself the cause if something goes wrong?

Feel more angry than is warranted by the situation?

Let others know abruptly of your feelings?

Say little about your feelings, hoping the other person will guess how you are feeling?

Feel reluctant to act in an unfamiliar situation without permission or encouragement from someone?

Feel confident in unfamiliar situations and take charge of things if it is indicated?

Encourage others to do their best work possible?

Consider that others are unlikely to do the job as well as yourself?

What do you find best relieves your tension (eating, smoking, drinking, drugs, sleep, activity, etc.)?

VI. *Use of Leisure*

What activities do you enjoy for recreation or relaxation?

How often do you engage in these activities?

How do these activities affect your health?

VII. *Communication Pattern (Observe and Listen for)*

Ability to express thoughts and feelings (talks freely or hesitantly, writes, draws, uses nonverbal behavior primarily):

Describe vocabulary (variety of words used, repetition of words, slang, or correct grammar):

Enunciation of words:

Rate of expression of speech (how quickly answers, rapidity in flow of speech, hesitations, smooth vs. uneven rate, urgency of speech):

Ability to express ideas (coherent, logical, confused, circumstantial, tangential, poverty of ideation):

VIII. *Cognitive Status (Observe and Listen for)*

Level of consciousness (alert, lethargic, confused, stuporous, comatose):

Orientation to time, place, person:

Educational level:

Ability to recall far past, immediate past, and present events (What brought you into the hospital/residence? Tell me about the events that led to your hospitalization/admission to nursing home/residence. Tell me some major things about yourself and your past life.):

Attention span (attends to immediate stimuli; length of concentration or attention span; is not distracted by extraneous stimuli, how capable of following train of thought, what stimuli distracts, how long interview proceeded before person showed fatigue, preoccupied with self or some event):

Speed of response to verbal stimuli (answers immediately, quickly, or slowly; hesitates; ignores certain statements):

Remains in reverie state or in primary process (daydreams, fantasizes, talks about material that seems nonsensical or is difficult to follow):

Ability to do logical thinking or problem solving (or unable to do cause-effect associations; states loose, magical, or nonsensical logic):

Ability to grasp ideas or follow directions:

Ability to abstract (answers questions literally, is able to elaborate or explain, can give meanings for behavior situations):

Presence of delusions or degree of reality in belief system:

Apparent insight into problem/situation (What have you been told about your illness? What do you think is the cause of your problem? Why do you think you have been admitted to the hospital/nursing home/residence?):

Aware of need for more knowledge about illness situation (What questions or concerns do you have about your illness, hospital stay, admission to nursing home/residence?)

IX. *Ego Functions*

Interviewer should note the following during the interview:

What was the primary emotion? Was it appropriate to the situation?

During the interview, what nonverbal behavior accompanied statements?

What questions elicited behavioral manifestations of discomfort or anxiety?

Was there accentuated use of any one pattern of behavior during the interview?

Did the person use "they" instead of "I" when responding to questions? Was he aware of body parts and functions without excessive preoccupation with himself?

Was the person realistic or did he show disturbed reality testing? For example, is the person adapting to reality? Does he show poor judgment? Does he understand the consequences of his behavior? Does reality interfere with creative behavior? Presence of delusions? Hallucinations?

Has the person learned the socially acceptable method of dealing with drives and feelings?

What defense mechanisms are apparently commonly used? What defense mechanisms were used during the interview?

Does behavior appear overcontrolled, undercontrolled, or without control? Describe.

Does the person appear able to have the various aspects of his personality integrated? What aspects of his behavior appear fragmented or lacking in unity or autonomy?

Summary of Impressions

(Note any discrepancies between the patient's/client's perception and that of the interviewer/care-giver.)

Intrapersonal Factors:

> Physical (appearance; posture; facies; dress; hygiene; range of body functions; physical findings that evidence anxiety):

> Psychological (cognitive and perceptual abilities; thought processes; emotional status; ego functions; adaptive/defensive mechanisms used; feelings about self and body image; values; attitudes; needs; expectations; aspirations; behavior patterns; creative expressions; needs; strengths; limits):

> Developmental (degree of apparent normalcy; apparent stage of behavior and coping/defensive mechanisms; past learning history; perception of environment and family values; goals and ideas and the influence of these; how current level of functioning and life-style relate to culture/ethnicity, age, and sex of person):

> Social (super ego functions; behavior/socialization pattern; use of language and communication skills; activities of daily living; perception of relations to others; value system; customs; taboos or superstitions; understanding of own roles and roles of others):

> Interpersonal Factors (family structures; relationship with family, friends, and others; communication ability; socialization level; expectations of family, friends, care-givers, and others in present situation; ability to anticipate consequences of behavior; resources):

> Extrapersonal Factors (cultural factors; social class level; occupation; work-related resources; environmental or work-related stresses; residence and geographical location; financial resources; relationship to community; community resources; effect of time of day, temperature, and weather on behavior; use of space and privacy):

Recommendations:

Short-term goals:

Long-term goals:

Note: This tool could be adapted by the nurse who is working in the home health care agency.

the helping relationship with nurse and elderly client

3

ROLES OF THE NURSE

As you use the nursing process daily with the person/family in later maturity, you will be functioning in a variety of nursing roles. You will be responsible for physical care, technical procedures, and for creating an environment that is safe, comfortable, stimulating, and health promoting. You will often be called upon to teach informally and formally to enable the person/family to manage self-care, learn about his illness or response to a situation, or better cope with his condition. Referral to other sources of help may be necessary, for no one health team member can meet all the client's needs. You may serve as counselor, and you can always serve as a source of emotional and social stimulation and support. Depending upon your behavior and the senior's needs, you may be seen as a parental figure.

All of us need loving contact with other people in order to stay human in the fullest sense. From the moment of birth the infant cannot survive unless he is cared for by a nurturing person. But the elderly person cannot survive either, emotionally or physically, unless someone cares about him. Caring is essential to a relationship.

How the senior reacts to you, your attitudes, appearance, and behavior will be influenced at least initially by past experiences with people. If experiences have been pleasant with others, he will respond more quickly to your caring. If he has felt primarily anxiety and tension in his contact with others, he is likely to be distant, to respond slowly, or even to tell you to go away. He may test your intentions with overtly obnoxious behavior, but under his apparent rejection of you will be strong interpersonal needs. Knowing this should stimulate you to continue to reach out, to care.

Important in the total care of the senior is the establishment and maintenance of a relationship. Your goals may be limited because you cannot always change the person's pathology and you cannot reverse the aging process, but you can help him to accept and understand his situation, find meaning in it to the degree possible, and grow from it. This total care involves not only physical care but also genuine concern for the client's self-worth as a human, regardless of his social value or capacity for achievement.[11]

WHAT IS A RELATIONSHIP?

Definitions

Relationship can be defined as *an interpersonal process in which one person facilitates the personal development or growth of another over time by helping him to mature; become more adaptive, integrated, and open to his own experience; or to find meaning in his present situation.*

There are different types of relationships: parent-child, husband-wife, teacher-student, friend-friend, and nurse-client.

The **nurse-client relationship** *results from a series of interactions between a nurse and client over a period of time, with the nurse focusing on the needs and problems of the person/family while using the scientific knowledge and specific skills of the profession.* This helping relationship develops through interest in, encounter with, and commitment to the person.

The Social Relationship

The nurse-client relationship differs from a social or personal relationship. The social relationship consists of the following characteristics:

1. The contact is primarily for pleasure and companionship.
2. Neither person is in a position of responsibility for helping the other.
3. No specific skill or knowledge are required.
4. The interaction is between peers, often of the same social status.
5. The people involved can, and often do, pursue an encounter for the satisfaction of personal or selfish interests.
6. There is no explicit formulation of goals.

Certainly you can have an association with another for a long time and not have a relationship. Many associations do not promote growth or a sense of security and they do not reduce feelings of helplessness and loneliness.

CHARACTERISTICS OF THE HELPING PERSON

The capacity to be a helping person is strengthened by a genuine desire to be responsible and sensitive to another person. In addition, experience with a variety of people increases your awareness of others' reactions and feelings, and the feedback you receive from others will teach you a great deal on both the emotional and cognitive levels.

Characteristics of a helping person include being:

1. Congruent—being trustworthy, dependable, and consistent.
2. Unambiguous—avoiding contradictory messages.
3. Positive—showing warmth, caring, and respect.
4. Strong—maintaining separate identity from the client.
5. Secure—permitting the client to remain separate, respecting his needs and your own.
6. Empathic—looking at the client's world from his viewpoint, being open to his feelings and beliefs.

7. Accepting—enabling the client to change at his pace.
8. Sensitive—being perceptive to feelings, avoiding threatening behavior.
9. Nonjudgmental—refraining from evaluating the client moralistically.
10. Creative—viewing the client as a person in the process of becoming, not being bound by his past, and viewing self in the process of becoming or maturing as well.[47]

Other characteristics that correlate highly with being effective in a helping relationship are being open instead of closed in interaction with others, perceiving others as friendly and capable instead of unfriendly and incapable, and perceiving a relationship as freeing instead of controlling another.[5]

Establishing and maintaining a relationship or counseling another does not involve putting on a facade of behavior to match a list of characteristics. Rather, both you and the client will change and continue to mature. As the helper, you are present as a total person, blending potentials, talents, and skills while assisting the senior client to come to grips with his needs, conflicts, and self.[38]

Working with another in a helping relationship is challenging and rewarding. You will not always have all the characteristics just described; at times you will be handling personal stresses that will lower your energy and sense of involvement. You may become irritated and impatient while working with the elderly. Accept the fact that you are not perfect and that you are always in the process of becoming. Analyzing your behavior in relation to the person/family can help you determine your effect on them and can help you to be more effective. Just as you help the senior to develop, you will also continue to expand your personality to better gain the above characteristics. As you open a panorama of possibilities to another, your own potential unfolds. Remember that the most important thing you can share with a client is your own uniqueness as a person.

Nursing experience in itself can bring about a cool efficiency, an overt indifference, and an impersonal attitude and environment for the client. The distant behavior that may result when the nurse is not rewarded by the work system for demonstrating helping characteristics seems to be an occupational hazard of nursing. Yet, in an increasingly mechanical world we have to remain human and treat our clients as human.[15]

CHARACTERISTICS OF THE HELPING RELATIONSHIP

The nurse-client relationship depends primarily on your experience, your attitudes toward self and client, and the nature of your involvement. The relationship develops out of what you and the other person are. Set techniques or rules exist to ensure a relationship, but the following discussion may help you understand the components that enhance its achievement.

Rapport

A relationship begins with the ability to establish *rapport, creating a sense of harmony between individuals.* To establish rapport quickly, you must have the following social skills:

1. A warm, friendly manner, appropriate smile, and comfortable eye contact.
2. Ability to treat the other as an equal, to eliminate social barriers, to convey acceptance, and to promote a sense of trust.
3. Ability to establish a smooth, easy pattern of conversation.
4. Ability to find a common interest or experience.
5. Ability to show a keen, sympathetic interest in the other, to give him full attention, to listen carefully, and to indicate there is plenty of time.
6. Ability to accurately adopt his terminology and conventions and to meet him on his own ground.[1]

Trust

Trust is the firm belief in the honesty, integrity, reliability, and justice of another person without fear of outcome, the inner certainty that the other person's behavior is predictable under a given set of circumstances.[19,47]

The capacity to develop a trusting relationship is built upon your attitude toward people, your flexibility in responding, and what you are personally. Techniques and knowledge are not enough. You will learn through experience what aspects of your personality are more effective with and helpful to others. Trust is based on consistency rather than compatibility. The senior cannot reveal himself nor share important information unless he can rely on you and believes that you will react with the same behavioral characteristics each time he meets with you and that you will keep content from the interview confidential, as mutually agreed upon. You may have to delay obtaining certain information until a sense of trust is established because the elderly client may feel very threatened by an interview or examination.[5,47] In addition, you must feel that you can predict the person's behavior because you have an understanding of the person.

Unconditional Positive Regard and Acceptance

Two qualities often described as essential to a relationship are positive, warm feelings and acceptance.[47] Is it possible to give expert and truly professional care and not feel positively toward your client? Most texts and most clients would say "NO." The human spirit loses its sense of vitality and sometimes even the will to live when surrounded by hostile persons.

Realistically, it is not possible to like everyone, just as it is not possible to establish and maintain a relationship with everyone. But you will find some clients you will be genuinely interested in and can feel affection for; other nurses will respond that way to other clients. There are the few cantankerous or repulsive people whom no one seems to feel any rapport with or interest in. Perhaps your willingness to reach out, to stimulate a more likable behavior in that person, to learn more about his uniqueness will be the result of your *unconditional positive regard, belief in the dignity, worth, and importance of the person, regardless of his behavior.*[47]

Every senior, when the outer mask is removed, has something likable and interesting about him—either for what he is or was. The rewards of your efforts to become involved with the difficult client will be to learn about him and his life, and in the process learn something about yourself, your persistence, beliefs about people, commitment to nursing, and interactional skills. Anyone can respond to someone who is attractive and gracious. The challenge, and the measure of the nurse, lies in the ability to relate to the person everyone else has given up on, such as the wrinkled 90-year-old man who pinches every female, the grotesque alcoholic, and the wobbly old lady who bites and spits.

Some people are hard to accept. *Acceptance means interest in and concern for another because he is a human being with dignity, avoidance of moralistic judgment, and the feeling that this person is worth all the attention, skill, understanding, and energy you can focus upon him.*[47] Acceptance means to relate to the inner core of the person, understanding but not agreeing with nor necessarily permitting inappropriate behavior. Acceptance means not to show your feelings of shock or disapproval aroused by the person's behavior and not to feel a need to control that behavior.

Acceptance means recognizing the right of another to have his own beliefs, values, and standards, even when they contradict your own. You do not condemn the person for his behavior; you do not zealously insist that he change his behavior just because it displeases you. Instead, you *assist* the person, if possible, to change his behavior to become more acceptable to others. The senior feels accepted if he feels neither above you nor below you, neither dominated by you nor alone without needed guidance. He senses you are not bored by him. If the person feels that you accept him, he feels free to disclose private information about himself and to call for your assistance without fear or embarrassment. He feels at ease with you. He feels good about himself in your presence.

Empathy

Unconditional positive regard and acceptance are easier to achieve if you have developed empathic understanding of people. *Empathy is feeling with the person and simultaneously understanding the dynamics of his behavior.*[47] As you and the senior feel and think together, your feelings for him impels you to act.

Empathy is the ability to sense the client's private world as if it were your own without ever losing the "as if" quality; to sense the client's anger, fear, or confusion as if it were your own without your own feelings getting bound up in the interaction.

You are empathic to the degree that you are able to abstract from your own life experience, by way of recall or generalizations, common factors that are applicable to the client's problems.

Certain qualities enhance empathic skills. The ability to empathize varies with the client, time, and nurse. Certainly a general interest in people, basic knowledge of human behavior, and a warm, flexible personality encourages empathy. Other characteristics that enable you to be more empathic are:

1. Similarity in values, experiences, social class, culture, occupational and economic level, religion, age, personality traits, or sameness of sex.
2. Ability to be alert, to listen with the "third ear," to become involved in another, to abandon self-consciousness.
3. Ability to cope with egocentricity, anxiety, fears, other feelings or various stresses that might interfere with listening to and feeling with another.
4. Variety of life experiences that help you to acquire a broad understanding of people, flexibility, and spontaneity.
5. Ability to maintain an adequate health and energy level.
6. Ability to interpret correctly and to avoid distorting perceptions.[55]

Empathy involves the following dimensions:

1. Tone—expressing warmth and spontaneity nonverbally and verbally.
2. Pace—timing remarks or behavior appropriate to the client's feelings and needs.
3. Perception—abstracting the core or essential meaning of the client's concerns and discussing them with him in acceptable terms.
4. Leading—being resourceful in formulating questions or statements that move the interview in the direction of the client's concerns.[6]

Empathy is not the same as sympathy or pity. The sympathetic person becomes stricken with emotion because he projects himself into the other person's place. The empathic person shares the experience but maintains objectivity.[30] The sympathizer may be secretly happy that a certain situation has not occurred to him or he may feel guilty in his luck. Empathy can be found in any situation, in grief and in joy.

Pity is contrary to helping. To cause another to feel like a victim debases the person now and conveys that he will remain debased and helpless. Pity conveys that the other person receives help because you are obligated and pseudoaltruistic. Spontaneous and genuine helping is done by one human being with another simply because you are both human.[5]

How do you communicate empathy? Use verbal and nonverbal communication so that the senior experiences a feeling of being understood. Your statements serve as an emotional mirror or as a reflection of his feelings without distorting or giving him advice. For example, you may say: "It seems as if you are very discouraged with P. T." or "It sounds as if you are quite concerned about whether you made a right decision." Avoid a response like, "I know how you feel." Such a response makes the senior unsure about your truly understanding him. It is a rote response and is not based on a genuine understanding of his current feelings.

Talk on the senior's level of understanding and adjust your tone of voice to his. For example, if you use a declarative, harsh tone of voice, it will seem as if you are telling the client what he thinks and how he feels and *not* reflecting *his* feelings. Using language that he does not understand will convey a lack of respect regardless of the accuracy of your interpretation.

Evaluate the elderly person's true feelings. Sometimes he is not ready to admit certain feelings and needs time to be allowed to deny them.

Reflect the senior's feelings to him frequently for correction, disapproval, or approval, and remain open to his response. A client who is free to correct you moves on to a higher level of self-understanding. If he cannot refute your reflection, he builds up defenses and then withdraws, thereby defeating the primary purpose of the relationship. Some examples of how to begin your reflections are: "If I understand you correctly, you feel . . . ." "Is this right?"

Respond actively and frequently enough to the client, without interrupting him, to indicate that you are focusing on his speech and feelings.[30]

The ultimate purpose of the empathic response is to convey to the person a depth of understanding about him and his predicament so that he can expand and clarify his understanding of self and others.[8] The client receives relief from loneliness and overcomes feelings of isolation and aloneness with his problems. Your willingness to understand how the senior feels about his world implies that his point of view is valuable. Also, the focus of evaluation is within the client, so that he becomes less dependent on the opinions of others and grows to value himself. Empathetic understanding is not a passive process, and it will not happen without effort. You must concentrate intensely on the person; since intense concentration allows you little time to reflect on personal needs, values, and ideals, it prevents judgmental thoughts or behavior.[30]

Improvement of patients is correlated with empathic response, regardless of their diagnoses. Not only are high empathic levels correlated with improvement, but low levels of empathy contribute to increased disturbance in patients. The lack of empathy displayed by nurses could, therefore, be hindering their patient's recovery.[28]

Purposeful Communication

A helping relationship involves careful listening to the client's total message rather than selective listening to the parts that are most enjoyable or easy. There are times when you will have to ignore your own needs; listen to ideas, values, or attitudes contradictory to your own; listen to offensive language; or observe behavior that makes you uncomfortable. If you ignore these stimuli, you will not be able to be helpful. Be prepared for such communication at some point in any relationship; work through your own feelings; and respond to the senior so that underlying feelings and needs can be handled.

Effective ways to communicate verbally were discussed in relation to the nursing process. Various sources also give useful techniques.[18,23,32,41,44,45,47,49]

Knowledge of interviewing techniques will increase your potential to be helpful to the client. The techniques should be thoroughly learned and internalized so that they become a part of your spontaneous behavior. These techniques are most effective when you are minimally aware of using them because they are so fully a part of you. Techniques are only aids that provide you varied and flexible ways of responding. They are useless unless they are based upon accurate perceptions of the client's communication.[5]

Goal Formulation

A helping relationship differs from a social relationship in that in the helping relationship there is explicit formulation of goals. You may have certain goals that you hope to accomplish, but the senior must actively participate with you in setting mutual goals. As the relationship progresses, new problems or concerns will be identified and new goals will have to be set. The relationship is structured in that you share with the client what he can expect and you listen to what the client expects of you. Together you determine the course of the relationship; intentions and expectations are verbally and nonverbally conveyed to each other, and the expectations change as the relationship progresses.[5]

General goals of the nurse-client relationship include:

1. Increasing the senior's self-esteem and promoting a positive self-concept and sense of security.
2. Decreasing the senior's anxiety to a minimum.
3. Providing a gratifying, positive experience.
4. Assisting the senior in improving communication skills and in participating comfortably with others.
5. Providing the opportunity for the person to grow emotionally.
6. Helping the person find meaning in his life situation.
7. Maintaining and stimulating the person biologically, mentally, emotionally, and socially.
8. Gathering data in order to gain in-depth assessment and provide individualized care.[51]

Humor

Intense interaction between two or more people cannot endure unless a sense of humor surfaces at times. *Humor is the ability to see the ludicrous or the incongruities of a situation, to be amused by one's own imperfections or the whimsical aspects of life, to see the funny side of an otherwise serious situation.*[19] Humor does not necessarily mean joking and teasing. It does not involve the put-down of another, and it does not always evoke laughter. Humor may be expressed as a tiny smile that lingers or the mental chuckle that occurs when you are sober-faced.

The purposes of humor include releasing tension, anxiety, or hostility; cautiously distracting from sadness, crying, or guilt; decreasing social distance; conveying a sense of empathy to another; expressing warmth and affection; encouraging learning or task accomplishment; and denying painful feelings or a threatening situation.

The elderly person often has an experienced use of humor beneath those steely eyes and tight lips. He may test you with a few dry statements to see if you are really alert and if you can make the cognitive connections he insinuates. Too often these dry statements receive only a grunt in reply, or worse, they are ignored and the person is labeled senile, confused, or crazy. If you do not respond to his humor, the senior loses emotional and social input and self-esteem, although underneath he may consider you his inferior—less educated, less experienced, less wise. You lose when you cannot expand your mind with the humorous. You dry up emotionally, and you have lost an opportunity to learn, to mature, and to enjoy.

UNDERSTANDING BEHAVIOR IN THE RELATIONSHIP

Principles of Human Behavior

Basic elements of human behavior to consider in the nurse-client relationship include the following ideas.

The person is an open system and maintains the self through exchanges with other people and various environmental stimuli. Input and output are required for life maintenance and reproduction. Since man is not self-sufficient, he must remain open to the ministrations of others in order to have certain needs met.[46]

Change in one part of a system produces change in all parts. Helping another produces effects not anticipated by the helper or person receiving help because of the resultant changes in the client. Helping another, that is, forming and maintaining a relationship, does not provide total freedom from discomfort, but it often changes the discomforts or the person's ability to cope with them. The essence of life is change, not bliss. Helping—relating—affirms and stimulates a person's power to change, to overcome helplessness in adversity. People who do not ask for help may bring about behavioral change in themselves.[46]

Human behavior has purpose. Therefore, the behavior is commonly preceded by imagining the desired result. The person visualizes the future and tries to bring it about. The helper tries to understand the client by understanding his goals or purposes so that he can encourage the client to pursue them if they are realistic. The senior's behavior may seem purposeless, but he is trying to meet his needs, even if these needs are not apparent at first. The goals or satisfactions sought are based on recall of earlier satisfactions and how they were obtained. Because of the tendency to regress under stress, the senior who needs help will be hoping to have things done for him, just as satisfactions were brought to him in his earlier life. Yet, receiving help from a stranger or impersonal caretaker is difficult. If you do not have a good relationship with your client, you may not be aware of his deep-felt need for help. Further, when you have a helping, trusting relationship with the elderly person, you can expect him to make extra demands on you when he feels great need, for he feels secure with you. In response, you may feel impatient or irritable. Your goals and the client's goals may differ, and these differences need to be resolved.[46,47]

When one need or goal is met, the person has energy to pursue another need, interest, or goal. Behavior changes direction, but it does not come to an end. Consequently, loss is implied even in successful behavior. In later life, when it is too late to reassign priorities, the person becomes more time-conscious in relation to gaining multiple satisfactions. You can help the senior use his time constructively so that he can meet the goals that have priority for him.

Most human behavior is learned and is based on past experiences. Behavior that had a satisfactory outcome is likely to be repeated; behavior that brought pain is likely to be extinguished. However, people go through different developmental levels, and the conditions under which they have to apply learning change over time. Human learning can become obsolete; the elderly person may behave in a situation in a way that was appropriate in the past but is inappropriate in the present situation. Thus, he needs your help to understand how to change his behavior. Whether or not he can unlearn behavior is questionable. Can something once learned ever be extinguished? If what was learned in the past seemed good or brought gratification, it might interfere with learning something new and supposedly better. Additionally, people seem to seek gratification in times of stress by reverting to earlier, more comfortable kinds of behavior. Thus, as a helper, you enable the person to acquire additional learning so that he has alternatives in coping. A feeling of being able to choose among alternatives improves the self-image because the person feels less helpless.[46]

If behavior is unsuccessful, tension increases; self-esteem falls. The unsuccessful person creates a new need, a need for psychological repair. Because the elderly person often feels less successful now than he did earlier, you can help him return to his former level of maturity and find new coping patterns that improve his self-evaluation.

Loneliness is a very basic and common feeling in people, especially in the elderly. People in distress may have many acquaintances, but they seldom have anyone who has the time, interest, understanding, or skill to help alleviate the suffering. The distressed person feels lonely. You can help to offset the loneliness through an individual relationship. Involvement in a group, as described in the next chapter, also offsets loneliness.

Humans develop, mature, and decline. They grow from helplessness into strength and then they return to some degree of helplessness. The person throughout life needs some experiences of being strong. You can help the elderly person to combat the helpless feelings that result from a slowdown of activities or decline.

At times the elderly client seems to hold on to helplessness, dependency, or passivity. An infant never completely has all the dependency needs met. In times of stress this form of dependency is again sought. The helper, with the usual personal stresses, may develop regressive tendencies and unconsciously and defensively become an ally of the client's regression. Dependency and helplessness in the client may be used vicariously by the helper to increase feelings of omnipotence and satisfaction or to enhance self-evaluation.[46]

The primary psychological needs of the person, based on his experience of dependency, are the need for association and sense of decreasing helplessness, which can be accomplished through your notice of and your involvement with him.

Guidelines for Your Behavior

When you relate to and work with a senior, you should consider the following guidelines.

The total complement of nonverbal clues should be observed; facial expression alone is not a good indicator of the senior's feelings. For example, cheerfulness can be a mask for anxiety, fear, uncertainty, or anger.

The quiet, cooperative person has as great a need to talk and to receive attention as does the outgoing, uncooperative, or demanding person. This senior is popular, but his cooperation may be his way of bargaining for security and your attention. Underneath the behavior may be feelings of doubt, anger or suspicion.

Some seniors will be hard to accept and will cause you anxiety because they are demanding, regressed, uninhibited in action or speech, stubborn, or generally unpleasant to be with. Such behavior is the best the person can demonstrate at that point; his behavior is the result of trying to handle his feelings and maintain his identity and integrity. Often such behavior is difficult to tolerate because it reminds you of characteristics you do not like within your own personality, or it reminds you that you could also behave like that when you are under stress, ill, or old. The elderly person may be embarrassed by his behavior even though he cannot control it. Without belittling or punishing the person you can convey that the nature of his behavior is temporary, that he is accepted even though the behavior is unacceptable, that you trust his capacity to grow and evolve more appropriate behavior as you work with him.

If tears make you uncomfortable, consider that the crying client is giving you a great compliment. He feels secure enough with you to permit himself to cry in your presence. He senses your acceptance and caring. The elderly person knows the social sanctions against crying and often will feel embarrassed when tears come spontaneously. Yet, mood is often more unstable in the elderly; the person cries more easily, but not necessarily in front of just anyone. Crying is usually brief and is a means of relieving tension. Convey that it is all right to cry, that you do not consider the person a baby or less of a man or woman. Give the person time to regain composure before continuing the conversation or activity.

Clients of different ethnic or racial backgrounds may react differently with you because of their past experiences with people. If the person has suffered much rejection or persecution during his life, he may be suspicious of your intentions and behavior as you try to establish a relationship. He may have learned that one way to avoid hurt was to remain unresponsive to contacts from others. Yet, he has a need for care, attention, respect, and security. Do not be rebuffed by this initial apathy or withdrawal. Consistent availability for short periods that does not push or probe will be accepted over time. Sometimes it takes months before the rejecting person senses and responds to your interest.

You may become attached to, or possessive of, a client and be unwilling to relinquish him to the family when he is ready for discharge from the hospital or home health care agency. (This frequently happens in care of children, but it can happen with clients of any age.) There is nothing wrong with liking a client. In fact, it helps, but your emotional involvement with that person will be different from that with a friend or relative. Except in the nursing home or long-term residence for the aged, your relationship is temporary; you begin as strangers and you are in a service role to the person. The best way to show that you like someone is to accept him as he is, meet his needs promptly, and help him to expand his relationships to others. Termination means that you have achieved a goal. Further, the most significant people to the client are usually his family. Helping the client and his family to relate more comfortably to each other may be necessary.

Constraints in the Helping Relationship

Certain limits exist for both you, the helper, and the client. Relationship means involvement and commitment; it takes time. The senior's dependency may create demands for extra time, advice, or responsibility. You will have to consider his feelings and needs, meet important demands, and set limits whenever necessary.[5] An honest response about your limitations of time and energy is most helpful. The elderly person usually accepts the fact that you have other demands placed upon you if they are explained objectively. Such honesty often stimulates the person to try to do all he can for himself. If you can respond without anger or without a sense of excessive obligation, the person will not feel rejected. Thus, undue dependency will be avoided.

Differences between you, the helper, and the client can be an obstacle to a satisfactory exchange. Perceiving each other as different prevents two people from coming closer. All helping is an overcoming of distance and difference between helper and client. You cannot empathize or engage in sharing if the real differences of two unique persons, such as age, sex, educational level, or sociocultural background, are not worked through.[45]

Inequity in a relationship in which the client's needs are sufficiently met but there is insufficient gratification for the helper may cause the ending of a relationship. If you feel depleted and cannot feel a sense of doing good, being worthwhile, learning about people and life, developing professional skills, or maturing, you can no longer meet the dependency needs of the other. Certainly this sense of depletion or inequity can be prevented if you have other relationships—with friends and colleagues—to support you. You should not expect to have personal needs, other than those just listed, met by the senior. Instead, focus on his needs. There isn't much tangible payoff. You must have considerable ego strength if you are to interact in a therapeutic way with a number of elderly clients. You cannot live out your problems and find answers by listening to the client.[46] This may be one reason why some nurses never form relationships with clients.

Yet, you may have certain needs, as a helper, met through client relationships. Loneliness in the client is relieved by the security of being attended to; your loneliness may be relieved by people seeking your help. The client's sense of helplessness needs hope that things will get better, that there are other ways of handling his situation, and that it won't cost too much in time and money. You may have a need to convey hope, optimism, and confidence and to use your imagination and skills to meet the challenge of stimulating another to handle a situation. You may need to convey what you have learned by overcoming obstacles.[46]

While encouraging a senior, you must control ambitions for his improvement. The senior may not be able to give up discomforts; they may be a core part of his identity. He may not be willing to change sufficiently to resolve his problem.[46]

As a helper, you may use the professional role to resolve developmental difficulties that remain from earlier life. The risk is that as the senior talks, you will relieve your own conflicts and fears of past developmental eras. In that case, the senior's problems may not be resolved; they are likely to be maintained unconsciously by you as you work out your problems through the client. You must be aware of any inappropriate feelings and overreactions. Keep your personal life out of the reaction to and concern with the client. You will also need a change in your professional and personal life at times so that you will be able to remain helpful and feel revitalized. Continuing education and seeking help from a friend or counselor by talking through your reactions and the possible causes can serve this purpose.[45]

As a helper, you may treat the client or his problems as trivial. It is important for anyone in distress to feel that his existence has meaning. If the client does not have a philosophical, religious, or political affiliation that permits him to transcend his personal destiny, the helping experience can be his only chance to gain such meaning. Treating the client as insignificant in the formative stages of the relationship increases his burden of loneliness and helplessness, and it decreases the chance of a working relationship.[46]

Your inability to recognize or handle transference phenomenon will hinder progress in a relationship. Arising most likely during the identification phase of the relationship, **transference** *is the process whereby the client inappropriately, unrealistically, but unconsciously displaces onto you or invests in you, the helper, the patterns of behavior and emotional reactions that originated with authority figures in the senior's childhood, usually with his parents.* Transference may be positive, that is, all the attitudes, emotions, or responses to you are loving or happy because the client sees in you his parents who fostered such responses. Positive transference also includes expression of unmet needs or desires, or delegated omnipotence, that is, the person repeatedly states how wonderful you are and how he wishes to be like you. Negative transference occurs when the client responds to you with anger or hate, such as he felt toward his parents earlier.[32]

Transference is not simply positive or negative, and it is not age or sex related. It is a recreation of the various stages of the emotional development or a reflection of his complex attitudes toward others who were important earlier in his life. Transference is triggered because you are developing a closeness to the senior. Realistic characteristics about you can trigger transference: your appearance, age, sex, personal manner, social, and ethnic background. Desire for affection, respect, and gratification of dependency needs also trigger transference. The senior seeks evidence that you can or will love him, often through making demands upon you. Legitimate or realistic requests should be met early in the relationship. Later, refusals to meet requests that are unnecessary or that the person can meet himself, along with discussion and interpretation of the significance of this behavior, are warranted.[32]

Questions about your personal life may involve a different kind of transference. Most often these questions are concerned about your status or ability to understand the person. Occasionally a direct answer to the question is appropriate. Usually it is more appropriate to inquire, "What leads to your question?" or "What did you have in mind?" It may be helpful to interpret, for example, "You ask about my age because you are unsure of me?"[32]

Competitive feelings resulting from earlier relationships with siblings or parents may be expressed toward you in transference. Such a client clearly strives to be one jump ahead of you; makes belittling, and disparaging remarks about you; challenges your statements or abilities; or constantly interrupts you. When the person is obviously competitive, it is helpful to make a remark about it, for example, "I didn't know we were having a race" or "You feel that you are competing with me?" At times, it is best to ignore competitive behavior; often such behavior is motivated by feelings of inferiority.[32]

Male patients may show interest in the power, status, or economic success of a male nurse, whereas they may be concerned about the motherly, seductive, or domineering behavior of the female nurse. Female clients are frequently concerned about the male nurse's attitude toward the role of women, whether he can be seduced, what his wife is like, and what sort of father he is. The female client may feel competitive toward the female nurse and be interested in her career and adequacy as a woman and mother.[32]

Older patients may treat you as a child, for example, by bringing food or other gifts, cautioning you about health or hard work, or reprimanding you. Elderly male clients may offer fatherly advice about financial matters, home, or cars; elderly females may give maternal advice.[32]

As the helper, you may experience **countertransference,** *inappropriate emotional response to the client as if he were an important figure in your past.* The helpful measure would be to respond to the client realistically, as he really is. Countertransference works in much the same way as transference does for the client. You may become dependent on the senior's praise or affection; unconsciously invite gifts or favors; offer excessive reassurance or help that is not really necessary; suppress his need to show anger; display knowledge, social, or professional status in order to solicit affection or admiration. Persons in the healing professions have a desire to be all-knowing and all-powerful, but if you assume such a role, the senior cannot overcome his feelings of inferiority and helplessness. Countertransference includes overidentification with the client; you exert pressure on him to improve and attempt to make him over in your own image. Countertransference can be overcome through guidance from a supervisor and a willingness to examine personal behavior and comments.[32] The countertransference response of wishing to be the senior's child, grandchild, or younger sibling may occur with older people, especially if they actually resemble your parents, grandparents, or siblings.[32]

Resistance is likely to occur at some time during a relationship. Your inability to recognize or handle it is the main obstacle. *Resistance is an attitude on the part of the client that avoids exploring symptoms, changing behavior, or otherwise feeling anxiety in the relationship.* Resistance is the client's way of protecting himself when you are touching painful areas of his life. Content that is basic to the problem and that is kept out of awareness or repressed prevents development of understanding on the part of the client, but repression also wards off threatening impulses. Resistance may occur when the senior is willing to give up the secondary benefits his illness or behavior provides.[32]

Either positive or negative transference can cause resistance. If the senior expresses only affection for you, you may reply, "You spend so much time talking about your feelings for me that you haven't talked about yourself." If a senior becomes silent after initial talkative sessions, you may remark, "Perhaps you're not talking much because of some feelings concerning me?" The senior may expect a cure or to have his life situation improved by identifying with you or telling you information that he thinks would please you. Transference can be used as resistance; it can be a motivating factor for the client to work to solve his problem.[32]

Resistance is commonly expressed by silence. The senior says, "I have nothing to say." Although this may be uncomfortable, sit quietly and wait for him to talk unless this is early in the relationship. He may be testing your sincerity. He may not trust you. Or he may think more slowly than the younger person. Initially, after waiting in silence, it may be more helpful to use open-ended, explorative questions to promote a fuller assessment. It can be helpful to state interest in why he is silent, saying, "Perhaps there is something that is difficult for you to discuss" or "You seem to be holding back."[32]

Silence can be provoked in the senior if you are too active; asking too many questions that can be answered with "yes" or "no," or providing him with the answers. This discourages spontaneity, constricts the flow of ideas, and may encourage a negative transference.[32]

Intellectualization, when the person talks as if he understands himself and his problems, but then cannot go on to act on that supposed understanding, may be a form of resistance. Usually there is an absence of appropriate emotion with the intellectual constructs. Intellectualization may include learning and using your professional jargon. You can discourage the resistance that comes with intellectualizing in several ways. Avoid "why" questions. Ask him instead to elaborate and give more details. Avoid questions that seem to seek an answer that pleases you or that you specifically want. Avoid using technical terms or professional psychological jargon.[32] As the person feels safe in the relationship, he may be able to drop this defense with you.

Preoccupation, persistently focusing on certain symptoms, problems, one phase of life or trivial details, is another form of resistance. You can demonstrate to the person that such behavior is not helpful and that it prohibits finding solutions. You may say, "You seem to have difficulty talking about anything except _____" or "Tell me first about _____, and then you can tell me the other details."[32]

Emotional displays as well as apathy, stoicism, or apparent boredom are forms of resistance. One emotion may be used to defend against deeper, more painful ones. Frequently, "happy sessions" indicate that the client obtains sufficient emotional gratification during the session to ward off anxiety, but this reduces motivation to change behavior. It is important to explore the process with the person.[32]

Frequent requests to change the time or date of the interview, arriving late, or using minor physical illness to avoid the interview may be unavoidable for the senior or they may be forms of resistance. Explore the senior's feelings about your interactions and the meaning of his behavior, and avoid giving undue attention to the behavior.[5,32]

Several problems arise in handling resistance. As a helper, you may feel hurt, impatient, angry, inadequate, or unaccepting to the client when he is resistant. Working through these feelings with another professional and with the senior will avoid a crescendo of feelings that may be damaging to the relationship. You may also think that the resistance results from your lack of expertise or misperception. Remember that the client may talk about irrelevant matters or may not fully trust you, not because of what you are doing, but because of earlier experiences with people. Again, an open, honest discussion with the senior will be useful. Security and concern will be transferred to the client in the closeness of the relationship, which in turn will help him become more secure and confident.

If the above constraints are ignored, the helper-client relationship is likely to deteriorate.[5]

Characteristics of a Nontherapeutic Relationship

There may be people with whom you cannot form a helpful relationship. There may be situations in which it would be best for the client if someone else were to work with him. You need to be aware of your own feelings of discomfort with a client, and you should be able to accept the fact that you cannot work with a certain person. Often the reasons will be obscure; you may want to work through the reasons with a counselor or supervisor for your own personal growth.

How can you or other colleagues know if an interaction is detrimental to the client? The following examples will help you analyze your affect upon the client.

You may increase the client's anxiety or feel increased anxiety with him. Often anxiety is manifested by anger, inappropriate laughing or humor, or withdrawal. Anxiety is always present when two strangers first begin to interact, but the anxiety should not be overwhelming. With time, support of colleagues and continued contact with the person, your anxiety should diminish. The more comfortable you become, the more comfortable the client will become. If this does not happen, unconscious forces may be operating. If neither you nor the client can cope with the discomfort, you must analyze the situation instead of pushing ahead blindly. Often the situation is resolved by the client's withdrawing from you—physically and emotionally. If such withdrawal persists, you should talk over the situation with an experienced colleague so that the final outcome will be best for both the client and you. Every helper who works with dependent or helpless people has the responsibility to stop when he is unable to function, whether in physical or emotional care. There is no substitute for knowledge, skill, and a compassionate attitude.

You may feel anger toward the client. The anger may be a reaction to his being old and your fear of becoming old. The anger may be a counterreaction to the client's anger that is related to something else, but directed toward you.

You can stop the cycle by recognizing your feelings and the helplessness felt by the senior, by talking with him to determine possible sources of anger, and by avoiding either a hostile or too sweet response. Do not belittle him by joking about his anger and do not reject or punish him for his anger. Make sure that you are not the cause of his anger because of actions that demean, aggravate, or neglect him. If the senior arouses anger in you, seek help from a skilled colleague to work through possible reasons for your anger, to talk about how you demonstrate anger in your behavior, and to work out how to handle the feelings. Anger prevents understanding the senior and seeing him as a unique person of worth. If your anger overpowers him, he will either withdraw or attempt to defend himself in other ways. A barrage of anger keeps the client from growing, or perhaps even surviving, especially if the anger is expressed through sadistic behavior.

You may think you are the only person who can care for the client or that you can solve all his problems. Such omnipotence is usually unfounded. Although nursing can meet some of your needs for approval, gratification, security, esteem, and achievement, do not rely only on the job and your clients to meet your needs. You cannot meet all of his needs, even when you are very important to him. In a relationship that encourages growth, you help the person reach out to others, and vice versa. Work with the health care team for the client's benefit.

You may have difficulty with dependency and independency within a relationship. You may want to have others depend on you. Therefore, you do things for the senior that he can do for himself. Such smothering discourages independent behavior in the senior. On the other hand, you may not be able to tolerate the senior's dependency, clinging, helplessness, or need for total assistance. Seek help to work through your own feelings. Accept the client as he is. Recall the behavioral principle that the person cannot become independent emotionally or physically unless his dependency needs are first met. Also remember that the elderly person values whatever independency he is capable of, fears dependency, and hates being infantilized.

You may want to treat the client as a social friend or look for companionship in him. The result is that you usually meet your personal needs but at the client's expense. Avoid using the senior as a confidante to solve your own problems or as an audience for talks about your personal life or to get attention or praise. Avoid using the senior to promote your own political, religious, or philosophical views, even when he uses you as a sounding board for his views. Talk about yourself and your activities with friends, family, or colleagues, not with the client.

Sometimes the elderly person may ask you questions about yourself and show an interest in you as a person. Some information may be important so that he has a feeling of knowing you and a sense of personal contact. However, experience has proven that a brief answer about yourself generally is sufficient for his curiosity or it takes care of the senior's idea of the social graces, that is, showing an interest in the other. In fact, after your brief answer, he will frequently interrupt and begin talking about himself. Your reply may have stimulated his thoughts, and the person in later maturity enjoys sharing ideas with someone who will listen.

*You may place the senior client in a **me-you pattern,*** perceiving and interacting with him as grandparent, parent, aunt, uncle, or someone else whom you know. Although you may feel affection for and interest in the client because he reminds you of someone you like (or feel dislike or repulsion for the opposite reason), the person deserves to be seen as the unique being he is. If you talk to him the way you would to someone you know personally, or have unrealistic expectations, the client will not perceive your affection or interest. Instead, he will sense that you are talking to someone else. He will feel used and he may withdraw. At best, a distorted relationship results from interacting with someone as if he were someone else. You are likely to miss important cues during assessment and are likely to intervene in a way that does not meet his needs.

You may consciously or unconsciously use intimidation to control the client. ***Intimidation** is making another afraid, forcing or deterring behavior with threats or violence, or overpowering another with awe.*[19] Rituals and policies can also intimidate. A common practice that is sometimes used as part of a behavior modification program is isolation: The nurses stop going to the patient's room, they answer the lights slowly or not at all, and they generally withhold services from someone whom they consider a nuisance.[42] The patient conforms; he does not ring the bell or ask for services. He also loses any sense of self-worth he had because he realizes that others think that his needs are unimportant. Furthermore, his fears of neglect are verified. And the staff may evaluate their behavior modification program as effective!

Intimidation certainly occurred in the following situation.

A resident of a nursing home called to the aide, saying that she thought the roommate was going to fall out of bed. The aide's answer, as she towered over the tiny old lady, was, "Now you sit in this chair before you fall down." The woman replied, "No, help me. I take care of her." The aide grabbed the woman by the arm and shoved her into a wheelchair. "Now sit there, and you stay." The aide walked away, but not in the direction of the woman's roommate. The old woman replied softly but clearly, "You think you're better than me. We're nothing here just because you can shove us around. There is no one else to care for her but me. She's my baby." The aide guffawed and replied, "Your baby? Sure! She's 93 and you're 75 years!"[17]

If you always have to win in an interaction, you set up the other person to lose. Competition in a nurse-client relationship is destructive; the client ends up losing, and so do you. If the client senses that you must come out on top and be the authority in every conversation, he will feel intimidated. And he will run emotionally, if not physically. And you also lose an opportunity to be helpful, to learn something from another person, and to learn about yourself.

If you joke or tease in a harsh or belittling manner, if you use jestful sarcasm, if you laugh at the elderly client's appearance or behavior, if you play childish games to get him to cooperate or be pleasant, if you use him as a scapegoat, you will be the cause of the elderly client's anger, hate, despair, hopelessness, and finally complete withdrawal and regression. A good example of the inhumanity of such behavior was written after a visit by a family member to a nursing home.[17] The following scene was described:

A very old lady repeatedly begged a young male aide, "Please, a cigarette." The aide replied in a joking, mocking manner, "You know you gotta cry first. Now cry for me." The lady whimpered. The aide jested, "Aw, you can do better than that." "Please—one cigarette," the lady begged in a high-pitched voice. Teasingly the aide replied, "No, you show me how you can cry." A few tears came to her eyes, along with a look of total frustration and humiliation. To which the aide replied, "See, you're just a crybaby! You're not old enough to smoke." And he laughed and then walked away.[17]

That such destructive communication with the elderly occurs is known and, unfortunately, is tolerated. A sense of repulsion and rage is felt as this incident and others like it are described by the reporter.[17] The aggression, hostility, and sadism that can underlie "joking" is well known. The pity is that the public neither knows nor cares how often such incidents occur in institutions or in supposedly helping relationships, and that people who are destructive to clients are hired and retained as employees.

You may use nontherapeutic communication techniques that will reduce the chance of forming or maintaining a relationship. To probe, challenge, offhandedly ask questions about very private matters, or ask "why" is threatening. Interrupting, speaking too rapidly, or talking too loudly to the elderly person who hears well or too softly to the hearing-impaired conveys a lack of interest. Controlling the conversational topic according to your needs or interests is rude, egotistical, and unprofessional, and it is frustrating to the senior. If you control the conversation, you will never learn what is really most important to the person. Asking a barrage of direct questions will get a nod, a "yes" or "no" answer, or a blank stare. Direct questions are appropriate at times, but too often health professionals think they know what information is needed and ask questions accordingly. The result is assumptions, not data. Using jargon, standing at a distance, or conveying by your posture that you are in a hurry will cause the senior to say very little or nothing at all. Falsely reassuring him or using glib clichés when he knows all is not well will cause him to be quiet. The feelings he was trying to express will remain inside, drain his energy, cause anger or irritability, or even cause confusion and disorientation as a means of avoiding the reality he faces. Never tell the elderly person to be cheerful when he doesn't feel cheery. In trying to cheer him, you may create a new problem for him. You may create guilt feelings because he is not living up to your expectations.

PHASES OF THE NURSE-CLIENT RELATIONSHIP

Working with the person in later maturity to establish and maintain a relationship is similar to working with any other client. The difference is that the length of hospital stay or agency contact may be longer for this person who often has several chronic illnesses than for the younger person with an acute illness. If you work in a nursing home, extended care facility, or residence for the elderly, the person's stay may extend for years, until he dies. In either case, because you usually have an opportunity to know this client in greater depth, you form a more meaningful relationship. That is one of the rewards of geriatric nursing.

The nurse-client relationship is usually divided into four phases: (1) orientation or establishment, (2) identification, (3) working or exploitation, and (4) termination.[25,43] Because of the long-term contact that is typical with the aged, another phase has been identified and inserted, that of maintenance, which differs from and follows the working phase.

Orientation, Initial, or Establishment Phase

This phase of the relationship begins when you first meet the client, when he seeks assistance, or is brought for care. You may carry out essential interventions simultaneously, or shortly thereafter, as indicated. However, for a relationship, your main tasks are to introduce yourself; learn who he is; become oriented to his expectations, health needs, and goals through assessment. Orient him to your role, to admission procedures, general aspects of the agency, your health care goals, and his role in the health care system. Formulate a tentative care plan and determine whether or not it matches the client's impression of his problem. Explore how long you will care for him and how you will work together.

You are strangers to each other. The senior is anxious about his illness or problems and your reaction to him. Your anxiety centers on the client's reaction to you and your ability to help him. Establishing rapport and showing unconditional positive regard and acceptance are vital for assessing and orienting the person and for beginning a relationship. The client should begin to sense that you are trustworthy. He may test you with various behaviors or questions in order to learn if you can be trusted, if you are congruent, or consistent. While you are assessing and getting acquainted with the person, you are also examining your own thoughts, feelings, actions, and expectations. During this time the senior may be assessing you as carefully as you are assessing him: He observes and listens for your voice tone, the words you say and how you say them, your facial expressions, mannerisms, posture, and dress. He watches carefully for your response to him; do you act bored, inattentive, hurried, or rejecting. Such behavior may slow or prevent a relationship.

This phase has been likened developmentally to that of infancy because the client depends on you. If you demonstrate that you are a caring, nurturing, safe person, the client will begin to feel more secure. During the days or weeks that follow, he will disclose more of himself so that you get to know new facets of him as a person. Answers to questions on the nursing history or assessment form may change as he learns that he can trust you enough to give you the true answer or as you help him to better know himself. Throughout this period you are also giving him more information about his situation, yourself, and the health care system.

Identification Phase

This phase has been compared developmentally to the childhood phase. During this period the client responds selectively to the person who seems to offer the help he needs. If you have been perceived as accepting, congruent, trustworthy, and empathetic, you become his identification figure. He chooses to actively enter the relationship.

This is the time when the senior and you become better acquainted as you mutually explore his deeper feelings, needs, and goals. He trusts your decisions and actions, works closely with you, follows your suggestions, and claims you as "his nurse who has all the answers." Because of the time you spend with him and your response to him, you may become an ego-ideal for the client. This is a positive transference in which he imitates your speech, mannerisms, dress, or ideas. He will make admiring statements about you. It may be helpful to explore with the client why he wants to emulate you, for in the process you can help him better understand himself and further establish his own identity.

If his earlier experiences with people were traumatic, he will take longer to feel trust and to move into this phase. He may isolate himself, withdraw, act independent, or not accept needed help. If you wish to form a relationship with him, you will have to remain available and carry out the behaviors of the orientation phase for a longer period of time, that is, until you see a response from the client.

You may feel uncomfortable during this phase because the senior is so compliant but also so dependent on you. Accept this dependency without fostering it unnecessarily. This is a time when you can teach him a great deal, a time when you can guide him to learn much about himself and to better cope with his situation. Because he feels close to you, your responsiveness and empathy can help him mature emotionally. You continue the steps of the nursing process throughout this phase, guiding him but also providing opportunities for self-care and increasing emotional security and independence.

Working, Therapeutic, or Exploitation Phase

Developmentally this phase is similar to adolescence. During this phase the senior becomes more independent and uses all of the services and resources offered by the health team that meet his needs. He becomes more assertive and self-reliant as he tries out self-care measures, insists on doing things his own way, or tries new ways of behaving with others. By now he is usually regaining physical and emotional health. He is functioning optimally. Therefore, his behavior changes as he becomes more involved in making decisions about certain aspects of his situation. Although the senior seems more independent, explorative, manipulative, and even self-centered and demanding, you can now work as partners in meeting his health care goals. If you enjoy the dependent client, you will feel uncomfortable during this phase. You should explore why you feel uncomfortable.

During this phase you gain an even better understanding of the senior and the meaning of his illness and life situation to him. You help him work through problems at his own pace; you offer support, and you help him gain insight to the greatest degree possible.

During interviews in this phase, the main responsibility for speaking rests with the senior; he must exercise his options on what he wants to talk about. You listen carefully and are silent more of the time than he is. Interpretation and feedback are indicated. Ultimately interpretation will be considered and the meaning integrated, which will convey a feeling of self-control and self-worth to the senior only if he himself discovers the connection between his thoughts, feelings, and resultant behavior, with your validation, of course.

You point out options of behavior and experiences to the senior that he does not see for himself. You convey hope that something can be done, inject optimism into the situation, and provide an element of confidence that the required changes will not be too expensive in pain, money, or time. You stimulate the senior to change, to lessen this feelings of helplessness, and to increase his ability to cope. You enable the senior to acquire additional learning so that he has alternatives in coping, which in turn will improve his self-image. You encourage expression of feelings, recognizing the importance of each person experiencing, understanding, and sharing his feelings with a confidant.

At the same time, you do not make decisions about his life-style for the client.[46] Your self-image should not depend on how the senior uses your help. You are accepting and nonpunitive if the person does not aspire to your every suggestion or if he does not use your help the way you anticipated. You recognize the client is not a carbon copy of you.

The helping process does not always proceed smoothly. Sometimes all you can do is relieve the senior's loneliness until conditions change and coping seems possible. This method of helping requires patience, a defense against becoming irritated by an apparent lack of success, humility regarding one's own powers of intervention, and at best, being satisfied with contributing to survival.[46]

If the senior was admitted to an acute care setting or a home health agency, he is now preparing for convalescence and discharge from your services. He has made the most of the services offered and is ready to resume his former life-style to the greatest degree possible. He is ready to move into the termination phase. If the client was admitted to a long-term care setting or geriatric residence, or if you work with elderly clients in the community through an independent practice, your relationship is not terminated. The nature of the relationship does change after a while, however. You enter into a maintenance stage with the client.

Maintenance Phase

Often the nurse who works in an acute care setting does not really experience the rewards of a relationship with the patient. The short stay typical of hospitalization or even the few visits given by a home health nurse allow nothing more than establishing rapport, if that.

Nurses often talk glibly about nurse-client relationships, but in many settings a relationship may never exist for any client.

"You can have instant coffee, and instant tea, and instant potatoes, but you can't have instant relationships. . . . We can't measure out a portion of ourselves to each other, and stir once, and be friends."[9]

Relationships are possible in the setting in which a client is followed by the same nurse over a period of time, for example, in a rehabilitation center, nursing home, senior residence, or psychiatric/mental health agency. Primary nursing, carried out as intended in an acute care setting, would allow for relationship formation. Some home health agencies provide care over a long period of time; they do not insist on a rapid turnover of cases. The nurse in independent practice or in an ambulatory care clinic is likely to see the same clients over a period of years.

The relationship that pertains to total health care and that extends over years is different from the nurse-patient relationship that is usually described in books. There is no termination, or at least not for a long time. Often termination comes with death of the senior. The active, working, exploitation stage goes on until the senior has reached his potential. But in this case, the senior reaches a plateau where only support and maintenance are essential for daily living. The senior may live at home, following your directions for health promotion measures, and may call on you for assistance only when chronic illness becomes uncontrolled or when he suffers a new condition of pathology or of aging. The senior may be in an institution and need maximum or minimal assistance with daily physical care. What characterizes this phase is that you must actively pursue interventions in order to maintain emotional and social well-being, depending, of course, on the senior's condition.

The kinds of activities that you may implement are described further in another article by this author.[40] Some nurses would not include making regular phone calls, bringing a bouquet of flowers, tidying a room, sharing a meal, or taking the person for a ride to see autumn leaves as part of nursing. But if these and similar activities are the result of your assessment of the person's psychological needs, if they are part of a systematic care plan, if they are performed to meet the client's needs and not your own, and if they are performed with the principles of human behavior and communication in mind, then their effectiveness can be evaluated. Then they are nursing interventions. Such activities will be a part of maintaining the life, spirit, and biopsychosocial well-being of the senior. Doing these extras when the senior is depressed or under stress will take time and effort, an investment of yourself, gasoline if driving is necessary, and minimal cost for materials. The reward will be the gratification of seeing a person reassert his will to live, to become creative in coping with problems or making "ends meet," and to remain independent.

This author has carried out the maintenance stage for years with elderly people who wanted to remain living in their own apartments but who could not manage without a helpful relationship because they were alone, without family, and with few resources. Thus, a number of elderly clients have remained as physically intact as possible, mentally alert, socially aware, and independent because this nurse does not define nursing in a narrow sense.

"A depth relationship has a mutual history of shared joy and anguish. It is a mellowed blend of caring and being cared for, of listening, of removing masks (which is seldom easy), of openness and honesty. . . . All of this takes time. And effort. And expenditure of self."[9]

Termination Phase

This phase is marked by the client's becoming as fully independent as possible. Old needs have been adequately met, goals have been accomplished, and he is ready to be discharged from the health care system. This is a time of impending separation as you plan together the management of his health situation. This phase is likened developmentally to adulthood; the client is freeing himself from the helping person and is generating strength and ability to stand alone. He is integrating his illness and any changes in his body into his total self-concept.

Termination is an important phase and it should be planned for. Unfortunately, in the acute care setting the elderly client is sometimes discharged so abruptly that neither thought nor time is given to how he will manage at home or who will care for him. The person may be sent to a nursing home when more careful planning could have kept him at home, with the aid of a home health agency.

During this phase you and the senior must work through feelings about separation—sometimes past ones as well as the present termination. Mutual attachment develops between you and someone you care for over a period of time. Each of you has invested something of the self into the other. Either one or both of you may feel uncertain about the person's ability to manage without you, especially if the elderly person's finances and resources are limited and if he has little in the way of family and other associations. Together you need to talk about your confidence in his ability to manage. Avoid increasing his dependency on you at this time just to meet your own needs. The senior may feel very insecure and stressed about termination. When the client leaves the health care system, both you and he should feel no regret about the discharge, since follow-up care, either physically or emotionally, should be planned for if it is necessary.

At times the senior may either consciously or unconsciously try to delay discharge and termination. He may think of many reasons why he cannot manage or new symptoms may develop, either as a result of his anxiety or in the form of malingering. The symptoms and excuses tell you of his inner feelings—his lack of trust in himself, his loneliness and helplessness, his need for a continued relationship.

These feelings will be magnified if you do not prepare the senior for termination, if you try to quietly slip out of the picture when you feel that he is improving and no longer needs you. He may not need your assistance with physical care, but he will need you emotionally. He needs an opportunity to resolve the feelings he is experiencing, or he will feel rejected and abandoned. He needs to go through a mourning process in relation to this separation so that when future separations and losses occur, he will be better able to cope with them.

Other feelings the senior may experience during the termination phase include ambivalence or anger about the loss of the relationship and care, a sense of rejection by you, grief and depression, or guilt about having done something wrong or about not having met your expectations. He may perceive the discharge and termination as being pushed out. He may feel that you no longer like him. He may have realistic fears about what will happen to him after discharge. He may deny that termination is near by not entering into discharge plans, decision making, and self-care, or by talking about how your relationship will continue.

Preparation for termination should begin early in the relationship when you tell the client about how long he can expect you to care for him and to remain in the health care agency. As the time for discharge approaches, talk about feelings—yours and his—as well as realistic discharge and teaching plans. Let him know that caring for him has been a meaningful experience for you. Help him see the gains he has made during the relationship. Talk about separation, loss, and termination as part of the life cycle, about the worth of past relationships, and about the anticipation of future relationships. This talk can involve valuable reminiscing for the elderly client and renewed hope for the future.

Relationship with the Verbally or Sensory Impaired

The elderly person may be aphasic because of organic pathology, mute because of emotional illness, too physically ill to talk, or blind, deaf, or regressed to the point that he cannot carry on a logical conversation. Nevertheless, you can have a relationship with such a client. All that has been discussed so far would also be applicable to some extent to this client.

The most essential aspect of a relationship with the verbally or sensory impaired person is your attitude and approach. You can convey that you are trustworthy, dependable, interested in, accepting of, empathic, and respectful by your posture, tone of voice, use of touch, and thoroughness of physical care. If you are repulsed by the client, you convey this feeling both nonverbally and vocally. The verbally and sensory impaired person is very vulnerable to the hostility, aggression, or sadism of his caretakers; often he cannot defend himself physically and he cannot call for help because of his immobility.

The principles of communication discussed earlier would also apply to a considerable extent here. You may use more direct questions, for the client might only be able to nod yes or no. But the attitude that your communication techniques convey would be equally important with a person who could not reply. You should talk to the person as if he could reply. Countless cases exist in which the mute patient finally talked because therapeutic communication techniques were used. If the aphasia is reversible, the senior will be better motivated to try to talk. If the senior is regressed, he will sense your caring and respect, and, as a result, his behavior may change in a positive direction. If the senior is deaf, he will see your caring. If he is blind, he will hear your caring voice.

Touch is a key communication technique with many elderly persons, but especially with the verbally and sensory impaired. Tactile sensations originate in utero, are essential for the infant's survival, and are important to the person for reality contact throughout life. After early childhood we touch the person less in our culture. Thus, adults are often uncomfortable about being touched or touching one another. With regression related to illness or age, touch is often appreciated by the person.

Touch in the form of a gentle stroke, a backrub, or handholding can convey any or all of the following:

1. Availability of the nurse; the person is not alone.
2. Empathy for his situation, gestures, or statements.
3. Concern, caring, interest, and warmth.
4. Encouragement and approval.
5. Direction to be followed.
6. Commitment to the person.
7. Rapport and trustworthiness.

If touch is rough, harsh, or jerky, it is likely to convey attack, aggression, or punishment. The senior feels more anxious after such encounters.

The nurse-client relationship is an integral part of the nursing process. You will need to assess the senior in order to determine which needs can be met through a helping relationship. Your therapeutic approach is a nursing intervention and is important in combination with any other nursing intervention. Understanding the phases of the relationship will help you understand the senior's changing behavior. Evaluation of the nursing process must include evaluation of the approach you use and its effectiveness in promoting wellness. You may be very skillful in relating to people generally, and those skills may be useful in the professional, helping relationship. However, you will want to evaluate your helpful characteristics and whether or not you use constraining or nontherapeutic approaches.

REFERENCES

1. ARGYLE, MICHAEL, *The Psychology of Interpersonal Behavior.* Baltimore: Penguin Books, 1967.

2. BAUMGARTNER, M., "Empathy," *Behavioral Concepts and Nursing Intervention,* ed. C. Carlson. Philadelphia: J. B. Lippincott Company, 1970, pp. 29–39.

3. BENDER, R. E. "Communicating with the Deaf," *American Journal of Nursing.* 66: No. 4 (1966), 757–60.

4. BENJAMIN, ALFRED, *The Helping Interview.* Boston: Houghton Mifflin Company, 1969.

5. BLOCKER, DONALD, *Developmental Counseling.* New York: The Ronald Press Company, 1966.

6. BUCKHEIMER, A., "The Development of Ideas About Empathy," *Journal of Counseling Psychology,* 10: No. 1 (1963), 61–71.

7. BURKHARDT, M., "Response to Anxiety," *American Journal of Nursing,* 69: No. 10 (1969), 2153–54.

8. CARKHUFF, ROBERT R., *Helping and Human Relations.* New York: Holt, Rinehart and Winston, 1969.

9. CARR, JO, and IMOGENE SORLEY, *Mockingbirds and Angel Songs and Other Prayers.* Nashville, Tenn.: Abingdon Press, 1975.

10. CASHAR, LEAH, and BARBARA DIXON, "The Therapeutic Use of Touch," *Journal of Psychiatric Nursing and Mental Health Services,* 5: No. 5 (1967), 442–51.

11. COWLEY, MICHELE, "No Cure, Just Care," *American Journal of Nursing,* 74: No. 11 (1974), 2010–12.

12. DEJEAN, SHERRILYN, "Empathy: A Necessary Ingredient of Care," *American Journal of Nursing,* 68: No. 3 (1968), 559–60.

13. DURR, CAROL, "Hands That Help—But How?" *Nursing Forum,* 4: No. 4 (1971), 393–400.

14. EHMANN, VIRGINIA E., "Empathy: Its Origin, Characteristics, and Process," *Perspectives in Psychiatric Care,* 9: No. 2 (1971), 72–80.

15. "Gentle Be Present," *American Journal of Nursing,* 74: No. 9 (1974), 1611.

16. GOLDSBOROUGH, JUDITH, "Involvement," *American Journal of Nursing,* 69: No. 1 (1969), 66–68.

17. GREENE, BOB, "Home Is a House of Despair," *St. Louis Post Dispatch,* January 4, 1977, Sec. D, p. 7.

18. GREENHILL, MAURICE, "Interviewing with a Purpose," *American Journal of Nursing,* 56: No. 10 (1956), 1259–62.

19. GURALNIK, DAVID, ed., *Webster's New World Dictionary,* 2nd college ed. New York: The World Publishing Company, 1972.

20. HALE, S., and J. RICHARDSON, "Terminating the Nurse-Patient Relationship," *American Journal of Nursing,* 63: No. 9 (1963), 116–19.

21. HARDIMAN, M., "Interviewing or Social Chit-Chat," *American Journal of Nursing,* 71: No. 7 (1971), 1379–81.

22. HARDY, JEAN, "The Importance of Touch for Patient and Nurse," *Journal of Practical Nursing,* 25: No. 6 (1975), 26–27.

23. HAYS J., and K. LARSON, *Interacting with Patients.* New York: Macmillan Publishing Co., Inc., 1963.

24. HEWITT, H., and B. PESZNECKER, "Blocks to Communicating with Patients," *American Journal of Nursing,* 64: No. 7 (1964), 101–3.

25. HOFLING, CHARLES, MADELEINE LEININGER, and ELIZABETH BREGG, *Basic Psychiatric Concepts in Nursing,* 2nd ed. Philadelphia: J. B. Lippincott Company, 1967.

26. INGLES, THELMA, "Understanding the Nurse-Patient Relationship," in *Issues in Nursing,* eds. Bonnie Bullough and Vern Bullough. New York: Springer Publishing Co., Inc., 1966.

27. JOHNSON, BETTY, "The Meaning of Touch in Nursing," *Nursing Outlook,* 13: No. 2 (1965), 59–60.

28. KALISCH, BEATRICE J., "Strategies for Developing Nurse Empathy," *Nursing Outlook,* 19: 11 (1971), 714–18.

29. ———, "An Experiment in the Development of Empathy in Nursing Students," *Nursing Research,* 20: No. 3 (1971), 202–11.

30. ———, "What Is Empathy?" *American Journal of Nursing,* 73: No. 9 (1973), 1548–52.

31. KREIGER, DOLORES, "Therapeutic Touch: The Imprimatur of Nursing," *American Journal of Nursing,* 75: No. 5 (1975), 784–87.

32. MacKINNON, ROBERT, and ROBERT MICHAELS, *The Psychiatric Interview in Clinical Practice.* Philadelphia: W. B. Saunders Company, 1971.

33. MANASER, JANICE, and ANITA WERNER, *Instruments for Study of Nurse-Patient Interaction.* New York: Macmillan Publishing Co., Inc., 1964.

34. MANSFIELD, ELAINE, "Empathy: Concept and Identified Psychiatric Behavior," *Nursing Research,* 22: No. 6 (1973), 525–30.

35. McCORKLE, RUTH, "Effects of Touch on Seriously Ill Patients," *Nursing Research,* 23: No. 2 (1974), 125–32.

36. MEADOW, LLOYD, and GERTRUDE GASS, "Problems of the Novice Interviewer," *American Journal of Nursing,* 63: No. 2 (1963), 97–99.

37. MONTAGU, M., *Touching: The Human Significance of the Skin.* New York: Columbia University Press, 1971.

38. MOUSTAKAS, CLARK, *Creativity and Conformity,* New York: Van Nostrand Reinhold Company, 1967.

39. MURRAY, JEANNE, "Self-Knowledge and the Nursing Interview," *Nursing Forum,* 2: No. 1 (1963), 69–79.

40. MURRAY, RUTH, "Caring," *American Journal of Nursing*, 72: No. 7 (1972), 1286–87.

41. ———, and JUDITH ZENTNER, *Nursing Concepts for Health Promotion*, 2nd. ed. Englewood Cliffs, N.J.: Prentice-Hall, Inc., 1979.

42. NEHRING, VIRGINIA, and BARBARA GEACH, "Patients' Evaluation of Their Care: Why They Don't Complain," *Nursing Outlook*, 21: No. 5 (1973), 322–24.

43. ORLANDO, IDA, *The Dynamic Nurse-Patient Relationship.* New York: G. P. Putnam's Sons, 1961.

44. PEPLAU, HILDEGARDE, *Interpersonal Relations in Nursing.* New York: G. P. Putnam's Sons, 1952.

45. ———, *Basic Principles of Patient Counseling*, 2nd ed. Philadelphia: Smith, Kline, and French Laboratories, 1969.

46. POLLAK, OTTO, *Human Behavior and the Helping Professions.* New York: Spectrum Publications, Inc., 1976.

47. ROGERS, CARL, *Client Centered Therapy,* Boston: Houghton Mifflin Company, 1951.

48. ROSENDAHL, P., "Effectiveness of Empathy, Non-Possessive Warmth, and Genuineness of Nursing Students," *Nursing Research,* 22: No. 3 (1973), 253–57.

49. RUESCH, J., and GREGORY BATESON, *Communication.* New York: W. W. Norton & Co., Inc., 1951.

50. SPEROFF, B. J., "Empathy Is Important in Nursing," *Nursing Outlook,* 4: No. 6 (1956), 326–28.

51. TRAVELBEE, JOYCE, *Intervention in Psychiatric Nursing.* Philadelphia: F. A. Davis Company, 1969.

52. TRIPLETT, JUNE L., "Empathy Is . . . ," *Nursing Clinics of North America,* 4: No. 4 (1969), 673–82.

53. VENINGA, ROBERT, "Communications: A Patient's Eye View," *American Journal of Nursing,* 73: No. 2 (1973), 320–22.

54. WIEDENBACH, ERNESTINE, "The Helping Art of Nursing," *American Journal of Nursing,* 63: No. 11 (1963), 54–57.

55. ZDERAD, LORETTA, "Empathetic Realization of a Human Capacity," *Nursing Clinics of North America,* 4: No. 4 (1969), 655–62.

group work
with the person
in later maturity

Study of this chapter will enable you to:

---

1. Define *group* and differentiate between *primary* and *secondary* groups.

2. Discuss how the historical development of group work methods has influenced present-day group work with the elderly.

3. Discuss the purposes and benefits of group work for the elderly.

4. Discuss the behaviors of an effective group leader.

5. Describe the responsibilities of the group leader in preplanning group work with the elderly.

6. Explore behavioral principles and forces related to group process.

7. List and define task and maintenance functions that characterize group process.

8. List the phases of group development and describe characteristic behaviors of group members and the leader's responsibilities in each phase.

9. Compare effective versus obstructive behaviors of group members.

10. Contrast various types of groups that are effective for the elderly, purposes and format of each group, and characteristics of eligible persons for each group.

11. Initiate and maintain group experience for selected seniors, utilizing knowledge gained from this chapter and the guidance of a skilled supervisor.

12. Evaluate your leadership style and ability to fulfill responsibilities in each phase.

13. Work with the recorder, observer, and group members to analyze the effectiveness of members in the group process.

14. Evaluate benefits of the group experience to the seniors.

15. Explore how group work with the elderly differs from group work with other age groups.

4

Group life is essential to the existence of every person. Since the beginning of mankind, humans have banded together to form small groups for safety, protection, and physical maintenance. Later, groups were formed for sociability and companionship. Today the human is a member of many groups. Some group experiences are fleeting and superficial; others fulfill belonging and intimacy needs and stimulate personal growth.

The **group** is defined as *an assembly of people, separate from the environment, who meet face-to-face over a period of time to accomplish a task or activity or to form an association, and who have their own identity.*[1,32] Groups are either primary or secondary, depending on the importance of the group to the person. *A **primary group** is like a family; it has considerable influence on the person, especially in emotional aspects.* A **secondary group** *is like an organization; people react to each other more as role occupants or in a formalized manner, have specific goals, and are narrow in influence.*[1]

BENEFITS OF GROUP WORK

The elderly person with whom you work is vulnerable to isolation and loneliness and is especially in need of human contact. During later maturity the person may be less involved in intimate group experiences than he was earlier. Increasingly, we find the elderly alone behind apartment doors or alone in the mass of institutional life. Certainly the elderly person with whom you work could benefit from a group experience.

Silver noted improvement in morale, cleanliness, and general behavior after group work with 17 psychotic elderly patients.[62] Linden worked over a 2-year period with 51 institutionalized elderly women and found that lost values regained importance; hunger for social relationships returned; regression was halted, and an urge to contribute to group cohesion emerged.[39] Goldfarb and Turner treated 150 elderly residents in a nursing home; 49 percent improved with an average of 8.5 sessions.[29] A group psychotherapy program instituted for the elderly at Michael Reese Hospital aided resocialization and helped to increase self-esteem and self-worth.[35] Shere reported that colleagues scoffed at her choice to conduct groups with the very old, but she reported the following improvement in group members: (1) reduced loneliness and depression, (2) increased self-respect, (3) returned pleasures of earlier life, (4) regained social interests, (5) reawakened intellectual interest, and (6) renewed readiness and ability for resuming community life. One of the patients reported, "You are the girl who kept me from sorrow . . . you gave me courage."[61] Nurses have also reported the effectiveness of group work.[11,13,16,24,51] Yalom and Terrazas reported that group work with psychotic elderly patients is effective if realistic goals are set, focus is on patient strengths and similarities, and group cohesiveness is built.[26]

Some health workers feel that group work is wasted on the person in later maturity because he is too rigid to change or because there is little lifetime left in which to change. Certainly group experience has been proven just as beneficial for the elderly as for any other person. Your *positive attitude* and *personal belief* that the elderly person can change will help him feel that living every day is important and that opportunities for change can be found within each day.

You will work with other groups of people, for example, professional team members and other personnel, as well as elderly clients and their families. Group work is done in educational, administrative, and practice settings. Groups may be formal, such as structured team conferences or a weekly support group, or they may be informal, such as a discussion with a dying patient's family or an on-the-spot discussion with a group of patients concerning the day's activity. You might work with groups in an intensive experience as consultant to a self-help group or you might help citizens work through environmental or social issues. Previously the nurse was primarily concerned with the individual; however, today you must be concerned with the person within the group and with the total group as well. You will frequently need knowledge and skill to effectively use group process as part of the nursing process.

This chapter will help you to understand general group development and process and to adapt that general knowledge to group work with the elderly. Thus, you will be able to accomplish some of the purposes for group work.

PURPOSES OF GROUP WORK WITH THE ELDERLY

Although a one-to-one relationship as described in Chapter 3 provides many benefits, group interactions supplement the benefits of the one-to-one relationship. Purposes of helpful groups include to:

1. Strengthen the sense of identity and self-esteem appropriate to the later stage of life and to increase feelings of happiness and comfort.
2. Increase awareness of reality, others, and the environment.
3. Enhance understanding of personal feelings, underlying reasons for behavior, and how behavior appears to others.
4. Gain greater control over life and a sense of personal responsibility and satisfaction.
5. Increase ability for and enjoyment of socializing with others by fostering friendships, thus reducing feelings of isolation, loneliness, or rejection.
6. Become less self-centered and dependent, become more flexible and considerate of others' feelings and ideas, and recognize similarities between self and others.
7. Learn to state ideas, concepts, and feelings more clearly.
8. Learn alternative methods and gain practice in handling daily problems and feelings in ways other than to withdraw, regress, or act out.

9. Review and learn from past experiences, see the meaning of life, and gain a broader view of life.

10. Accept life: what it has been, is, and will be.

HISTORICAL PERSPECTIVES

Study of group function has interested many philosophers, scientists, sociologists, psychologists, and educators. But group work began in the twentieth century; in 1905 Joseph Pratt, a physician, gathered together a group of patients with tuberculosis in order to teach them self-care and at the same time elevate their morale and mood. Many leaders and varieties of group techniques have evolved since then. Table 4.1 summarizes the major group approaches, many of which can be used with the elderly.

TABLE 4.1   Evolution of Group Work

Date	Founder	Group Method	Description
1912	Joseph Moreno	Psychodrama	The person expresses feelings by acting out various roles on a stage. The audience participates vicariously and makes comments and interpretations to the individuals acting the roles.
1920	Trigant Barrow S. H. Foulkes	Group Psychoanalysis	Theories of individual psychoanalysis are applied to a group. Concepts of transference and resolution of resistances are emphasized.
1935		Alcoholics Anonymous	Alcoholics are directed, cared for, and admonished by leaders and group members who themselves are former alcoholics. With 12 steps toward abstinence, dependence on God and fellow man, and inspiration from the group, the individual struggling with alcohol addiction is treated.
1937	Abraham Low	Recovery, Inc.	Groups of former hospitalized psychiatric patients are led by the members with directions from Abraham Low's book, *Mental Health Through Will-Training.*
1930– 1940	Leo Festinger Kurt Lewin R. White	Group Dynamics	Group Dynamics Theory, which is based on scientific study of groups, is used to promote cohesiveness and expression of feelings.
1940	Maxwell Jones	Therapeutic Community	Environment is used as an agent for treatment (milieu therapy), and individual needs are considered in relation to the group needs. Staff members and patients participate in ward government, make policies, and share responsibilities for the total environment and each other.

TABLE 4.1 (*Continued*)

Date	Founder	Group Method	Description
1950	Martin Buber	Existential Groups (based on existential philosophy)	Lonely, alienated people meet to seek meaning in life, gain spontaneity, and increase sense of community.
1950	W. R. Bion	Tavistock Conference (named for the Tavistock Clinic in England)	Focus is on a common problem within members of the group, such as trust, loss, hopelessness, or dependency.
1960	Nathan Ackerman Theodore Lidz Carl Whitaker Donald Jackson	Family Dynamics (theory of family systems and "double bind" theory related to schizophrenic families evolved from research with family groups)	Family communication and process is analyzed in the group.
1960		Training Group Movement	Intense group method to train mental health workers to become more sensitive and capable as group leaders. Encounter, sensitivity and other groups have developed from this group method.
1960	Eric Berne	Transactional Analysis (T.A.) (based on psychoanalytic theory)	Member's participation is analyzed according to adult, child, and parent roles, since members symbolically reenact former problems by relating to others in the role of parent or child. Behavior is altered by choosing the adult role.
1960	Lawrence Tirnauer	Encounter Group	Person learns to overcome distance from others through emotionally intense, short-term session that focuses on group process.
1960	Carl Rogers	Basic Encounter	Sensitivity training that emphasizes the nondirective, empathic approach to expressing feelings and relating to others. The person within the group is the focus rather than the group as a whole.
1960	Fritz Perls	Gestalt	The individual within the group is the focus. Role playing, personal experimentation, exploration of individual feelings, fantasies, dreams, and "the hot seat" are used in this group to concentrate on a person's problems and help him make changes in his life.

Group work is now diverse in leadership, purpose, and approach, and it is done by a variety of people. A physician or a housewife might be found leading the same kind of group. Objectives might include personality reconstruction, promotion of insight, remotivation, problem solving, reality orientation, support, or education. Outcomes depend on the skills and interest of the leader and the needs of the group members.[44]

Although group leaders use a variety of methods, approaches, and philosophies, the approaches can be divided into three major groups:

1. Evocative—to encourage spontaneous expression of feelings in an atmosphere of acceptance and understanding.
2. Directive—to indoctrinate or give advice, with the emphasis on proper attitudes and conduct, using an authoritarian approach.
3. Didactic—to educate through a class or seminar.[64]

THE GROUP LEADER

The leader is the key to a successful group. To be a leader, you must first understand the principles of leadership as they apply to a group, behavior and its meaning, the goals and functions of group members, and the phases of group work. Just reading this chapter or only understanding theory will not be sufficient for you to become an effective leader. You will need to be involved in a group. Skills are improved with practice in leading groups, and more so with the assistance of a supervisor. Also, as the leader, you should be an effective role model for the members, relatively free of unreconciled emotional conflicts and able to tolerate intense emotional reactions.

Characteristics of an Effective Leader

No leader is perfect. But certain characteristics combine to help a person be a good leader. Certainly all the characteristics of the helping person discussed in Chapter 3 are equally important whether you are helping one person or a group. Several qualities are worth reemphasizing. The more secure you are as a person, the more secure the group members will be with you. The better you understand yourself, the better you can understand and accept others, and in turn help members accept people as they are. You cannot wear a facade; group members will recognize your strengths and limits, and they will know whether or not there is consistency between what you say and who you are. The more of life you have encountered and dealt with successfully, the more you will help the group members mature. What you are outside the group influences what you bring to the group, and what you learn within the group will influence your behavior outside the group.

Your ability to be an accepting, empathic leader enables members to express feelings, deal with them honestly, and then to profit from the experience. If you can feel with others' problems, feel a sense of concern, but also maintain an objectivity and sense of humor about human nature, you will be better able to tolerate the intensity of group experience and to help members feel unique, worthwhile, and understood.

You will also need to be perceptive, that is, to listen with the third ear for unspoken messages. The sigh, the frown, the tight lips, the eyelid tic can say as much as any eloquent sentence. At times your intuition will be useful. Although intuition cannot be measured, it can be accurate.

Further, you must have the capacity to love, laugh, and cry; spontaneity, yet restraint; compassion, yet objectivity; the capacity to be assertive and yet to be cautious and listen; a perception of reality, and yet a creativity and openness to change.

If the above characteristics are present, you may not change life or its struggles and pain, but you can cope, and help others to cope, with them more successfully.

Leadership Style

As the leader, you may set a democratic, autocratic, or laissez-faire climate. Studies about the effects of these three styles on group performance indicate that the democratic style results in increased friendliness, group-mindedness, motivation, and originality.[72] Different leaders have different styles; be aware of the kind of leader you are, and be sensitive enough to observe the results of your methods.

Regardless of the style you use, you will need to maintain your own position without superiority, live up to group norms, and avoid giving orders that cannot or will not be obeyed. Use established channels to give directions, and listen attentively to each member and the group as a whole. Demonstrate that you know what you are talking about and acknowledge the expertise of others. These rules are especially important with the elderly.

Responsibilities of the Leader

Desired characteristics are not enough. You must also be responsible. You are accountable for the group from its beginning through its last day and termination. You have the responsibility to share with the group what you are personally, but you also have the responsibility to fulfill certain objectives to the best of your ability.

As a leader, you are responsible for careful planning before the group begins. The following questions should be asked before you make any decisions about the group:

1. What kind of group do I want? One that focuses on activity, support, insight, discussion, or reality orientation?
2. How does my agency regard group therapy? Will the group have agency support?
3. What are my strengths and weaknesses? Am I prepared to do group work? How can I learn more about leading groups?
4. Do I need a co-therapist? What are the advantages of having a co-therapist? Do I need validation or support from another person? Do I need another role model for the group?
5. Would I benefit from a supervisor or counselor who could help me validate group processes, rethink my leadership style, and help me become more effective in the group experience?
6. How will I choose group members? Should the group be homogeneous with all members having a similar problem? Should the group be heterogeneous with the members presenting a variety of problems? Can I handle the heterogeneous group which is more life-like? Certain elderly persons are not likely to function in a talking group but may function in a nonverbal or activity group.
7. What are the members' needs? Will I have the time and opportunity to interview each one before the first meeting?

The leader should orient the selected group members to the general purpose and plan of the group sessions and expectations of the members before the first meeting. This is essential for the elderly so that they have time to anticipate group meetings instead of rebel against a change thrust upon then. Although this information must be repeated at the first session, the members have some understanding about why they were chosen; they have the right to make the final decision about attending. The first session will be less disorganized if members have received information previously about the group before the session begins.

You are responsible for the physical and structural arrangements. Determine if sessions should be held daily, weekly, or more frequently. Starting time, duration of the session, and place should be consistent. Whether the sessions are open or closed often depends on the type of group and kind of clients and agency. In an *open format new members are continually added and other members leave.* In a *closed format, the membership remains the same for the duration of the group.* The elderly often feel less confused by a closed format; newcomers to the group may be viewed competitively. The elderly prefer the closed format because it creates less overt change. Since visitors to the group sessions are usually discouraged, members should not bring family or friends. Ideally, the size of the group should be between 8 and 12 people so that all have an opportunity to participate and receive your attention. The group may need to be smaller if the patients are handicapped or in wheelchairs. The seating arrangement during the meetings should allow all members to see each other face-to-face; a circular arrangement is usually best. Mechanical equipment, such as movie or slide projector or tape recorders, is used for certain groups. Equipment should be obtained in advance and should be in working order.

The group's surrounding area becomes very much a part of the group itself and influences the effectiveness, activity, and life of the group. Factors such as uncomfortable temperature or furniture, disturbing noises, repugnant odors, and physical discomfort of any kind decrease group efficiency. How the members sit around the group, where the leader sits, how small or large the room is, and whether or not members are facing one another all influence the group's functioning.[6] Consider the physical and emotional environment and the members' comfort and safety to encourage group growth.

Decide whether or not to have a group recorder and observer. The recorder takes notes of the session proceedings; these notes give a content summary and frees members from taking notes. *The observer does not participate but analyzes the group process with the leader.* The observer objectively evaluates group atmosphere, participation of members, effectiveness of leadership, group cohesiveness and productivity, and general flow of discussion. These two service team members can validate with you about the group process and thus enable the group to function more productively. The need for a recorder and observer will depend on the size, type, and goals of the group and your expertise.

Now you are ready to begin your plan for group work. Be as prepared as possible, but once you begin, the best way to become more expert is to plunge ahead. Trust the group process. You are human and you will make mistakes, but that will only draw you closer to the group.

Other responsibilities of the group leader that relate to the phases of group development are summarized in Table 4.2.

PRINCIPLES RELATED TO GROUP PROCESS

Behavior Has Meaning

Everything that goes on in a group has some meaning. All activity of each member has significance: everything that is said and every movement that is made have meaning. Be aware not only of the obvious but also of the covert behavior. But to analyze or interpret every word and gesture is ineffective; it is even destructive. Look at the group as a whole entity. Choose the patterns of behavior that are important to the group to further question or to interpret.

Behavior Occurs on Different Levels

Behavior within a group occurs on two levels simultaneously: the cognitive and the affective levels. *Cognitive behavior refers to intellectually understanding goals; discussion of facts, issues and topics about members or others, and*

TABLE 4.2   Leader Responsibilities During Group Work

Formation Phase	Change Phase	Termination Phase
1. Help the group get acquainted by defining the problem or reason for meeting.	1. Call on the group to clarify, analyze, and summarize problems.	1. Prepare the group for separation.
2. Establish a group *contract, an agreement between leader and members,* if agreeable to you and the members. The contract can be general or specific, depending on how it is established. The contract covers attendance and completion of group experience. Confidentiality should be clearly understood.	2. Permit verbal rebellion or expression of negative feelings to help the member gain comfort, insight, and tools for relieving pent-up feelings of anxiety, guilt, and anger. Through this release and the mutual sharing of feelings, thoughts, fantasies, and experiences, group members become better acquainted with one another, learn to care about each other, and feel more positive.	2. Help the group review, summarize, and evaluate growth.
3. Help the group establish ground rules about appropriate behavior.	3. Provide for members' security and safety of property.	3. Help the group to separate physically and let go emotionally from each other and from you.
4. Invite trust gently; allow distance when necessary.	4. Clarify feelings; encourage all members to state feelings.	
5. Help members discuss feelings and thoughts about their expectations, misconceptions, or group experiences generally.	5. Help the group to operate with little direction. (Seniors may need more support than other groups.)	
6. Redirect questions so that they are answered by members.	6. Encourage involvement, cooperative activity, and mutual support so that *cohesiveness, a sense of belonging and togetherness,* and loyalty develop.[77]	
7. Help all members participate. Call on each member if necessary.	7. Observe for forces that block change or growth in the members and engage the group in helping the member grow.	
8. Keep members' attention on goals; evaluate group process.		
9. Clarify issues as they arise.		
10. Assist the recorder and observer in their roles and clarify their roles to the group.		

attention to procedural questions. Cognitive behavior relates to the following questions: How shall the group get started? What is the agenda for group sessions? What are the general rules for operation?[5]

Affective behavior refers to feelings, group morale and participation, influence of members upon each other, nonverbal responses, group atmosphere, styles of leadership, and degree of conflict, competition, and cooperation.[5] Group members seldom deliberately notice the affective level of group functioning, yet the affective level of the group frequently makes or breaks a group's effectiveness. For example, during group discussion the senior may know why he has to be in a nursing home. But his feelings of loss and despair will come through and may silence the entire group from pursuing the subject.

Cognitive level of functioning is relatively easy to recognize; you must be perceptive to observe affective behavior. When you are analyzing affective behavior, ask yourself the following questions:

1. What is the feeling generated within the group?
2. What feelings am I detecting within myself and the group generally? Do I detect interest, boredom, anger, hopelessness?
3. What are my clues? Voice tone, facial expressions, body posture, or gestures?
4. What expressions of anxiety are present in myself and others? Blushing, restlessness, excessive talking, withdrawal, increased smoking?

Group Climate Affects Function

A constructive group climate refers to the feeling within the group which enables the leader and members to disclose or expose self, share with others, and allow others freedom to talk or be quiet.

Fear of talking about self is often great because of past experiences, patterns of relating, or insecurities; the person is unwilling to take the chance even though he wants to. The group must convey acceptance and wait until the member can share about himself without undue pressure. Rapid self-disclosure does not necessarily mean progress or growth; often too early self-disclosure achieves nothing except bruised feelings.[73]

The security of a constructive, accepting climate encourages risk-taking; the material to be talked about may be of a highly personal nature that possibly has never been said aloud before. The speaker must feel sure that the leader and members will at least listen even if they don't understand, that they will not ridicule, condemn, probe, or break confidentiality. If the speaker is respected, then other members will also risk self-disclosure.

Dynamic Forces Exist

Certain forces—drives, feelings, ideas, and maneuvers—exist within the person (intrapsychic), between people (interpersonal), and in the environment, and these forces affect the person's behavior and therefore the entire group. The irritability or concern that members feel for each other and the degree of willingness to listen, share, compromise, and work with each other create a group atmosphere that is either disruptive or smooth. External events cannot be kept outside the group, such as the sick child, loss of job, hazardous weather, or relocation of home. Noise in a surrounding area; room temperature or decor; appearance, behavior, smell of another group member; or number of group members also influence members' behavior and group spirit.

Other forces come from within the group itself.

1. Attitudes of the person have anchorage in groups. You can more easily change the person's attitudes by changing the group climate than by attempting to directly change the person.
2. Groups demand a certain degree of conformity from members. The more cohesive (close) the group, and the more the person feels his needs are met by the group, the more power it has over his behavior.
3. Decisions made by a group obtain greater commitment from members than arbitrarily imposed decisions from outside the group.
4. Opinions and behaviors that are deviant from the rest of the group are likely to be ignored, rejected, or punished by other members.
5. Efforts to cause members to deviate from group norms will encounter strong resistance from the person.
6. People tend to be more effective learners when they are acting as group members than when they are acting as individuals.
7. The more closely a person's attitudes, values, or behavior fit the group's purpose, the more influence the group will exert on him.
8. The greater the member's prestige in the eyes of the other members, the greater the influence he can exert.
9. Cooperation and communication are increased in groups in which goals are mutually defined, accepted, and understood by the members.
10. Group climate or style of group life has an important impact on the personalities of members. The behavior of members may differ greatly from one group to another.[20,69]

Group Goals

All groups are trying to reach at least one *primary goal, a target, aim, or long-range task that gives direction.* The goal may be to develop a product or an idea or to promote personal development. The major goal may be as simple as companionship or as specific as planning a party. Goals depend on the leader's abilities and the members' needs. Do not consider your goals so important that they overwhelm the members' goals. The goals should be known, attainable, rational, and directed toward change. Additionally, the group might set up *secondary goals, short-term objectives that must be reached in order to accomplish the overall task.*[41] For example, the specific goal is for the nursing home residents to prepare a visitor's handbook. Secondary goals include (1) setting up a time schedule, (2) planning an outline, and (3) preparing pictures.

Group Functions

If a group is to achieve its goals, it must carry out two functions: task functions and maintenance functions. *Task functions are behaviors directed toward selecting and achieving the primary and secondary goals of the group. Maintenance functions are activities that support the welfare, morale, harmony, and relationship of the group.*[41]

Task functions, which get a job done, include the following behaviors:

1. Initiating activity: The person suggests new ideas, solutions, or ways of organizing the group.
2. Seeking information: The person asks for clarification or facts pertinent to the discussion.
3. Seeking opinion: The person asks for a description of feelings, values, or ideas.
4. Giving information: The person offers facts to push what he thinks should become the group's view.
5. Giving opinion: The person states a belief about a suggestion or piece of information that is based on personal values or experience instead of on facts.
6. Clarifying or elaborating: The person gives examples or develops meanings in order to help the group envision how a proposed solution might work.
7. Coordinating: The person shows relationships among various ideas or suggestions and pulls together new ideas or various activities.
8. Summarizing: The person restates ideas or proposed solutions after the group has discussed them.
9. Testing: The person examines the practicality of ideas, applies suggested solutions to real situations, and reevaluates.[41]

Maintenance functions, which increase feelings of security, include the following behaviors:

1. Encouraging: The person is warm, friendly, and responsive to others, praises others and their ideas, and pushes for group solidarity.
2. Expressing group feelings: The person summarizes group feelings and reactions.
3. Harmonizing: The person mediates differences between other members or relieves tension and conflict through the use of humor or pleasantries.
4. Compromising: The person yields, admits error, or moves his original position in order to work out a conflict in which he is involved.
5. Gatekeeping: The person makes it possible for another member to contribute to the group by calling on him or by suggesting a time limit for talking to another. Thus, he keeps communication channels open.

6. Setting standards: The person states standards for the group to use in choosing a task, procedure, or solution. He reminds the group to avoid decisions which conflict with group standards.[41]

PHASES OF GROUP DEVELOPMENT

Every group, like the persons who make up the group, is unique and develops an individual style and identity through several phases. Responsibilities of the leader during the phases of development are summarized in Table 4.2. The group's pattern of development is divided into the following phases: formation of the group (Phase I), change within the group (Phase II), crisis within the group (Phase III), and termination of the group (Phase III or IV).

Phase I: Formation of the Group

Initially people come together with varied experiences and backgrounds, with or without previous contact, and having little concern or affection for each other. Each person responds in his own way and makes a decision about the degree of involvement based on his desire to be included. The group may be perceived as threatening to the person, and he is likely to respond with his usual pattern of behavior to stress, such as aggression, withdrawal, competition, or vacillation.[1]

Carl Rogers describes five steps or patterns that make up the first major phase. They are:

1. *Milling around*—a period of initial frustration; confusion; awkward silence; polite, superficial, or irrelevant conversation; self-preoccupation; intellectualization; and lack of continuity. The person may search for status or power, resist authority, or pair off with another.
2. *Resistance to personal expression or exploration*—most members will not risk open disclosure. A few reveal rather personal attitudes initially, which in turn causes great ambivalence in the other members.
3. *Description of past feelings*—expression of private feelings gradually begins to assume a larger proportion of the discussion.
4. *Expression of negative feelings*—anger directed toward the leader or members is usually the first significant expression of feelings. Deeply positive feelings are more difficult and dangerous to express. The member may feel that no one is interested in his problem at this early stage.
5. *Expression and exploration of personally meaningful material*—at this point some member begins to talk about his problems and related feelings, a painful process to which the entire group may not be receptive.[56]

During Phase I, members discuss the group structure, what "freedom" means in this group, and how each member interprets what the leader says. Each person struggles for security, to regain equilibrium, and to adapt to the new situation. Members gradually share more about themselves. Agreement among members that feelings, thoughts, and behaviors are to be tolerated is essential to begin open discussion and move toward an identity and a subculture.[1]

Phase II: Change Within the Group

In this phase the emphasis shifts from personal needs, desires, and goals to more collective identity. The person's mood changes. The members engage in more genuine conversation. Each member attempts to find a place within the group, the power he has, and what expectations the group has of him. The members gradually become more patient, respectful, cooperative, and supportive, and they are able to work together. Members may seek or offer assistance.[1]

Every senior begins to deal with trust of self and others. Most people want to trust each other, but they are blocked by fears of rejection, betrayal, and exposure, depending on difficult past experiences and lack of self-esteem.

As members begin to risk and share important and private feelings and ideas about themselves, a change occurs within the group. Members become close emotionally. The facades crack as they show the real self, which results in further expressions of positive and negative attitudes. Each member begins to perceive others more accurately. Members show more feeling for each other, are more at ease with one another, become more productive, and experience behavioral and attitudinal change. Feedback from others helps the senior increase in self-acceptance and self-esteem.[56]

During this phase the seniors want the group to exist. They create an atmosphere in which work can be done, develop guidelines for making decisions, and help each member make his unique contribution. Members give and receive help and can discuss the processes within the group and improve its functioning. Now the group members are socialized into the group; they accept and internalize norms of caring and expression of feelings and move toward a goal. Outsiders are emotionally and physically rejected by the group because of the closeness that has developed among the members.

Phase III: Crisis Within the Group

This phase is a turning point in the life of the group. It may occur at any time in the group's phases or it may never occur.

If members are expressing their deepest feelings with honesty, forcefulness, and spontaneity, and if members experience accepting feedback, the working phase deepens. Members experience healing. Behavior changes. But if negative feelings are not accepted, conflict emerges and regression or disintegration of members or of the group occurs.

Conflict emerges when members feel that they are not getting what they want from each other and the leader.[1] Group conflict emerges for various reasons:

1. The leader or other members harshly confront the person who is honestly discussing feelings. The rest of the group feels uneasy or rejected.
2. Members may seek out each other between group sessions to show concern or share experiences. Too much outside contact that is not discussed in the group will break up the group.
3. The member may refuse to move toward the group goal, such as listening to others, talking honestly about feelings, or participating in an activity.[1]

When conflict occurs, the group responds in various ways. The deviant may be forced out or be dominated by another to quiet his view. Alliances may form as members speak for or against one another. Ideally, members collectively arrive at a satisfying compromise or solution and regain a sense of solidarity.[56] The leader is responsible for helping the group avoid or overcome disruption and for providing for the emotional and physical safety of the members.

Phase III or IV: Termination of the Group

Separation or termination occurs when goals are met or when it is no longer feasible to meet. Termination must be planned for in advance. If the group experience has been satisfying and has helped members to feel better about the self and others, there will be feelings of separation anxiety, loss, rejection, and abandonment. Members may doubt their ability to get along without each other; the leader may be reluctant to let the group go. Greater hostility is likely to be felt by the members and the leader if the group must terminate for some reason beyond their control or before they feel that they have resolved the problems of the group or individual members. Hostility directed at the leader may be demonstrated in open anger or through increased dependency. Ideally, the leader recognizes the accomplishments of the group, helps members to recognize their growth, and realizes that optimal function of members was the original goal of the group. As feelings about separation are talked through and as other difficulties are dealt with, personality maturity and ability to cope with stress and life itself are strengthened.[1] If the group experience has been effective, the members leave feeling increased self-esteem and positive about their behavioral change.

The group experience is difficult to describe; so much of it is in the realm of feelings. Only a positive group experience can help the person know the warm, safe emotional climate that encourages a deeper sharing, a broader scope of thinking, and attitudinal and behavioral changes.

Committed, working group members are essential to an effective group. The members' activities and behaviors contribute to group maintenance, move the group to its goals, help each member achieve personal goals, or block the group's performance.

Each member must feel a sense of obligation to and involvement in the group. He must be dependable, trustworthy, and willing to maintain confidentiality. The group member should prepare carefully before the group meeting so that he can do his own thinking, come to a conclusion, and then speak clearly and concisely about his ideas. He should question if he does not understand and should listen attentively when others are speaking. Observation of the group process and maintenance of an accepting climate are the responsibility of members as well as of the leader, recorder, and observer. Each member must support the total functioning of the group while he is meeting his own needs.

Obstructive Maneuvers in the Group

A group member may be unable to contribute satisfactorily to the group function for a number of reasons. The member then uses obstructive behavior that may be pursued as individual goals.

Individual goals serve the member's immediate self-interest or protect him from the group process, often at the expense of overall personality growth. The following individual roles are irrelevant or destructive to the group function:

1. Aggressor: The person expresses disapproval of other members' feelings, ideas, or behavior; takes credit for others' ideas; shows envy; overreacts to others' statements.
2. Blocker: The person opposes without reason; is resistant and stubborn; goes off on a tangent; argues; rejects others' ideas without consideration; maintains an angry silence if he does not get his way; may frequently be late or absent.
3. Help-seeker: The person tries to get a sympathetic response by expressing insecurity, personal confusion, or self-depreciation without reason or empathy for another's problems.
4. Playboy: The person displays lack of involvement in the group; is cynical; engages in horseplay, clowns and mimicks.
5. Self-confessor: The person uses the group as an audience to express personal points of view, feelings, or themes irrelevant to the group. Often the person reveals self prematurely in order to gain attention.
6. Dominator: The person asserts authority or superiority by monopolizing or

manipulating group members through flattery, interruptions, changing the subject, or giving directions.

7. Special interest pleader: The person introduces or supports suggestions related to personal concerns or philosophy.
8. Competitor: The person competes with others to produce the best idea, talk the most, play the most roles, or gain the leader's favor. He may try to assume the therapist's role.
9. Blackmailer: The person intimidates others into going along with personal schemes; he threatens that confidential content will be discussed outside the group or that the members will suffer harm in some way if they do not go along.[41]

Obstructive behavior may be caused by the person's lack of self-esteem, negative self-concept, inability to communicate appropriately with others, faulty patterns of relating, or anxiety related to the group situation.

You will have to help the senior recognize his behavior and its effects, support other members when they are the recipients of the obstructive behavior, and work with group members to encourage behavioral change to promote group cohesiveness.

Other common forces that obstruct group function or block change are resistance, transference, and countertransference. These are discussed at length in Chapter 3 and are similar in a group setting as they are in a one-to-one relationship. *Resistance is any psychological maneuver on the part of the group member to resist self-awareness, personal growth, change, or relationships with the group and other group members.* Feelings of apathy, hostility about past groups, or fear of change may be the cause. Defense mechanisms such as denial, projection, or isolation are used. Resistance may result in a person's breaking away from the group or destroying its progress if he refuses to go along with group goals. *Transference refers to unconscious attachments directed at leader or group members whereby feelings, attitudes, and experiences will be expressed that are appropriate to parental or other authority figures from the past.* The member may be overaccepting of or hostile toward the leader, or he may distort the leader's or member's statements because he is reminded of a dominating parent or boss. *Countertransference relates to the leader's unconscious or conscious emotional reaction to the individual group members. The leader may respond to certain members as he did to others in his past life.* These feelings may be positive or negative and often are in response to transference feelings from a member. You may give a member extra privileges because he reminds you of a favorite uncle. Or you may feel boredom, anxiety, apathy, or hostility toward the group or individual members. Countertransference may be demonstrated by authoritarianism or overprotectiveness if you sense helpless feelings in a member. You can use transference as a tool toward change and growth; transference is inevitable, but you must become aware of and eliminate countertransference feelings. Ask yourself the following questions: What am I doing to cause these emotions? Do any of the group members remind me of anyone I know? What do I feel about the individual group members? What can I do about these feelings?

As a leader, you are responsible for helping the obstructive member. You may be able to confront the offending member about his behavior. You may encourage other group members to work with you in bringing forth more appropriate behavior. Feedback from the group may stimulate the member to change. You may have to counsel the person individually or refer him to another counselor. It may be especially difficult for you to work with a resistant elderly person because of your own countertransference feelings about old people. In this case, you should seek help from a skilled counselor or supervisor. By providing an emotionally safe climate you may be able to reduce the senior's need to use individual roles; friendship and respect from you and other members may help him become group-oriented.

EVALUATION

Evaluation of group progress is a continuous part of group work. It is as essential as evaluation is in the nursing process.

As the leader, you are responsible for evaluating yourself throughout the duration of the group. The following checklist can be used:

1. Am I successful in reducing the member's anxiety about participating in this group?
   (a) Do I encourage a warm-up period with members before the meeting begins?
   (b) Do I convey warmth, support, and nonthreatening humor?
   (c) Do I arrange for a comfortable meeting environment?
   (d) Do I use a matter-of-fact, pleasant approach if there are many suspicious or unfriendly members in the group?
2. Do I reward participation and promote progress toward group goals by verbal statements, smiling, or nodding my head?
3. Have I conveyed to the members during the orientation phase that participation is a group norm? Or do I talk too much and for too long?
4. Do I encourage each member to participate? Do I accept statements and work them into the group discussion so that they have meaning to the group? Do I make reluctant members feel that their ideas are wanted and needed and do I prevent talkative members from monopolizing or dominating without conveying rejection of them? Do I keep the discussion and activity moving? Do I protect members from attack but accept disagreement if it is expressed reasonably?

5. Do I keep quiet during pauses so that group members realize that they have a responsibility toward the group discussion?
6. Do I hear ideas and feelings expressed by members and restate them accurately in a more concise, clear form, thus conveying acceptance, attention, respect, and understanding, without agreeing with the stated ideas or feelings?
7. Am I sensitive to nonverbal communication from group members? Am I empathic to sadness, apathy, hostility, or intense concentration?
8. Do I stimulate problem solving by asking questions, clarifying situations, inquiring about feelings, raising alternative choices, and remaining nonthreatening?
9. Did I learn enough about each member before the group started? Do I keep sufficient contact with members between group sessions so that I can promote a sense of trust and group cohesiveness and be able to ask pertinent questions about a member's behavior?
10. Do I summarize periodically so that I can move the discussion forward, indicate progress, restate the problem in a new light, or point up differences that exist in the group?
11. Do I receive genuine feedback verbally or do members tell me what they think I want to hear?
12. Do I keep the group interested by asking questions that are difficult enough, encouraging tasks that are neither too easy nor too hard, using a variety of techniques and formats for meetings, and encouraging members to perform tasks rather than personally doing all the work?
13. Do I use every possible opportunity to give the group real power to make choices? Do I recognize that patient groups tend to be more conservative than staff in decisions and can usually be trusted about matters related to themselves?
14. Do I turn responsibility over to the group as soon as possible but regain it from them whenever necessary?
15. Am I relating wisely to group deviants? Do I convey respect, provide for their emotional safety, and prevent scapegoating by members? When scapegoating appears, am I comfortable enough to look for and deal with the members' feelings of worthlessness, fear or weakness, and fear of similarity to the deviant?
16. Am I contributing to group cohesiveness by encouraging members to make choices; agree on goals, norms, and the means to achieve them; talk out differences; and review and alter goals as necessary so that the group remains helpful?
17. What is my leadership style?
18. Am I developing and rewarding qualities of leadership among the members? Do I support members who have the ability to draw out others? Do I encourage members to direct statements and questions to each other instead of to me? Am I quiet when I should be?

19. Is the group moving toward its goals? Do I help the group remain aware of its goals and the gains made by members?
20. Am I flexible enough to revise goals as members progress or as circumstances change?[66]

As a group leader, you will probably never be able to anwer "yes" to every question on this list. But if your answers progress from "sometimes" to "often" to "usually," you will experience the rewards of observing growth in group members and realizing your own increasing effectiveness as a group leader. Working with a supervisor also helps to evaluate yourself. Clarifying with the group recorder and observer can further help you to evaluate your skill.

The group member benefits from evaluating his activity in the group and

---

Evaluation of myself before group:

Evaluation of where I would like to go:

    Long-range goal:

    What can I do to achieve this goal?

Evaluation of group goals:

My participation in the group (rate each behavior on the following scale):

    1. always
    2. usually
    3. often
    4. sometimes
    5. never

1. Make clear open statements.

2. Paraphrase others' comments.

3. Direct my comments to group members.

4. Encourage others to participate.

5. Listen attentively to other members.

6. Share openly my feelings with the group.

7. Give feedback.

8. Help summarize.

9. Work toward productivity.

10. Check out perceptions.

11. Support others in group.

12. Stay actively involved.

Figure 4.1. Group member self-evaluation form.

```
┌─────────────────────────────────────────────────────────────────────────┐
│                                                                           │
│   Leader's name:                    Observer's name:          Group:      │
│                                                                           │
│   Date:                             Number of sessions:                   │
│                                                                           │
│   Group size:                       Meeting time:                         │
│                                                                           │
│   Physical facilities:                                                    │
│                                                                           │
│   Group atmosphere:                                                       │
│                                                                           │
│        Accepting    1   2   3   4   5   Rejecting                         │
│                                                                           │
│        Cohesive     1   2   3   4   5   Individualistic                   │
│                                                                           │
│   Group stage of development:                                            │
│                                                                           │
│   Group goals:                                                           │
│                                                                           │
│        Movement in the direction of goals:                               │
│                                                                           │
│        Clarity:                                                          │
│                                                                           │
│        Commitment to goals:                                             │
│                                                                           │
│        Content toward goal achievement:                                  │
│                                                                           │
│   Leadership style:                                                      │
│                                                                           │
│        Democratic:               Autocratic:           Laissez-faire:    │
│                                                                           │
│   Leader effectiveness:                                                  │
│                                                                           │
│        Participation   1   2   3   4   5   Resistance                    │
│                                                                           │
│   Communication pattern:                                                 │
│                                                                           │
│   Observer response:                                                     │
│                                                                           │
└─────────────────────────────────────────────────────────────────────────┘
```

Figure 4.2. Report of group process.

his performance of various roles. The Group Member Self-Evaluation Form, Figure 4.1, can assist him in evaluation.

The function of the group observer is to help the leader, and at times the members, evaluate overall group function and individual participation. The Report of Group Process, Figure 4.2, can be used by the observer for evaluation purposes.

TYPES OF GROUPS FOR THE PERSON IN LATER MATURITY

Whether you are knowledgeable about group process and accustomed to group work or are reading about group function for the first time, you should approach the task of group work with elderly patients as a new experience. Certainly all of your past knowledge is important, for it strengthens and deepens your ability to build a group. However, any group you work with, in any setting, is unique. Each group is a different experience in spite of similarities, because the group responds out of its own inner resources and experiences and has its own objectives. This is especially true in groups of elderly persons. Therefore, the group you will be working with will be a new and challenging experience. If you work with more than one group of elderly patients over a period of time, you can use your knowledge and experience to react perceptively to the similarities and differences of each group you work with. In addition, you should keep notes, do research, and share your insights so that you can help others do group work with the elderly.

Reality Orientation Group

The purpose of reality orientation is to maintain reality contact and to reverse or halt the confusion, disorientation, social withdrawal, and apathy characteristic of residents in institutions.[31] Reality orientation should be not only a technique to prevent confusion or disorientation but also a philosophy—a way of thinking about care of the elderly. As a philosophy, reality orientation helps the staff recognize that regressive phenomena are not natural concomitants in old age and that expecting regression in the elderly and treating the person as an infant will reinforce such behavior.

Reality orientation has three components that can be used simultaneously: (1) a 24-hour daily routine, (2) supplementary classroom experience, and (3) attitude therapy.[31]

Twenty-four-hour reality orientation involves using every staff-patient contact to help the patient know who and where he is, the time of day, the day of year, and who the people are around him. Basic, current, and personal information is presented repeatedly to the person. Clocks with large numbers are in plain view. Calendars with big print are displayed and checked off. Each person wears a readable name tag. Large lettering on doors and color codes on floors, walls, and doors help the person find his room and other areas on the ward. Any realistic response is reinforced with a smile, praise, or supportive statements. Staff members state what they are doing in all activities with the person. Repetition of information and reinforcing the person are essential. A sense of constancy and familiarity is maintained in order to help the senior cope with daily living and unusual stressors.[25,31]

Supplementary classroom reality orientation is a simple form of small group work for severely confused and disoriented persons. A group of 4 to 6 residents meet daily for 30 minutes with a staff person who is familiar with their total nursing care plan and needs. The immediate goal is to teach them basic person–time–place information and establish group participation in a structured setting. The classroom setting provides for personal attention in a firm, supportive environment. Classroom reality orientation for 6 weeks is effective in reversing signs of memory loss, confusion, and disorientation in patients, including those over 80 years.[31]

Attitude therapy is basic to all reality orientation. A consistent attitude and approach maintained by all staff members when they care for the person or lead the group is essential to convey to the resident what is expected of him. One or a combination of the following five attitudes is prescribed as part of the treatment: active friendliness, passive friendliness, matter-of-fact, kind firmness, and no demand.[31]

Reality orientation is effective. After one year of treatment, patients have markedly improved in behavior by showing more self-pride, greater socialization, improved manners, more interest in radio or television, and more concern with general appearance. Several studies have shown that 76 percent of the regressed patients improved.[25,31]

Reality orientation programs are useful in that some residents improve considerably in behavior; all can be maintained at the functioning level observed on admission to the institution; regression typical of institutionalization is prevented.

One reality orientation program with women in a state hospital helped them to again respond to their names, increase conversational and socialization skills, call other residents and attendants by name, follow directions, and increase accuracy of time orientation.[31]

Reality orientation programs show that the elderly are capable of more physical and mental activity than commonly believed. A relationship certainly exists between expectancies and behavioral change. The attention given to residents through this kind of program reinforces appropriate behavior as well as the desire to be appropriate.[31]

Staff involved in reality orientation programs usually consider themselves, and are considered, to be a special group, which increases their morale and thus improves their performance with and care for the residents.[21,31]

The reality orientation program was first proposed and implemented by Veterans Administration Hospital, Tuscaloosa, Alabama. Further information and training material may be obtained from them.

Sample Session: Four patients are taken to the classroom by the nurse aid responsible for their care. She shakes each patient's hand, calls each patient by name, and looks each patient in the face for a short period of time. Each patient is asked, "What is your name?" Names can be printed on cards in large letters and set in front of the patients. Each correct response is praised and supported. Much repetition is used. The leader asks, "How are you today?" and allows time for each person to answer. After slow, simple orientation to time, day, and place (using visual material such as calendars, clocks, newspapers, or pictures) a comment is made about the weather and other important current affairs. "John, it is raining outside." "Today is one week before Christmas (or Hanukah)." After approximately 30 minutes the patients are returned to their rooms with a hand shake and a good-by.[25] To get results, such sessions should continue on a regular basis for as long as necessary.

Remotivation Group

Remotivation is a simple form of group work that can be used in a nursing home, hospital, or senior center. It is often used in combination with reality orientation groups. The goal of this therapy is to prevent disengagement, increase interest in reality, and stimulate thinking as the person focuses on simple, objective aspects of everyday life. Institutionalized patients may suffer the effects of emotional, social, and sensory deprivation, withdrawal, depression, loneliness, alienation, confusion, disorientation, or disturbed thinking resulting from the loss of familiar faces and the new setting.

Remotivation sessions involve five specific steps:

1. *Creating a climate of acceptance.* About 5 minutes are spent greeting each person by name, expressing pleasure at his presence, and making encouraging remarks.
2. *Creating a bridge to the world.* About 15 minutes are spent talking about a topic of general interest which was chosen by the group at the previous session. Each patient is encouraged to respond.
3. *Sharing the world we live in.* About 15 minutes are spent in further developing the topic just discussed. Visual aids are used in this step.
4. *Appreciating the work of the world.* About 15 minutes are used to discuss jobs that relate to the topic, how a commodity is produced, and the types of related jobs done by the patients in the past.
5. *Creating a climate of appreciation.* About 5 to 10 minutes are spent expressing pleasure in the patient's attendance and in his contribution. Plans are made for the next meeting, which provides continuity and something to look forward to.[46]

This group is usually limited to 12 sessions, one hour per session, with as many as 15 patients in a group. The leader can be an attendant, although a professional nurse leader can add to the depth of the group. The sessions are held in a comfortable setting; patients sit in a semicircle. The leader stands in the center and conducts the group in an organized classroom style. A warm, accepting climate is maintained and the session is structured around the discussion of a specific topic. The topic for the day may be centered around an animal, nature study, a poem, or game, any topic that is of interest to the group. These contacts with reality serve to interest and involve the patient in living again. Nurses working with the elderly have reported a change in life satisfaction after a series of remotivation groups.[49] Remotivation Kits may be obtained from the American Psychiatric Association, Washington, D.C.

Sample Session: Fifteen patients are escorted into the activity room where tea and cookies are being served. Each person is greeted by name and is welcomed. This creates a Climate of Acceptance. The leader starts the group by commenting, "Today we are going to talk about picking apples." A poem is read several lines at a time so that each patient has a turn reading. Apples are passed from patient to patient to feel, see, smell, and touch. Questions are directed to the group with much feedback given after each response. The leader moves around the room touching and talking to individual patients, thus creating a Bridge to the World. Patients begin to talk more to one another after a session or two. John may recall how he picked apples on his father's farm when he was a child. Mary talks about making apple butter. Cora shares her favorite recipe for apple pie. Henry states he worked in a canning factory. (This is Sharing the World We Live In.) Under the leader's guidance, the discussion continues on a related subject—making apple products, commercial or home canning, caring for an orchard. Patients are encouraged to talk about their past experiences or jobs. Pictures or an object, such as an apple doll, may be passed around the group to elicit responses. (This is Appreciating the Work of the World.) As patients share the experiences of their lives, today's world becomes less frightening. Interest in living in renewed. The leader comments on the responsiveness of each person, tells the patients he appreciates their coming, and reminds each patient of the next session. Goodby's are said. Each person is called by name as he leaves. Patients leave with a feeling of being accepted and restored. (This creates a Climate of Appreciation.)

The use of staff to lead discussion groups on current topics with patients or nursing home residents may not be possible because of the time limits. The St. Cloud Veterans Administration Hospital in Minnesota successfully used elementary school children to assist with remotivating patients. The students were prepared by attending sessions to orient them to the aged person. Each student was assigned to meet with an individual patient. Then groups of students and seniors met twice weekly; the groups were led by nursing students. The group discussions were centered on a variety of reality-oriented topics. During the group session, the school child and the patient also spent some time talking with each other. The patients showed significant positive change in appearance, neatness, and interest in surroundings and others and a decrease in irritability, isolation, and inappropriate behavior. Some behavioral change remained for a long time after the 20-week session, but benefits lessened after the program was discontinued. Additionally, school children learned positive characteristics about the elderly.[67]

Activity Group

The goal of the activity group is to set up the structure and provide the direction of task accomplishment. The leader of this group, through support and encouragement, helps patients cope with stress through an activity. Reality awareness, physical ability or dexterity, and learning abilities are enhanced.

The activity should also enable the patients to experience accomplishment, sensory and cognitive stimulation, and encounters with people. The needs, characteristics, and interests of the patients, instead of those of the therapist, must be considered in planning the group. How often have you seen the activity director engrossed in making a doll or having a party while the group of patients seem bored or uncomfortable? It is helpful for the leader to have a consistent group so that relationships can be developed. The leader can then plan activities based on his knowledge of the group. The activity groups might be involved in such tasks as having a party, modeling with clay, doing exercises, or sketching a large picture together.

Activity groups can be useful with regressed, withdrawn, and immobilized patients when tasks are planned to meet specific needs. Not all patients need an activity group, however. These groups are often very popular in institutions for the elderly, but the emphasis is often only on the physical task. Every group has to be *doing* something, even if it is only physical exercises. Every group has to be a happy, cheery group. Staff members like to see the overt changes that doing and happy groups can achieve. Unfortunately, staff members may not realize the feelings of pain, resentment, and frustration that can underlie the happy facade, especially when the leader treats the members like children and uses a saccharin sweet manner and a strained, cheery voice. Patients learn not to talk about feelings in such a group; most likely the leader is not able to tolerate the pain, loneliness, and suffering. The patient's feelings will come out in physical complaints, or the resulting hopelessness may result in death. No one will bother to analyze how the milieu, including the activity group, contributes to either. After all, physical illness and death are considered part of the package of aging. Such results can be avoided, however, if activity groups are planned to meet emotional and social, as well as physical, needs.

Support Group

The primary goal of the support group is to present information about normal changes in old age and through informal group contact bring about individual growth and the ability to cope with these changes. A pilot Geriatric Arthritis Program was set up at University Hospital, University of Michigan. Four support groups were formed; in all four groups such themes as depression, social isolation, and sensory losses were discussed repeatedly. Brainstorming covered such topics as memory, vision, hearing, interpersonal relationships, health management, housing and relocation, dying and death, and how to anticipate or cope with various situations. Role playing, group techniques, and group exercises were used to encourage expression, experience, and problem solving.

Sample Session: The leader introduces the topic of loss and asks members to share their ideas and feelings. As members speak, the leader jots some of the basic ideas on large pieces of paper. After some discussion related to the topic, an exercise is used to illustrate feelings. Two people representing husband and wife hold a long board. Other group members are added to help hold the board; they represent important aspects in the life of the husband and wife, such as jobs, homes, health, siblings, children, friends, and income. One by one the group members are told to let go of the board. In a symbolic sense, the members are able to envision the experiences many of them have lived through. They share their feelings with the group.

A major benefit of a support group is to help members realize the universality of their problems. Most older people begin to feel that no one has the same difficulties as they experience. When they hear that others share in the same dilemma, it can be a "discovery of not being alone" or "welcome to the human race." Also, as the topic is discussed and solutions to the problem are given, many people might be able to find answers to some of their own problems.

Loss is a universal theme. A group of elderly patients led by this author for 1½ years discussed the theme of loss repeatedly. At one session there were two empty chairs: one member had died and one had been discharged. No one would sit in the two chairs normally occupied by the two lost members. But the other members immediately spoke of the two missing persons. As the group discussed the two men, experiences associated with them, and jokes told by them, the group members appeared more and more depressed. Apparently they were allowing themselves to experience the feelings they had previously tried to deny. One man stated, "Well, it's like when you are in the Army. Your buddy goes to the front line and never comes back. You learn never to have a buddy again." In essence, he was saying, "It hurts to lose a friend. Rather than be hurt again, I'll protect myself; I won't become involved again." After much discussion the members agreed it was unwise to withdraw. As one 80-year-old man said somberly, "Without others, you are very lonely." Another gave the group hope when he said, "As one door closes, others will open up."

Closely related to loss is the subject of death. This subject comes up over and over again. One of the author's groups began with 12 patients. Over the course of 2 years six patients died. Certainly every group member was aware of the decreasing size of the group. Several times members voted not to allow new members to join. One patient said to the leader, "One day you'll be the only one left." This statement indicated that he thought death was only for the elderly. Death is the end, a wrap-up of what life has meant, a closure, and a judgment. One patient, almost 95 years old, stated, "Death is like summing up the column of numbers and coming up with a total." Contrary to the attitude of younger people, older people realize that their chances are few to redo life or give life new meaning. One patient said, "To give my life meaning, I need something to do, someone to love, something to look forward to." From this statement we can understand the sense of hopelessness and worthlessness that most elderly are likely to experience.

Discussion Group

The major goals of the discussion group are to encourage learning and involvement with other people. Although education is the major goal, the group can be helpful by emphasizing individual strengths and increasing self-esteem.

Sample Session: The elderly clients come into a room and seat themselves around a large table. Each one writes his name on a large card and places it in front of himself on the table. The leader begins by saying, "This is your group. Where should we start?" A common aim is drawn from the group. Each member states what he would like to discuss in the group, for example: "I would like to know what to do about my arthritis." "My husband died last month, and I wonder about banking and taxes." "I am living alone and I wonder what I would do if I needed help." Problem solving, information seeking, and involvement in the group are explored. An agenda for the next few meetings is prepared. A relationship between the leader and members is begun. Each member leaves knowing that the topic for the next meeting will be "loss." Several members plan to read some background material on the subject.

The level of functioning in a discussion group is fairly high. The discussion will be based upon theory, but through the discussion, members may move to deeper insights. The leader will always be looking for an opportunity to deepen the discussion, to validate with the group members, to acknowledge and support, and to remain objective so that the members will be able to see a balance in the topic and will be able to accept the opinions and statements of others.

The discussion group can help the elderly to make friends. Most persons in later maturity feel that they cannot make new friendships. They dwell on their losses and seem unaware of opportunities to make friends, perhaps because of low self-esteem or decreased emotional and physical energy.

Within therapy groups the primary tie for the member is often with the leader. The leader can balance this by promoting cohesiveness among members. This is not easy, especially for institutionalized patients who often relate with each other as small children. Activities done together may resemble parallel play. The patients' irritations with each other resemble sibling rivalry. Their dependency on staff is pronounced, but the resentment of authority and striving for independence comes through.

As a leader, encourage members to talk *to* each other instead of through you. Wait for them to share problems and their skills in solving them. Solutions will be better accepted because they are given by someone who has lived through them. The leader can be a friend without having all the answers.

Reminiscing Group

The goal of the reminiscing group is to allow its members an opportunity to share their thoughts and feelings about the past life. Butler spoke of the life review as a common process in the elderly, especially as death becomes more imminent. As this process occurs, the past is considered and dealt with in preparation for death.[18] The reminiscing process is natural, universal, and adaptive. It is a response to various crises.

A reminiscing group is useful to the aged because members share experiences and participate with one another, gain a new perception of self and others, and review historical and significant events of their time.[24]

Reminiscing groups may be long-term or short-term, formal or informal, structured or spontaneous. A democratic climate is essential. The leader might plan a topic for the session, such as travel, foods, animals, or historical eras. Pictures, records, music, or various old objects could be used to stimulate discussion. Or members could spontaneously discuss whatever topic is of interest. As the group grows in trust, conversation moves from superficial to more intimate, emotionally loaded levels.

For example, one 89-year-old man in a reminiscing group told the author, who was the group leader, about five short events; each event related to rejection by or loss of a loved one. As he reminisced, he became more tearful. The leader responded by asking if he was concerned about what would happen to the relationship within the group. The discussion that followed centered on trusting the leader and the group.

If you truly accept the senior, you will acknowledge and be interested in his past life. Most of what the person is lies in the past and present, for not a great deal of future remains. Encouraging the person to talk about the past helps him to better accept himself and his current situation. The sense of self-worth increases as the leader acknowledges his experience and wisdom.

Sample Session: The leader begins the group by asking, "What comes to your mind for discussion today?" The members are accustomed to the broad opening and are comfortable with the leader and with each other.

One petite lady with beribboned, silver gray hair begins by telling the group she saw a robin that morning. This is a fairly neutral topic. An Italian man replies, "That means Spring is on the way." This leads into a discussion of previous springs. Jerry, a spry Irish man, laughs and replies, "It was the spring of 1892 when I was working through New England selling violins. I was a pusher of instruments, just like Music Man." As he tells the group about his lucrative position, the other members laugh, and he joins in. He obviously enjoys telling the story.

Feelings of joy, pleasure, humor, and sadness are evident in the group. The group sits quietly and the leader asks if anyone could say what they are feeling. Mary answers, "It was good to hear, but the sadness is that it's gone." Jerry states, "Yes, but there is each day to be lived." The group ends the session with coffee or tea and cookies. With the sharing of events and memories, a closeness prevails.

The sharing of memories is adaptive and promotes a bonding with others. It reaffirms individual identity, position, and personal worth, and in turn reduces loneliness and isolation.

Growth Group

The goal of this group is to increase the personal growth of the group members, depending on personal needs and the level of group experience. At times the thrust of intervention is supportive in order to encourage acceptance and understanding of self and others. At other times intervention is based upon the human relations approach and emphasizes conscious phenomena and emotional expression. The leader encourages members' self-awareness, expression of feelings, sense of trust, and increased behavioral skills with and sensitivity to others. Various verbal and nonverbal methods are used to accomplish these goals.

Leading a growth group is not easy, for as members share their deeper feelings, the leader is likely to experience fatigue and sadness. However, talking about feelings of loneliness, isolation, dependency, and worthlessness allows a release and a resolution. The primary goal of the group is not to keep pain hidden but to share it, deal with it, and grow from having encountered it.

Insight Group

The major goal of the insight group is to stimulate members' involvement, and through this, exploration and interpretation of behavior in the group. The elderly are capable of transference, which over time promotes self-awareness of behavior.[40] Regression in behavior may occur when requests or overt needs are gratified too hurriedly or reassurance is given too quickly. Some elderly persons, those in firm contact with reality and who have the ability to abstract, respond better to clarification, confrontation, and interpretation.[40] Some therapists report that elderly persons can achieve insight into how their present conflicts with people are a result of past relationships with important people.[18,35,40] A sense of importance, increased awareness of the world, ability to confront reality and others, a greater sense of responsibility for the enjoyment and personal satisfaction of others, and insight into personal behavior result from the insight group.[27,40]

Nurses with advanced preparation in psychotherapy are knowledgeable and experienced to do insight group therapy with the elderly. This approach can be especially helpful in treating elderly persons suffering with neurotic and depressive conflicts. The authors believe that this approach is also useful in helping the elderly work through the developmental tasks of aging and death. Through exploration of past experiences, the senior can resolve some of the hidden conflicts and face the remaining life more openly and realistically.

Discharge Group

The major goals of the discharge group are to retrain elderly patients who have been institutionalized for a long period of time but who can resume life in the community, or to help the hospitalized patient gain information and skills to better cope with his situation after discharge. The group experience involves discussion of feelings and fears concerning discharge and role playing of some of the real problems associated with discharge. Role playing the experiences and skills of daily living, such as, shopping, banking, cleaning house, cooking, or even using the phone can help the person act more appropriately in the community. Group meetings might also include discussion of current events and general information about coping with the everyday world. Information about Golden Age Clubs and Senior Citizen Centers, their purpose, and how to join, would be appropriate. Often this group is open; membership changes as some patients are discharged and patients awaiting discharge join the group. Discharge groups may include families if the patient has any family members alive and interested.

How Group Work Differs with the Elderly

The type of group you establish for the elderly client will be different from the group you establish for younger people. There are other distinctions as well.[13,14,16]

Touch is used more with clients in later maturity than with other clients, except children. Touch used spontaneously and in combination with sincere affection compensates for the emotional, social, and sensory deprivation that many older people endure. They will reach out to you; you should be comfortable with touch.

People who are different are better tolerated by elderly clients. For example, they are more likely to understand the needs of the person who is monopolizing, silent, or different in behavior. The members will let you focus on an individual member for a time; if they trust you, they know that you will also give them attention. Groups of youthful members are more likely to show impatience with you and the deviant member, be sarcastic to another, or compete to get attention.

The content of discussion in groups of elderly members is more likely to deal with the theme of loss and center on reminiscing, regardless of the type of group you are leading. Younger groups talk more about their present activities and concerns and future aspirations. Also, older people will talk more about their physical complaints. Listening to him talk about his arthritic joints, constipation, and jittery heart is essential to convey caring.

Elderly group members who are alert are more concerned about the state of the world generally than are younger members, who are more concerned with their own problems. The person in later maturity has lived long enough to have a perspective about the life cycle and a historical sense for the world situation.

Elderly group members react to the leader differently. They warm up to you quickly but will be slow to trust. Yet, they will let you be yourself. You don't have to parade professional behavior; they see through a facade. They do not expect you to have all the answers; they recognize the collective wisdom in the group and are willing to learn from each other. They will perceive when you do not feel well or are very worried and will be as supportive, warm, and understanding as possible. The elderly have a need to be needed; they will give as much to you—or more—than you give to them. Little gifts brought to you should be graciously accepted. You will have to be open to them, however. They will test you in various ways and will assess your personal security, ability to cope, and feelings about life, death, and them. In their wisdom they are likely to perceive more than younger clients would.

Group work with the elderly can be an opportunity for both you and the members. The experience will be stimulating and enjoyable but also demanding. At times you will feel distressed as you observe and listen, as you experience vicariously their debility and losses—of things and of people. Yet, you will find great rewards as you provide opportunities for touching, closeness, encountering, and sensory and emotional stimulation between the group members and between them and yourself. The group experience can make a real difference in the lives of elderly clients—and in your life.

REFERENCES

1. ANDERSON, RALPH, and IRL CARTER, *Human Behavior in the Social Environment.* Chicago: Aldine Publishing Company, 1974.

2. ARNHART, EMELIA A., "Establishing Group Work in a Psychiatric Unit of a General Hospital," *Journal of Psychiatric Nursing and Mental Health Services,* 13: No. 1 (1975), 5–9.

3. BAINES, J., "Effects of Reality Orientation Classroom on Memory Loss, Confusion, and Disorientation in Geriatric Patients," *The Gerontologist,* 14: (1974), 138–42.

4. BALGOPAL, P., "Variations in Sensitivity Traning Groups," *Perspectives in Psychiatric Care,* 11: No. 2 (1973), 80–86.

5. BLOCHER, DONALD, *Developmental Counseling.* New York: The Ronald Press Company, 1966.

6. BORMANN, ERNEST, *Discussion and Group Methods: Theory and Practice.* New York: Harper & Row, Publishers, Inc., 1969.

7. BOUCHER, MICHAEL, "Personal Space and Chronicity in the Mental Hospital," *Perspectives in Psychiatric Care,* 11: No. 5 (1971), 206–10.

8. BOYLIN, WILLIAM, S. GORDON, and M. NEHRKE, "Reminiscing and Ego Integrity in Institutionalized Elderly Males," *The Gerontologist,* 16: No. 2 (1976), 118–24.

9. BRADFORD, L., and DOROTHY MIAL, "When Is a Group?" *Educational Leadership, 21: (1963),* 147–51.

10. BROWNE, LOUISE, and JENNIE RITTER, "Reality Therapy for the Geriatric Psychiatric Patient," *Perspectives in Psychiatric Care,* 10: No. 3 (1972), 135–39.

11. BURGESS, ANN, and AARON LAZARE, "Nursing Management of Feelings, Thoughts and Behavior," *Journal of Psychiatric Nursing and Mental Health Services,* 10: No. 6 (1972), 7–11.

12. BURNSIDE, IRENE M., "The Patient I Didn't Want," *American Journal of Nursing,* 68: No. 8 (1968), 1666–69.

13. ———, "Group Work Among the Aged," *Nursing Outlook,* 17: No. 6 (1969), 68–71.

14. ———, "Group Work with Aged," *The Gerontologist,* 10: (1970), 241–46.

15. ———, *Psychosocial Nursing Care of the Aged,* New York: McGraw-Hill Book Company, 1973.

16. ———, "Overview of Group Work with the Aged," *Journal of Gerontological Nursing,* 2: No. 6 (1976), 14–17.

17. ———, *Nursing and the Aged.* New York: McGraw-Hill Book Company, 1976.

18. BUTLER, ROBERT, "Intensive Psychotherapy for the Hospitalized Aged," *Geriatrics, 15: (1960),* 644–53.

19. ———, *"The Life Review: An Interpretation of Reminiscence in the Aged,"* *Psychiatry,* 26: No. 1 (1963), 65–76.

20. CARTWRIGHT, D., "Achieving Change in People: Some Applications of Group Dynamics Theory," *Human Relations,* 4: (1951), 381–92.

21. CITRIN, RICHARD, and DAVID DIXON, "Reality Orientation—A Milieu Therapy Used in an Institution for the Aged," *The Gerontologist,* 17: No. 1 (1977), 39–43.

22. CULBERT, S. A., "The Interpersonal Process of Self-Disclosure: It Takes Two to See One," *Explorations in Applied Behavioral Science.* New York: Renaissance Editors, 1967.

23. DURKIN, HELEN, *The Group in Depth.* New York: International Universities Press, 1964.

24. EBERSOLE, P., "From Despair to Integrity Through Reminiscing with the Aged," in *A.N.A. Clinical Sessions.* New York: Appleton-Century-Crofts, Inc., 1975.

25. FOLSOM, J. "Reality Orientation for the Elderly Mental Patient," *Geriatric Psychiatry* (Spring, 1968), 291–307.

26. GIAMBRA, LEONARD, "Daydreaming About the Past, The Time Setting of Spontaneous Thought Intrusions," *The Gerontologist,* 17: No. 1 (1977), 35–38.

27. GIFFIN, KIM, "Adulthood and Old Age," *The Gerontologist,* 9: No. 4 (1969), 286–92.

28. GOLDBERG, CARL, *Encounter: Group Sensitivity Training Experience.* New York: Science House, Inc., 1970

29. GOLDFARB, A., and H. TURNER, "Psychotherapy of Aged Persons—Utilization and Effectiveness of Brief Therapy," *American Journal of Psychiatry,* 109: (1953), 916–21.

30. HARRIS, C., "The Florida State Hospital Patient Behavior Rating Sheet," in *Behavior Assessment: New Directions in Clinical Psychology,* eds. J. Cone and R. Hawkins. New York: Brunner-Mazel, 1976.

31. HARRIS, CLARKE, and PETER IVORY, "An Outcome Evaluation of Reality Orientation Therapy with Geriatric Patients in a State Mental Hospital," *The Gerontologist,* 16: No. 6 (1976), 496–503.

32. HOMANS, GEORGE C., *The Human Group.* New York: Harcourt Brace & World, Inc., 1950.

33. KALKMAN, MARION, and ANNE DAVIS, *New Dimensions in Mental Health—Psychiatric Nursing.* New York: McGraw-Hill Book Company, 1974.

34. KASTENBAUM, ROBERT, *New Thoughts on Old Age,* New York: Springer Publishing Company, Inc., 1964.

35. LAZARUS, LAWRENCE W., "A Program for the Elderly at a Private Psychiatric Hospital," *The Gerontologist,* 16: No. 2 (1976), 125–31.

36. LEWIN, KURT, "Frontiers in Group Dynamics: Concept Method and Reality in Social Science; Social Equilibria and Social Change," *Human Relations,* 1: (1947), 5–42.

37. LEWIS, C. N., "Reminiscing and Self-Concept in Old Age," *Journal of Gerontology,* 26: (1971), 240–43.

38. LIEBERMAN, M., and J. FALK, "The Remembered Past as a Source of Data for Research on the Life Cycle," *Human Development,* 14: (1971), 132–41.

39. LINDEN, M., "Group Psychotherapy with Institutionalized Senile Women," *International Journal of Group Psychotherapy,* 3: (1953), 150–70.

40. ———, "Transference in Gerontologic Group Psychotherapy," *International Journal of Group Psychotherapy,* 5: (1955), 61–79.

41. LIPPITT, GORDON, and EDITH SEASHORE, *The Leader and Group Effectiveness.* New York: Association Press, 1962.

42. LUFT, JOSEPH, *Group Process: An Introduction to Group Dynamics.* Palo Alto, Calif.: National Press Books, 1970.

43. MANASTER, AL, "Therapy with the 'Senile' Geriatric Patient," *The International Journal of Group Psychotherapy,* 22: (1972), 250–57.

44. MARRAM, GWEN, *The Group Approach in Nursing Practice,* 2nd ed. St. Louis: The C. V. Mosby Company, 1978.

45. MATHESON, WAYNE E., "Which Patient for Which Therapeutic Group," *Journal of Psychiatric Nursing and Mental Health Services,* 12: No. 3 (1974), 10–13.

46. MCCLELLAND, LUCILLE, *Textbook for Psychiatric Technicians.* St. Louis: The C. V. Mosby Company, 1971.

47. MCMAHON, A., and P. RHUDICK, *Psychodynamic Studies on Aging: Creativity, Reminiscing, and Dying.* New York: International Universities Press, 1967.

48. MEERLOO, J., "Modes of Psychotherapy in the Aged," *Journal of the American Geriatrics Society,* 9: (1961), 225–34.

49. MOODY, LINDA, VIRGINIA BARON, and GRACE MONK, "Moving the Past into the Present," *American Journal of Nursing,* 70: No. 11 (1970), 2353–56.

50. MORRISON, MALCOLM, "A Human Relations Approach to Problem Solving," *The Gerontologist,* 16: No. 2 (1976), 185–86.

51. MUMMAH, HAZEL R., "Group Work with Aged Blind Japanese in the Nursing Home and in the Community," *The New Outlook for the Blind,* 69: No. 4 (1975), 160–64.

52. NORDMARK, MADELYN, and ANNE ROHWEDER, *Scientific Foundations of Nursing,* 2nd ed. Philadelphia: J. B. Lippincott Company, 1967.

53. OHLSEN, MERLE, *Group Counseling.* New York: Holt, Rinehart, and Winston, 1970.

54. PETTY, BERYL, T. MOELLER, and R. CAMPBELL, "Support Groups for Elderly Persons in the Community," *The Gerontologist,* 15: No. 6 (1976), 522–28.

55. ROGERS, CARL, *On Becoming a Person.* Boston: Houghton Mifflin Company, 1961.

56. ——, *Carl Rogers on Encounter Groups.* New York: Harper & Row, Publishers, Inc., 1970.

57. ——, "Carl Rogers Describes His Way of Facilitating Encounter Groups," *American Journal of Nursing,* 71: No. 2 (1971), 275–79.

58. ROUSLIN, SHEILA, "Relatedness in Group Psychotherapy," *Perspectives in Psychiatric Care,* 11: No. 4 (1973), 165–71.

59. SCOTT, M. LOUISE, "To Learn to Work with the Elderly," *The American Journal of Nursing,* 73: No. 4 (1973), 662–64.

60. SHEPHERD, CLOVIS, *Small Groups.* San Francisco: Chandler Publishing Company, 1964.

61. SHERE, E. "Group Therapy with the Very Old," in *New Thoughts on Old Age,* ed. R. Kastenbaum. New York: Springer Publishing Co., Inc., 1964.

62. SILVER, A., "Group Psychotherapy with Senile Psychotic Patients," *Geriatrics,* 5: (1950), 147–50.

63. SMITH, E. FRANCES, "Teaching Group Therapy in an Undergraduate Curriculum," *Perspectives in Psychiatric Care,* 11: No. 2 (1973), 70–74.

64. SOLOMON, PHILIP, and VERNON PATCH, *Handbook of Psychiatry.* Los Altos, Calif.: Lange Medical Publications, 1971.

65. SPOTNITZ, HYMAN, *The Couch and the Aide.* New York: Alfred A. Knopf, Inc., 1961.

66. SWANSON, MARY, "A Check List for Group Leaders," *Perspectives in Psychiatric Care,* 7: No. 3 (1969), 120–26.

67. THRALON, JOAN, and CHARLES WATSON, "Remotivation for Geriatric Patients Using Elementary School Students," *Nursing Digest,* 5: No. 4 (1975), 48–49.

68. TOFFLER, ALVIN, *Future Shock.* New York: Bantam Books, Inc., 1970.

69. TROW, W., S. ZANDER, W. MORSE, and D. JENKINS, "Psychology of Group Behavior: The Class as a Group," *Journal of Educational Psychology,* 41: (1950), 322–88.

70. WATER, JANE, *Group Guidance, Principles and Practices.* New York: McGraw-Hill Book Company, 1960.

71. WERNER, JEAN, "Relating Group Theory to Nursing Practice," *Perspectives in Psychiatric Care,* 5: No. 6 (1970), 248–61.

72. WHITE, R., and R. LIPPETT, "Leader Behavior and Member Reaction in Three Social Climates," in *Group Dynamics,* eds. D. Cartwright and A. Zander. Evanston, Ill.: Row Peterson, 1953, Chapter 40.

73. WICKS, ROBERT J., *Counseling Strategies and Intervention Techniques for the Human Services.* Philadelphia: J. B. Lippincott Company, 1977.

74. WOLFF, K., "Group Psychotherapy with Geriatric Patients in a Mental Hospital," *Journal of the American Geriatrics Society,* 5: (1957), 13–19.

75. ——, "Treatment of the Geriatric Patient in a Mental Hospital," *Journal of the American Geriatrics Society,* 4: (1956), 472–76.

76. YALOM, IRVIN, and FLORENCE TERRAZAS, "Group Therapy for Psychotic Elderly Patients," *American Journal of Nursing,* 68: No. 8 (1968), 1690–98.

77. YALOM, IRVIN D., *The Theory and Practice of Group Psychotherapy.* New York: Basic Books, Inc., 1970.

78. YEAWORTH, ROSALEE, "Learning Through Group Experience," *Nursing Outlook,* 18: No. 6 (1970), 29–32.

SOCIETY AND LATER MATURITY:
Implications for Nursing Process

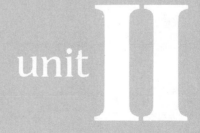

unit **II**

sociocultural influences on the person in later maturity

Study of this chapter will enable you to:

---

1. Compare personal with societal values, attitudes, myths, and stereotypes about the elderly person.

2. Discuss how various cultures and societies view aging and relate to the elderly.

3. Identify value orientations in the United States that negatively affect attitudes toward the elderly and, in turn, the senior's self-concept.

4. Explore how myths and stereotypes held by the health worker influence care given to the senior and his family.

5. Discuss aging-group-consciousness and the aged subculture, the usefulness of this phenomenon to the senior, and your role in promoting aging-group-consciousness in the elderly.

6. Assess the elderly person/family considering how sociocultural influences affect self-concept and health status.

7. Intervene with elderly persons from various sociocultural backgrounds, using information presented in this chapter and the bibliography in the Appendix.

5

In Chapter 1 you explored your values, attitudes, and feelings related to the elderly person. In this chapter sociocultural values and attitudes are explored.

CULTURAL PERSPECTIVES ON LATER MATURITY

Cultural Level Related to Attitudes Toward the Aged

The value placed on the elderly and attitudes toward them vary with the culture's level of sophistication.

The aged in a nomadic or semipermanent society are held in low regard because the sick and elderly may be unable to contribute labor or transport themselves. The harshness of dry or cold climates occupied by most nomadic groups and daily foraging for food place a high value on youth and vigor. Physical survival is the main preoccupation; building an intellectual or cultural life is a low priority. Relatively little folklore is transmitted to the young, a minimum of religious thought links them to the gods, and a paucity of *rites de passage* exist through which the elderly can exercise control.[30]

Tribes are more attached to land, inhabit friendlier ecologies, number more persons per village, and possess real and movable property. They have complex family and kin networks to govern every aspect of interaction, believe in complicated religions or mythologies, and practice a formally ritualistic life. Stability and tradition give seniors more social role and status. The population lives longer, and a larger number of aged compete among themselves, which may keep the senior alert and sharper at life skills.[30]

In peasant communities economic sophistication is greater. Financial exchange is based on land and offers opportunities for developing skills, fortunes, and control over persons through division of labor. The aged are likely to have more land and related status; land is inherited from the elderly.[30]

Pastoral and agricultural economies have a more complex, social organization and economic development, combined with security of a relatively productive and peaceful environment. Thus, cultural and religious traditions flourish. The aged are involved in preserving a heritage; they have prestige and power. The greater the number of grandchildren, the greater their economic importance. Parents of the grandchildren defer to the aged. The frustration of intergenerational conflict is sublimated, displaced indirectly, or given vent downward in the age pyramid.[30]

Generally, the lowest esteem for the aged is found in the simpler society with the smallest socioeconomic structure and with the fewest material resources and human relationships for control.[30]

However, a technological society that does not adhere to traditional mores reverses the trend of upward esteem for the elderly. Technology apparently takes over aspects of society for which the aged were responsible. Social and geographic mobility and individual autonomy are again valued, as they were in nomadic societies. Technologically complex jobs promote financial and social separation from traditional restraints and the extended family. The elderly lose their family ties, decision-making power, security, and special status or esteem. Encoded information in books, libraries, and data banks make the senior's experience less valuable for transmitting traditions, values, or information. Instead, the aged must depend on younger people for their well-being and activity roles.[30]

A study of aged persons in three geographically distant agrarian cultures indicates that when the aged are esteemed, longevity is increased. Studies of villages in remote regions of Vilcabamba in Equador, Hunza in Kashmir, and Abkhazia in the Soviet Union reveal that many persons are 100 years and older.[18]

In Vilcabamba, Catholic baptismal records confirmed ages, as did the number of generations of offspring. Hunza has an oral tradition which is transmitted; no written records exist. The ruler verified the ages of some of the people from knowledge of his state's history. The best documentation has been done by a gerontologist in Abkhazia who used church and state records, age at marriage, time until birth of children, present ages of offspring, and memory of outstanding national events. Heredity may contribute to longevity, since gene purity (absence of genes increasing risk of fatal disease) would be possible in isolated Vilcabamba and Hunza. In Abkhazia the aged are a mixture of ten ethnic groups. However, in all three areas the aged had parents who also lived more than 100 years. The common characteristics of these distant cultures are as follows: (1) Old people are esteemed; they occupy a central and privileged position and their wisdom is elicited. (2) No forced retirement exists; old people continue to do satisfying but hard labor. (3) The sense of family continuity is strong. (4) A stable mode and rhythm of life exist. (5) The diet is low in calories, fat, and protein. In spite of the scant diet, by American standards, the villagers were not malnourished, and they engaged in vigorous exercise and work that fatigued the Western researchers. (6) The aged people felt that their longevity was related to being happily married and to remaining sexually interested and vigorous past the childbearing years, since only married people attained extreme age. (7) Further, the aged died quickly once they lost their useful role in the community.[7,18]

Although the number of centenarians is increasing in the United States, perhaps fewer people reach extreme old age because they are not esteemed; they feel useless and roleless; and our technological society expects them to die in the seventies or eighties. Certainly dietary and hereditary factors may also contribute, but some of our oldest citizens featured in our media describe how they have engaged in drinking, smoking, and dietary excesses all of their lives.

Religious Cultural Influences on Attitudes

Religious teachings about life, the value of the person, and the meaning of death affect values and attitudes even when the person is no longer actively practicing a religion.

The Jewish religion regards long life as good and as a reward for righteous living. Old age is associated with wisdom and good judgment. Respect for parents is a primary duty; care of the aged is assumed by the family whenever possible. Otherwise, the elderly person is cared for in an institution that is as homelike as possible.[24]

Christianity developed in a Greco-Roman culture and was influenced later by Germanic culture, neither of which regarded its aged very highly unless they had achieved unusual power. Christians traditionally and generally have shown less respect and feeling of responsibility to their aged than have Jewish people. Of the Christian population, Catholics have traditionally shown more concern by developing services and institutions to care for the elderly. Protestants are a diverse group but tend to be Calvinistic; they traditionally have considered misfortune to result from the person's lack of responsibility and planning. With less sympathy for the elderly who could not care for himself, they regarded the state and local community responsible for the aged who had no family to care for them. The Protestant Ethic, which emphasized independence and achievement, was dominant in the United States earlier in this century. This work ethic had an effect on the kinds and locations of institutions that were built, and it created an attitude of rejection toward the senior members who could no longer be productive.[24]

Racial and Ethnic Cultural Influences on Attitudes

In the rural Appalachian, Black, and Spanish-American communities, old age is considered an achievement. Intergenerational ties are strong. The senior is given higher status and security and feels accepted and respected. The person is expected and is allowed to be of assistance to the extended family for as long as possible; in turn, the senior is cared for by the family if at all possible.

Oriental cultures here and abroad have traditionally valued and cared for their aged. The elderly person is a source of wisdom and often exerts considerable power. Ancestor worship is not uncommon.[36]

Caucasian ethnic groups vary. Traditionally, the aged were respected; in families of European descent family ties were close. Thus, close ties between the generations are still seen in some European ethnic populations. However, most immigrant families were assimilated into the United States culture, and extended family ties changed to nuclear family relationships. For example, elderly Polish-Americans resent the lack of respect shown them by their children and feel anger at the changing norms.[19,28]

A study of Italian-American and Polish-American ethnic attitudes revealed that respondents who had higher earnings (above $10,000 annually), had at least a high school education, and were second or third generation favored independent living arrangements for elderly relatives. Second- and third-generation respondents had less preference for intergenerational families. Yet, most respondents wanted to keep the elderly relative in their homes, regardless of the person's physical status. Second- and third-generation members were more likely to prefer home care rather than institutional care for the bedridden elderly, a finding which might not be present in ethnic groups who traditionally have less close-knit families. Those who preferred institutional care for the elderly preferred an institution that was Catholic or of the same ethnic background and staff who were of the same ethnic background because of their language skills and knowledge of customs.[8]

Americans are not the only aged who feel devalued. A cross-cultural study of students' attitudes toward old people revealed negative stereotypes in India, Japan, Puerto Rico, Sweden, Greece, and England. Indian students have more negative feeling than United States' students do. Greeks consider older people more conservative, less active, and more interfering than do Indians. Apparently, many cultures have generally negative stereotypes of aged.[29]

Changing Cultural Values Which Affect Attitudes Toward Later Maturity

The historical era in which the person was born and in which he lives affects his development through the life cycle, his health status, available opportunities, social status, problems to be confronted, and how his needs are met.

The population which is currently in later maturity and which spans two generations, was born in the late 1800's or early 1900's when the United States was in a period of peace and isolated from world conflict. These people in young adulthood were at the forefront of industrial expansion. Rugged individualism, hard work, and thrift, rather than educational degrees, enabled the person to achieve and progress.

Current value orientations in the United States that negatively affect the senior include emphasis on:

1. Speed, change, progress, activity, and efficiency.
2. Personal achievement, occupational success, and upward mobility.
3. Youth, beauty, and health.
4. Reliance on science, machines, and various social institutions.
5. Materialism, consumerism, and disposable items, which imply that to be old is worn out and worthless.
6. Conformity to the majority and to the group, which can become a kind of tyranny.

7. Personal pleasure and happiness as an actively pursued goal. Responsibility and commitment are not nurtured and are not even expected at times.
8. Scientific knowledge and the latest research findings. Wisdom gained from experience is not considered important.
9. Competitive and aggressive behavior instead of cooperation and contemplation.
10. Geographical mobility, which loosens family and neighborhood ties. Family property may not exist and smaller family size and homes imply no room for the senior.

The values conflict is self-evident and is most intensely felt by rural or small-town elderly. However, most elderly have lost power and responsibility and are given a lower social status. Economic position is often precarious in spite of their earlier hard work and thrift. Socioeconomic status is more important than age in determining position in the United States, since socioeconomic status is related to life-style, residence, and power in the community.[17]

The transition to aging in many respects resembles the adolescent period in the United States; the person is in a marginal position of having lost an established status without having acquired a new one. Twentieth-century trends in technology and urbanization have created new role expectations for which the elderly person is unprepared.

STEREOTYPES AND MYTHS ABOUT LATER MATURITY

A number of negative stereotypes or myths about the person in later maturity persist in American society.[20,25,26] Some of the common ones are as follows.

Age 65 is a good marker for old age.

Fact: Factors other than chronological age cause the person to be old. Many people are more youthful than their parents were at age 65. With increased longevity, perhaps 70 or 75 should be the chronological marker.

Most old people are in bed or in institutions and are ill physically and mentally.

Fact: About 5 percent are institutionalized; 95 percent are living in the community. While 67 percent of older persons outside institutions have one or more chronic conditions, 14 percent do not. Chronic conditions range from mild and correctable to more severe. About 81 percent of the aged living in the community have no mobility limitations; 8 percent have trouble getting around; 6 percent need the help of another person; and 5 percent are homebound. The average number of restricted activity days is only twice that for young adults. A small percentage show signs of mental deterioration and senility or become mentally ill; most of these seniors can be treated to some extent.[25,38,41] In one study of septuagenarians, one-third reported no physical disease, and only one-half of those with physical disease considered themselves ill. Hypochondria was observed in only 3.9 percent of the subjects.[32]

Retirement is disliked by all old people and causes illness and less life-satisfaction.

Fact: Although this may be true for some people, many older people look forward to retirement and are retiring before 65 so that they can continue other pursuits. Most are not sick from idleness and a sense of worthlessness. Over three-fourths of the seniors have satisfying lives.[16,23,25]

Special health services for the aged are useless because the aged won't live much longer anyway.

Fact: At age 65 the average person can look forward to 15 more years of life. The elderly have fewer acute illnesses and accidental injuries, and these are correctable although older people take longer to recover than younger people do. Common chronic conditions are cardiovascular disease, cancer, arthritis, diabetes, and sensory impairments, which can be treated so that the person can achieve maximum potential and comfort.[25,39]

The elderly are slow to learn, less intelligent, and more forgetful.

Fact: Research refutes this statement (see Chapter 10). Further, many professionals continue their work after 65.[39]

The elderly are self-pitying, apathetic, irritable, and hard to live with.

Fact: Research shows that mood is related to the present situation and past personality. The older person is as likely as a younger one to have an interesting and pleasant personality.[25,26,41]

The elderly are inactive and unproductive.

Fact: Many young children have working grandparents. Thirty-six percent of men over 65 years are employed in some type of job. Older women often do their housework into their eighties or nineties. Older workers have a job attendance record that is 20 percent better than young workers, and they also sustain fewer job-related injuries.[26,41]

The elderly do not desire and do not participate in sexual activity.

Fact: Recent research refutes this (see Chapter 11).[41]

The elderly are isolated, abandoned, and lonely, and they are unlikely to participate in activities.

Fact: Many elderly prefer to live in a separate household. In one study 80 percent of the elderly lived with someone and did not feel lonely. Another study indicates that 8 percent of people over 65 years never married and were adjusted to living alone. Elderly people who do not have children often have siblings or friends with whom they live.[25,33] Other elderly live in institutions or residences for the aged where they make friends. The percentage of purposefully abandoned elderly is small; often the person who is a loner in old age has always been a loner.[33,41]

Attitudes of professional health workers toward older people are often negative and stereotypical. The aging process is viewed as deterioration and as concomitant with disease changes; the elderly are viewed as rigid, unadaptive, and slow to respond to treatment. Many consider that treatment should be custodial or palliative; they do not consider conditions associated with late life as correctable.[5,15]

Recent studies indicate that younger people, including school children, may feel more positive toward the elderly and that education about aging can make a difference in attitudes. Younger women and adolescents were more positive and less cynical about aging, less socially distant from the aged, and had fewer negative stereotypes toward the aged.[10,11,34,35] In-service training of women in geriatric health care and social service agencies resulted in less cynical feelings, stronger endorsement of family and public responsibility, and less anxiety about aging.[10]

Providing learning experiences for students in health care fields with older people who are healthy, living in the community, capable, and alert will help our future health practitioners gain a different perspective on aging. Too often students have their only contact with very old people who are debilitated and dependent, need total care, have multiple diagnoses, and are institutionalized. Further, the student may have no one to help him work through feelings about old age and dependency. No wonder health workers' fear and have negative feelings about growing old. Certainly health workers with such attitudes are in no position to teach anyone in society about positive aspects related to aging.

ATTITUDES TOWARD THE SELF IN LATER MATURITY

Attitudes toward aging and about the self as an older person vary with age, the rural and urban elderly, and between working and retired population. In one study retired urban dwellers ages 75 and older felt a sense of personal gratification and favorable community attitudes. They were satisfied with their housing, financial status, and family relationships. Urban dwellers who were under 75 years, one-fourth of whom were still working, had the opposite attitudes toward retirement. Rural persons who were retired, regardless of age, felt dissatisfaction with their housing and health status and were generally less happy, but they perceived favorable community attitudes. Apparently the urban old-old population in this study, those who had survived and coped with a variety of stresses, were the psychological elite. The urban young-old (65 to 74 years) apparently made more demands on their environment that were not fulfilled; hence, they felt negative and were not as well-adjusted. The rural population may also have had higher expectations of their environment, based on their earlier life experiences, and more difficulty in coping with the social changes that have affected the elderly.[40]

Implications of this study are that the young-old will soon become the old-old and may carry the same expectations and attitudes with them. As this population becomes older, they may remain dissatisfied, which may affect their emotional health, or they may demand more opportunities for fulfillment and community services.[40]

Ageism is the term used to refer to the *social disdain and avoidance of elderly persons and discriminatory practices in employment.*[1,11] The elderly person is very aware of ageism, negative stereotypes and myths, and that he is frequently considered a burden on society even though he is competent. He may feel rejected, isolated, lowered self-esteem, anger, self-hate, and dependent. A negative self-concept may result from the negative societal feelings which are manifested directly, such as in forced retirement and segregated housing, as well as indirectly, such as in jokes about aging. Institutionalized and dependent aged are more likely to hold negative attitudes toward old age.[6,20,24,38]

Persons with high self-esteem, who are independent, educated, and had a socially valued occupation have positive, or at least ambivalent, rather than negative, attitudes toward old age. For some older people, the symbols of old age, for example, retirement, increased leisure, acquisition of new roles, and changing appearance, are accepted and even bolster self-evaluation.[14,16,21,30,37] These people are likely to be aging-group-conscious and belong to the subculture of aging.[22,24,27]

THE ELDERLY PERSON'S INFLUENCE ON SOCIETY

Aging-Group-Consciousness

Aging-group-consciousness is an adaptive emotional response to social influences, stereotypes, and stresses in an attempt to salvage some positive affect toward the self by joining the subculture of the aged."[27]

The elderly person increasingly realizes that he has the ability and flexibility to cope with change, or else he would not have survived at all. Elderly people are living much longer than they thought they would, and they have developed a new awareness of themselves as people who count in society.

The aging-group-conscious consists of elderly people who feel vulnerable and subject to certain deprivations because of age. Although they react to these deprivations with some resentment, they work to overcome the deprivations. They identify with other elderly persons. A sense of unity and belonging develops as they become involved in senior citizen clubs, work collectively on problems, unite to form a political force locally or nationally, socialize with peers, try new leisure pursuits, and generally stave off a negative self-concept. They react to the losses of old age, including loss of accustomed roles, by seeking to develop new roles.[27,37]

These seniors are as busy as they were before retirement, contrary to the Cummings' and Henrys' Disengagement Theory. They do not disengage. Growing old—reaching later maturity—is considered a satisfying experience to the people who are aging-group-conscious, since they develop new interests, new friends, and a special subculture.[12,27] Because of their concerns for the aged, they want more legislation and organizations to specifically assist the aged. The Gray Panthers is an example of elderly people who are aging-group-conscious.[25]

Subculture of Later Maturity

A subculture may be expected to develop whenever members of a group interact more with each other than with other groups of people because of common backgrounds, interests, problems, or mutual friendships and assistance.[26]

Society has segregated the elderly. Development of social and welfare services especially for the elderly has increased their identification with each other.[26] This separateness gives them the opportunity to act and think independently in their own behalf. The elderly are pursuing activities formerly denied them in an effort to create a quality of life consistent with personal wishes.[25,27]

Thus, certain elderly persons can collectively be said to constitute a subculture; they are aging-group-conscious and they interact primarily with each other under a set of values distinctive and meaningful to them.[26,27] This is apparent in the self-segregating trends among older people as they move to retirement residences, villages, or towns. The rural elderly also establish a subculture as more youth move to the city. The elderly make up a major population in the inner city as younger people move out to the suburbs.[27] As the subculture of the senior citizen emerges, older adults are becoming increasingly active politically in their own behalf, influencing legislation that will affect them. For example one organized group in Arizona successfully worked to legalize adult communities in the state.

Since the person ages gradually, he continues to carry on roles and behavior typical of the general culture and to be socialized gradually into the aged subculture. Most elderly will not lose touch with the general culture even though they immerse themselves in peer activities. Some people are also physiologically and psychologically younger than their chronological years, and they resist being considered old or joining the elderly subculture.[27]

Certainly the efforts of the elderly to improve their situation will also benefit us in our later years. The aged subculture and their activities will have more impact as our elderly population increases in proportion to the rest of the population. This increase is a universal trend.

Demographic Trends

A cross-national survey of eight industrialized countries (Canada, England, Federal Republic of Germany, France, Israel, Poland, United States of America, and Yugoslavia) reveals the following trends:

1. More people are living longer.
2. Birth rates are declining but increased longevity has led to the present high percentages of aged people in these countries.
3. Social and economic trends contribute to create a social problem out of a normal process. Older workers are defined as nonproductive or too expensive to retrain or as redundant when technological changes cause reductions in certain categories of workers. Early retirement is thus mandated.
4. Children are less likely to live near elderly parents because of increased geographic mobility, and daughters are less likely to be at home to care for parents because they have careers.
5. Inadequate resources constrain the elderly to cope with extensive periods of enforced retirement, greater isolation, and increased needs as time passes.
6. Seniors are becoming increasingly politicized; they are better educated, are more articulate, and have more time to organize and pursue issues. They vote and have increasing influence and power; local and national governments will increasingly respond to their needs.[13]

Social change sometimes goes a full circle. In the future the later years may again mean a time when the person has more influence and time for leisure, politics, education, or other pursuits. The magic age of 65 will not mean mandatory retirement; the senior may engage in a late-life career until the mid-eighties simply because the manpower is needed. Housing, social services, and other programs may be increasingly designed for the elderly citizen. The predicted energy crisis may be offset by using the energy and wisdom of the senior citizen.[15] Conditions can be improved for the senior population if today's young and middle-aged adults work with the elderly to bring about the change. You have an important role as a citizen and a professional to be involved in making legislative and policy changes. Otherwise, rejection and alienation of the elderly may increase, which will directly affect today's young and middle-aged adults.

THE NURSING PROCESS AND SOCIOCULTURAL ASPECTS

As a nurse, you must keep abreast of the impact of sociocultural influences on the elderly, especially as they relate to health problems and services. You can help shape public thinking about and health care policy for the senior members of our society. You can do research to better understand the social environment of the elderly, its effect on them, and the seniors' perception of society and their own needs. As you care for the person in later maturity, consider their sociocultural backgrounds (ethnic, religious, geographical) in order to determine and meet the needs and preferences of the person and his family.

The sociocultural assessment tool in Chapter 2 can help you better understand the aged person and family—the values, needs, problems, and preferences. Patient care goals should be individualized and should depend on assessment of the person's unique background. You will wish to explore numerous references to add to your knowledge about specific cultural groups. The bibliography in the Appendix at the end of this chapter will help you in your pursuit of knowledge to individualize care.

Overcoming your myths and stereotypes and maintaining a positive attitude toward the elderly are essential when you work with them or you will contribute to a negative self-concept in the elderly. This does not mean that you deny or do not assess realistic problems, illness, or limits in an individual. Developing a reaction formation, viewing old age as only a time of pleasure, is not realistic nor helpful to the senior either. Maintain a balanced viewpoint. Old age means different things to different seniors, and how they perceive themselves and their condition will also vary from time to time. Stay open to *present* feelings and behavior of the senior.

REFERENCES

1. ANDERSON, WM., and N. ANDERSON, "The Politics of Exclusion: The Adults Only Movement in Arizona," *The Gerontologist,* 18: No. 1 (1978), 6–12.

2. BUTLER, ROBERT, *Why Survive? Being Old in America.* New York: Harper & Row, Publishers, Inc., 1975.

3. CHRISTENSON, JAMES, "Generational Value Differences," *The Gerontologist,* 17: No. 4 (1977), 367–74.

4. CLARK, MARGARET, and MONIQUE MENDELSON, "Mexican-American Aged in San Francisco," in *Human Life Cycle,* ed. Wm. Sze. New York: Jason Aronson, Inc., 1975, 671–90.

5. COE, RODNEY, "Professional Prospectives on the Aged," *The Gerontologist,* 7: (1967), 114–19.

6. DAVIES, LELAND, "Attitudes Toward Old Age and Aging as Shown by Humor," *The Gerontologist,* 17: No. 3 (1977), 220–26.

7. "Diet and Longevity in Abkhazia," *American Journal of Nursing,* 75: No. 10 (1975), 1810.

8. FANDETTI. DONALD, and DONALD GELFAND, "Care of the Aged: Attitudes of White Ethnic Families," *The Gerontologist,* 16: No. 6 (1976), 544–49.

9. HAVIGHURST, ROBERT, "Perspectives on Health Care for the Elderly," *Journal of Gerontological Nursing,* 3: No. 2 (1977), 21–24.

10. HICKEY, TOM, W. RAKOWSKI, D. HULTSCH, and B. FATULA, "Attitudes Toward Aging as a Function of In-Service Training and Practitioner Age," *Journal of Gerontology,* 31: No. 6 (1976), 681–86.

11. IVESTER, CONNIE, and KARL KING, "Attitudes of Adolescents Toward the Aged," *The Gerontologist,* 17: No. 1 (1977), 85–89.

12. KAHANE, EVA, J. LIANG, B. FELTON, T. FAIRCHILD, and Z. HAREL, "Perspectives of Aged on Victimization, Ageism, and Their Problems in Urban Society," *The Gerontologist,* 17: No. 2 (1977), 121–29.

13. KAMERMAN, SHEILA, "Community Services for the Aged," *The Gerontologist,* 16: No. 6 (1976), 529–37.

14. KAPLAN, H., and A. POKORNY, "Aging and Self-Attitude: A Conditioned Relationship," *International Journal of Aging and Human Development,* 1: (1970), 241–50.

15. KEITH, PATRICIA, "An Exploratory Study of Sources of Stereotypes of Old Age Among Administrators," *Journal of Gerontology,* 32: No. 4 (1977), 441–50.

16. KIMBROUGH, MARY, "65th Year—No Longer a Sad Magic Marker," *St. Louis Globe-Democrat,* June 19–20, 1976, Sec. J, p. 12.

17. KIMMEL, DOUGLAS, *Adulthood and Aging.* New York: John Wiley & Sons, Inc., 1974.

18. LEAF, ALEXANDER, "Every Day Is a Gift When You Are Over 100," *National Geographic,* 143: No. 1 (1973), 92–119.

19. LOPATA, H., *Polish Americans: Status Competition in an Ethnic Community.* Englewood Cliffs, N. J.: Prentice-Hall, Inc., 1976.

20. McTAVISH, D., "Perceptions of Aging," *The Gerontologist,* 11: (1971), 90–101.

21. MILLER, S., "The Social Dilemma of the Aging Leisure Participant," in *Middle Age and Aging,* ed. Bernice Neugarten. Chicago: The University of Chicago Press, 1968.

22. NEUGARTEN, BERNICE, "Grow Old Along with Me, The Best Is Yet to Be," *Psychology Today,* 5: No. 7 (1971), 45ff.

23. ———, "Patterns of Aging: Past, Present, and Future," *Social Science Review,* 47: (1973), 4.

24. PALMORE, ERDMAN, "Sociological Aspects of Aging," in *Behavior and Adaptation in Later Life,* eds. Ewald Busse and Eric Pfeiffer. Boston: Little, Brown & Company, 1969, 33–69.

25. ———, "Facts on Aging," *The Gerontologist,* 17: No. 4 (1977), 315–20.

26. RANDALL, OLLIE, "Aging in America Today—New Aspects of Aging," *The Gerontologist,* 17: No. 1 (1977), 6–11.

27. ROSE, ARNOLD, "The Subculture of Aging. A Framework for Research in Social Gerontology," in *Older People and Their Social World,* eds. Arnold Rose and Warren Peterson. Philadelphia: F. A. Davis Company, 1965, pp. 3–16.

28. SANDERS, I., and E. MORAWSHA, *Polish-American Community Life: A Survey of Research.* Boston: Boston University Press, 1975.

29. SHARMA, "Cross-Cultural Comparison of Stereotypes Toward Older People," *Indian Journal of Social Work,* 32: No. 3 (1971), 315–20.

30. SHEEHAN, TOM, "Senior Esteem as a Factor of Socioeconomic Complexity," *The Gerontologist,* 16: No. 5 (1976), 433–40.

31. SMITH, MICKEY, "Portrayal of the Elderly in Prescription Drug Advertising," *The Gerontologist,* 16: No. 4 (1976), 329–34.

32. STENBACK, A., M. KUMPULAINEN, and M. VAUHKONEN, "Illness and Health Behavior in Septuagenarians," *Journal of Gerontology,* 33: No. 1 (1978), 57–61.

33. STREIB, GORDON, "Older Families and Their Troubles: Familial and Social Responses," in *Human Life Cycle,* ed. Wm. Sze. New York: Jason Aronson, Inc., 671–90.

34. THOMAS, E., and K. YAMAMOTO, "Attitudes Toward Age: An Exploration in School-Age Children," *International Journal of Aging and Human Development,* 6: (1975), 117–29.

35. THORSON, J., L. WHATLEY, and K. HANCOCK, "Attitudes Toward the Aged as a Function of Age and Education," *The Gerontologist,* 14: (1974), 316–18.

36. THUY, VUONG, *Getting to Know the Vietnamese.* New York: Frederick Ungar Publishing Co., 1976.

37. WARD, RUSSELL, "The Impact of Subjective Age and Stigma on Older Persons," *Journal of Gerontology,* 32: No. 2 (1977), 227–32.

38. WEG, RUTH, "Aging and the Aged in Contemporary Society," *Physical Therapy,* 53: No. 7 (1973), 749–56.

39. Workbook on Health for Participants in Community White House Conferences on Aging. Washington, D.C.: January, 1971.

40. YOUMANS, E. G., "Attitudes: Young-Old and Old-Old," *The Gerontologist,* 17: No. 2 (1977), 175–78.

41. ZINBERG, NORMAN, and IRVING KAUFMAN, *Normal Psychology of the Aging Process.* New York: International Universities Press, Inc., 1963.

CHAPTER APPENDIX: BIBLIOGRAPHY. CARING FOR THE PERSON IN A PLURALISTIC SOCIETY

AICHLMAYR, RITA, "Cultural Understanding: A Key to Acceptance," *Nursing Outlook,* 17: No. 7 (1969), 24–28.

AILINGER, RITA, "A Study of Illness Referral in a Spanish-Speaking Community," *Nursing Research,* 26: No. 1 (1977), 53–56.

American Nurses' Association, *Becoming Aware of Cultural Differences in Nursing.* Kansas City, Mo.: American Nurses Association, 1972.

ANDERSON, GWEN, and BRIDGET TIGHS, "Gypsy Culture and Health Care," *American Journal of Nursing,* 73: No. 2 (1973), 282–85.

BACA, JOSEPHINE, "Some Health Beliefs of the Spanish Speaking," *American Journal of Nursing,* 69: No. 10 (1969), 2172–76.

BECHER, MARSHALL, *et al.,* "A New Approach to Explaining Sick-Role Behavior in Low-Income Populations," *American Journal of Public Health,* 64: No. 3 (1974), 205–15.

BOUWS, BETH, "Working with Albanian Families," *American Journal of Nursing,* 74: No. 5 (1974), 902–5.

BRANCH, MARIE, and PHYLLIS PAXTON, *Providing Safe Nursing Care for Ethnic People of Color.* New York: Appleton-Century-Crofts, 1976.

BRAXTON, EARL, "Structuring the Black Family for Survival and Growth," *Perspectives of Psychiatric Care,* 14: No. 2 (1976), 165–73.

BRINK, PAMELA, ed., *Transcultural Nursing.* Englewood Cliffs, N. J.: Prentice-Hall, Inc., 1976.

BRENTON, D., "Health Center Milieu: Interaction of Nurses and Low-Income Families—Value Differences Between Nursing and Low-Income Families," *Nursing Research,* 21: No. 1 (1972), 46–52.

BROWN, ESTHER L., *Newer Dimensions of Patient Care, Part III: Patients as People.* New York: Russell Sage Foundation, 1964.

BRUHN, JOHN G., *et al.,* "Social Aspects of Coronary Heart Disease in a Pennsylvania German Community," *Social Science and Medicine,* 2: (June, 1968), 201–13.

BULLOUGH, BONNIE, and VERN BULLOUGH, *Poverty, Ethnic Identity and Health Care.* New York: Appleton-Century-Crofts, 1972.

BURNETT, IMODALE, and GARY WALSH, "Caring for Single Room Occupancy Tenants," *American Journal of Nursing,* 73: No. 10 (1973), 1752–56.

CAMPBELL, T., and B. CHANG, "Health Care of the Chinese in America," *Nursing Outlook,* 21: No. 4 (1973), 245–49.

CASSEL, JOHN, "An Epidemiological Perspective of Psychosocial Factors in Disease Etiology," *American Journal of Public Health,* 64: No. 11 (1974), 1040–43.

DAVITZ, LOIS, Y. SAMESHIMA, and J. DAVITZ, "Suffering as Viewed in Six Different Cultures," *American Journal of Nursing,* 76: No. 8 (1976), 1296–97.

DI ANGI, PAULETTE, "Barriers to the Black and White Therapeutic Relationship," *Perspectives of Psychiatric Care,* 14: No. 4 (1976), 180–84.

Ethnicity and Health Care. New York: National League for Nursing, 1976.

GLENN, MAX, *Appalachia in Transition.* St. Louis: Bethaney Press Co., 1970.

GLITTENBERG, JOANN, "Adapting Health Care to a Cultural Setting," *American Journal of Nursing,* 74: No. 12 (1974), 2218–21.

GREELY, ANDREW M., *Ethnicity in the United States: A Preliminary Reconnaissance.* New York: Wiley-Interscience, 1974.

GREER, COLLIER, ed., *Divided Society: The Ethnic Experience in America.* New York: Basic Books, Inc., Publishers, 1974.

GREGG, ELINOR D., *The Indians and the Nurse.* Norman: University of Oklahoma Press, 1965.

GRIER, MARGARET, "Hair Care for the Black Patient," *American Journal of Nursing,* 76: No. 11 (1976), 1781.

HARDY, MARY, and MARGARET BURKHARDT, "Nursing the Navajos," *American Journal of Nursing,* 77: No. 1 (1977), 95–96.

HONGLADAROW, GAIL, and MILLIE RUSSELL, "An Ethnic Difference—Lactose Intolerance," *Nursing Outlook,* 24: No. 12 (1976), 764–65.

HOWARD, ALAN, *Ain't No Big Thing: Coping Strategies in a Hawaiian-American Community.* Honolulu: The University Press of Hawaii, 1974.

HYMOVICH, DEBRA, and MARTHA BERNARD, *Family Health Care.* New York: McGraw-Hill Book Company, 1973.

IRELAN, LOLA, ed., *Low-Income Life Styles.* Washington, D. C.: U. S. Department of Health, Education, and Welfare, 1966.

"Issues on Poverty and Health Care," *Nursing Outlook,* 17: No 9 (1969), 33–75.

JACO, E. GARTLEY, *Patients, Physicians, and Illness,* 2nd ed. New York: The Free Press, 1972.

JANZEN, SHARON, "Psychiatric Day Care in a Rural Area," *American Journal of Nursing,* 74: No. 12 (1974), 2216–17.

JOYCE, SR. CAROL ANNE, and BARBARA, LYSO, "People Who Need People," *Nursing Outlook,* 19: No. 7 (1971), 470–72.

KADUSHIN, CHARLES, "Social Class and the Experience of Ill Health," *Sociological Inquiry*, 34: (Winter, 1964), 67–80.

KEGLES, S. STEPHEN, "A Field Experimental Attempt to Change Beliefs and Behavior of Women in an Urban Ghetto," *Journal of Health and Social Behavior*, 10: (1969), 115–24.

KLUCKHORN, FLORENCE, "Family Diagnosis: Variations in Basic Values of Family Systems," *Social Casework*, 32: (February-March, 1958), 63–72.

LAFARGUE, J., "Role of Prejudice in Rejection of Health Care," *Nursing Research*, 21: No. 1 (1972), 53–58.

LEININGER, MADELINE, *Nursing and Anthropology: Two Worlds to Blend.* New York: John Wiley & Sons, Inc., 1970.

LEONARD, SISTER M., and SR. CAROL JOYCE, "Two Worlds United," *American Journal of Nursing*, 71: No. 6 (1971), 1152–55.

LIEBERMAN, HARRY M., and RODNEY M. POWELL, "Health Services for the Poor," *Public Health Reports*, 85: No. 4 (1970), 284–94.

MCCABE, GRACIA, "Cultural Influences on Patient Behavior," *American Journal of Nursing*, 60: No. 8 (1960), 1101–4.

MCGREGOR, FRANCES, "Uncooperative Patients: Some Cultural Interpretations," *American Journal of Nursing*, 67: No. 1 (1967), 88–91.

MCKENZIE, JOAN, and NOEL CHRISMAN, "Healing Herbs, Gods, and Magic: Folk Health Beliefs Among Filopino-Americans," *Nursing Outlook*, 26: No. 5 (1977), 326–29.

MUECKE, MARJORIE, "Overcoming the Language Barrier," *Nursing Outlook*, 22: No. 4 (1970), 53–54.

MURILLE-ROHDE, ILDAURA, "Family Life Among Mainland Puerto Ricans in New York City Slums," *Perspectives of Psychiatric Care*, 14: No. 4 (1976), 174–79.

NAIL, FRANK and JOSEPH SPELLBERG, "Social and Cultural Factors in the Responses of Mexican-Americans to Medical Treatment," *Journal of Health and Social Behavior*, 8: (1967), 299–308.

NAIMANN, H., "Nursing in Jewish Law," *American Journal of Nursing*, 70: No. 11 (1970), 2378–79.

PARKER, S., and R. J. KLEINER, "The Culture of Poverty: An Adjustive Dimension," *American Anthropologist*, 72: (1970), 516–27.

PAYNICH, MARY, "Cultural Barriers to Nurse Communication," *American Journal of Nursing*, 64: No. 2 (1964), 87–90.

PHOTODIAS, JOHN D., and HARRY SCHWARZWELLER, *Change in Rural Appalachia.* Philadelphia: University of Pennsylvania Press, 1970.

PRIMEAUX, MARTHA, "Caring for the American Indian Patient," *American Journal of Nursing*, 77: No. 1 (1977), 91–94.

RAINWATER, LEE, "The Lower Class: Health, Illness, and Medical Institutions," in *Among the People: Encounters with the Poor*, eds. Irwin Deutscher and Elizabeth J. Thompson. New York: Basic Books, Inc., 1968.

ROSE, PETER I., ed., *Nation of Nations: The Ethnic Experience and the Racial Crisis.* New York: Random House, Inc., 1972.

SABSHIN, M., H. DISSENHAUS, and R. WILKERSON, "Dimensions of Institutional Racism in Psychiatry," *American Journal of Psychiatry*, 27: No. 6 (1970), 787–93.

SACHMAN, E. A., "Sociomedical Variations Among Ethnic Groups," *American Journal of Sociology,* 76: (1970), 319–31.

SCHULMAN, SAM, and ANNE SMITH, "The Concept of 'Health' Among Spanish-Speaking Villages of New Mexico and Colorado," *Journal of Health and Human Behavior,* 4: (1963), 226–35.

STANDEVAN, M., "What the Poor Dislike About Community Health Nurses," *Nursing Outlook,* 17: No. 9 (1969), 72–75.

SYME, S. LEONARD, et al., "Social Class and Racial Differences in Blood Pressure," *American Journal of Public Health,* 64: No. 6 (1974), 619–20.

"Syndrome of Poverty," *American Journal of Nursing,* 66: No. 8 (1966), 1750–62.

WALLACE, LOUELLA, "Patient Is an American Indian," *Supervisor Nurse,* 8: No. 5 (1977), 32–33.

WEISS, O., "Cultural Shock," *Nursing Outlook,* 19: No. 1 (1971), 40–43.

WELLER, JACK E., *Yesterday's People: Life in Contemporary Appalachia.* Lexington: University of Kentucky Press, 1965.

WESTWICK, J., "On the Road in Alaska," *American Journal of Nursing,* 74: No. 9 (1974), 1674–75.

WHITE, ERNESTINE, "Health and the Black Person: An Annotated Bibliography," *American Journal of Nursing,* 74: No. 10 (1974), 1839–41.

WIGGINTON, ELIOT, *The Foxfire Book.* Garden City, N.Y.: Doubleday & Co., Inc., 1972.

ZBOROWSKI, MARK, "Cultural Components in Response to Pain," *Journal of Social Issues,* 8: (Fall, 1952), 16–30.

————, and ELIZABETH HERZOG, *Life is with People.* New York: International Universities Press, Inc., 1952.

————, *People in Pain.* San Francisco: Jossey-Bass, Inc., Publishers, 1969.

ZOLA, IRVING KENNETH, "Culture and Symptoms: An Analysis of Patients Presenting Complaints," *American Sociological Review,* 31: (October, 1966), 615–31.

social stresses and their management in later maturity

Study of this chapter will enable you to:

1. Consider the rights and needs of the elderly person from his perspective.

2. Discuss how social stresses affect obtaining of rights, meeting of needs, and the health status of the senior.

3. Explore the crisis of retirement and advantages and disadvantages of mandatory retirement.

4. Describe factors that influence reaction to retirement and how the senior may be helped to adjust to retirement.

5. Explore community resources that can give financial assistance to the senior.

6. Discuss ways to stretch the budget with a person who is on a limited income.

7. Determine the kinds of housing arrangements that are available to the elderly.

8. Assess the senior's home environment and plan for suitable housing, considering his preferences for comfort, safety, and convenience.

9. Analyze the leisure activities available to the senior in your community and their accessibility to the elderly.

10. Discuss factors that influence the senior's ability to pursue leisure or recreational activities.

11. Work with an elderly person to help him better enjoy his leisure time and to engage in enjoyable activities.

12. Explore your responsibilities as a professional and as a citizen to reduce social stresses for the senior by working with him individually.

6

Late life becomes more stressful for many citizens because of the sociocultural influences, changes, and stereotypes discussed in Chapter 5. In addition to the negative status associated with being old, other negative statuses may also be present: being poor, a member of a minority group, or a woman. All of these are complicated by illness.

The American dream is to retire comfortably, to enjoy late life, and to feel secure. Too often after 45 or more years of hard work the dream is shattered.

A Harris Poll on Attitudes Toward Aging and the Elderly indicated that Americans think that (1) no one should be forced to retire as long as he is able to work, (2) government funds should help support older people, (3) Social Security payments should be increased as the cost of living increases. Increasingly, the public apparently feels ambivalent instead of negative about old age. The public generally respects old people, wants late life to be a conflict-free time, and is worried about the problems related to old age.[27] Middle-agers, and even young adults, are concerned that today's stressful situation for the elderly may not be corrected by the time they reach late life.

Even the emotionally mature, flexible senior will feel the pinch of social stresses discussed in this chapter. Coping abilities depend to a great extent on the inner resources of the person, but the lack of adequate income or external resources and various social stressors can cause him to feel less than satisfied with life.[18]

It is hoped that this chapter will sharpen your awareness of the day-to-day problems that exist for a large number of our population in later maturity. Then you can consider these stressors as you give health care.

BASIC REQUIREMENTS FOR LIFE

Basic Rights

The White House Conferences on Aging in 1961 and 1971 reaffirmed that the person in later maturity has certain basic rights. These rights include to:

1. Have basic necessities, such as food and decent housing.
2. Feel useful and respected.
3. Have adequate medical care.
4. Obtain employment based on merit.
5. Share in the community's recreational and educational resources.
6. Have moral and financial support from the family or community.
7. Have access to knowledge on how to improve later life and the resources which enable improvement.
8. Live independently as possible, depending on health status.
9. Live and die with dignity.[37]

Often the elderly cannot secure these basic rights, regardless of past planning or the emotional or spiritual resources they may have. Unless the senior is aging-group-conscious and is successfully involved in the subculture of the aged, current misfortunes and trends in the social system may work together to cause him to live precariously. When these rights are not achieved to some degree, stress is experienced.

Basic Needs

What the senior needs is often perceived differently by health workers, lawmakers, clergy, and the seniors themselves. In one study the elderly ranked their ten greatest needs as follows:

1. Transportation.
2. Legal services.
3. Visitation program to homes, hospitals, and nursing and retirement homes.
4. Program of reassurance by regularly scheduled telephone calls.
5. Meal services such as group meals or home-delivered meals.
6. Assistance in finding housing.
7. Handyman services.
8. Homemaker or home-health-aid services.
9. Visiting nurse services.
10. Information and referral services.[33]

Interestingly, public health nurses in this study also listed the same two top priorities and six out of the ten needs.[33]

The elderly value services that help them stay independent, remain in contact with others, and meet the needs of daily living. The general public is often concerned with the elderly's having some form of institutional living, recreation centers, and community and interpersonal involvement outside the home. The nurses in this study reflected the current gerontological theories; they gave higher priority to social and recreation centers, church relationships, employment services, and education.[33] Clearly, the elderly may perceive their needs differently and must be involved in planning for ways to provide for their felt needs.

A cross-national survey of eight industrialized countries* identified the following services as significant for older people in need of help: (1) income maintenance, (2) health services, (3) housing, (4) socialization, (5) education, (6) employment, (7) counseling, and (8) access to other services. All countries identified the first three as primary categories of need.[32]

---

*The countries surveyed were Canada, Federal Republic of Germany, France, Israel, Poland, United Kingdom, United States, and Yugoslavia.

England has been the international leader in promoting a comprehensive national aging policy that is designed to keep the elderly in the home as long as possible. All of these countries are now learning that the senior prefers to live in his own home and that home-based care is less expensive than institutional care. These countries also have some form of economic assistance and insurance benefits; only the United States and Israel do not supplement financial benefits with comprehensive health insurance.[32]

In a study of over 900 seniors in Canada the main problems were loneliness and the lack of transportation and home maintenance programs. Many seniors could remain in their homes if help were given with periodic house cleaning, odd jobs, grocery shopping, or transportation to medical care. Because of loneliness and lack of transportation, the elderly were less likely to respond to encouragement to make their own arrangements for social contact. Basic to all of these problems were the meager monthly income and inflation.[55]

The major social stresses on most elderly can be divided into the following categories: (1) mandatory retirement and postretirement roles, (2) income changes and securing essentials to live, especially food, (3) housing, and (4) transportation. Other concerns include safety, obtaining health care, consumer protection, use of leisure time, opportunities for educational and social pursuits, and legal aid.[37] Securing necessary health care and legal aid for the elderly will be discussed in Chapters 7 and 8.

The priority of stresses differ for people in various geographic areas. In urban areas, the advantages of activities, programs, and presence of other people exist, but the senior may still be isolated and alone. Disadvantages of living in an urban area include vulnerability to crime and physical injury. In rural areas the environment tends to be safer, but there are the problems of transportation, housing maintenance, lack of nearby medical care, absence of activities for seniors, and physical and social isolation.

MANDATORY RETIREMENT

When the Social Security Act of 1935 was passed by Congress, the age of 65 was arbitrarily set to determine old age and eligibility for economic benefits. Congress did not poll elderly people to determine if they were ready for retirement, but many elderly people had been working for 50 or more years. They were worn down by hard labor and harsh life situations. The Great Depression had adversely affected the elderly. The age of 65 seemed old. Further, retirement age did not affect all people.[63]

Over the years a fixed retirement age assisted business and insurance companies in planning for worker benefits, forced personal preparation for retirement, and assured increasing numbers of young adults of potential jobs and job advancement.[6]

Today, many 65-year-olds prefer to remain at work but cannot. Often the person could continue to work longer if allowed, since in some jobs, such as secretarial, little change in work output or performance is needed. Retirement may come earlier if work skills become obsolete, and in certain positions retirement is possible after 20 or 30 years of service. If the person is self-employed, he often chooses not to retire at age 65.[63]

Legislation to prohibit mandatory retirement for some categories of workers before age 70 has been passed. In the future the retirement age may even be 75 years instead of 65 in order for society to benefit from the seniors' productivity.[10,63]

The Crisis of Retirement

Retirement is a crisis because it is a major turning point in adult development, marking the shift from middle age and work to old age and sometimes unwanted leisure. It is a crisis because it threatens feelings of identity, integrity, and self-esteem. For most people, loss of work means loss or reduction of income, influence, authority, status, social relationships, professional skills, creativity, activity, and control over the environment.[6,18] All of this, combined with aging physical changes, causes the person to feel less like the same person. He mourns because of these changes. Other areas of life, including the emotional and sexual relationship with the spouse, may be affected by the mourning and crisis resolution.

Retirement may be less of a crisis for the woman. She has been constantly undergoing role modifications and crises as she entered different life stages.[24] The woman has had to remain flexible. She has worked through the meaning of productivity in relation to childrearing and children leaving home, especially if she has combined career and homemaking. Further, she is more likely to be able to keep busy with household tasks after retirement and to begin new friendships.[25,31,39]

Retirement has three aspects: (1) it is an event, (2) it denotes a status, and (3) it involves a process.[57] Retirement is an event, like a *rite de passage,* with the banquet and token of appreciation on the last work day being inadequate for the economic and life-style implications. Usually, preparation for retirement has also been inadequate, especially since this period of life is gradually becoming longer as life expectancy increases.

Retirement denotes a status, a new social position with new roles, expectations, and responsibilities. The roles and responsibility decrease; the standard of living gradually declines or at least is tightened; expectations must be changed. As the number of retired persons continues to rise and the amount of time spent in retirement lengthens, it is likely that the retired status may become more positive and evolve a more rewarding set of activities. As our society places more value on leisure, and as more retired people provide meaningful community service, the social position of retired persons is likely to rise.[57]

Retirement involves a process of anticipating new status and of consciously and unconsciously working through conflicts and resocialization involved in the status change. The biological, social, and emotional changes simultaneously occuring affect the person's reaction to and resolution of retirement.[57]

Factors Influencing Reaction to Retirement

Retirement does not affect everyone the same way. Several variables contribute to adjustment.[20]

Accumulated savings and pensions may enable the senior to pursue desired activities that promote adjustment to retirement. Lack of economic security means permanent impoverishment. Most retirees, even those who have some economic stability, view retirement as a time to be cautious about spending.

Lifelong attitudes about work are crucial. The senior was raised in a society with an almost religious devotion to work. The self-concept and sense of worth may be tied to the job. Leisure activities may have little meaning. Retirement may mean isolation from the valuable, productive mainstream of life and being passive, weak, and disorganized.[40] The retired person may be referred to as someone *who was* instead of someone *who is*. Statements like this threaten identity.[62] If work was an unpleasant burden and meant little more than a paycheck, then retirement may be anticipated.[40]

The person who has difficulty accepting himself, his life status, and accomplishments; who is obsessively tied to work to structure his life; who has a rigid, angry, self-depreciating personality; and who has failed to develop hobbies, interests, or friends will have difficulty organizing the retirement years and will feel a sense of loss. Further, he now has time to think. He can no longer use activities as a means of keeping conflicts under control. The person who is mature and has high self-esteem and high life satisfaction will maintain such feelings.[40]

Preretirement planning—financially, emotionally, and socially—and gradually tapering off from full-time to part-time work promote a better adjustment than abruptly ending work and the associated life-style. The gradual move into retirement also helps the person look upon retirement as a change to a new status instead of losing a prized status. Now he has time to make new social contracts and develop new interests. The person's attitude before retirement is crucial for satisfaction, or lack of it, after retirement. If he feels that retirement is the final step in a progressive, sequential career in which there is a sense of fulfillment and completion, retirement is less traumatic than if it occurs after a disruptive pattern.[9,21,50,52]

Ill health, which may have forced retirement, often causes ambivalence. The person gains time to take care of himself but he loses the advantages of a job and higher income. Health insurance benefits may no longer be available when they are needed. Ill health is an additional financial drain and limits the enjoyment of leisure activities.

The person who has a lower level of education, a lower economic status, and little organizational association has more difficulty adjusting to retirement. Higher socioeconomic status and education enable the person to come to retirement with relatively superior community involvement, interpersonal competence, and financial resources. The more social and personal resources available to the retiree, the more options he can choose from to develop a satisfying life-style that facilitates higher morale in retirement.

Relationship to spouse and ability to rework the shared living affect happiness after retirement. The older woman often becomes dominant and enjoys being the decision-maker and leader in the home after many years of being submissive. After her mate's retirement, she has to adjust to having him home all day. Her household or work schedule is no longer dependent on his work schedule. He may assume some household tasks, which may be viewed as either threatening or helpful. They may do things together more spontaneously. The relationship becomes more intense. They may enjoy each other's company; each may feel constrained by the other's presence, activities, and wishes. Often it takes months to adjust to spending so much time together and to each other's irritating traits.

If the retired couple is responsible for aged parents or relatives, either at home or in an institution, the financial burden and lack of independence can be trying. Getting assistance with care of the aged person is difficult; the alternative is to have no time for themselves while they are still able to do things together. Their limited income may also force them to swallow their pride and accept help from welfare agencies.

Realization of the rewards and compensations of retirement can aid adjustment. The person is freed from routine; he is no longer governed by the clock. There is time to putter around without purpose (which can also be difficult to adjust to). The person is no longer inhibited by the boss or the company from saying what he thinks. New learning adventures or community services can be entered because there is time for them.

In one study little evidence of a wide range of negative consequences of retirement was seen. Instead, retired persons seemed to adapt to the changed role requirements and to tolerate the related negative aspects in much the same way that they adapted to earlier changes.

The person who led an active, meaningful life continues his life-style into retirement. If life was disordered and had little central meaning, retirement is likely to be unsatisfying and dehumanizing.[17,19,25,31,37,57,62]

Post-Retirement Work and Service Roles

Evidence shows that satisfied retirees are more rather than less active in post-retirement, especially in volunteer work, leisure activities, and social interaction with friends and relatives, thus refuting Disengagement Theory.[5] Because work provides considerable meaning in life, some seniors will continue to work part-time after retirement. Extra income and feeling needed and competent are achieved.

The senior is usually an effective worker and worth hiring in a second career or keeping past retirement age. He does better in a job that requires judgment, experience, and quality of performance instead of speed. Although the senior does not work as fast, he gets as much done in a week as a younger person who works rapidly but does not sustain the pace. He makes fewer mistakes and spoils less material. Slowing the pace, relying on individual speed instead of external pacing, is adaptive for the physical-chemical-neural changes that occur. He does the task with less wasted motion, which with his caution and slower pace helps him to be a very safe worker; he is less likely to sustain injury on the job. He is less likely to be preoccupied with personal life problems as the younger worker, and he is less likely to be dissatisfied or want to change jobs. He is dependable and is absent less because of his desire to keep the job he has. Disabling injury and illness and accident proneness are less frequent than commonly thought and less frequent among older than younger workers. Most older workers get along as well with fellow workers as do young ones.[3,13,31]

Older persons can work as school-crossing guards, meter patrolmen, babysitters, receptionists, secretaries, sales personnel, consultants, caterers, watchmen, or tutors.

The American Association of Retired Persons (AARP) has established an employment service called Mature Temps for members who wish to work on a part-time basis.[2] Information can be obtained by writing Mature Temps at 521 Fifth Avenue, New York, N.Y. 10017.

The Foster Grandparents Program, which is federally funded, takes a number of seniors off the welfare rolls and provides a much needed service. The elderly share their patience, love, and concern with children in hospitals, centers for the retarded or disabled, and in day-care centers.

A group of retired business executives in New York City, called Executive Volunteer Corps, provide business advice to younger persons in business.[34] A similar group is the Service Corp of Retired Executives who volunteer to help small businesses and community organizations with management problems.

Other retirees may prefer to become involved in volunteer work through a church, community center, day-care center for children or senior citizens, hospital or clinic, sick or residential child's center, nursing home, or VISTA (Volunteer in Service to America). The experiences and wisdom gained through a lifetime can be shared with others while the senior remains alert and healthy through contact with others. Women are more likely than men to volunteer, partly because they are accustomed to this type of work and are more willing to be unpaid.

For some people, participation in a senior citizen center or in leisure activities, such as bingo or card games, is adequate. Even then variety and emotional involvement with others are likely to be desired to some extent.

The retiree may also become active in a local or state political organization or assist in teaching crafts or other noncredit adult or child education courses. The senior may be a skilled craftsman, a competent first-aider, or an artist, musician, golfer, or gourmet cook who is willing to teach others formally or informally. He can serve as a teacher's aid, assisting students and the teacher in the classroom.

The retiree may join fraternal organizations or specialized clubs for nature study, birdwatching, stamp or coin collecting, gardening, photography, travel, or bridge. Such clubs meet emotional, social, and cognitive needs.

The retiree may return to academic or noncredit courses to gain knowledge or skill in a certain discipline, either for personal growth reasons or in turn to engage in volunteer or paid service. The American Association of Retired Persons conducts an Institute of Lifetime Learning and offers home study courses to members.[2]

INCOME ADJUSTMENT AND BUDGET BALANCING

Income is the most basic concern of persons in later maturity in the United States. After retirement, little income may be available except for savings, Social Security, and pensions, unless the person has a part-time job or receives gifts of money from family or friends. Inflation makes their few dollars worth less. The cost of all services continues to rise. Social Security was never intended to be the sole income, and in the past many workers were ineligible for participation, such as farm, domestic, or certain self-employed workers. As a result, some elderly live in poverty.

Some persons have expressed that they feel guilty receiving Social Security, even though they know that they have contributed to the fund. Because the check comes from Washington, D.C., they feel that it is welfare. However, most people perceive the monthly Social Security check as if it were the monthly wage.

The aged who receive an income below poverty level may apply for Supplemental Security Income (SSI) at the local Social Security Administration office. But many of the aged have too much pride to do so. Further, lack of information, bureaucratic complexity, and desire for privacy hinder the full use of existing benefits.

Inadequate income has repercussions for everything the elderly wants or needs and is at the core of the social problems that confront the person. Inadequate income affects availability and maintenance of housing; health care; transportation to shopping areas that offer lower prices; and pursuit of cultural and recreational interests. Consumer fraud, exposure to crime, and lack of knowledge or availability of a variety of services are indirectly and directly related to low income.

Economically, the elderly must be very adaptive to be able to stretch the limited income. Unless the person is in an upper-income bracket, housing takes about one-third of the monthly income, either in rent or in taxes and maintenance on the self-owned home. Food is the next highest budget expenditure if adequate nutrition is maintained.[37] Often the person deliberately eats less because of inadequate funds. Yet often the senior will indulge in one food that is special to him and that symbolizes a luxury, such as beer, wine, a special kind of cheese or bread, ice cream, or snack foods. Having enough of his favorite food means that he feels less deprived and is able to tolerate other privations. Medication is also an expensive item if the person is chronically ill or becomes ill. Medications may be taken less frequently than prescribed in order to save money. Often there is little or no money for clothes, grooming aids, recreation, or organizational memberships. Often the car is given up a few years after retirement because of the expense. At first, the senior goes places he can reach by walking, bicycle, or bus. When he becomes homebound, his recreation becomes the newspaper or other reading material, television, radio, and the telephone.

Financial planning for retirement should begin at least 10 to 15 years before retirement so that the person can investigate and use various means to supplement retirement pensions and Social Security. Annuity funds should be started sooner.[45] Various resources are available to help the middle-ager plan for retirement or to help the retiree budget wisely.[44] If the person plans wisely for retirement, the monthly income can sustain a more comfortable living, even if the standard of living is reduced somewhat.

You can encourage the senior to explore all avenues of income and various resources available to him. You can teach him about nutritious foods that are economical. In turn, you can give him the pleasure of teaching you how to stretch the dollar. Also encourage the senior to accept financial benefits which help defray costs of health care. Details about Medicare and Medicaid can be obtained from the local Social Security Administration office. The American Association of Retired Persons has low-cost health care insurance and a drug service available to members. The drug service saves considerable money for the person taking regular prescriptions and it is helpful to the homebound person. The doctor's original prescription is sent to one of five locations in the country, is filled with the generic named drug, and is mailed to the person. No postage is charged; the person is billed at a price lower than most local pharmacies charge. Nonprescription drugs can be purchased from a catalog. If the person has the AARP insurance, a partial refund on medication purchase is given at the end of the year.

HOUSING AND LIVING ARRANGEMENTS

Housing is strongly related to income and life-style. A variety of alternate housing arrangements should be available so that senior citizens may have esthetic and economic choices and may live comfortably and independently but not be isolated. Finding a suitable place that can be afforded is not easy.

Current Arrangements

A disproportionate number of elderly reside within the central cities, and considerable age segregation occurs in all metropolitan areas. The trend is for greater age segregation in younger, growing cities and less age segregation in declining cities as the aged are displaced by demolition of deteriorating areas. Age segregation appears to be part of the urbanization process.[35]

Community health nurses often find the urban elderly living in deplorable conditions. Most cities of any size have the bag ladies, elderly women who have no place to live, carry all of their possessions in a large shopping bag, wander in stores or sit in a park by day, and find shelter in a cheap, rundown hotel or abandoned building at night. Other elderly, called rag ladies and men, spend their days rummaging for discarded papers and rags which they collect and store in abandoned buildings. Although the accumulated material is a fire and pest hazard, they use it as insulation and covering to keep warm in cold weather. (Such collecting may also serve the need to keep busy or to fulfill various emotional needs.) The lack of housing for these people is compounded by other problems: inadequate food; various health problems; rats, roaches, and other vermin biting or causing disease; lack of sanitation and hygiene; exposure to violence because they are easy targets; and lack of anyone who cares. These elderly persons are no better off than the hobos who once roamed the countryside getting food handouts from farm women and sleeping in haylofts. In fact, the hobo's existence may have been more secure.

Other elderly rent lodging, but the place may be structurally unsound, dirty, overcrowded, and generally unpleasant. There may be no hot or running water or indoor plumbing, even in urban areas. A hotplate may be the only thing available for cooking. Sometimes the person lives in a small apartment. In many cities numerous elderly are classified as SRO's (single-room-only tenants) who rent a room in a rundown, inner-city hotel until they are forced to move because the building is to be demolished. Typically, the rent is too high for the accommodations and landlord services are negligible. These people may prefer to stay downtown, but they need decent living quarters and support services. Either the local or federal government needs to be responsible for designing and building alternative housing. Because community nurses commonly encounter such clients, they can work with other community leaders to upgrade existing hotels, build new facilities if needed, and provide the necessary social, health, and welfare services.

147

Public housing projects may offer the senior adequately constructed housing for low rent, but location, noise, and fear of crime may be deterrents to living there. In some cities managers of low-rent, high-rise apartments have the tenants actively involved in providing self-government, maintenance, security, ambulatory health care, and peer activities, so that the apartment houses become inviting places to live for a sector of the elderly population. The elderly tenants can also band together to provide a look-out service for each other to compensate for their slower pace and physical inability to escape or resist attackers; thus, they avoid becoming the victims of crime.

If the senior owns his own home, he may live in an older, rundown section of the city or on an isolated homestead. Sometimes retired couples want to continue living where they made their homes through the years, especially if neighbors and the environment have remained relatively unchanged. They may enjoy the architectural, ethnic, and cultural background of the area. In addition to the cost of taxes and maintenance of house and lawn, the senior becomes physically unable to do maintenance tasks eventually. The couple/person must move, giving up treasured space and possessions in the process. Sometimes the move is forced because the familiar neighborhood is in a deteriorating section of the city where crime is also a problem.

The couple/person may consider moving to a retirement village, often in a warmer climate. Before making such a move, these people ought to visit for a lengthy period in the new area during different times of the year. Other factors in the locale need to be considered before any move: year-round climate; topography; noise and air pollution; general safety; cost of living; housing arrangements; health care facilities; churches; parks; social groups; transportation; shopping areas; grocery delivery; and recreation and work opportunities. Preference for age segregation versus variety of ages in a neighborhood must be considered. The *National Directory of Retirement Residences: Best Places to Live When You Retire,* by N. Musson, published by Frederick Fell, Inc., may assist decision making.

In some instances the widow(er) or couple must move in with their children. The degree of adjustment for all generations involved depends considerably on previously established relationships, amount of space, and amount of activity in the younger family's life-style.

Other living arrangements are also seen. Elderly siblings or two or more seniors who are not married may live together. The senior may choose to live alone in a small apartment near his children rather than in the children's home. If the person is alone and in poor health, he may move into an institutional setting for care and companionship.

Housing Alternatives

For some elderly, an alternative to moving to more compact quarters without giving up personal possessions or a sense of space is to purchase a mobile home. The mobile home may be permanently located on a lot in a mobile home park especially for senior citzens or on a half-acre in the countryside, or it may become the home-on-wheels for the couple who wishes to travel. Mobile homes vary in size, can usually be purchased for less than regular homes, and may come partly or totally furnished or unfurnished.

Increasingly, in urban areas, small villages or high-rise apartments are being built for the elderly which permit age-segregated living without moving to a different geographical area. Often they have inviting names, such as Friendship Village or Park View Towers. The elderly person or couple has his own apartment and possessions. Some of the apartments have kitchen galleys. Or the senior may have just a refrigerator to keep snacks and eat in a central dining room with everyone else. Each apartment has an emergency button so that the resident feels more secure in getting help in case of illness or injury. Many have a special health care facility as part of the building; others have a nurse, nutritionist, and podiatrist who come at regular intervals to do assessment, primary care, and teaching. Often a social director arranges a variety of activities for the residents, and provisions are made for self-initiated activities such as crafts, woodworking, billiards, reading, or swimming. Sometimes a garden area is provided; residents can plant flowers or vegetables in a small plot. A small balcony adds to the feeling of space. Maid and laundry service may be available for an extra charge. Transportation to various shopping centers and cultural, civic, and sporting events is usually provided, often at no extra charge. The cost for such a living arrangement varies with the location, sponsorship, type of facility, and number of services offered. Such living arrangements provide for privacy, security of a 24-hour watchman, convenience of no maintenance work, enjoyment of activities, and companionship of peers. In such a setting, aging-group-consciousness is enhanced, and a subculture forms.

In England smaller homes for 25 to 40 people are built. Family groups of eight persons are accommodated in one apartment or cottage. Each resident has the use of a kitchenette, pavilion or porch, sitting area, and storage. The bathrooms have shower cubicles with hand-operated sprays, slatted seats, and grab rails. Showers are preferred to a tub because the elderly can use them more independently and with less hazard. Long corridors are avoided because the residence is built on the cottage plan, and residents are not under the constant surveillance of the health care staff who are on the premises.[41] Such a model would be useful for the United States.

Ideally, the elderly are involved in planning for their living arrangements. Hartman *et al.* describe how residents in an inner city—the commercial, low-rent, and hotel area—were organized when the Redevelopment Agency of San Francisco wanted the land in the central district. The ideas of the elderly were solicited through many meetings and many of the ideas were used in relocation plans.[26]

The residents gave the following guidelines to architects to decrease the sense of vulnerability:

1. Develop a street area into a mini-neighborhood for the elderly and leave an active pedestrian way.
2. Build modern looking structures that are cleaner, more prestigious looking and comfortable than the old hotels, which reflected negatively on the status of the residents.
3. Include a commercial establishment on the ground floor, such as a cooperative neighborhood food store staffed by resident volunteers, but exclude bars, massage parlors, and liquor stores in order to keep out undesirable outsiders.
4. Build a safe street entry that provides quick entry instead of an esthetic courtyard where a mugger could hide.
5. Design the lobby so that the elderly do not have to run a gauntlet of people and so that unruly or inebriated tenants or outsiders cannot loiter.
6. Place mailboxes in the lobby instead of by apartment doors for security reasons.
7. Include individual apartment balconies to provide a view, exposure to sunlight, a place to grow plants, a sense of space, and a way to get outdoors.
8. Provide wall-to-wall carpeting for soundproofing and prestige; good television reception; and easily-opened entry doors.
9. Provide phone booths for residents who cannot afford private phones.
10. Provide roof areas for sitting, visiting, and sunning.[26]

Other suggestions made by seniors to make housing more comfortable for them include:

1. Temperature should be individually controlled and equal from floor to ceiling because the elderly person frequently feels chilled as a result of lower metabolism and poor circulation.
2. Windows should be large and there should be many conveniently placed electric lights to enhance impaired vision.
3. Storage space should be adequate and conveniently reached. Often shelves and cupboards can be reached by the 6-foot-tall architect, but the senior was not as tall in his adult years as young adults are today, and he has shrunk 2 inches or more in height. Thus, in many housing units built especially for the aged the senior often must climb to reach even frequently used supplies.
4. Floors should be nonskid and level for safety.
5. Adequate wall space uninterrupted by doors or windows allows the older person to keep some of his own furniture, which is often taller and larger than furniture manufactured today.
6. Ramps that slope gently are essential in public areas; stairsteps should be minimum.
7. Handrails along walkways and hallways are an essential safety factor.
8. Outer doorways should provide security from intruders but not be so heavy that older, frail people must use undue effort to open them.

9. Fire protection devices should be in a prominent place and maintained regularly.

In 1968 Congress passed the Architectural Barriers Act which states that buildings that are constructed, rehabilitated, or leased with federal funds, including housing for senior citizens, must meet certain barrier-free criteria. These criteria consider the physical limitations of aging, but hearing loss is seldom considered. Further legislation may be needed. Electronics and telecommunications could be used to send messages when audio messages fail to get a response from the resident in his home. A flashing light could be a fire alarm signal; a blinking light could indicate a ringing telephone. Helping the person stay in control in his environment helps him to maintain a positive self-concept and self-esteem and to remain active at a high level of competence.[18]

Improved living environment does affect the social and psychological well-being, as well as the health status, of the person. In one long-range study comparing seniors who moved to a low-cost, high-rise apartment for the elderly with a sample of similar seniors who did not move, the results showed that those who moved were healthier over a period of years and were better satisfied with life.[11] Apparently coping, in terms of meeting basic needs, was facilitated by the improved living environment and planned housing for late life. Basic physiological processes of eating, sleeping, elimination, and regulation of heat and cold were easier to achieve in a clean, well-built, temperature-regulated apartment that had a well-equipped kitchen, bathroom, laundry room, and a garbage chute. Safety and security needs were met because undesirable outsiders, burglars, and muggers could be kept out; elevators eliminated using dangerous stairways, and groups could unite for activities. Interpersonal needs could be met by contact with compatible people, and the living arrangement was attractive for entertaining friends and relatives. The new environment enhanced self-esteem, and self-actualization needs could be met through the activities at the senior center.[11]

LACK OF TRANSPORTATION

The myth exists that the elderly person is too slow and too impaired to drive an automobile. In our fast-paced society the older driver is considered a nuisance. A study by the University of Denver College of Law indicates that the senior driver averages 40 percent fewer accidents; seniors are the least likely of all age groups who drive to be involved in an accident. The normal caution of the elderly becomes an asset on the road.[23,51]

However, the senior eventually has to sell his car, if he owned one, because of his limited budget. If vision, hearing, and reflexes become impaired, he either realizes that he is no longer a safe driver or he is unable to renew his driver's license. Often younger family members encourage the senior to sell the car because of expense and safety factors. Giving up the automobile is not an easy decision; the car is often a part of self-concept, and it facilitates an independent, more youthful life-style. Giving up the car is yet another signal of old age and incompetence, even if the person is not old and is not incompetent.

Some active seniors solve part of their transportation problem by using bicycles for short shopping trips and other errands. In addition, they benefit from the exercise.

Without available transportation, the elderly person becomes dependent on others for the simplest errands. Often public transportation is lacking, inconvenient, or too expensive. Without adequate transportation, the person cannot shop in distant shopping centers; participate in spiritual, cultural, social, or recreational interests; and cannot seek medical services.

Some housing units for the elderly provide bus service for free or at a low fare for shopping on certain days of the week. Some cities have buses with reduced fare during nonrush hours. This permits the senior to take advantage of community activities and shop at a time when streets are reasonably safe. But bus steps are high and bus rides are jerky. Therefore, many of the elderly find a bus trip an uncomfortable experience, especially if they have packages to hold. Certainly adequate transportation and the removal of physical and spatial barriers are necessary in order to help the elderly retain an active role in the community.

USE OF LEISURE TIME

Leisure is defined as *freedom from obligations, the paid work role, or formal, obvious duties. Leisure is any activity pursued for enjoyment—a state of mind rather than an activity.*[38,49]

Recreation is activity, such as sports, hobbies, or vacation, that renews the mind and body by relieving tension or boredom.[49]

During the busy young and middle years the person may wish for some free time to pursue hobbies or to do nothing. People in the United States today generally have more time away from work than did earlier generations. The work week is shorter and there are paid holidays and vacations. After retirement, when leisure time is available without end, it may be perceived as a stress.

The person approaching 65 is encouraged to adjust by spending more of his time in leisure activities, and after 65 he is encouraged to spend his leisure time in activities that have special meaning for him. Supposedly, the problems of retirement are then resolved. This view takes little note of associational aspects and social needs and may actually encourage withdrawal. The identity that can be established with leisure is more limited than was the identity established with an occupation. Then, too, leisure is not highly valued in our society and was even less so when the older person was growing up. That which is not valued is not pursued happily for very long. Enforced leisure may contribute to feelings of worthlessness, apathy, anger, and depression.[43,51]

The person in later maturity tends to remain interested in the activities he previously enjoyed if he can physically do them and if he can afford them. In one study most retirees pursued activities alone rather than in a group, a pattern that had begun preretirement.[49] Isolate-type activities are not necessarily the result of retirement.[38,49] Often the elderly remains very active physically into the seventies or eighties—golfing, hiking, swimming, gardening, doing calisthenics, jogging—if he has always been active.

Participating in systematized leisure activity, such as birdwatching, photography, stamp or coin collecting, genealogy study, or woodworking, accomplishes several purposes, which include (1) entering the aged subculture, (2) maintaining reality contact, (3) participating with others who have similar interests, and (4) meeting social, emotional, cognitive, and physical needs. Some hobbies also provide a source of income, even if it is a limited one.[43,51]

Various factors cause the senior to change his pursuit of recreational activities, for example:

1. Declining health, strength, energy, endurance, sensory, and cognitive abilities.
2. Reduced income after retirement so that he cannot afford the cost of membership, transportation, the event itself, or appropriate clothing.
3. Living arrangement, whether he is in a residence for seniors that provides recreational activities or lives alone.
4. Extent to which past activities related to his occupation; occupation-oriented activities are less likely to be continued.[18,31,37,38,49]

In old-old age sedentary and mental forms of recreation are preferred. Television, radio, reading, playing cards or bingo, visiting with others, attending church, or just sitting and rocking are preferred when the person is physically unable to be as active, to travel, or to attend cultural or civic events. If the person is mentally alert, he tends to develop an enjoyable pattern of leisure regardless of health, income, or other restrictions.[49]

Residents of senior housing or members of senior groups usually are more active in pursuing many interests and social events than are seniors who live in isolated housing because the activities and social events are available and the seniors do not have to be concerned about transportation, cost, and safety. Nevertheless, the senior may tire of the planned, structured recreation and prefer solitary activities. Retirees who participate in favorite activities have a higher life-satisfaction score and a more positive self-concept.

Watching television is a popular leisure time activity for many elderly persons (in spite of the youth-oriented programs) because of less physical energy, their sedentary life-style and free time. Further, television is free entertainment once the set is paid for. It provides contact with the outside world almost 24 hours a day; it helps to distract from life's problems and boredom, and it helps to impose some structure to a structureless life through a rigid time schedule of programs.[43]

Most seniors need help to adjust to a schedule that is not constrained by full-time employment, to resolve feelings related to use of leisure, and to settle into a schedule that is neither too empty nor too full. Sometimes the elderly are exploited by family, organizations, or even the church after retirement; others may feel that the person wants and needs to stay busy. Sometimes the person is kept so busy that he has no rest and no free time. Helping the person continue or find an activity suited to his interests and situation is useful for his physical and emotional health.

CONSUMER PROTECTION

In spite of legislation, the work of the Better Business Bureau, and federal, state, and local consumer advocate groups, the senior is often a victim of fraud. A wide range of important services can be presented in a confusing or seductively attractive way. Since the elderly are perceived as not being very alert or well educated, unscrupulous businesses try to solicit door-to-door, by telephone, or by mail. They offer unnecessary or slipshod services and often they play on the fears or incapacities of the elderly.

You can teach the senior about these practices and the importance of identifying and avoiding fraud in banking, budgeting, insurance, retirement or funeral planning, home maintenance, and real estate. Teach them about medical quackery and how to distinguish quack cures or food faddism from reliable medical care, effective public services, and effective health practices.

STRESSES FOR THE MINORITY PERSON IN LATER MATURITY

The elderly person suffers the problems of a minority group in many ways in the United States. The problems are compounded when the person is a member of a minority group.

The minority aged have had more serious problems throughout life. Nearly one-half of the Black elderly are below the poverty level compared with one-fourth of elderly whites. The Native Americans, Asian-Americans, and Spanish-speaking Americans are also more likely to be in poverty than are white Americans.

The average life expectancy for the Black man is 61 years, 7 years less than for the white man. Average life expectancy for the Native American is 46 years and 57 years for the Spanish-speaking American.[37]

The minority person often does not live to collect Social Security, if he even qualifies for it. Because of the kinds of jobs he has held, the check will be smaller if he does receive one. He is often forced to apply for welfare payments and food stamps in order to live.

A lifetime of inadequate nutrition, medical care, and shelter, and a limited choice in life-style compounds the stresses of old age. The person often has difficulty being admitted to a nursing home when family or self-care can no longer be managed. Isolation, language barriers, poor transportation, lack of knowledge of resources, and lack of social services add to the distress. Often family and kinship groups are not utilized as fully for the person's welfare as they could be.[37]

Asian-Americans have been overlooked as a group in need of help because of the stereotype that all aged Orientals are revered and cared for in the extended family. Further, they have too much pride to ask for help or admit that their neighborhoods are eligible for aid.[37]

Bilingual students could be educated to work with the minority elderly. They could staff institutions, mobile clinics, and welfare offices, assist in community programs for the elderly, work with families, and provide health education.

FUTURE DIRECTIONS

The current problems of the elderly in the United States reflect our basic assumptions as a free society. Every person is entitled to freedom of association and expression, privacy, individual choice, dignity, and use of community resources. But many persons in later maturity cannot exercise these rights for various reasons. Many of today's elderly population are:

1. Foreign-born who had difficulty as immigrants in becoming assimilated into our society as participative citizens.
2. Rural in background and transplanted to an urban society without the preparation needed to cope with the fast-changing, twentieth-century technology and bureaucracy.
3. Less well-educated than today's citizens and less aware of how to secure the aid of resources.
4. Ill with health problems related to lack of earlier medical or dental care.
5. Women, since fewer men live past 65 years of age; the elderly woman was socialized in a different historical era to be dependent and submissive and to pursue home and childrearing roles; this has prepared her poorly to cope with today's society, its norms, and its expectations.[60]

All of these factors have compounded the social stresses felt by today's seniors.

It is predicted that future generations in later maturity may be able to better prepare themselves for late life so that they may encounter fewer stresses or may be able to cope more adequately. Further, social advances may reduce the stress for late-life citizens in the future. Thus, they should be able to live their last years in better health and have more income, education, and status than the present generation.[37,47,60]

Use of the nursing process is incomplete unless you apply knowledge about society and its stresses to the client/patient/family you assess and work with. You have a responsibility to work as a professional and a citizen to reduce the social stresses to the extent that basic needs and rights can be met. Further, you can encourage the senior to become active in his own behalf by working with other senior citizens, the appropriate organizations, and legislators. Encourage the elderly to vote; help them get to a polling place or use an absentee ballot. Encourage seniors to visit each other and to share their wisdom with younger generations. Encourage aging-group-consciousness and joining the subculture of aging so that they can feel greater self-esteem and worth. Help the senior plan not only for present needs but for the future as well.

Each of us can begin now to prepare emotionally, spiritually, physically, and financially for late life as well as to continue to improve conditions for today's generation of seniors. Whatever we do for today's senior ensures our future security to a greater degree. Certainly much of what we see around us we would not want to experience. Further, our own preparation may help us to better cope with different and unknown future stresses.

REFERENCES

1. Administration on Aging, *HEW Fact Sheet,* N (OHO) 77-20229, December, 1976.

2. American Association of Retired Persons, "Here Is the Most Positive and Realistic Approach to Growing Older You Have Ever Heard About," Washington, D.C.: American Association of Retired Persons Directory, n.d.

3. ANDERSON, J., "The Use of Time and Energy," in *Handbook of Aging and the Individual,* ed. J. Birren. Chicago: The University of Chicago Press, 1959, pp. 769–96.

4. ANTUNES, GEORGE, *et al.,* "Patterns of Personal Crimes Against the Elderly," *The Gerontologist,* 17: No. 4 (1977), 321–27.

5. BARFIELD, R., and J. MORGAN, "Trends in Satisfaction with Retirement," *The Gerontologist,* 18: No. 1 (1978), 19–23.

6. BISCHOFF, LEDFORD, *Adult Psychology.* New York: Harper & Row Publishers, Inc., 1969.

7. BRADSHAW, B., *et. al.,* "Community-Based Residential Care for the Minimally Impaired Elderly: A Survey Analysis," *Journal of the American Geriatric Society,* 24: No. 9 (1976), 423–29.

8. BROTMAN, HERMAN, "Income and Poverty in the Older Population in 1975," *The Gerontologist,* 17: No. 1 (1977), 23–26.

9. BUCK, K., "The Ambiguity of Retirement," *Behavior and Adaptation in Late Life.* Boston: Little, Brown & Company, 1969, pp. 93–114.

10. BURKHAUSER, RIEHARD, and G. TOLLEY, "Older Americans and Market Work," *The Gerontologist,* 18:No. 5 (1978), 449–53.

11. CARP, F., "Impact of Improved Living Environment on Health and Life Expectancy," *The Gerontologist,* 17: No. 3 (1977), 242–49.

12. CHATFIELD, WALTER, "Economic and Sociologic Factors Influencing Life Satisfaction of the Aged," *Journal of Gerontology,* 32: No. 5 (1977), 593–99.

13. CLEMENTE, F., and J. HENDRICKS, "A Further Look at the Relationship Between Age and Productivity," *Gerontologist,* 13: (1973), 106–10.

14. COHEN, ELIAS, and S. POULSHOCK, "Societal Response to Mass Dislocation of the Elderly," *The Gerontologist,* 17: No. 3 (1977), 262–68.

15. COOK, FAY, WESLEY SKOGAN, THOMAS COOK, and GEORGE ANTUNES, "Crime Victimization of the Elderly," *The Gerontologist,* 18: No. 4 (1978), 338–49.

16. COSTA, FRANK, and MARNIE SWEET, "Barrier-Free Environments for Older Americans," *The Gerontologist,* 16: No. 5 (1976), 404–9.

17. CRAIG, GRACE, *Human Development.* Englewood Cliffs, N. J.: Prentice-Hall, Inc., 1976.

18. CURTIN, SHARON, *Nobody Ever Died of Old Age.* Boston: Little, Brown & Company, 1972.

19. DAVIDSON, WAYNE, and KARL KUNZE, "Psychological, Social, and Economic Meanings of Work in Modern Society: Their Effects on the Worker Facing Retirement," in *Human Life Cycle,* ed. Wm. Sze. New York: Jason Aronson, Inc., 691–700.

20. DEBEAUVOIR, SIMONE, "Old Age: End Product of a Faulty System," *Saturday Review,* April 8, 1972, 38–45.

21. DIEKELMAN, NANCY, "Staying Well While Growing Old: Pre-Retirement Counseling," *American Journal of Nursing,* 78: No. 8 (1978), 1337–38.

22. DOWD, J., and V. BENGSTON, "Aging in Minority Populations," *Journal of Gerontology,* 33: No. 3 (1978), 427–36.

23. "Driving Skills of Senior Motorists," *More Years for Your Life,* 8: No. 5 (1969), 1.

24. FOWLER, ELEANOR, "What Price Aging?" *Women's International League for Peace and Freedom,* 37: No. 2 (1977), 3.

25. FOX, JUDITH, "Effects of Retirement and Former Work Life on Women's Adaptation in Old Age," *Journal of Gerontology,* 32: No. 2 (1977), 196–202.

26. HARTMAN, CHESTER, JERRY HOROWITZ, and ROBERT HERMAN, "Designing with the Elderly," *The Gerontologist,* 16: No. 4 (1976), 303–11.

27. HAVIGHURST, ROBERT, "Perspectives on Health Care for the Elderly," *Journal of Gerontological Nursing,* 3: No. 2 (1977), 21–24.

28. HAYNES, S., A. MCMICHAEL, and H. TYROLEY, "Survival After Early and Normal Retirement," *Journal of Gerontology,* 33: No. 2 (1978), 269–78.

29. HEFLIN, THOMAS, "Social Security: Individual or Social Equity?" *The Gerontologist,* 16: No. 5 (1976), 455–57.

30. HEUMANN, LEONARD, "Estimating the Local Need for Elderly Congregate Housing," *The Gerontologist,* 16: No. 5 (1976), 397–403.

31. HURLOCK, ELIZABETH, *Developmental Psychology,* 4th ed. New York: McGraw-Hill Book Company, 1975.

32. KAMERMAN, SHEILA, "Community Resources for the Aged," *The Gerontologist,* 16: No. 6 (1976), 529–37.

33. KEITH, PAT, "A Preliminary Investigation of the Role of the Public Health Nurse in Evaluation of Services for the Aged," *American Journal of Public Health,* 66: No. 4 (1976), 379–81.

34. KELL, D., and C. PATTON, "Reaction to Induced Early Retirement," *The Gerontologist,* 18: No. 2 (1978), 173–79.

35. KENNEDY, J., and G. DEJONG, "Aged in Cities: Residential Segregation in 10 USA Central Cities," *Journal of Gerontology,* 23: No. 1 (1977), 97–102.

36. KILTY, KEITH, and A. FELD, "Attitudes Toward Aging and Toward the Needs of Older People," *Journal of Gerontology,* 31: No. 5 (1976), 586–94.

37. KIMMEL, DOUGLAS, *Adulthood and Aging.* New York: John Wiley & Sons, Inc., 1974.

38. KLEEMEIER, ROBERT, "Leisure and Disengagement in Retirement," in *Human Life Cycle,* ed. Wm. Sze. New York: Jason Aronson, Inc., 1975, pp. 661–69.

39. KLINE, CHRYSEE, "Socialization Process of Women," *The Gerontologist,* 15: No. 6 (1975), 486–92.

40. LIDZ, THEODORE, *The Person.* New York: Basic Books, Inc., 1968.

41. LIPMAN, ALAN, and ROBERT SLATER, "Homes for Old People," *The Gerontologist,* 17: No. 2 (1977), 146–156.

42. McLEAN, JANET, "Creative Recreation Makes the Difference Between Growing Old and Getting Old," *Modern Nursing Home,* 22: No. 4 (1968), 65ff.

43. MILLER, STEPHEN, "The Social Dilemma of the Aging Leisure Participant," in *Older People and Their Social World,* eds. Arnold Rose and Warren Peterson. Philadelphia: F. A. Davis Company, 1965, pp. 77–92.

44. MORK, LUCILE, *A Guide to Budgeting for the Retired Couple.* Home and Garden Bulletin No. 194, Washington, D. C.: U. S. Government Printing Office, 1973.

45. MORRISON, MALCOLM, "Planning for Income Adequacy in Retirement," *The Gerontologist,* 16: No. 6. (1976), 538–43.

46. NEWMAN, SANDRA, "Housing Adjustments of the Disabled Elderly," *The Gerontologist,* 16: No. 4 (1976), 312–17.

47. PALMORE, ERDMAN, "The Future Status of the Aged," *The Gerontologist,* 16: No. 4 (1976), 297–302.

48. PLONK, MARTHA, and MARY PULLEY, "Financial Practices of Retired Couples," *The Gerontologist,* 17: No. 3 (1977), 256–61.

49. REPPERS, LARRY, "Patterns of Leisure and Adjustment to Retirement," *The Gerontologist,* 16: No. 5 (1976), 441–46.

50. "Retirement to Age-Segregated Communities Facilitates Social Adjustment of Elderly," *Geriatric Focus,* 8: No. 9 (1969), 2–3.

51. ROSE, ARNOLD, "Group Consciousness Among the Aging," in *Older People and Their Social World,* eds. Arnold Rose and Warren Peterson. Philadelphia: F. A. Davis Company, 1965, 19–36.

52. ROSENFELD, ALBERT, "The Willy Loman Complex," *Saturday Review,* August 7, 1976, 24–26.

53. SCHULZ, RICHARD, and GAIL BRENNER, "Relocation of the Aged: A Review and Theoretical Analysis," *Journal of Gerontology,* 32: No. 3 (1977), 322–33.

54. SHINKLE, FLORENCE, "Profiles in Aging," *St. Louis Post-Dispatch,* May 25, 1975, Sunday Pictures Section, 4–14.

55. "Sociomedical Students Involved in Problems of Elderly," *Canada's Mental Health,* 24: No. 2, (1976), 38.

56. STIRNER, FRITZ, "The Transportation Needs of the Elderly in a Large Urban Environment," *The Gerontologist,* 18: No. 2 (1978), 207–11.

57. STREIB, GORDON, and CLEMENT SCHNEIDER, *Retirement in American Society: Impact and Process.* Ithaca, N. Y.: Cornell University Press, 1971.

58. STRUYK, RAYMOND, "The Housing Situations of Elderly Americans," *The Gerontologist,* 17: No. 2 (1977), 130–39.

59. "Study Shows Older People Are Nations' Safest Drivers," *Geriatric Focus,* 8: No. 8 (1969), 3–4.

60. UHLENBERG, PETER, "Changing Structure of the Older Population of the USA During the Twentieth Century," *The Gerontologist,* 17: No. 3 (1977), 197–202.

61. WEILER, P., P. KIM, and L. PICHARD, "Health Care for Elderly Americans," *Medical Care,* 14: (August, 1976), 700–10.

62. WOLFF, ISLE, "Retirement: A Different Season," *Nursing Outlook,* 21: No. 12 (1973), 763–65.

63. WOODRING, PAUL, "Why 65? The Case Against Mandatory Retirement," *Saturday Review,* August 7, 1976, 18–20.

community resources for the person/family in later maturity

Study of this chapter will enable you to:

---

1. Discuss types and importance of community resources available to the senior.

2. Share information about the American Association for Retired Persons.

3. Visit a local senior citizen center and discuss its activities with senior members.

4. Discuss purposes of a geriatric day-care center and services for the senior.

5. Describe the purpose of adult foster home care and placement criteria.

6. Contrast the types of agencies that provide home health services, the variety of services provided, and the advantages of these services to the senior and his family.

7. Contrast the types of short-term and long-term care institutions in your community.

8. Compare advantages of primary to hospital care for the senior and his family.

9. Visit a long-term care institution in your community, and ask questions or make observations as if you were admitting an elderly family member.

10. Discuss problems for the senior related to long-term care institutions and ways to improve conditions and the care given.

11. Explore future trends in the care of senior citizens and the nursing implications.

12. Assess the needs of the elderly you work with for additional services so that they can maintain independence to the degree possible.

13. Discuss your role in promoting adequate number and variety of community resources and in obtaining quality service from these agencies.

14. Refer the person/family as indicated to community resources.

7

INTRODUCTION

Various health and social welfare agencies and services exist to assist the senior population, and more options are needed to meet needs. Sponsorship may be by the federal or state government or by voluntary groups within a local community or region.

Information on federal legislation that provides for Medicare, Medicaid, Supplemental Security Income, pensions, jobs, nutritional programs, housing, transportation, and referral services for the elderly is discussed in Chapter 8.

Federal Administration on Aging (AoA) programs filter down to the state and local levels. Plans and priorities for each geographic area differ according to the needs of the older persons who live there; therefore, programs sponsored through each Area Agency on Aging may differ. Programs offered through Area Agencies include: (1) multipurpose senior centers; (2) transportation assistance through mini-bus service or volunteers who use their own cars; (3) shopping assistance; (4) handyman services in the form of small repairs done for a minimal fee; (5) hot, nutritious noon meals served at a low cost in various easily reached community facilities; (6) friendly visitors for the homebound; (7) library services for the homebound; (8) information and referral services to help the elderly find the services they need; and (9) home health and homemaker service by home health agencies so that the senior can remain in his home instead of being institutionalized.

In many cities, the Mayor's Office for Senior's Citizens and other local organizations combine to offer a variety of services. These services may include hot midday meals; a place for socializing, recreation, and reading; meals brought to the homebound (meals-on-wheels); protective and legal services; health screening, teaching, and sometimes direct care. Usually these services are given in a variety of sites throughout the city: churches, neighborhood senior citizen centers, apartments for the elderly, schools, libraries, or other public facilities.

Unfortunately, often the planning for and creation of agencies and services are poorly coordinated, with governmental and voluntary groups overlapping certain areas and completely missing others. Even worse, many elderly persons remain nearly unaffected by efforts of all such groups, since they either do not learn what is available, cannot understand how to secure what is needed, or are overwhelmed by the bureaucracy involved.

This chapter focuses on services and resources that help to more directly meet health and psychosocial needs of the person/family in later maturity. For purposes of discussion, services will be divided into the following categories: (1) voluntary organizations that provide religious, recreational, associational, educational, advocacy, or informational services, (2) community support services outside the home, (3) community support services in the home, and (4) long-term care institutions for the isolated, frail, ill, or disabled aged who require personal, medical, or nursing care.

Future populations of older persons may participate in voluntary organizations to a greater extent than elderly persons currently do because of more leisure time resulting from early retirement, possible improvements in health and economic security, and increasing levels of education.[19,20]

Voluntary associations serve several important functions. They bring together people who have common concerns or interests, and they heighten social interaction. They expand life space, meet socioemotional needs, and add purpose to life. Because of the strength in numbers and collective resources, members are in a better position than uninvolved persons to acquire and exert influence, including political; obtain needed services; and serve as a locus for the dissemination of opinion.[19,20] Often the person can support former interests by maintaining membership in certain kinds of organizations, for example, the Wildlife Federation or Sierra Club. Or he can support a cause dear to his heart, such as a membership in the local art or science museum. Increasingly organizations that are under the direction of the elderly are also assisting the elderly to obtain part-time employment.

Membership Profiles

Membership in fraternal groups is lowest among younger age groups and it is highest among the oldest age groups; more men than women belong. Apparently membership in fraternal organizations and lodges was more common in the past, and the same population group continues to belong.[20]

Church membership is more prevalent in older age groups, more characteristic of women than men, and related to other aspects of religiosity.[20]

Men of all age groups are more likely to participate in sports groups, but more younger than older persons belong, possibly because of health differences.[20]

Fewer elderly persons belong to professional and academic societies because of: (1) lower level of education generally than the younger population, (2) greater likelihood of having been a blue-collar rather than a professional or white-collar worker, and (3) retirement, so that the person is less likely to belong to professional or academic associations. The number of women who belong is the same or in excess of males who belong to these associations.[20]

Membership in service clubs peaks in middle age and trails off for both younger and older populations. Men belong to service clubs to a greater extent than do women. Membership in political clubs does not differ by age.[20]

More men over 75 years belong to veterans' clubs than men 65 to 74 years, probably because of the age of present seniors when World Wars I and II occurred.[20]

Older people are also likely to belong to age-related associations, such as the American Association of Retired Persons (AARP), senior citizen centers, or golden age clubs.

Belonging is not equated with participation, which can range from token membership to active involvement. The following chart compares types of associations to which persons in later maturity belong and their order of preference:[20]

Men		*Women*	
Church-related	43%	Church-related	56%
Fraternal	25%	Other	12%
Labor	18%	Fraternal	12%
Veterans	12%	Literary, art, discussion, study	10%
Other	12%	Hobby or garden clubs	10%

Types of Organizations

The two associations discussed below are presented as examples of the many organizations that are available for the senior to join. Many other local, state, or national associations are not as multipurpose as AARP and are not as single-purposed as ACCORD. Probably every community has some kind of group that the senior can join if he desires; for example, church-related organizations usually exist even in isolated, rural areas. Some organizations, such as AARP, can keep a member involved by mail.

The *American Association for Retired Persons* (AARP), was founded by Dr. Ethel Andrus in 1958, has active chapters in over 1000 communities. A variety of services, some of which were discussed in Chapter 6, are offered to members who must be 55 years of age or older:

1. Pharmacy service, in which prescription and nonprescription drugs, medical appliances, and sickroom supplies can be ordered by mail for a reasonable cost and without postal charge. Pharmacies are located at St. Petersburg, Florida; Long Beach, California; Kansas City, Missouri; Hartford, Connecticut; and Washington, D.C.
2. Institute of Lifetime Learning, which offers a variety of educational courses and lectures in regional centers or for home study.
3. Health insurance plans for low cost without eligibility requirements, which cover hospitalization, drugs, nursing home, and home nursing care.
4. Life insurance plan at reasonable cost and without a preliminary physical examination.
5. Auto insurance plan with a guaranteed lifetime renewable feature and a limited cancellation feature.
6. Travel service that offers low-cost tours around the world.

7. Nursing home program at The Acacias in Ojai, California, which is a model for other nursing homes and offers modern nursing and medical facilities.
8. Mature Temps, Inc., which offers temporary employment for income supplementation.
9. *Modern Maturity* and the *AARP News Bulletin,* which are received automatically upon joining.
10. Legislative services that work with federal and state governments on legislation pertaining to the elderly.[3]

The main office is located at 1225 Connecticut Avenue, Washington, D.C., 20036.[3]

ACCORD (Action Coalition to Create Opportunities for Retirement with Dignity, Inc.), is an advocacy organization for aged persons which began in upstate New York.[24] A group of older people who realized that they were not alone with their problems of inadequate income, housing, transportation, and medical care organized and obtained federal funds for the development and staffing of the organization. They obtained state and federal funds for improved transportation, housing, and health care when local funds were insufficient. Older people, rather than professionals, defined their problems and suggested preferred solutions.[24]

Membership to ACCORD is free to people over 55 years of age; there are 19,000 people in the country who belong. All members receive a newsletter four times a year which includes questionnaires, information, and news designed to stimulate a sense of organizational identity and involvement even for the homebound. Over 400 members do routine work for the organization on a volunteer basis. Additionally, there are 55 affiliate organizations, ranging from labor union retirees to local executives, from church-related fellowship groups to housing groups, all which add to the power base in the community and facilitate public education, research, and political action.[24]

Advocacy for older citizens by ACCORD has resulted in the following accomplishments:

1. Buses with steps that hydraulically lower to desired height for persons unable to climb the high steps of ordinary buses.
2. Less expensive, limited telephone service options for those unable to keep a phone at regular service rates, since a telephone is a lifeline to the community.
3. Elevators in apartment houses that are long enough for stretchers so that people to not have to be carried in chairs to waiting ambulances.
4. Discounts for older persons from approximately 700 merchants.[24]

The organization has helped professionals to work with older people instead of making decisions for them. ACCORD has made a major educational impact on the community because it has made senior citizens more visible and it has changed the public's image of what it means to be elderly.[24]

Various services provided by the Area Agency on Aging or other organizations fall into this category, such as congregate meals, senior centers, legal assistance, information and referral services, transportation arrangements, day care, and vacation services for families with a senior member.

Some of these services have been discussed in Chapters 6 and 8. Senior centers will be discussed briefly, but the discussion will focus on two services that exist in some communities and are needed in most communities for the senior who needs some assistance: geriatric day-care and foster home care. It is possible that more of these services will be developed in the future to meet the varied needs of a diverse population in late life.

Senior Citizen Centers

Most communities of any size have a *senior citizen center, a gathering place for the elderly where a number of services are offered.* The center can be a separate building especially built, easily reached, and barrier-free, or it can be located in a public facility such as a library, community center, church, or apartment complex for elderly persons. Senior citizen centers have become common.

Some centers are maintained by a minimal staff and many volunteers; other centers are staffed by a variety of professionals and nonprofessionals, sometimes including retirees. The center may function primarily as a place to eat a hot noon meal and informally chat with friends. Many centers are multifunctional, for they offer social, recreational, and educational activities; social work services; health and counseling services; part-time employment opportunities; and attendance at cultural events.[41] The center often provides information about supplemental security income, homestead property tax relief, food stamps, income tax benefits, and other financial or legal matters.

Geriatric Day-Care Programs

Day Care is a program of services provided under health leadership in an ambulatory care setting for adults who do not require 24-hour institutional care but who are usually incapable of full-time independent living because of physical or mental disability.[31,74]

Purposes of day-care programs include the following:

1. Assisting in daily care and supervision of the senior in order to relieve family tensions.
2. Serving elderly and disabled persons who can benefit from a program of medical and psychosocial rehabilitation.
3. Keeping the person in his home as long as possible in order to avoid the effects of environmental change.

4. Serving applicants who are waiting for nursing home placement or reducing the number of applicants.
5. Acting as a liaison between an isolated home life and the activities of community organizations.
6. Providing otherwise independent aging persons with a nutritionally balanced meal and an atmosphere conducive to social rehabilitation.[31,74]

Because of the spiraling costs of health care, the needs of working families, and concerns about long-term institutionalization, day-care programs are gaining nationwide interest. A day-care program may be incorporated into services offered by a hospital or nursing home, or limited day-care services may be provided in a senior citizen center or apartment for the elderly.

A variety of services are provided: (1) physical maintenance and rehabilitation; (2) nursing care; (3) socialization activities to overcome isolation and depression and foster a sense of well-being, independence, self-worth, and responsibility for self; (4) recreational and occupational therapies; (5) dietary services; and (6) spiritual care.[31,94] Usually the person is transported to the center by the family; some day-care programs provide a special vehicle to pick up the participants.[31,74]

Single or married offspring, elderly spouses, and often elderly siblings will care for the less independent senior as long as possible. Day-care programs are a way of getting additional help and assuring the senior's safety while family members are out of the home at work or at school or when other elderly caretakers cannot manage care for 24-hours daily, 7 days a week, because of their own physical or mental status.

This program is also useful if the family wishes to take a vacation or short trip or attend to extended business, and it is especially useful if the day-care program is housed in an institution that provides 24-hour service.[74] Leaving the senior for several days and nights in a familiar setting is an alternative to hiring a sitter. Usually a sitter cannot be obtained for an extensive period. One of the disadvantages of keeping a frail senior family member in the home is that often the family cannot get away as a unit for business or vacation. A well-run day-care program in the right setting provides an alternative in care.

Foster Home Care

Adult foster home care, where the senior lives with and is cared for by an *unrelated family,* continues to be a service needed by most communities. More and more older people, often without family, are too frail to live alone but are not so physically or mentally impaired that they need to be institutionalized. This more unrestrained life allows seniors to experience the cheer and companionship of a family instead of the depersonalization and rules of an institution.[29]

The concept of foster care for the senior is similar to that of foster care for

children. Foster families must be chosen carefully; the home must be structurally sound and safe, and it must provide adequate space and privacy for
each guest. The foster family must be able to assist the senior with hygiene
measures and provide transportation for treatment, if necessary.[29,63] Of primary importance is that the foster family likes elderly people and can relate to
them with warmth and patience.

Payment to the foster family comes from Social Security or public assistance funds, although some people do pay for the foster care themselves. The
foster family must give evidence that it is not merely trying to earn money but
is truly interested in older persons and their welfare.[29]

In matching guests and the foster family, the following must be considered: (1) cleanliness and comfort of the home, (2) permission and area for visitors, (3) adequate quarters, usually on the first floor, and (4) temperament of
the persons involved. Ideally, the senior has a choice of foster homes.[29,63]

To offset the growing need for homelike facilities for the elderly, a number
of senior-citizen communes, Share-A-Home, have been started in Florida. The
living plan is similar to that of the youthful communes.[48]

COMMUNITY SUPPORT AND HEALTH SERVICES IN THE HOME

The person/family in later maturity usually prefers to remain in his own home
rather than to go to an institution such as a nursing home. Because of his advanced old age, frailty, and illness, this desire may not be realized unless assistance is given. Assistance may be in the form of a caring family member, relative, neighbor, or friend who helps the senior meet basic needs. Unfortunately,
caring for the ill person in the home can create various problems for the family,
such as (1) performing physical care inadequately or with difficulty because of
lack of instruction, support, or equipment; (2) maintaining regular family
functions and responsibilities; (3) coping with emotional and financial burdens
imposed by the ill member; or (4) transporting the ill person for treatment.[77]
Thus, other services provided by the community are also useful, for example,
(1) homemaker or handyman services to assist with household chores, shopping, or home repairs; (2) transportation to medical facilities and church; (3)
telephone visitation; (4) meals-on-wheels; and (5) home health care services.

Telephone Services

*Telephone services, whereby the elderly person calls a designated number
daily,* have been organized in some communities for homebound persons. If
the person does not call, the volunteer who is with the service first calls the senior, then a neighbor or friend. If they know nothing about the senior's situa-

tion, the police are called to check on the older person. The senior knows that if something were to happen to him, at least once within 24 hours a routine check would be made. One of the concerns of many homebound, partly incapacitated elderly is that a fall, a stroke, or even death might go unnoticed by others for some time.

Equally effective to a daily telephone call is a plan by West Germany, where the local postman is being trained to serve as friend and helper to elderly people on his route. In his daily stop at the senior's home, he can check on the person's well being, report anything unusual, or transmit the senior's needs to the proper authority.

Meals-on-Wheels

Many communities have *meals-on-wheels, a service that delivers meals to the homes of seniors who cannot or do not feel able to prepare a major meal daily.* Most programs are sponsored by public or private organizations, including churches, or senior citizen programs. Cost of the meals is low, or the charge is based on the person's ability to pay. Often the amount of food that is brought for one meal actually serves the senior two meals because many elderly people eat smaller amounts at one time. Some programs serve seniors on alternate days, for example Mondays, Wednesdays, and Fridays, with food portions large enough for leftovers on alternate days.

Some seniors enjoy the program; they enjoy the surprise menu and are not too limited in their food preferences. Others may try a meals-on-wheels program but then discontinue it for various reasons: (1) Hot and cold foods do not arrive hot and cold, respectively. (2) The foods served may not be liked; therefore, they are thrown away and the money is wasted. (3) The meal may arrive at a time of day that the senior does not associate with eating. (4) The cost may be more than the senior can either afford or wishes to spend for food. For example, we think a full meal for $1.75 or $2.00 is inexpensive. The elderly person may be living on a budget too slim for such luxury, as discussed in Chapter 6.

Home Health Services

Skilled home nursing and other health care services, such as physical and occupational therapy, nutritional assistance, or mental health counseling, are important services for the elderly person/family who need follow-up care after hospitalization, have chronic or terminal illness, or are incapacitated but wish to remain at home. This form of care is less expensive than institutional care, and the client adjusts and recovers better. The client has someone who cares for him; he enjoys familiar surroundings and preferred food; he is seen as a unique person with a life history and future. While not all ill elderly can be cared for at home, more families could keep their senior members at home if adequate home care services were available. Further, the taxpayer could be saved money.[35,42,60,97]

Skilled health care in the home is usually given by visiting nurse associations or designated home health care agencies. In New York City, however, physicians, nurses, and social workers from a hospital, the Department of Health, and the Visiting Nurse Service combined their efforts to reach a group of elderly persons who are often neglected: the derelict, isolated men and women living on Skid Row and in single rooms of welfare hotels. Visits were made to the rooms of those who were unable to leave because of fear or illness. Others who wanted care appeared at a clinic that was set up in one of the ghetto hotels. No fee was charged, and there was no regular registration procedure. A history, physical examination, and necessary treatment were done by a doctor or nurse; concise records were kept.[12]

The nurses were more successful than were the other team members in case finding and long-term treatment, often against initial client resistance. The nurse was clearly the key member of this team, for the nurse is usually the person who is generally known and trusted in the community and is in a position to find and solve many difficult human issues.[12]

One project by graduate students in nursing began with blood pressure screening in a high-rise apartment for the elderly to gain the confidence and interest of the residents as well as secure a basic health history. The nurses learned that the residents were more concerned about their living conditions than with their physical problems. The residents listed the following problems:

1. Infestation by vermin in the apartments.
2. Inability to get help in an emergency, although a call system was in working order.
3. Lack of phone service for some residents who felt they saved money by not having a personal phone.
4. Difficulty in getting around the apartment because of a poorly designed floor plan and accumulated clutter.
5. Fear that belongings would be tampered with or taken from the apartment during the resident's absence.
6. Lack of communication between the people offering services and the residents.
7. Lack of visitors and loneliness.
8. Fear of going to a nursing home or hospital.[49]

In order to promote emotional as well as physical health and to become the residents' advocate, the nurses undertook various projects. Regular staff meetings were held with the staff of the building to share information about identified needs and to do joint planning. These meetings proved helpful in improving residents' living quarters, for residents would not voice complaints directly to the building administrator.

Residents were organized into a committee to be responsible for knowing who needed help and giving help if possible. Shopping, mail pick-up, preparing a light meal, and other small tasks could be done by able-bodied residents for those who were more dependent. This group of residents also oriented new residents, assumed responsibilities delegated by a residents' council, and organized social functions.

Safety education, including how to maintain a safe apartment, was presented to the residents by the nurses. Information included: (1) storage and use of drugs and poisons, (2) proper use of electrical appliances, (3) proper use of step stools, (4) methods to discourage vermin from collecting, (5) accident prevention, and (6) what to do in case of an emergency. Firemen gave a program on how to prevent and put out a small fire and how to call for help.

Group coffee klatches among the residents were initiated to help decrease social isolation, encourage reminiscing, and promote visiting.

The nurses made a door-to-door survey to get a current list of residents, a more comprehensive health history, and teach about nearby community and health services as well as services that were provided by the nurses. Many residents were in need of but were not receiving health care. Dental services were arranged because most residents needed dental care. A program presenting information to the women on cancer and how to make arrangements for a free Pap test was well attended.[49]

You can readily imagine how many apartments or hotels housing the elderly could use a program like this one. Such programs are as important as the traditional visiting nurse home health care because these programs would be preventive as well as therapeutic.

Various other approaches are being tried to promote home care. In one city the hospitals combine resources to maintain a Hospital-Home Health Care organization (HHHC) to serve their patients. The program provides home nursing; home delivery of a hot meal daily; physical and respiratory therapies; transportation to the doctor's office after hospitalization; and homemakers to help with chores. These services have enabled many elderly, sick people to live at home safely and with dignity and comfort. Staff members of the program also work with families to teach them how to care for their senior members. Most of the visits by the HHHC are paid for by Medicare or Medicaid.[75]

At the University of Southern California Medical Center (Los Angeles County), physicians have been assigned to make house calls on a 24-hour basis to 500 chronically ill patients.[75] This program may be an exceptional one, but it certainly is an indication that home-based care is currently seen as an important alternative to institutional care.

Increasingly, we see programs like the Outreach Health Care Program sponsored by St. Mary's Extended Care Center in Minneapolis. In addition to the usual institutional services, the Center provides home health care and related personal services to elderly so that they may remain in their own homes/communities as long as they are in relatively good mental and physical health. The facility offers an alternative to isolation and institutionalization.[22]

Emergency services are typically hospital-based and are often needed by, but lacking for, elderly persons. Most housing projects for the elderly could have a night emergency service. Since more emergencies occur at night, staff could live in during the night to answer calls (obtaining emergency help during the day is not as difficult). Emergency services provided by one housing project helped the elderly to remain independent and feel safe. The elderly may define emergency differently from the way most health professionals do.[30] The word emergency conjures up visions of a coronary attack to you; to the elderly it may mean falling out of bed, locking oneself out of the apartment, or periods of dizziness or disorientation. In one project, when the resident pulled an alarm cord located in the bathroom, bedroom, or kitchen, a light went on above his door, the door lock opened, and a bell rang in the hall. A team of two staff members were present at night to answer calls. Usage of the alarm system was as follows: (1) 40 percent for physical difficulties, (2) 9 percent for psychological difficulties, (3) 6 percent for interpersonal reasons, (4) and 45 percent for maintenance and security reasons. The call system was not abused.[30]

The passage of Medicare stimulated expansion of home health care services. Unfortunately, Medicare limits the type of illness covered and the number of visits permitted, and it is dependent on the physician's referral.[96] More physicians need to become aware of the existence and value of home health care. The various insurance companies need to explore the economy of this type of program. More preventive and health-related services, rather than just medical services in the home, should be covered by third-party payers. With an increasing number of senior citizens in the future, some of whom will become ill, more home health agencies and qualified staff will be needed. Certainly clients who wish to remain at home, and who have families who want them at home, should have the services available.

In Oregon the Department of Human Resources operates Project Independence, which gives elderly citizens a choice between living at home or in a nursing home. The elderly person who remains at home receives a variety of services, depending on need. These services may include: housekeeper, visiting nurse, driver to take the person shopping, participation in a day-care center, and meals-on-wheels service. Many elderly choose to remain at home because they feel that they have more freedom, fewer constraints, and greater satisfaction. The governor considers the program an economical one; the cost per person averages $180 monthly compared to $500 to $700 for maintaining a person in a nursing home. If a person needs the assistance provided by a nursing home, he may choose to enter one.

The elderly often resist going for health care as long as possible. They attribute their symptoms to old age, when in fact the symptoms may be related to a treatable condition. For example, many seniors have a mild anemia that causes symptoms of fatigue, apathy, tachycardia, chilliness, and dizziness. With treatment, the symptoms clear.

Yet, for either correctable or chronic illness, such as colds, anemia, hypertension, digestive disorders, arthritis, diabetes, and cardiovascular and renal disease, the person may resort to home remedies first and for some time. He goes to the hospital only when he is severely ill. Lack of convenient primary or ambulatory care services contributes to this situation. Delay of treatment is also related to fears about the cost of health care but, even more so, to the dehumanization and lack of control the senior suffers in the hospital. Further, he perceives that the diagnostic and treatment measures may be as painful as the condition. He may also fear that the hospital is the first step to the nursing home or to death itself.

Primary Health Care

Primary health care services include care given on initial contact and in the ambulatory setting, providing treatment for acute diseases, managing chronic diseases, providing for continuity of care, using preventive measures, counseling, teaching, and employing an understanding of emotional and social factors in assessment and intervention.[85]

The nurse is ideally suited to give primary care. The nurse practitioner is one who (1) provides traditional nursing care, (2) assesses normality and abnormal conditions or minor disorders, (3) performs a general physical and behavioral examination, (4) orders or performs basic laboratory tests, (5) treats minor ailments, and (6) counsels or teaches patients with chronic, emotional, or psychosomatic disorders. The nurse practitioner works independently or collaboratively with other health professionals.[28,85]

Studies repeatedly show that nurse practitioners are accepted by patient/clients because they give satisfactory care (or more effective care than the physician gives), can save the doctor time that can be directed to more seriously ill patients, and can work in various settings, including geriatric, psychiatric, medical-surgical, or community settings. The elderly can be found in any of these settings. No negative effect on morality rate, physical function capacity, or social or emotional functioning has been shown to result from patient care by nurse practitioners rather than physicians.[28,85]

Use of more nurse practitioners in ambulatory care settings appears to be one way to improve health care for the population in later maturity and to avoid complications and institutionalization.

172

Hospitalization

Admission to the hospital is a crisis for the elderly person: a crisis related to physical illness, to loss of a familiar environment and routine, and to separation from loved ones. Often he must cope with the crisis alone; he may have no living relatives and few friends young enough to visit or do extras. Or the elderly spouse may be homebound and unable to visit and share the stress. The spouse may not even be able to hear well enough to converse with the hospitalized person over the phone, if he is able to talk on the phone. Unfortunately, the hospital worker—professional or nonprofessional—cannot be relied upon to offer support, or to even be aware of this patient's crisis.

Further, the elderly person is often overwhelmed and confused by the hurried pace, the plethora of personnel, the battery of tests and treatments, the strange sounds, and ever-changing routines. He soon becomes smothered by the patient role. No wonder that he develops the symptoms and behavior of acute brain syndrome described in Chapter 21. Further, he is likely to develop nosocomial infections, adverse reactions to medications and procedures, or suffer an accidental injury. The thorough diagnostic work-up given younger patients may be unnecessary and may give false positives, for the norms are often more appropriate to young adults than to seniors.[85] This author's experience has been that the elderly person tends to become sicker physically and emotionally if he is left in the hospital environment too long. The Utilization Review Committee may seem cruel with its dogmatic approach to discharge (for governmental and financial reasons). However, the best approach seems to be to physically treat the elderly person in as short a time and as thoroughly as possible and then discharge him to the home setting, if possible, so that he can recuperate and regain his lost abilities and potential.

If the person cannot be discharged quickly for whatever reason, and if he is not bedridden, a therapeutic group may be one way to help him remain alert and motivated and to help him work through the crisis of hospitalization. If the patient has little contact with other significant people, the group can become an oasis in an otherwise alien environment.[51] Some of the types of groups discussed in Chapter 4 are useful in the acute care setting as well as in a long-term or psychiatric setting.

Long-Term Institutional Care

Although only 5 percent of the senior population reside or are patients in an institutional setting, often laymen and health professionals alike equate old age with dependency and institutionalization. Yet, most persons in later maturity wish to remain at home and avail themselves of the services described above rather than to go to a long-term care institution. Women (because they live longer), whites, those who live alone, and the very old are more likely to be institutionalized than are men, Blacks (because they are more often cared for by family), those living with someone, and the not-so-old. One study revealed that a person has about a 25 percent chance of being institutionalized before death because of chronic disease or disability.[68]

There are protective personal resources against institutionalization or the emergence of disorders that force institutionalization. These resources are interrelated and include: (1) economic condition, (2) education, (3) maintenance of physical health throughout life, (4) adaptive mental and emotional mechanisms throughout life, and (5) social relationships.[33]

Nursing and extended care homes developed because of the increasing institutionalization of health care services in society; the increasing numbers of elderly; and the problems of caring for sick and infirm elderly persons who could not manage self-care, could not be cared for by a changing family structure, or were not wanted in the home. These institutions have become a major business in the United States as the result of Medicare and public assistance, societal trends, and the profit motive. Some institutions meet the needs of their residents well; others deserve condemnation. Some offer innovative programs and a variety of services given by professional staff; others offer minimal custodial care by nonprofessional staff. Some are licensed by the state and accredited by the Joint Commission on Hospital Accreditation; others do not meet these minimal standards.

Institutionalization is necessary and helpful for some people in late life, but research indicates some problems with it; therefore the following discussion will explore the many facets of this mode of care.

Selecting a nursing home or extended care facility should be done carefully by the family and senior member. The following questions should be asked:

1. Is the institution licensed by the state and accredited by the Joint Commission of Hospital Accreditation?
2. Does the institution require or give a complete physical examination shortly after admission?
3. Does the institution offer progressive stages of care—acute to ambulatory—and what is the cost of each stage?
4. What services are available if the person becomes acutely ill? What are the policies about keeping acutely ill persons?
5. What is the staff-resident ratio?
6. Does the institution have a dietitian to plan regular and special diets; occupational, recreational and physical therapists; and a social worker?
7. What pharmacy services are available? Where are drugs obtained?
8. How often does a physician come to the home? Can the person retain his own physician?
9. Do staff members inquire about unique characteristics, needs, interests, preferences, and hobbies of their residents?
10. What is the daily routine like? Are religious services provided?

11. Where are the residents? Sitting in the day room or their own rooms, lying in bed, or walking around without constraint?
12. What does the person have to pay to enter, remain, and receive full care? Must all personal and real property be given to the institution?
13. Does the owner require entrance contracts? Do these contracts fail to promise a return of property if the person leaves the home?
14. Is there an extra charge for shaving, cutting hair or nails, shampoos, laundry of personal clothes, or receiving snacks?
15. What is the total cost per month? What services are included? What do additional services cost?
16. How many residents are in the institution? What is the average space per resident?
17. Are there emergency buzzers in bedrooms, bathrooms, and activity areas?
18. What do the residents eat? Do bedridden patients receive hot food? Are they fed? Is there a charge for feeding?
19. Is there a sprinkler system and are there fire extinguishers? Is there a heat and smoke sensor system and is an automatic direct line hooked to the local fire station?
20. What is the staff turnover rate? What is the apparent staff morale?
21. Is there an in-service program for staff? What is included in the offerings?

The local Better Business Bureau can be called to determine if it is aware of any problems between the facility and past residents or if the answers you received were realistic or appropriate.

Certain observations are as important as the questions asked and should be made during several visits. Visit unannounced and at different times of the day to gain a comprehensive picture.

1. How are the residents addressed? By title and last name, first name, or general terms like "Grandma"? Do staff members refer to the persons as patients or as residents? (If they use the term patient, often the institutional philosophy or practices do not include restorative or rehabilitative services.)
2. How many persons are out of bed? When? What are they doing? How are they groomed and dressed? (Too many persons in bed may reflect a lack of staff or a philosophy of custodial care unless the institution has a large number of acutely ill persons.)
3. How do staff members react to spontaneous questions or the presence of the residents in the area of the nurse's station? To visitors? To you?
4. How do staff members react to each other?
5. What is the general condition of the institution? Is it clean but not so meticulous that it is apparent that residents do not engage in activities? Are the inside and outside environments pleasing in appearance? Are there

apparent safety hazards? How does the institution smell? What is the noise level?

6. How do the bedrooms appear? Does the resident have personal belongings in his room?
7. Are there handrails in the halls and bathrooms?
8. How quickly do staff members respond to the emergency buzzer or resident's request?
9. Do residents talk freely with each other?
10. When are visiting hours? What is the staff's response to people who visit in early morning or late evening?

If the institution is carefully explored by the family and client, unhappy situations are usually avoided. In addition, thorough exploration shows care of and interest in the senior. The family is more likely to remain involved if care is used in selecting a nursing home.

Good homes are likely to be expensive and have a waiting list. Available choices may be limited by lack of money, desire for a specific religious affiliation, family concerns, or physical or mental status of the senior. Further, the kind of facility chosen for the senior will depend on whether or not he needs total physical care. The facility may serve only the very dependent or may combine services for those who are (1) ambulatory, needing a protected environment, some supervision, and minimum nursing care, (2) up and about with assistance, needing some help with hygiene and daily activities, and (3) totally dependent, primarily bedfast, needing all basic care done for them, and needing skilled nursing care.

A survey of nursing homes in 16 states revealed that homes giving higher quality of care demonstrated the following characteristics: (1) licensure or certification; (2) beds for over 100 residents; (3) proportionately higher number of staff to the number of patients; (4) physical, occupational, and speech therapies available, and (5) high occupancy rates. The physical plant could be old or new. Reimbursement from Medicaid was based on need, not calculated as a flat rate. Individualization of care for both ambulatory and less mobile residents was apparent.[95]

But, finding an ideal home is not easy. In one study of 288 nursing homes the following characteristics were apparent:

1. Residents are old, with a median age of 82 years, and poor; 68 percent have an income of less than $3,000 annually, and 22 percent have no income at all.
2. Most need help with personal hygiene. The most common primary and secondary diagnoses, in order of frequency, are heart disease, chronic brain disease, generalized arteriosclerosis and hypertension, musculoskeletal diseases, stroke, fractures, and neurological disease.
3. Residents who have been in a home less than 4 months have probably seen

their doctor within the month; the long-term residents are less frequently seen by a physician.

4. Drugs are administered by licensed personnel 93 percent of the time; pharmacists make only monthly reviews of the residents' drug orders in 68 percent of the cases. Often drug prescriptions are outdated.

5. Nutrition is often poorly managed in nursing homes. Most facilities have the services of a part-time dietitian, ranging from ½ day to 20 days monthly. In 30 percent of the facilities, too few nutrition staff are on duty in a 12-hour period to permit adequate preparation of meals. No dietary information was found in 60 percent of the care plans. Special diets are often not available, and residents often go for 14 hours from the evening to the morning meal. If the person rejects his meal, he is offered no appropriate substitute in 73 percent of the facilities. A considerable number of nursing home residents may be slowly starving because often the food that is served is unpalatable to the senior or he needs, but does not get, assistance with feeding.

6. While nursing services may be inadequate, other therapies are lacking to an even greater extent. Only 30 percent receive needed physical therapy; only 11 percent receive appropriate occupational or speech therapy. Often such health care workers are hired on a part-time basis; they can accomplish little, and nursing home aids are not prepared to carry on such treatments when the professionals are not present. Social workers are available, usually part-time, in about one-half of the facilities, and social activity programs are conducted in 72 percent of the facilities, with staff working part-time in about 30 percent of the homes.[39]

Elliott, Greene, and Moss also describe the deplorable conditions which exist in many institutions for the elderly.[26,34,62]

Thus, too little is being done for the residents of long-term care facilities; the extensive treatment and continuity of care cannot be adequately carried out by part-time professionals.

Involving the elderly person in selection of a nursing home or extended care facility is crucial for several reasons. The person remains in control. The person can better cope with the crisis of relocation if he knows what is facing him and can predict when he will move and where he will go. There is less uncertainty. Also, if he has helped select—even visited his new home, if possible—he can anticipate what it will look like, fantasize what his life will be like, and think about how he will act. Anticipatory mental work enhances crisis resolution; a potentially harmful event can be interpreted to be emotionally tolerable, even acceptable. He can choose what seems best for him; having been able to avoid something makes the chosen place seem more acceptable. The greater the choice, the less negative the effect of relocation. The more predictable the environment, the less the stress. The most negative outcome results when the person is moved involuntarily from his own home to an institution without having any choice in the decision about the institution. Often death results shortly after institutionalization; death rates are highest for the first 3 months. Even relocation within the same institution increases the likelihood of death.[1,11,50,51,52,55,80]

Results of institutionalization in many cases represent family rejection; loss of home and possessions; loss of privacy, decision making, and independence; loss of self-identity, self-esteem, and individuality; increased frustration, insecurity, and anxiety because of the strangeness of new surroundings as well as their own expectations; and loss of personal control over destiny. The mental well-being of the elderly, already impinged upon by personal and social losses he has experienced, and occurring at a time in life when physical and psychological capacity for coping with stress is diminished, is further threatened by the losses and stress of institutionalization.[8,23,76] Admission to an institution—even the best—constitutes a crisis.

Institutions vary in type, and thus in effects on the residents. Some institutions are more open; they allow more freedom for the residents. Others are closed; they are classified as total institutions.

In total institutions, all aspects of life are tightly scheduled, conducted in the same place, under the same single bureaucratic authority, and in company of a large group of other people. Such a structure results in an almost castelike split between those being treated—the patients (or inmates) and the caretakers or staff. Little cross-communication exists between the two groups.[16,34]

A peculiar characteristic of total institutions is that they devalue the person before he is even admitted, which then justifies manipulation of the person to fulfill the aims and routines of the institution.[8] The consequences of such attitudes, policies, and procedures upon those who enter is to cause: (1) depersonalization, (2) loss of self-identity, (3) loss of control over self and meager personal resources, (4) restriction of physical, emotional, or social mobility, and (5) loss of attachment to society. This person is written off by society and himself. He is all but biologically dead.[16]

When a person finds himself in a hostile environment in which he cannot find satisfaction, he creates a substitute world mentally, where his lot is better. Such fantasy may become his only source of security; thus, the fantasy and accompanying withdrawal and hallucinations are maintained at any cost. No wonder that confusion, disorientation, and psychosis (organic brain syndrome) are frequently present in the patients who live in total institutions. Their identity has become false—crazy by social standards—but it is the only identity that can be maintained.[4,16]

The person who in the past viewed himself as controlling his own fate is more devastated by a total or controlling institution than the person who perceived himself without control.[80]

Studies consistently show that persons admitted to institutions have a higher death rate than do those who remain outside. Perhaps they are sicker than the control group. Perhaps the admission screening and procedures do great harm as they strip the person to nothingness. Perhaps the patient receives no crisis therapy to help work through feelings of loss related to relocation.[33] Perhaps he gives up life because he perceives that others have given up on him.

Even the more enlightened administrators and staff are hard put not to have a constraining environment in any kind of home for elderly people because of the size of the facility, numbers of residents, and work that must get done. Further, the person may have functioned well in his own home with a territorial separation from other people, but when he is placed in close proximity with others, he feels overwhelmed and threatened. He may become withdrawn or suspicious and need more help.

It is difficult to operate an institution unless meals are served and treatments are given at specified times. That means that the senior cannot very easily stay up late and arise in midmorning as he could in his own home. He gets no breakfast if he does not arise early enough. If he is not hungry and purposefully misses breakfast, he will either be awakened or queried about why he did not go and will be made to feel guilty. Staff members will prevent him from walking outdoors, which can be an enjoyable experience for the old and young, because they fear he will fall and fracture brittle bones. He may have been admitted to recuperate from a serious illness, but he probably will not be able financially to leave, for often the senior has to sign away all his assets when he enters the institution.

The institutionalized elderly are dependent because of disability, emotional and economic need, and institutional policies. They must depend on staff and volunteers, which is debasing even when they are kind and well-intentioned. Often staff members are sadistic and infantilizing in their care.[34,46]

The best way to avoid the minor or major negative effects of institutionalization is to keep the elderly person out of an institution unless he really needs to be in one. The criteria should be: Does the senior need the home? What alternatives are available?[66]

Institutional care can be humanized. Admission to an institution, as such, does not decrease self-esteem or cause emotional or mental deterioration.[6] Permanent changes from dependence and loss of self-identity to independence and maintenance of self-identity and esteem in institutionalized populations can be produced when administrative and nursing staff members change their attitudes toward residents and recognize that behavior is learned. Residents will learn either independent, alert behavior or dependent, apathetic behaviors, depending on the rewards and structure in their environment.[8,73]

One way to humanize care is to provide an opportunity for the person to give of himself, to share his inner resources or experience, to do something for another, to be in the role of giver rather than only that of receiver. Without being able to give, the person becomes lonely, depressed, and isolated and feels useless. To give to another is a potent healing force. One program provided for the elderly to be in the role of parent, grandparent, counselor, or friend to a group of mentally retarded adults, participating with them in recreational and social activities. A bond was formed between the senior and the adult retardate; each helped the other in his own way. The increased attention and inter-action improved morale in both groups.[46] Chapter 6 discusses various ways that the elderly can remain participants, even if they are institutionalized.

Institutionalization can be a positive experience if the following criteria are met:

1. The person enters the home of his choice voluntarily.
2. The home is located close to where he lived before so that family and friends can visit.
3. The person is accustomed to being with people, and some of the residents in the home are similar to him in activity and alertness levels.
4. The person recognizes that he needs assistance with physical care or super-vision in activities.
5. Quality interaction is maintained with at least one staff member and other loved ones. The closeness of the relationship is more important than the number of relationships.
6. Social affiliations between residents are encouraged because they promote positive group identity.
7. Adequate environmental stimuli and space are provided by the home.[5,45]

Some people's conditions improve after admission to an institution, espe-cially if:

1. The institution encourages independence, decision making about personal use of time and space, learning new skills, and developing new relationships.
2. The institution maintains contact with the community. Various groups or volunteers come in and interact with the residents, and residents regularly attend functions in the community, such as sports or cultural events, asso-ciational meetings, or a senior citizen center. Thus, the residents receive so-cial and intellectual stimulation through interaction with relatively healthy peers, experience creative expression, remain aware of the community and in better reality contact, and feel increased independence, self-sufficiency, and self-esteem.
3. The person moves from a cold, hostile, dependency fostering, dehumanizing environment to one that is warm and autonomy fostering and that gives in-dividualized care.[40,75]

FUTURE PROJECTIONS

Levels of Care

Health care is designated at three levels of prevention: primary, secondary, and tertiary. These levels will be more carefully considered in the future to determine needed services. *Primary prevention is care designed to reduce the risk of illness* and includes social welfare programs, group activities, transportation, home delivered meals, and homemaker services. *Secondary prevention involves early diagnosis and prompt treatment* in in-patient, clinic, or emergency room settings, consequently shortening the duration of illness. *Tertiary prevention focuses on rehabilitation after illness* to reduce residual effects of illness and encourage reentry into the community at an optimal level of functioning.[15]

Physical and mental health services will mesh. Community health services will treat not only the senior's physical and psychological problems but also help him handle problems of poverty, inadequate transportation, lack of food, and inadequate housing. Securing extermination, sanitation, or homemaker services may also be involved. Doing any one or several of the above may cause a definite improvement in physical and mental health.[15]

Trends

Most communities with increasing numbers of older citizens could use more of the following services:

1. Complexes that combine a range of separate but related services, such as housing, congregate meals, health care, shopping, church, and recreation.
2. Home health services that complement hospital and institutional services, utilizing the family practitioner, public health nurse, physical therapist, social worker, nutritionist, and chiropodist.
3. Day-care programs and neighborhood recreational centers.
4. Meal delivery to homes on a regular basis.
5. Homemaker services to assist with chores, household tasks, and shopping.
6. Short-stay beds to take infirm aged to relieve a family situation or permit a family to take a vacation or have a free weekend or holiday.
7. Transportation or escort assistance.
8. Reassurance, visitation, counseling, information, and spiritual services for individual or families.[25,86,87,88,89,96,97]
9. Self-help, educational, and advocacy centers for more independent, less needy elderly.
10. Protective and legal services and foster care placement for the frail, neglected, or abused elderly.

Crucial to attainment of the above services is thorough planning and coordination to prevent repetition of some services and omission of others.[25] Whether or not the more innovative services will be provided depends on social values, consumer demands, and funding.

As a nurse, you can use the information presented in this chapter in various ways. You may be involved in any one or all three levels of care—primary, secondary, or tertiary.

Refer to Services

You have a responsibility to know about a variety of resources and services in your community so that you can help the client/family better understand and use them. Whether you work in a hospital or the community, you will at times need to refer clients to another agency or service. Many larger communities publish a *Community Service Directory* that lists and describes the agencies and organizations that help a person in need. One city published a special section in the yellow pages of the telephone book entitled "Senior Citizen Services," which enabled both lay people and professionals to know about the community agencies and their services for people in late life.[90] Better use of various information and referral services and of the resources is essential; the importance of reducing stress for the senior was discussed in Chapter 6.

Encourage the elderly client/family to secure help from various resources on their own, as indicated by their needs, so that they can remain independent as long as possible. Collaborate with agency personnel and other health providers to achieve this goal. Attention must be paid especially to the needs of the aged couple so that they can remain together as long as possible. Often minimal assistance from yourself and selected agencies, including home health care services, will prevent institutionalization.

Participate in the Community Health and Social System

Whether or not you work directly with the elderly, you have a responsibility to the profession and the community. Work within the system to improve the system. There are many ways to serve the elderly.

For example, become involved in the Agency on Aging in your area so that you can help determine needs and influence the types of programs that will be developed. Become involved in local or state PSRO committees in order to help set the best possible standards and change the review process from looking at the facility to looking at the person in the long-term care facility. Help develop outcomes of patient care that are achievable and person-centered. Serve on teams that survey nursing homes for state licensure.[59]

Help educate the state and federal legislators and the public about the need for services other than nursing homes and the purposes and costs of different types of services. Work for better coordination among existing services. Become involved with any one of the various organizations that serve the elderly in your community. Every organization needs committed volunteers as well as paid staff if it is going to meet its clientele's needs.[58,59]

Become an advocate for the elderly in the following ways:

1. Keep up-to-date on programs that benefit the elderly.
2. Review and evaluate community resources.
3. Help a senior client or patient/family to file a complaint, if necessary.
4. Share community responsibility with other providers of health care.[58]

Promote Home Health Care

Helping the older person/family remain at home must be done with tact, patience, and finesse. Suggest rather than state what must be done. Let the senior decide how much help he really needs and wants. Often he resents outsiders coming in to do the tasks he has always done. He may regard the homemaker or handyman with suspicion, as if they are strangers who will steal. Often the outside helper will not be able to do any task well enough to please the senior. If the senior trusts you, he is more likely to trust and use other helpers who are available to do essential tasks and save him physical energy. Often you can interpret the senior's preferences to the other home health team members so that they can do a more effective job. If the senior feels that you and others are working *with* him instead of manipulating or doing *for* him, he will be better satisfied and feel that he is in control of the situation.

Additionally, you may work as a community health nurse and give direct patient care in the home.

Promote Quality Institutional Care

Whether you choose to work in a primary care setting, hospital, nursing home, or facility for the elderly, you have a responsibility to become as knowledgeable about and skillful in gerontological nursing as possible. The elderly client/family typically has many complex physical and psychosocial problems. Creative, not custodial, care is needed.

The nurse practitioner who has advanced preparation in gerontological nursing can do total health assessment, deliver a major portion of primary patient care, and assume leadership in consulting with and educating the nursing home staff. You may be the specially trained geriatric nurse practitioner. As such, you do not replace the physician with his medical services, but you can upgrade considerably the quality of nursing care while working with other professional health team members, such as the social worker, physical therapist, pharmacist, chaplain, physician, and others.[18,70]

Functions of nurse practitioners in some settings include to:

1. Meet the resident in the nursing home shortly after admission and explain the nursing role.
2. Make a thorough initial and ongoing assessment of each patient/resident.
3. Compile and maintain problem-oriented medical records, insuring a complete medical and personal record on each person.
4. Confer with other team members to assure comprehensive services without omission or unnecessary overlap.
5. Teach residents, answer their questions, and maintain whatever strengths and health are present.
6. Assess the medications that the person receives in order to avoid drug overdose or interactions, gradually reduce or eliminate tranquilizers, and reverse side effects and complications of long-term therapy.
7. Evaluate each person's progress in relation to each problem or change in condition. Consult the physician about any senior who does not progress as anticipated.
8. Determine the need for, perform, and interpret additional diagnostic procedures, such as urine, guaiac, electrocardiogram, or various blood tests.
9. Request basic radiology studies, and after receiving the report, decide on therapy, further evaluation, or referral.
10. Work with the other professional team members to evaluate and alter the prognostic expectation.
11. Manage selected medical-surgical or psychiatric patients within a general protocol.
12. Initiate and alter certain drug therapies for a group of chronic and acute conditions for as long as the patient's status remains within predicted limits. For example, the patient may do better with a mild tranquilizer in the early evening than in the morning; he is less likely to be confused or agitated at night and daytime drowsiness will be avoided. The physician reviews and cosigns changes in drug regimens.
13. Assess personal and family relationships, patient and staff relationships, and life situations that affect the senior's health status.
14. Provide for continuity of care when the senior moves from one setting to another or is referred to other practitioners.
15. Care for emergency calls as needed.
16. Instruct the nursing home staff formally and informally.
17. Assess and use a variety of resources (state and federally funded) programs, service groups, professional and special interest groups to help residents and staff.[17,18,70]

Working with the elderly involves a slower pace to accommodate to their reaction speed and comprehension. During data collection redirect the person to the necessary questions patiently and repetitively, but allow him to relate thoughts, repeat, and reminisce. As you listen, sort out pertinent data. Do not tune out repeated statements or apparent verbal meanderings; often such verbalizations contain much information about the unique person that cannot be obtained by direct questioning.

A health history can be accomplished in one or two sessions of 30 to 40 minutes each, depending on the person's attention span and endurance. Physical assessment is best done at a separate session to avoid fatigue. When the person is sitting, do the assessment that can be accomplished in that position, sequential or not. When the person lies down, finish the assessment.[18]

Various therapeutic approaches can be used to maximize normal living in an institutional setting, decrease personnel isolation, and convey a sense of esteem. Most of the following seem simple enough to do, but initiating them into a system of care may take time, persistence, and a sense of commitment to your clients. Helpful interventions include:

1. Integrating male and female divisions.
2. Holding residents responsible for special, designated tasks in the ward community.
3. Using self-government by the residents to promote decision making and self-determination.
4. Permitting family and friends to visit at any time.
5. Making available to the elderly the treatment modalities used with younger people, when these are appropriate.
6. Promoting social and affectional interactions among residents and between staff members and residents. Often the predinner cocktail hour (serving grape juice, wine, and mild cocktails); the afternoon beer and pretzel party; or the parties, dances, and sing-a-longs planned by recreational therapy can be times for initiating harmony that continues to deepen into relationships. (Further, beer and wine have been shown to have helpful physical effects as well: appetite is increased, digestion is improved, and anxieties are reduced.)[4,92]

Patient advocacy is not done only in the community organization or in the voting booth. You may also be a patient/resident advocate on any unit in an institution for specific persons, for the frail, confused, disabled who are mobile. These are usually the ones who get less of their needs met because they cannot fend so well against the more able, aggressive, and rational members. These residents may get less to eat because more able persons grab food from their trays. They are likely to wear less attractive, ill-fitting clothing; they get what's left in the ward closet by the more active, rational residents. They are likely to occupy less desirable chairs and space on the unit. As a result, they become increasingly isolated from the group, out of contact with reality, and increasingly powerless in their own behalf. Observe ward activities closely; perceive yourself as protector and advocate for those who cannot negotiate in their own behalf. Interrupt interactions between residents when one is being bullied, pushed aside, or physically or emotionally harmed. Be aware of the total milieu, including position of furniture and chairs, to make sure that it is functional and comfortable for all persons who live there.[56] Developing a therapeutic milieu is an independent function and is an important nursing role.

Constantly work to individualize your intervention. Modify the routine to suit the senior's preferences whenever you can. The chapters that follow will discuss setting patient-care objectives and various interventions to maintain or restore health or optimal functioning for a variety of nursing diagnosis. Base your practice upon the information presented in those chapters and other references.

REFERENCES

1. ALDRICH, C., and E. MENDKOFF, "Relocation of the Aged and Disabled: A Mortality Study," *Journal of American Geriatric Society,* 11: No. 3 (1963), 185–94.

2. ALFANO, GENROSE, "There Are No Routine Patients," *American Journal of Nursing,* 75: No. 10 (1975), 1804–7.

3. American Association of Retired Persons, *Here Is the Most Positive and Realistic Approach to Growing Older You Have Ever Heard About,* Washington, D.C., n.d.

4. ANDERSON, CATHERINE, "Alienation in the Aged: Implications for Psychiatric-Geriatric Nursing," *ANA Regional Conferences.* New York: Appleton-Century-Crofts, 1967, pp. 115–22.

5. ANDERSON, NANCY, "Institutionalization, Interaction, and Self-Conception in Aging," in *Older People and Their Social World,* eds. Arnold Rose and Warren Peterson. Philadelphia: F. A. Davis Company, 1965, pp. 245–57.

6. ANDERSON, ODIN, "Reflections on the Sick Aged and the Helping Systems," *Journal of Gerontological Nursing,* 3: No. 2 (1977), 14–20.

7. AVERBACH, MARILYN, *et al.,* "Health Care in a Selected Urban Elderly Population," *The Gerontologist,* 17: No. 4 (1977), 341–46.

8. BALTES, MARGRET, and MELISSA ZERBE, "Independence Training in Nursing Home Residents," *The Gerontologist,* 16: No. 5 (1976), 428–32.

9. BARNEY, JANE, "The Prerogative of Choice in Long-Term Care," *The Gerontologist,* 17: No. 4 (1977), 309–14.

10. BATTISTELLA, ROGER, "The Right to Adequate Health Care," *Nursing Digest,* 4: No. 1 (1976), 12–17.

11. BOTWINICK, JACK, *Aging and Behavior.* New York: Springer Publishing Co., Inc., 1973.

12. BRICKNER, PHILIP, *et al.,* "Outreach to Welfare Hotels, the Homebound, the Frail," *American Journal of Nursing,* 76: No. 5 (1976), 762–64.

13. BRODEN, ALEXANDER, "Reaction to Loss in the Aged," in *Loss and Grief: Psychological Management in Medical Practice,* eds. B. Schoenberg, A. Carr, D. Peretz, and A. Kutscher: New York: Columbia University Press, 1970, pp. 199–217.

14. BRODY, E., and G. SPARK, "Institutionalization of the Aged: A Family Crisis," *Family Process,* 5: (1966), 76–90.

15. CARTER, CAROLYN, "Community Mental Health Programs and the Elderly," *Nursing Clinics of North America,* 11: No. 1 (1976), 125–33.

16. COE, RODNEY, "Self-Conception and Institutionalization," in *Older People and Their Social World,* eds. Arnold Rose and Warren Peterson. Philadelphia: F. A. Davis Company, 1965, pp. 225–43.

17. CRAIG, GRACE, *Human Development.* Englewood Cliffs, N.J.: Prentice-Hall, Inc., 1976.

18. CRAVEN, RUTH, "Primary Health Care Practice in a Nursing Home," *American Journal of Nursing,* 76: No. 12 (1976), 1958–60.

19. CUTLER, STEPHEN, "Membership in Different Types of Voluntary Associations and Psychological Well-Being," *The Gerontologist,* 16: No. 4 (1976), 335–39.

20. ———, "Age Profiles of Membership in Sixteen Types of Voluntary Associations," *Journal of Gerontology,* 31: No. 4 (1976), 462–70.

21. ———, "Aging and Voluntary Association Participation," *Journal of Gerontology,* 32: No. 4 (1977), 470–79.

22. DANIEWICZ, CATHERINE, "Outreach Program Minimizes Premature Institutionalization," *Hospital Progress,* 55: No. 12 (1974), 26–35.

23. DUDLEY, CHARLES, and GEORGE HILLARY, "Freedom and Alienation in Homes for the Aged," *The Gerontologist,* 17: No. 2 (1977), 140–45.

24. EASTER, MAUD, "Senior Power: A Case Study in Education for Aging," *Adult Leadership,* 23: No. 3 (1974), 81–84.

25. EHRLICH, PHYLLIS, "Protective Services Study Report for Metropolitan St. Louis," sponsored by National Association of Social Workers—Task Force on Aging; Community Professional Ad Hoc Committee on Protective Services; and St. Louis University—Institute of Applied Gerontology, October, 1974–June, 1975.

26. ELLIOTT, NEIL, *The Gods of Life.* New York: Macmillan Publishing Co., Inc., 1974, pp. 46–61.

27. ERICKSON, ROSEMARY, and KEVIN ECKERT, "The Elderly Poor in Downtown San Diego Hotels," *The Gerontologist,* 17: No. 5 (1977), 440–46.

28. FLYNN, B., "The Effectiveness of Nurse Clinicians' Service Delivery," *American Journal of Public Health,* 64: No. 6 (1974), 604–11.

29. "Foster Homes for Older People Help Solve a Growing Problem," Aging, OA No. 118, Washington, D.C.: Office of U.S. Department of Health, Education, and Welfare, August, 1964, 1–4.

30. GARROW, WM., "The Planning and Implementation of a Night Emergency Room Service for Elderly Living in Congregate Housing," *The Gerontologist,* 16: No. 5 (1976), 410–14.

31. GIBBONS, SR. KATHLEEN, "A New Era of Day Care Programs for the Elderly," *Hospital Progress,* 52: No. 11 (1971), 46–49.

32. GOLDFARB, ALVIN, "Institutional Care of the Aged," in *Behavior and Adaptation in Late Life,* eds. Ewald Busse and Eric Pfeiffer. Boston: Little, Brown & Company, 1969, pp. 289–312.

33. ———, "Some Issues in Caring for the Aged," *Canada's Mental Health,* 21: Nos. 3–4 (1973), 6–9.

34. GREENE, BOB, "Home Is a House of Despair," *St. Louis Post-Dispatch,* January 11, 1977, Sec. D, p. 7.

35. HABER, P. A. L., "Hospital-Based Home Care After Myocardial Infarction," *Geriatrics,* 30: (November, 1975), 73–75.

36. HANSSEN, A., et al., "Correlates of Senior Citizen Participation," *The Gerontologist,* 18: No. 2 (1978), 193–99.

37. HAREL, Z., and B. HARD, "On-Site Coordinated Services in Age-Segregated and Age-Integrated Public Housing," *The Gerontologist,* 18: No. 2 (1978), 153–58.

38. HAVIGHURST, ROBERT, "Perspectives on Health Care for the Elderly," *Journal of Gerontological Nursing,* 3: No. 2 (1977), 21–24.

39. "HEW Reports on Long-Term Care Study," *American Journal of Nursing,* 75: No. 9 (1975), 1432–34.

40. HEYMAN, DOROTHY, and GRACE POLANSKY, "Social Casework and Community Services for the Aged," in *Behavior and Adaptation in Late Life,* eds. Ewald Busse and Eric Pfeiffer. Boston: Little, Brown & Company, 1969, pp. 323–43.

41. HIRSCH, CAROL, "Integrating the Nursing Home Resident into a Senior Citizens Center," *The Gerontologist,* 17: No. 3 (1977), 227–34.

42. "Home Care Services Make Economic Sense," *Geriatric Focus,* 7: No. 20 (1968), 1ff.

43. HORN, MILDRED, "Hospital Based Home Care," *American Journal of Nursing,* 75: No. 10 (1975), 1811.

44. HUGHES, D., and G. PETERS, "Organizational Position and Perceptions of Problems in a Nursing Home," *Journal of Gerontology,* 33: No. 2 (1978), 279–87.

45. HURLOCK, ELIZABETH, *Developmental Psychology,* 4th ed. New York: McGraw-Hill Book Company, 1975.

46. KALSON, LEON, "MASH: A Program of Social Interaction Between Institutionalized Aged and Adult Mentally Retarded Persons," *The Gerontologist,* 16: No. 4 (1976), 340–48.

47. KANE, ROBERT, DONNA OLSEN, CONSTANCE THETFORD, and NANO BYRNES, "The Use of Utilization Review Records as a Source of Data on Nursing Home Care," *American Journal of Public Health,* 66: No. 8 (1976), 778–82.

48. KELLOGG, MARY, and ANDREW JAFFE, "Old Folks' Communes," *Newsweek,* April 19, 1976, pp. 97–98.

49. KICK, ELLA, "Delivering Health Care to the Elderly in a High Rise," *Nursing Clinics of North America,* 11: No. 1 (1976), 189–97.

50. KILLEAN, E., "Effect of Geriatric Transfers on Mortality Rates," *Social Work,* 15: (1970), 19–26.

51. LANGLOIS, PATRICIA, and V. TERAMOTO, "Helping Patients Cope with Hospitalization," *Nursing Outlook,* 19: No. 5 (1971), 334–36.

52. LAWTON, M., and M. YAFFE, "Mortality, Morbidity, and Voluntary Change of Residence by Older People," *Journal of American Geriatric Society,* 18: No. 10 (1970), 823–31.

53. ——, E. BRODY, and P. TURNER-MASSEY, "The Relationship of Environmental Factors to Changes in Well-Being," *The Gerontologist,* 18: No. 2 (1978), 133–37.

54. LEINBACH, RAYMOND, "The Aging Participants in an Area Planning Effort," *The Gerontologist,* 17: No. 5 (1977), 453–48.

55. LIEBERMAN, M., "Relationship of Mortality Rates to Entrance to a Home for the Aged," *Geriatrics,* 16: (October, 1961), 515–19.

56. LIPMAN, ALAN, and ROBERT SLATER, "Status and Spatial Appropriation in Eight Homes for Old People," *The Gerontologist,* 17: No. 3 (1977), 250–55.

57. *Missouri Office of Aging: Serving Missouri's Elderly,* Jefferson City: Department of Social Services, Missouri Office of Aging, May, 1975.

58. MCCAULEY, MARY, "Careers in Long-Term Care Scrutinized," *The American Nurse,* 7: No. 7 (1975), 9.

59. ———, "Alternatives to Institutionalization Offered Elderly," *The American Nurse,* 7: No. 6 (1975), 27.

60. MCGUIRE, KATHLEEN, "Skilled Home Health Care," *St. Louis Globe-Democrat,* January 5, 1977, Sec. A, p. 16.

61. MILLER, DULCY, and SUSAN BEER, "Patterns of Friendship Among Patients in a Nursing Home Setting," *The Gerontologist,* 17: No. 3 (1977), 269–75.

62. MOSS, FRANK, "It's Hell to Be Old in the U.S.," *Parade,* July 17, 1977, pp. 9–10.

63. NEWMAN, EVELYN, and SUSAN SHERMAN, "A Survey of Caretakers in Adult Foster Homes," *The Gerontologist,* 17: No. 5 (1977), 436–39.

64. O'BRIEN, JOHN, and GORDON STREIB, eds., *Evaluation Research on Social Programs for the Elderly.* DHEW Publ. No. (OHD)77-20120. Washington, D.C.: United States Government Printing Office, 1977.

65. O'DONNELL, J., J. COLLINS, and S. SCHULER, "Psychosocial Perceptions of the Nursing Home: A Comparative Analysis of Staff, Resident and Cross-Generational Perspectives," *The Gerontologist,* 18: No. 3 (1978), 267–71.

66. "Old Age Homes: Gilded Cages for Domesticated Canaries," *Geriatric Focus,* 9: No. 3 (1970), 3–5.

67. PABLO, RENATO, "Intra-Institutional Relocation: Its Impact on Long-Term Care Patients," *The Gerontologist,* 17: No. 5 (1977), 426–35.

68. PALMORE, ERDMAN, "Total Chance of Institutionalization Among the Aged," *The Gerontologist,* 16: No. 6 (1976), 504–7.

69. PAYNE, BARBARA, "The Older Volunteer: Social Role Continuity and Development," *The Gerontologist,* 17: No. 4 (1977), 355–61.

70. PEPPER, GINETTE, ROBERT KANE, and BARBARA TETEBERG, "Geriatric Nursing Practitioner in Nursing Homes," *American Journal of Nursing,* 76: No. 1 (1976), 62–64.

71. PIEROTTE, DORIS, "Day Health Care for the Elderly," *Nursing Outlook,* 25: No. 8 (1977), 519–23.

72. PINO, C., L. ROSICA, and T. CARTER, "The Differential Effects of Relocation of Nursing Home Patients," *The Gerontologist,* 18: No. 2 (1978), 167–72.

73. PROCTOR, PAM, "Nursing Homes Where Life Is Worth Living," *Parade,* April 25, 1976, pp. 9–12.

74. RATHBONE-MCCUAN, ELOISE, "Geriatric Day Care—A Family Perspective," *The Gerontologist,* 16: No. 6 (1976), 517–21.

75. ROBINSON, DONALD, "You Don't Have to Put Your Parents in a Nursing Home," *Parade,* January 23, 1977, pp. 22–24.

76. ROBINSON, KATHY, "Therapeutic Intervention," *Nursing Clinics of North America,* 9: No. 1 (1974), 89–96.

77. ROSE, MARY, "Problems Families Face in Home Care," *American Journal of Nursing,* 76: No. 3 (1976), 416–18.

78. ROSSMAN, ISADORE, "Options for Care of the Aged Sick," *Hospital Practice,* 12: (1977), 107–16.

79. SCHMANDT, JURGEN, V. BACH, and B. RADIN, "Information and Referral Services for Elderly Welfare Recipients," *The Gerontologist,* 19: No. 1 (1979), 21–27.

80. SCHULZ, RICHARD, and GAIL BRENNER, "Relocation of the Aged: A Review and Theoretical Analysis," *Journal of Gerontology,* 32: No. 3 (1977), 323–33.

81. SCHWAB, SISTER MARILYN, "Nursing Care in Nursing Homes," *American Journal of Nursing,* 76: No. 10 (1976), 1812–15.

82. SEELBACK, WAYNE, "Gender Differences in Expectations for Filial Responsibility," *The Gerontologist,* 17: No. 5 (1977), 421–25.

83. SHERMAN, SUSAN, and E. NEWMAN, "Foster Family Care for the Elderly in New York State," *The Gerontologist,* 17: No. 6 (1977), 513–20.

84. SIEGEL, BARRY, and J. LASKER, "Deinstitutionalizing Elderly Patients: A Program of Resocialization," *The Gerontologist,* 18: No. 3 (1978), 293-300.

85. SKIPPER, JAMES, "The Right to Adequate Health Care: Nursing Implications," *Nursing Digest,* 4: No. 1 (1976), 17–18.

86. SMITH, H., R. DISCENZA, and B. SAXBERG, "Administering Long-Term Care Services: A Decision-Making Perspective," *The Gerontologist,* 18: No. 2 (1978), 159–66.

87. "Socio-Medical Students Involved in Problems of Elderly," *Canada's Mental Health,* 24: No. 2 (1976), 38.

88. SPASOFF, ROBERT, *et al.,* "A Longitudinal Study of Elderly Residents in Long-Stay Institutions," *The Gerontologist,* 18: No. 3 (1978), 281–92.

89. "Study Shows Great Need for Medical and Social Follow-up After Elderly Patients Leave Hospital," *Geriatric Focus,* 8: No. 6 (1969), 2–3.

90. "Telephone Yellow Pages List Aids for Aging," *More Years for Your Life,* 7: No. 9 (1968), 3.

91. TOSELAND, RON, and JAMES SYKES, "Senior Citizens Center Participation and Other Correlates of Life Satisfaction," *The Gerontologist,* 17: No. 3 (1977), 235–41.

92. "Two Studies Reveal Physiologic and Psychologic Benefits to Geriatric Patients Who Inbibe Wine," *Geriatric Focus,* 6: No. 6 (1967), 2–3.

93. WEISSERT, WM., "Two Models of Geriatric Day Care," *The Gerontologist,* 16: No. 5 (1976), 420–27.

94. WESSON, ALBERT, "Some Sociological Characteristics of Long-Term Care," in *Older People and Their Social World,* eds. Arnold Rose and Warren Peterson. Philadelphia: F. A. Davis Company, 1965, pp. 259–71.

95. WILSON, SALLY, "Nursing Home Patients' Rights: Are They Enforceable?" *The Gerontologist,* 18: No. 3 (1978), 255–61.

96. WINN, SHARON, and KENNETH MCCAFFREE, "Characteristics of Nursing Homes Perceived to Be Effective and Efficient," *The Gerontologist,* 16: No. 5 (1976), 415–19.

97. *Workbook on Health for Participants of Community White House Conferences on Aging.* Washington, D.C.: January, 1971.

legal issues affecting the person in later maturity

Study of this chapter will enable you to:

1. Discuss major legislation that provides benefits and services for the elderly.

2. Explore legal concerns for the senior.

3. Determine legal services that are available locally for the senior.

4. Discuss medical and ethical issues of aging and effects of the legislation.

5. Assess the senior's needs for legal assistance, financial benefits, or various services that are available.

6. Inform the senior and his family of available benefits and services, their eligibility, and how to secure them.

7. Refer the senior and his family to specific agencies or services or assist him in securing help.

8. Work with other health team members, public officials, or interested lay persons over a period of time in order to determine the needs of the elderly, effectiveness of current legislation and services, and ways to improve legislation and benefits and services.

9. Continue study of the interrelationship of legal, moral, and ethical aspects of aging and death and their impact on nursing practice.

8

Programs and resources for the elderly, how they came about, and how they interrelate are confusing to many people. Considerable legislation affects the elderly, who can gain the intended benefits when someone helps them through the bureaucracy. This chapter will help you understand the major available programs and where to secure assistance.

Benefit Programs and Pensions

In 1935 the *Social Security Act* was passed, prompted by the rapidly growing numbers of unemployed and older workers separated from the labor force during the Great Depression.[12] Most American workers today can collect Social Security payments upon retirement because of age or disability. The wage earner's dependents and survivors are also eligible.[29]

The 1977 Amendments to the Social Security Act stipulate that the senior 65 years and over collecting social security can work and still collect full social security benefits if the amount earned is $4,000 or less per year. If earnings are above this amount, the Social Security Administration withholds $1 in benefits for each $2 earned over that amount. After age 72 the person can earn as much as he wants and still receive full benefits.[26,35] In 1982, the exempted amount will go to $6,000 and will apply to persons under 69 years rather than 72 years.[26]

Refer persons contemplating retirement to the local Social Security Office. A government publication entitled *You—The Law—And Retirement* is available from the United States Government Printing Office and provides useful information. A free Social Security Administration pamphlet entitled *Estimating Your Social Security Retirement Check* may help the senior figure his benefits if he retires at 62 or at age 65.

Since 1974, persons 65 and older, as well as the blind and the disabled with sharply limited income and resources, may receive federal payments. Supplemental Security Income (SSI) takes the place of the previous Old Age Assistance programs that were administered through state and county departments of public welfare. Application for SSI assistance is made by contacting the local Social Security Office. As of July 1, 1978, SSI, when combined with all other income, gives an individual a minimum monthly income of $189.40 and a couple $284.10.[35] States that were paying higher benefits under Old Age Assistance supplement the SSI payments. Instruct persons investigating SSI to ask about state benefits when they contact the Social Security Office.

Other federal benefit programs are administered by the Railroad Retirement Board, the Civil Service Commission, Bureau of Retirement Insurance and Occupational Health, and the Veterans Administration Benefits Office. If you feel that the potential retiree might qualify for benefits under these programs, refer him to the appropriate agency. Most major cities have a Social Security Administration Office and a Veterans Administration Office. The Railroad Retirement Board's address is 844 Rush Street, Chicago, Illinois. The Civil Service Commission's address is 1900 E. St. N.W., Washington, D.C.[29]

The person should begin seeking information on benefits well in advance of his retirement date; the Social Security Administration suggests at least 3 months. A birth certificate is often required for age and identity verification; locating it may take some time. Alternative documents may have to be secured if the birth certificate is not available. Without the 3-month leeway, the person's benefits may not start when he is eligible.

Encourage those persons who have problems about eligibility for benefits to seek legal advice. Even if they have been told that they are not eligible, the decision may be reversed. Persons who have problems with public agencies can demand a formal hearing. Those who are accompanied by someone with legal training fare better than those who attempt to handle their own cases.[29]

The *Employees Retirement Income Security Act of 1974* guarantees that employees can retain some pension rights if they work for one employer for as few as 5 years. The longer the person is employed, the higher the benefits when he reaches retirement age. The legislation has little impact on people who retired before the bill was enacted, except that their private pensions should be more secure.[29] The Act also gives tax exemptions to people who are not covered by a company pension plan but who deposit money each year into certain types of investments or annuities in order to have a pension when they retire. Any bank, savings and loan association, trust company, or credit union can supply information on these programs, usually referred to as IRA (Individual Retirement Account).

Since remarriage may affect social security pensions and any other benefits, the retiree should contact the agency or company administering the program or seek legal assistance to determine how to maintain benefits.

Health Care Legislation

Since 1966, amendments to the Social Security Law have made it possible for persons over the age of 65 to enroll in *Medicare insurance,* which is composed of Parts A and B.

Part A of Medicare provides *hospital insurance* and helps pay for certain medically necessary services when the senior is a bed patient in a skilled nursing facility or at home receiving services from a home health agency. Part A covers almost all services a person would ordinarily receive when he is a patient. There is, however, a deductible amount that is not reimbursed which must be paid by the senior in each benefit period. The amount is subject to change, depending on increasing medical care costs.[34] Further, certain services that are important to the elderly are not covered, for example, preventive services, prescription drugs used outside the hospital, eyeglasses and hearing aids, institutional care with skilled nursing care for more than 100 days, and long-term care in an institution providing custodial care.[33] Anyone 65 or older and who is entitled to Social Security or Railroad Retirement is automatically covered under Part A.

Part B of Medicare provides *medical insurance,* which is a voluntary plan in which the eligible person may enroll for a monthly premium. These premiums are subject to change as medical costs escalate, and they are automatically deducted from monthly checks for Social Security, Railroad Retirement, and Civil Service benefits. People who do not receive any of these benefits as part of their employment pay their premiums directly to the Social Security Administration.[34] Part B helps pay for doctor's and outpatient services, medical supplies, home health care, outpatient physical and speech therapy, and other services. A deductible amount must be met by the patient for each calendar year.[33] Routine checkups, outpatient services, and home health care without prior hospital care are not covered.[31]

A person approaching age 65 who has not received Medicare information should telephone the nearest district office of the Social Security Administration at least 3 months before his birthday even if the person does not intend to apply for Social Security benefits.[29] He can qualify for Medicare even if he continues to work. *Your Medicare Handbook,* a publication of the Social Security Administration, is invaluable in helping the person understand exactly what costs are covered.

As a result of the 1974 amendments to the Social Security Act, health facilities participating in Medicare funding must meet standards that assure that they provide high-quality health care. The Act outlines 14 Patient's Rights which must be in writing and implemented by skilled nursing facilities that receive Medicare funds. The patient, his guardian, next of kin, or sponsoring agency must be informed of these rights, which are briefly described in Table 8.1.[8]

Each hospital and skilled nursing facility has a Utilization Review Committee to assure the most effective use of facility services by Medicare patients. It reviews admissions on a sample basis and all long-stay cases.[34]

The senior may want to carry additional health insurance. A number of profit and nonprofit organizations offer policies that are designed for people covered by Medicare. The State Insurance Commissioner should be contacted before such insurance is purchased. That office can advise about a specific policy or company and may also be able to provide information on the necessity or advisability of purchasing such insurance.[29]

Medicaid may also be available to low-income persons, whether or not they are enrolled under Medicare. Medicaid often pays for services that are not covered by Medicare, such as eye glasses, dental care, prescribed drugs, and long-term nursing care at home. Medicaid pays for a wide variety of medical and hospital services for people who are ineligible for Medicare.[13] The person should contact the local Department of Social Services or Welfare Office or the state or Area Agency on Aging to learn whether or not he qualifies for Medicaid. The problem is that in almost one-half the states the person cannot qualify unless he is destitute, with so little money or possessions that he cannot meet daily living expenses, even with Medicaid.[33] Medicaid is administered by the state government according to federal guidelines. But each state sets its own requirements for eligibility, and states vary greatly.[31]

TABLE 8.1   Patients' Rights

The governing body of the institution formulates written policies about rights and responsibilities of patients. The institution, through the administrator, is responsible for development of and adherence to these policies. The staff are trained to implement these rights.

The patient admitted to the agency is:

1. Informed fully prior to, at admission, and during the stay of rights and regulations governing patient behavior and responsibility.
2. Informed fully prior to, at admission, and during the stay of services available and related charges, charges not covered by Social Security, or those above the basic per diem rate.
3. Informed fully by a physician of his medical condition, unless contraindicated, and invited to participate in planning his medical treatment. The person may refuse to participate in experimental research. Any contraindications to informing the patient are documented by the physician in the chart.
4. Transferred or discharged only for medical reasons, his welfare, or the welfare of other patients, or for nonpayment for his stay, except as prohibited by Titles 18 and 19 of the Social Security Act. The person is informed about the transfer or discharge in advance; this record documents informing the patient as well as the reason for transfer/discharge.
5. Encouraged and assisted to exercise his rights as a patient and citizen, to voice grievances, suggest changes in policies or services to staff or outside representatives, without fear of restraint, interference, coercion, discrimination, or reprisal.
6. Permitted to manage personal financial affairs. At least a quarterly accounting of costs for care should be given to him.
7. Freed from mental and physical abuse, chemical restraints, and physical restraints except as ordered by the physician to protect himself or others.
8. Assured confidentiality of his personal and medical records. He may or may not approve their release to someone outside the agency, except upon transfer to another health care institution or if required by law or third-party payers.
9. Treated with consideration and respect, as an individual with dignity, and accorded privacy in treatment and care of personal needs.
10. Not required to pay for facility services that are not included as part of his treatment plan.
11. Permitted to associate and communicate privately with persons of his choice, send and receive personal mail unopened unless medically contraindicated, as documented by his physician in the medical record.
12. Permitted to meet and participate with social, religious, and community groups at his discretion, unless medically contraindicated as documented by the physician in his record.
13. Permitted to retain and use personal clothing and possessions as space and his condition permit, unless medically contraindicated as documented by the physician in his record.
14. Permitted to visit privately with his spouse; if both are patients, they may share a room unless medically contraindicated as documented by the physician.[8]

Job Legislation

In 1965 the Older Americans Act was passed, creating the Administration of Aging (AoA) as an operating agency of the Department of Health, Education and Welfare. The agency works parallel with the Social Security Administration and the Public Health Service. The Administration on Aging cuts across all areas of federal programming and has three operating programs within itself: (1) grants to states for community service projects, (2) research and demonstration projects, and (3) training programs. Two of these objectives focus primarily on employment with no age discrimination and on meaningful activity within the widest range of civic, cultural, and recreational opportunities.[12] Initially, the act provided funds for the creation of an Agency on Aging in each state.

The purposes of the state Office of Aging include to:

1. Provide consultation and assistance to agencies and individuals in developing services for the elderly.
2. Conduct studies of problems, needs, and conditions of the elderly.
3. Develop and implement a statewide plan for programs for the aging.
4. Administer federal funds made available to the state under the Older Americans Act.
5. Provide fiscal and technical support to the Area Agencies on Aging.
6. Educate the public about concerns of the senior population.
7. Serve as a clearinghouse for exchange of information and ideas on aging.[28]

Each state is divided into geographical regions which have an Area Agency of Aging to plan and coordinate services and programs for the senior citizens in the specific area. These Area Agencies do not provide direct services but work through existing organizations, such as churches, public and private social service agencies, and community action groups.[28]

In 1973 amendments called for an Older Americans Community Employment Act to be administered by the Department of Labor. A new agency, ACTION, was created to handle the RSVP and Foster Grandparents Programs and administer the Domestic Volunteer Service Act. Employment opportunities through federally aided programs[12] are summarized in Table 8-2. Other employment programs for older people are sponsored by national voluntary organizations. They include:

1. Senior Aides, administered by the National Council of Senior Citizens, 1511 K. Street N.W., Washington, D.C. 20005.
2. Senior Community Service Project, sponsored by the National Council on the Aging, 1828 L Street N.W., Washington, D.C. 20036.
3. Senior Community Aides sponsored by NRTA/AARP, 1909 K. Street N.W., Washington, D.C. 20006.[29]

TABLE 8.2 Federally Funded Employment Opportunities for the Senior Citizen

Program	Agency Administering	Eligibility	Job Description	Compensation
Foster Grandparent Program	ACTION Foster Grandparent Program 806 Connecticut N.W. Washington, D.C. 20525	Low-income men and women 60 and over who are in good health.	Work for 4 hours a day 5 days a week. Devote 2 hours each day to each of 2 children who are physically, emotionally, and mentally handicapped in institutions or private settings.	Transportation allowance, $32 per week, hot meals while in service, accident insurance, and annual physical exam.
Retired Senior Volunteer Program (RSVP)	ACTION/RSVP Address as above.	Retired men and women over 60.	Service in a variety of agencies, organizations, and institutions designated as volunteer stations. These include courts, schools, libraries, day-care centers, hospitals, nursing homes, Boy and Girl Scout offices, economic development agencies, and other community service centers.	Reimbursed upon request for transportation to and from assignment, meals, and out-of-pocket expenses associated with their service.
Volunteers in Service to America (VISTA)	ACTION/VISTA Address as above.	Men and women of any age with particular talents and experience. Minimum one year commitment.	Work in impoverished urban or rural areas with migrant families, on Indian reservations, in institutions for mentally handicapped, or in Job Corp Centers. May help people with problems in education, day care, drug abuse, corrections, health, legal aid, and city planning.	Attend 4 to 6 weeks training as needed. Monthly food and housing allowance, $75 monthly for incidental expense, and $50 monthly readjustment allowance on completion of service.

TABLE 8.2 (*Continued*)

Program	Agency Administering	Eligibility	Job Description	Compensation
Peace Corps	ACTION/Peace Corps Address as above.	Older men and women actively recruited as well as others of all ages. Minimum 2-year commitment.	Work in developing nations with programs in agriculture, mathematics, and science teaching; teacher and manpower training; vocational trades; business and public administration; and natural resource development and conservation.	Attend 12 to 14 week orientation and training, mostly in country of service. Transportation provided to training, to and from assignment, and for home leaves and emergencies. Monthly allowance for food, travel, rent, and all medical needs. Readjustment allowance of $75 monthly payable on completion of service. A $10,000 optional life insurance coverage under the Federal Employees Compensation Act for disabilities incurred during training or service.
Senior Companion Program	ACTION/SENIOR COMPANION PROGRAM Address as above.	Low-income men and women age 60 and over.	Serve adults with special needs in their homes, nursing homes, or other institutions.	Patterned after Foster Grandparent Program.
Action Cooperative Volunteers	ACTION/Cooperative Volunteers Address as above.	People of all ages wishing to contribute one year of service.	Local projects that help communities tackle problems of poverty and environment. Service in public and nonprofit agencies involved in elementary and secondary education; adult basic education; human, social, and environmental projects, particularly those related to poverty; and economic development.	Biweekly living allowance. Medical insurance, $75 monthly for incidentals, $50 per month set aside for readjustment.

Program	Contact	Eligibility	Description	Benefits
Service Corp of Retired Executives (SCORE)	SCORE Small Business Administration, 1441 L Street, N.W. Washington, D.C. 20416	Retired businessmen and women with management expertise.	Work as counselors to owners or managers of small businesses and community organizations in need of management counseling.	Reimbursed upon request for out-of-pocket expenses.
Senior Community Service Employment Program (SCSEP)	Office of National Programs Employment and Training Administration, U.S. Department of Labor, Attn: Title 14, 601 D Street, N.W., Room 6402 Washington, D.C. 20213	Economically disadvantaged persons 55 years and older.	Serve in part-time community service jobs, such as in day-care centers, nutrition programs, and beautification, conservation, and restoration projects. Projects sponsored primarily by: Green Thumb, Inc. (National Farmers' Union), National Council of Aging, National Council of Senior Citizens, National Retired Teachers' Association (NTRA), American Association of Retired Persons (AARP), U.S. Department of Agriculture's Forest Service.	Receive $2.50 per hour. Yearly physical exam. Personal and job-related counseling. Sometimes placement in regular subsidized jobs.
Comprehensive Employment and Training Act	Department of Labor gives grants to state and local units to establish programs. Contact Manpower Office, Human Development Department, or the Employment and Training Administration of the local community or state.	Economically disadvantaged, the underemployed, and the unemployed of all ages.	Programs designed to help workers compete for, secure, and hold challenging, meaningful jobs.	

Nutrition Legislation

The National Nutrition Program for Older Americans is administered by the Administration on Aging. It is designed to provide inexpensive, nutritionally sound meals to older citizens, particularly those with low incomes or those in greatest need. The 1972 amendments to the Older Americans Act state why the Nutrition Program was considered necessary. Generally, many older persons do not eat adequately because they cannot afford to. Many cannot shop for or prepare well-balanced meals. Some feel too rejected and lonely to prepare and eat a meal alone. Other physiological, psychological, social, and economic changes that occur with aging result in malnutrition and further physical and mental deterioration.[19]

Nutrition Projects have been established throughout the country which provide at least one hot meal a day, at least 5 days a week, to Americans 60 years and over and the spouse of any age. The meal must provide one-third of the Recommended Daily Allowance of nutrients as published by the Food and Nutrition Board. Meals are usually provided for groups in public settings, such as schools, churches, community or senior citizen centers, or public housing. Escort and transportation service is also a part of the projects. Interested persons should contact their state Agency on Aging or the local Office of Aging. The Nutrition Program is not a home-delivered activity, but it will provide home-delivered meals to regular participants who from time to time cannot attend the meal service site.[19]

The Nutrition Program's sites act as centers of activity for participants. The senior can eat a meal and also receive health and other supportive services, such as information and referral, transportation, health and welfare counseling, consumer education, legal advice, shopping assistance, or information on housing, income maintenance, crime prevention, and the aging process.[19] Further, the program reduces isolation by combining food and friendship. This program serves a need, as shown by the number of participants. In 1975 an average of 228,000 meals were served daily at 4400 sites.[8] In 1976 these estimated figures increased by about 30 percent. However, many seniors do not know about or choose not to participate for various reasons, although these people are in need of better meals.

All participants are given an opportunity to pay for all or part of the cost of the meal. No one, however, may be turned away because of inability to pay; there is no means tests.[19] Each participant determines for himself what he is able to contribute.

Food stamps are available to low-income people. Eligibility is determined by the local welfare department; in rural areas the Agriculture Department Extension Agent may be able to provide eligibility information. The stamps can be used to buy home-delivered meals, meals served in a central place, or for groceries.[29]

Housing Legislation

Low-cost public housing units are available for elderly persons who have very low incomes. Moderate-cost housing is often sponsored by churches and other nonprofit agencies with help from the federal government. Waiting lists for low- and moderate-cost housing are usually very long. The Department of Housing and Urban Development (HUD) and the Farmers Home Administration of the Department of Agriculture are helping states and communities expand such housing. The local Office of Aging Information and Referral Service should be able to provide information about housing.[29]

Transportation Legislation

The Department of Transportation and the Administration on Aging have recently initiated a working agreement pledging mutual cooperation to achieve increased mobility for older persons by improving their access to public and specialized transportation systems in urban areas. About 1000 transportation projects exist for the senior in the United States; most are supported by the state Agency on Aging.

Some communities, with assistance from the federal government, make available coupons for transportation similar in concept to food stamps. The stamps may be used for any variety of public or private transportation.

The National Mass Transportation Act of 1974 requires that any public transit system receiving funds under the Act charge half-fare or less to the elderly.[29]

There is also a movement to make public transportation barrier-free through the use of specially designed vehicles that eliminate steps, narrow aisles, and other inconvenient features.[6]

Information and Referral Service Legislation

The 1973 amendments to the Older Americans Act required that state and area Agencies on Aging provide information and referral services to assist seniors in securing needed services. Coordination of information and referral services and government information services should enable the older citizen to obtain any and all types of information about aging and available nationwide resources that might be important to him.

In 1974 the Administration on Aging created the Clearinghouse on Aging. It focuses on a broad range of information about problems for the aged, their impact on the social system, and subjects such as nutrition, housing, and supportive social services. The Clearinghouse is charged with (1) collecting, analyzing, and disseminating information about the elderly and their needs; (2) providing information to agencies and organizations concerning problems for the aging; (3) encouraging establishment of state and area information and referral services to meet the needs of the elderly; and (4) stimulating other agencies to prepare and disseminate information.[4]

The Information and Referral Service in a particular locale may be provided by the area Agency on Aging. In many places, however, another local, public, or voluntary organization has this responsibility. If you or the senior are seeking information, look for "Area Agency on Aging" or "Information and Referral" in the telephone directory.[13] If neither is listed, then anyone who gives service to the elderly may be able to advise how to contact the local information and referral service.

Nursing Process and Federal Legislation

Federal legislation has been enacted that influences every aspect of the senior's life. Stay abreast of changing legislation and be aware of available programs and resources so that you can describe them to the senior and his family and help them to secure necessary and appropriate assistance. You may need to encourage the senior to collect benefits that he has earned. The senior may feel ashamed to take a "handout" from the government, for example, Social Security payments, which he has contributed to. If you work with people in late life, you will become aware of the needs that exist. Become involved in planning and advisory councils supported by local or state offices on aging, or contact local, state, and federal legislators and officials. Your ideas and work with public officials can make a difference.

LEGAL ISSUES AFFECTING THE PERSON IN LATER MATURITY

Wills

Everyone should have a *will, a declaration of what the person wants done with his property after his death.*[5] Often the senior puts off making a will; if he dies without one, his property will be distributed according to his state's law for intestate succession. This varies from state to state and may not provide for the same contingencies as if the person himself had made a will prior to death. The will should be reviewed periodically, since the passage of time can bring about changes in circumstances relative to persons and property which the senior may desire to provide for.

The senior's mental ability is a factor in making a valid will. He must be of sound mind, which for will making means that he can understand (1) the type and amount of property which is his to pass on to others, (2) the persons who are the natural objects of his generosity and their claims on him, (3) the disposition of property that he is making, and (4) the relationship between these factors and making an orderly bequest of the property.[5] Guardianship does not necessarily mean that the senior does not possess mental capacity to make a will. As long as the four requirements outlined above are met, illiteracy, moral depravity, extreme old age, severe illness, or great weakness will not invalidate a will. Fraud and duress, however, will invalidate a will.

Formalities of will making are determined by the statutes of the state. Generally, the will should be in writing and must be signed (a mark can suffice if properly identified by one who can write). Two competent witnesses are usually also required to sign the will.[5] An oral will is sometimes recognized, but it is frowned upon by the courts. States have certain restrictions that must be met before an oral will can be recognized as valid. Since statutes vary from state to state, emphasize that legal assistance should be secured before making a will to ensure that the senior's wishes are honored.

Gifts

Personal property, which includes everything owned by the person exclusive of real estate, may be disposed of by *gift.* In order for a gift to be valid, the donor must (1) have the mental capacity and intent to make the gift and (2) transfer control over the gift to the receiver. Further, the receiver must accept the gift. *The gift made in imminent expectation of death* is called a *gift causa mortis.* It is made on the condition that property shall belong to the receiver upon death of the donor but is revokable by the donor prior to death or if the donor recovers.[3]

Since mental competency is required for the making of wills and gifts, you must accurately assess the senior's mental functioning and record observations if he is involved in either of these legal activities. The record may become evidence if the will or gift is contested.

Incompetence to Manage Property

Mental incompetence means that a person is unable to take care of his business and legal affairs. In most states this is decided in a court of law, but in a few states a senior hospitalized for mental illness is considered to be mentally incompetent as well. The designation of mental incompetence carries with it the prohibition from (1) making contracts, (2) buying and selling property, (3) deciding what to do with money or estate, (4) marrying, (5) divorcing, and (6) implementing other rights of citizenship we take for granted. The label incompetent indicates that the person cannot enter into legal relationships with others. His signature is practically worthless. Before the person is declared to be incompetent, there should be a mandatory court hearing, notification of the person as to his rights, and representation by legal counsel. If the person is found to be mentally incompetent, a guardian, conservator, or committee will be appointed to take care of his legal affairs. The only legitimate purpose of an incompetency finding should be to preserve the person's assets. However, this is not always the case. If you suspect that some unscrupulous person is trying to gain control of the senior's assets by declaring him mentally incompetent, bring it to the attention of the administrator of the institution.[11] Or seek legal advice on how to proceed.

If you are caring for someone who has been declared incompetent, remember that he cannot give his own consent for procedures or surgery; his guardian must be contacted before acting.

Restoration of legal competence is possible, but in many states the law is vague, informal, or unduly burdensome. However, the person who has apparently recovered the ability to handle his own legal affairs should have the opportunity to have his legal competence restored.[11]

Commitment to a Psychiatric Hospital or Ward

Sometimes the elderly person who becomes cognitively impaired is admitted to a psychiatric hospital, usually by another party rather than voluntarily. The admission may or may not be an emergency.

Emergency procedures vary from state to state. In some states a person who is cognitively impaired cannot be hospitalized by a family member or guardian until after the person has had an opportunity to appear before a judge and be heard. The judge cannot order hospitalization until doctors have certified that the person is mentally ill and dangerous to himself and others. In some states the judicial hearing is not required. Emergency hospitalization is usually for a specific limited period of time; in almost all states the period is less than 30 days.

Involuntary nonemergency hospitalization is usually for an indefinite period or for long periods which can be renewed. The procedures governing involuntary hospitalization also vary from state to state. Most states require a court order after the opportunity for a judicial hearing.

If the hospital begins involuntary commitment proceedings while the senior is a patient, usually at the doctor's or family's request, the senior is not permitted to leave.[11]

A patient who is about to be involuntarily committed should know that in many states he has the right to a judicial hearing at which he can be represented by legal counsel. Also, he should know that he cannot be detained against his wishes after notifying the hospital that he wishes to leave, beyond the required time period following voluntary admission.

Patients who have doubts about their legal rights regarding hospitalization should obtain the services of a lawyer. Studies show that patients have a much better chance of opposing hospitalization and gaining release if they are represented by a lawyer. The court can appoint a free lawyer if the patient requests one and cannot afford to retain his own counsel. The appointment of a lawyer is not automatic; failure to request one will be presumed to be a waiver of the right to counsel.[11]

Protective Services for the Elderly

Often elderly citizens experience difficulty because of diminished physical or mental health or they are neglected and in need of special protection and support services. When the person becomes physically unable to care for himself or becomes confused about day-to-day routines, the community may have to make provisions for protecting and supporting him. If the person has family, it usually helps the person manage daily affairs. The senior who needs help is the one who has no relatives and no caring persons or whose relatives do not institute treatment in his behalf or may actually be abusive.

Protective services are defined as social, legal, physical, and counseling services for an older person living in the community who is so physically or mentally impaired that he is unable to manage his own affairs without serious consequences to himself or others and who has no relative or other person presently willing or able to act on his behalf.[9] Protective services are characterized by two features: the coordinated delivery of services to adults at risk and the actual or potential authority to make decisions about use of services for the person's benefit.[2] Communities that have recognized this need have attempted to organize community resources to work together, so that a single vital service, or a broad spectrum of aid, can be quickly mobilized to sustain the elderly person whose personal capabilities have faltered. For example, the Protective Services for the Aged project serving the near-northside of Chicago is organized by the Welfare Council of Metropolitan Chicago and funded by a National Institute of Mental Health grant. The project's purpose is to draw various community services into a supportive network that can reach out and befriend the community's aged who are no longer able to manage by themselves.[32]

Several problems are paramount. Getting the services to where they are needed is difficult. A detection or surveillance system through which needy cases can be found is a must. How often have we heard of an elderly person found frozen to death in his unheated housing because utility bills were not paid. Police, community health workers, neighborhood health aids, utility meter readers, postmen, clergy, and other community workers should all be aware of elderly persons residing in their areas of responsibility and should observe for and report suspicious conditions. A *telephone reassurance service, an organized program that calls elderly or incapacitated persons who live alone to check on their well-being,* can help with surveillance and detection of persons in need. If the person does not answer at the appointed time, an emergency life line goes into immediate action. As prearranged, a neighbor, nurse, or policeman makes a house call; if a crisis is discovered, the person's doctor and relatives, if any, are notified.

When the person in need is discovered, some way to remove him from his residence to a hospital or institution or to administer care on the premises must be available. But a legal problem is encountered. If the person refuses treatment or refuses to be removed from his residence, the caretaker leaves himself open to a charge of assault and battery or trespassing. In most jurisdictions today, it is necessary to go to court and have the person declared mentally incompetent. If the senior has no family, often no one is willing to do this. If family members refuse to go to court, little can be done to force them. Also, the time involved is often protracted; very often by the time the legal complications are finally overcome, the person is dead or so seriously ill that recovery is doubtful. An example of such a case was an elderly woman who broke her hip. She was able to get to a couch where she sat until she died. She refused to let her son take her to the hospital or to move her because of pain. The community health nurse worked diligently trying to get her to necessary care. When the nurse finally convinced the son to get needed care, it was too late.

Therefore, legal services are obviously one of the main resources needed for a protective service project.

Sources of Legal Service

The Bar Association or the Lawyer's Reference Service, listed in the local telephone directory, will usually provide information on available legal services. For a nominal fee, the reference service will review an individual's problem and suggest if the services of an attorney are needed. If they are needed, the reference service will contact an attorney for the person.

Free legal services on civil matters are available to low-income persons through the Legal Aid Society. Title XX of the Social Security Act provides funding for legal services for the elderly and disabled within certain income levels. The Area Office on Aging can give more information on this program. Free legal services for low-income people in some criminal cases are usually supplied by the public defender's office.

The American Civil Liberties Union defends and advances free speech, fair procedures, and equal protection under the law through court or legislative action. Other organizations may supply legal counsel in specific situations. For example, some trade unions have arrangements with attorneys to offer legal assistance to their members. The National Association for the Advancement of Colored People (NAACP) provides legal counsel and guidance in specific cases dealing with economic and political problems of Blacks. Other organizations should be checked to see if they offer legal services. Also, government agencies responsible for specific programs or services usually have a department or a person who handles complaints and problems brought to their attention. The Bar Association of the state or local community may have a listing, available upon request, of agencies, addresses, and phone numbers, and description of problems they handle.

Nursing Process and Legal Services

Anyone may experience situations that have legal repercussions, but the senior may have special needs and problems. He may also experience difficulty in getting needed legal help because of reduced mental or physical capacity, limited income, or lack of resources for contacting help, such as transportation or telephone. Be aware of the available legal services in your community and where and how they can be utilized so that you can teach the elderly person about them or encourage him to use them if necessary.

Be aware in your daily care of the elderly that *informed consent is a legal doctrine designed to protect a person from unwarranted medical intrusions upon his body.* Because aging processes can affect the senior's capacity to give voluntary, knowing, competent consent, you must make every possible effort to see that he does understand the medical diagnostic procedure or treatment or research experimentation to which he is consenting.[2,18,23]

MEDICAL, ETHICAL, AND LEGAL CONSIDERATIONS OF AGING

Death with Dignity and Living Wills

Prolonging life through mechanical devices has become possible as a result of resuscitative procedures and automatic respirators. In most states death is defined as the cessation of cardiac and respiratory activity.[3] Yet, these functions can be artificially stimulated and maintained. Thus, some authorities feel that a new legal definition of death should be adopted. The definition of death would be based on the Harvard University criteria established in 1968: the cessation of brain functioning determined by (1) total lack of response to external painful stimuli, (2) absence of spontaneous heartbeat and respirations, (3) absence of reflexes, with pupils dilated, fixed, and unresponsive to light, and (4) a flat encephalogram for two consecutive times within 24 hours when the test has been done by competent personnel with correctly functioning equipment.[6,24] Persons under the effect of hypothermia or suffering from an overdose of central nervous system depressants would be excluded from these criteria.[24] However, definitions of death attempting to incorporate these criteria, such as in Kansas, have met with criticism. The American Medical Association (AMA) suggests that death should be determined by the physician's clinical judgment, that is, based on currently accepted criteria. The AMA's position provides for changing medical technology and for broadening medical knowledge that a statutory definition could not provide. Some feel that the only one who will benefit from the new definition based on absence of electroencephalogram (EEG) activity is the transplant surgeon. He will know when it is safe to begin planning for taking transplant organs without the danger of legal accusations of homocide, negligence, or abandonment.[7]

This author feels that a new definition of death will not clarify the issue; if anything, it will probably cloud the issue more. By removing the pronouncing of death from the physician's clinical judgment and by basing it on the electrical impulses recorded by a machine on a piece of paper, we are effectively making death an impersonal, mechanical, and unemotional event. Theoretically, the physician would never have to see the patient if brain wave presence were the primary criterion. Death is not impersonal; it is not mechanical; and it is not unemotional. Therefore, the clinical judgment of the physician who examines the total patient (of course, using mechanical aids) should remain the primary determiner of when death has occurred.

Does a right to die exist? More and more people are asking this question. Certainly it is not a right guaranteed by the Constitution, although recently some court cases have spoken of a right to die. Some refer to this issue as death with dignity. Some confuse the issue with *euthanasia*, which generally means *to cause death painlessly to end suffering.*[14] The issue becomes more confusing when voluntary and involuntary and direct and indirect euthanasia are spoken of. *Voluntary euthanasia means that the person consents to another to have his life painlessly ended,* perhaps by an injection; *involuntary means that life is terminated without the person's consent. Direct euthanasia means that the person ends his own life* (suicide); *indirect refers to a request to another to terminate life when the self is dysfunctional or unable to participate in the act of termination. Direct or active involuntary* refers to *mercy killing,* which legally is murder. *Indirect or passive involuntary euthanasia means that certain measures are withheld that are essential for life.*[15] For example, oxygen is not started; antibiotics are not ordered for pneumonia; infection is allowed to take hold; or cardiac resuscitation is withheld from the cancer patient. Or large doses of narcotics may be given for pain control knowing that the patient's death is hastened. The latter form of involuntary euthanasia occurs most commonly in hospitals and nursing homes, but there is no legal support for it.

The Supreme Court of the United States has recognized a right to privacy, and many feel that when the issue of the right to die comes before it, the Court will include the decision to choose to die under the right to privacy.[25]

Today, most courts will not require that any one submit to *life-prolonging treatments or procedures, which are measures only intended to prolong life of a person suffering from a terminal illness. Life-preserving treatments, measures absolutely essential if the person's life is to be saved,* will be ordered for infants and incompetents, even against the wishes of a guardian, and for adults who have dependents. Competent adults who have no one dependent on them for support have been recently recognized by courts to have the right to choose what is to be done to their bodies, even if the refusal of medically indicated care may result in death. Health-improving measures generally have not been ordered by courts for infants or incompetents if their parents or guardians refuse.[25]

A very recent New Jersey case concerned a comatose adult whose life was being artificially supported by a respirator. Her parents sought to have the machine turned off. The physicians, fearing homocide charges or negligence litigation, refused. The parents went to court. The New Jersey Supreme Court held that the right to privacy could be asserted by her family in her behalf since she was unable to do it for herself. Further, if the attending physicians decided that there was no reasonable possibility of her emerging from the comatose state to a cognitive, vital one, the machines could be discontinued without any civil or criminal liability.[16]

Many adults in later maturity fear that when death approaches they will not be permitted to die but will have their lives prolonged by heroic measures and machines, at the expense of themselves and their loved ones. It is being suggested that this can be avoided by drawing up and signing what is referred to as a living will. The ***Living Will*** *is a document indicating that in the future the person does not want to have life unnecessarily prolonged if he becomes radically incapacitated by an accident or illness.* This document has no legal effect at present, but it does serve to make known the wishes of the one who is making the will.

Free sample copies of the Living Will can be obtained by writing the Euthanasia Education Council, 250 W. 57th Street, Room 831, New York, New York 10019.   A similar document, entitled Christian Affirmation of Life, is available for Catholics. It is available from the Catholic Hospital Association, 1438 S. Grand Ave., St. Louis, Missouri 63104. The person who signs such a document should be advised to give copies to his closest family member and also to his physician, lawyer, and clergyman.

California has passed a Natural Death Act and has become the only state to grant terminally ill patients the right to authorize withdrawal of life-sustaining procedures when death is believed imminent. The Act provides for a written directive in a specified form to be signed by the patient and instructs doctors to withhold life-sustaining procedures in the event of terminal illness. Life-sustaining procedures are defined by the law "as any medical procedure or intervention which utilizes mechanical or other artificial means to restore or supplant a vital function which . . . would serve only to artificially prolong the moment of death." Other conditions include:

1. A 14-day grace period between signing and taking effect.
2. Two witnesses are required (they may not be relatives, the physician, or employees of the health care facility where he is staying).
3. Women must agree to suspend the directive if they become pregnant.
4. The form must be renewed every 5 years, and it must become a part of the person's medical record.
5. The form is revokable by the patient's either marking on it or verbally expressing his views or directing his physician to revoke it regardless of the patient's mental state.
6. Failure of a physician to carry out the Living Will does not carry a penalty although it "shall constitute unprofessional conduct," which could lead to license suspension or revokation."[27]

We will probably see more of this kind of legislation in the future.

Euthanasia Legislation

Every year euthanasia legislation is introduced into various state legislatures. To date, none of this legislation has been passed.

Active intervention to terminate life is murder both legally and morally. Christians and Jews condemn any form of active intervention, but they do condone the withdrawal of any measure that may be artificially delaying death. Christian moralists distinguish between ordinary and extraordinary medical and surgical procedures. *Ordinary measures refer to whatever treatment a patient can obtain or receive without imposing an excessive burden on himself or others.* The senior undergoing treatment and those ministering to him are bound to use the ordinary means of preserving life and restoring health. *Extraordinary means are those that are very costly, painful, difficult, or dangerous.* One is not obligated to undergo extraordinary treatment, and the physician is not obligated to administer it when the patient cannot be consulted.[5,21]

Nursing Process and Medical, Ethical, and Legal Considerations

Medical, ethical, and legal questions are becoming more involved and more complex every day. Increasing depth of knowledge and advances in technology are making life-sustaining a possibility almost indefinitely, but the quality of that life may be little more than a vegetative existence. Multidisciplinary approaches to these questions will be required now and in the future. Medical technology needs to be studied for its moral and legal implications. Thus, ethics committees for hospitals and other institutions are being suggested. In their meetings all questions could be thoroughly reviewed, studied, and then rationally and objectively decided.[16,17] Yet, there may also be disadvantages to these committees.[17]

As a nurse, you will encounter many situations that involve decisions of an ethical, legal, and medical nature. The search for answers is constant and is not easy. Pursue formal and independent study of ethical and moral issues. Discuss your ideas with others; listen to the ideas of others. Base your practice on a moral, ethical, and clinically sound framework.

REFERENCES

1. "AoA Nutrition Program, From Small Start, Now Serving 228,000 Meals Daily," *Aging,* No. 247, AoA Publication No. (OHD) 75-20143 (May, 1975), 20–21.

2. BERKOWITZ, SANDRA, "Informed Consent, Research, and the Elderly," *The Gerontologist,* 18: No. 3 (1978), 237–43.

3. BLACK, HENRY CAMPBELL, *Black's Law Dictionary,* rev. 4th ed. St. Paul, Minn.: West Publishing Co., 1968.

4. "Clearinghouse on Aging: Its Goals and Functions," *Aging*, No. 247, AoA Publication No. (OHD) 75-20143 (May, 1975), 21–22.

5. CREIGHTON, HELEN, *Law Every Nurse Should Know*, 3rd ed. Philadelphia: W. B. Saunders Company, 1975.

6. CURRAN, WILLIAM, and E. DONALD SHAPIRO, *Law, Medicine and Forensic Science*, 2nd ed. Boston: Little, Brown & Company, 1970.

7. ———, *Law, Medicine, and Forensic Science* (1974 Supplement). Boston: Little, Brown & Company, 1974.

8. "Department of Health, Education, and Welfare, Social Security Administration. Skilled Nursing Facilities. Health Insurance for the Aged and Disabled; General Administration," *Federal Register*, 39: No. 193 (October 3, 1974), 35774–35778.

9. EHRLICH, PHYLLIS, "Protective Services Study Report for Metropolitan St. Louis," sponsored by National Association of Social Workers-Task Force on Aging; Community Professional Ad Hoc Committee on Protective Services; and St. Louis University-Institute of Applied Gerontology, October, 1974–June, 1975.

10. "Employment and Volunteer Opportunities for Older People," *HEW Fact Sheet AoA*. DHEW Publication No. (OHD) 76-20233. Washington, D.C.: U.S. Department of Health, Education, and Welfare, Office of Human Development, Administration of Aging, June, 1976.

11. ENNIS, BRUCE, and LOREN SIEGEL, *The Rights of Mental Patients—An American Civil Liberties Union Handbook*. New York: Avon Books, 1973.

12. "Federal Action for Aging Began in 1930's: What Has Happened Since," *Aging*, No. 247, AoA Publication No. (OHD) 75-20143 (May, 1975), 13–15.

13. "Federal Programs to Assist the Elderly," DHEW Publication No. (OHD) 77-20229, *HEW Fact Sheet AoA*. Washington, D.C.: U.S. Department of Health, Education, and Welfare, Office of Human Development, Administration on Aging, December, 1976.

14. GURALNIK, DAVID, ed., *Webster's New World Dictionary*, 2nd college ed. New York: The World Publishing Company, 1972.

15. HENDIN, DAVID, *Death as a Fact of Life*. New York: Warner Paperback Library Edition, 1973, pp. 60–82.

16. *In the Matter of Karen Quinlan*, 70 N.J. 10, 355 A. 2d 617, 1976.

17. LESTZ, PAULA, "A Committee to Decide the Quality of Life," *American Journal of Nursing*, 77: No. 5 (1977), 862–64.

18. MAKARUSHKA, JULIA, and ROBERT McDONALD, "Informed Consent, Research, and Geriatric Patients:The Responsibility of Institutional Review Committees," *The Gerontologist*, 19: No. 1 (1979), 61–66.

19. "National Nutrition Program for Older Americans," *HEW Fact Sheet AoA*. DHEW Publication No. (OHD) 76-20230. Washington, D.C.: U.S. Department of Health, Education and Welfare, Office of Human Development, Administration on Aging, April, 1976.

20. NEUGARTEN, B. L., and R. L. HAVIGHURST, *Extending the Human Life Span*. Report Prepared for National Science Foundation/RANN-Research Applications Directorate, Division of Advanced Productivity, Research and Technology. Washington, D.C.: U.S. Government Printing Office, 1977.

21. POPE PIUS XII, *Pope Speaks—Prolongation of Life for Osser Vatore Romano*, 1957, pp. 393–98.

22. REGAN, JOHN, "Intervention Through Adult Protective Service Programs," *The Gerontologist*, 18: No. 3 (1978), 250–54.

23. REICH, WARREN, "Ethical Issues Related to Research Involving Elderly Subjects," *The Gerontologist,* 18: No. 4 (1978), 326–37.

24. ROSNER, FRED, "The Definition of Death," *Archives of the Foundation of Thanatology,* 1: No. 3 (1969), 105–7.

25. SCHULTE, EUGENE, "With the Courts," *Quality of Life: A Goal of Long-Term Care Facilities.* St. Louis: Catholic Hospital Association, 1973.

26. SCHULZ, JAMES, "Liberalizing the Social Security Retirement Test, Who Would Receive the Increased Pension Benefits," *Journal of Gerontology,* 33: No. 2 (1978), 262–68.

27. SHERBERG, ELLEN, "Is There a Right to Die?" *St. Louis Post-Dispatch,* June 8, 1977, Sec. H., p. 3.

28. *The Missouri Office of Aging: Serving Missouri's Elderly.* Jefferson City, Mo.: Department of Social Services, 1975.

29. *To Find the Way to Opportunities and Services for Older Americans.* DHEW Publication (OHD) 75-20807. Washington, D.C.: U.S. Department of Health, Education, and Welfare, Office of Human Development, Administration on Aging, 1975.

30. WALES, JEFFREY, and D. TREYBIG, "Recent Legislative Trends Toward Protection of Human Subjects," *The Gerontologist,* 18: No. 3 (1978), 244–49.

31. WEIL, PETER, "Dominant Patterns of Older Persons' Health Status and Health Service Uses," *Journal of Gerontological Nursing,* 3: No. 2 (1977), 25–32.

32. *When an Older Person Needs Special Protection and Supportive Services Call 327-2101.* Chicago: Protective Services for the Aged, Welfare Council of Metropolitan Chicago, n.d.

33. *Workbook on Health for Participants in Community White House Conferences on Aging.* Washington, D.C., January, 1971.

34. *Your Medicare Handbook—Health Insurance Under Social Security.* DHEW Publication No. (SSA) 73-10050. Washington, D.C.: U.S. Department of Health, Education, and Welfare, Social Security Administration, 1973.

33. Social Security Office Telephone Interview, St. Louis, Missouri, June 14, 1978.

NORMAL AGING CHANGES IN LATER MATURITY:

Implications for Nursing Process

unit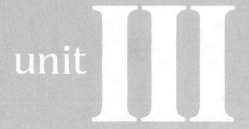

physical changes
in later maturity

Study of this chapter will enable you to:

1. Describe the physical changes that are normally present in later maturity.

2. Contrast normal physical changes with pathological changes in the elderly person.

3. Use assessment of physical aging changes as a basis for nursing diagnosis, patient care objectives, and a care plan for the senior in various settings.

4. Adapt nursing interventions to the normal aging changes presented by the senior.

5. Teach the senior and his family about the major expected physical changes.

6. Teach the senior how to cope with the major physical changes of aging.

7. Teach health promotion measures to the senior, family, and other staff members to prevent, whenever possible, pathological changes in later maturity.

8. Work with the senior, family, and other health team members to maintain optimal physical function and to prevent illness and related complications whenever possible.

9. Evaluate the effectiveness of your care.

9

Serious or crippling illness is not an inevitable part of normal aging and is not normal for the majority of persons in later maturity. Only 4 percent of people over 65 are confined to hospitals, nursing homes, or homes for the aged.[11]

Recent research has begun to differentiate illness changes from normal aging changes. Manifestations of normal aging are described as being "time-related, irreversible, and deleterious"; illness changes are also deleterious, but they are reversible and not necessarily time-related. Illness is preventable; therefore, many changes in later maturity caused by illness should and could be prevented. However, removal of all chronic disease will not prevent aging changes. Certain changes occur that cannot be explained on the basis of disease conditions.[10]

In a study of normal aging with 182 people over 60 years at Duke University, the most frequent disease conditions found were: (1) impaired vision and hearing, (2) arteriosclerosis, (3) cardiovascular disease, (4) hypertension, (5) emphysema/asthma, and (6) arthritis. In this study, differences in physical capacity were found in relation to socioeconomic status and age, but not sex and race. The conditions listed above, exclusive of impairment of hearing, were found more frequently and caused greater disability in the lower socioeconomic group. Although hearing acuity generally diminishes with increasing age, there is a substantial difference when sex and race are considered.[11]

Physical changes are also caused by environmental or individual factors. An example of an environmental factor is that of solar exposure and resultant skin wrinkling. An individual factor could be prematurely gray hair because of genetic cause.

Thus, changes demonstrated in later maturity are not absolutely predictable and may result from aging, illness, environment, and individual traits. The kind of life led, the illnesses or accidents experienced, the physical care obtained, and the genetic endowment all combine to cause the person to age in his unique way.

Although pathogenesis may not be important when assessing biological changes, it is important in the area of prevention and treatment. If you are aware that a change may be the result of a disease process and not an inevitable consequence of aging, you will be more likely to refer the patient for treatment to other health team members. You must also recognize signs of illness so that complications can be prevented.

This chapter will discuss physical changes resulting from the aging process and some related health promotion measures that you can implement. Later chapters will discuss changes resulting from disease, as well as aging, environment, and individual traits. Additional information on the physiological processes discussed in this chapter can be obtained from physiology texts.

Physical status of the senior may be assessed by using the methods and tools discussed in Chapter 2. When your assessment confirms the *nursing diagnosis* that the person demonstrates some or all of the *normal physical changes* of aging, your *long-range care goals* could include the following:

1. Tasks related to activities of daily living will be accomplished with as much comfort and effectiveness as possible.
2. Illness or complications of aging will be avoided through healthful living practices.

Short-range care goals could include the following:

1. Physical changes and related limitations of aging will be considered when physical activities that are pertinent to the life-style are planned.
2. Regular physical examinations will be obtained in order to prevent, treat, correct, or limit concomitant disease processes.
3. Health practices related to nutrition, exercise, rest, and elimination, specific for the physical changes, will be followed to prevent health problems.
4. Various aids, such as for vision or hearing, will be used as necessary in order to maintain communication and reality contact.

Intervention will include working with other health team members to give the best possible physical care. You can help the senior and his family adjust to normal physical changes through a variety of nursing measures. Teach them that these changes are normal and the changes that would indicate disease. Teach them the specific practices discussed in this chapter that will maintain activity and health. Listen to their feelings about aging; reinforce that aging characteristics are as worthwhile as the youthful characteristics commonly pictured in advertisements. Counsel family members so that they better understand the senior and what they can do to promote his health.

You may be able to *evaluate* the effectiveness of your care when your nursing interventions help the elderly person cope with his changing body. Further, the health promotion measures you initiate should help to prevent pathological changes or disease complications.

CELLULAR CHANGES

Study of performance changes during human aging shows a linear loss of work-performing ability with age, coupled with increased probability of death. Apparently death occurs when the challenge encountered requires a greater energy output than the stressed systems can generate.[40]

Aging is primarily the total result of the changed ability of individual cells to perform specialized, integrated functions. Aging occurs in individual cells because of disruption in cellular interaction and deterioration of extracellular components.[40]

Various cellular changes appear to be basic to all other aging changes. Lipofusion pigments accumulate in the nerve, liver, myocardium, and other cells. The cause and role of age pigments in the symptoms of aging have not been established; apparently, occlusion of a major portion of the cytoplasm by these seemingly nonfunctional pigments decreases the reserve function of aging cells.[44]

The nucleus of the cell changes with aging. The loss of gene function may be a key to senescence. Once many cell types, including central nervous system, muscle, and certain endocrine gland cells, have gone through their final developmental mitosis, the nuclear DNA is not replaced. Cell multiplication and tissue repair are reduced.[44]

Some researchers have suggested that aging may result from DNA deterioration. Given sufficient time, the following damage occurs: fragmentation of DNA, substitution of one base for another, and changed chemical reactions between DNA and substances in the environment. Whether or not the damage that occurs is great enough to cause functional impairment is unknown; all kinds of damage have not been examined sufficiently.[44]

A gradual loss of cells occurs; the total number of cells may decrease 30 percent between youth and old age. This loss is substantiated by reduced organ weights and total cell counts. When young and old people are compared, changes are found in the amount of cellular potassium, DNA, and nitrogen. In old age, body protein and intracellular water decrease, but extracellular water and plasma volume remain constant. Microscopically, the remaining cells are larger and the structural tissue patterns are increasingly irregular. Fat tends to increase in proportion to the decreased cell mass, thus leaving the total body mass relatively unchanged.[17]

Shock has demonstrated that a decrease in basal oxygen utilization is proportionate to the decrease in active cell mass. He assumes, therefore, that metabolic activity of the residual cells is essentially unchanged. Circulatory demands are also reduced, probably because of the reduced cell mass.[17,44]

Certain hormone-producing cells are less functional; the glucose tolerance of humans decreases with advancing age. An increased percentage of the population exhibits incipient diabetes on the glucose tolerance test at advanced age.[44] Stress intensifies glucose intolerance. Elderly patients undergoing stress from illness, injury, or surgery should be carefully assessed for the appearance of diabetic symptoms. Blood and urine glucose levels may become elevated. Glucose tolerance testing will probably be performed and appropriate therapy started. Removal of the stress may restore more normal glucose tolerance; the symptoms of diabetes disappear and specific treatment is no longer indicated. Therefore, the older patient who has recently been diagnosed as diabetic should be advised and reminded of the necessity for staying under close medical supervision.

Gonad function decreases; hormone output is reduced. The ovaries appear to decrease in sensitivity to gonadotropin. It has been shown in experimental animals that the developmental potency of öocytes produced later in life is greatly reduced. This occurs even if the ovum is transplanted into a young host.[44]

Red blood cell counts and hemoglobin content decrease gradually and significantly, and red blood cell life is shorter because of greater hemolysis. Fat content increases in the bone marrow, causing a slight reduction of hematopoietic cells. Hemoglobin and hematocrit tests should be routinely obtained at least once a year, so that anemia can be treated if necessary. Also, the diet of the senior should be high in meat, especially organ meats, green leafy vegetables, and whole grain or enriched breads and cereals. Maintaining an adequate dietary intake is a challenge, however, for the many reasons discussed throughout the book. Vitamin supplements with iron may be prescribed, but indiscriminate use of vitamins and so-called health foods should be discouraged.

A recent study of rats shows that lymphocyte and total white blood cell counts are subject to considerable variation; they decrease in the first two-thirds of life and increase in the last third. Neutrophils remain relatively stable, but they increase in older age. The percentage of lymphocytes decreases significantly in favor of neutrophils and a change in immune globulins also occurs.[27] A study of 1684 patients has shown that lymphocyte count drops precipitously from birth to age 20, remains stationary for three decades, and then declines at an accelerated rate to age 90.[28] These factors contribute to a decreased resistance to infection in the senior. Thus, prophylactic immunization for influenza should be encouraged, and the seniors should be warned against participating in large groups during the cold and flu season. Prompt treatment of infections is also necessary. Asepsis in caring for wounds or catheters or during procedures is paramount in elderly patients.

Cellular changes affect body function in the aged. Other changes, for example, changes in the musculoskeletal and integumentary systems, affect outward appearance as well as general function of the person.[51]

MUSCULOSKELETAL CHANGES

Among the earliest, progressive, most obvious changes are those of the locomotor system: decreased muscle strength, speed of motion, skeletal flexibility, and equilibrium. Yet, many of the changes in the musculature and skeleton in the elderly are caused by illness and not by aging. Differentiating an aging change from a change caused by illness is difficult. For example, is osteoporosis in postmenopausal women an illness or an aging change?

Height Changes

Height decreases for both men and women with advancing age; the reduction is primarily seen in the trunk. Disk thinning evidently is the cause for shrinking stature in the middle years, with reduction in the height of the vertebrae the prime reason thereafter. Elderly women show a larger amount of osteoporotic vertebral narrowing than do men. Thus, the characteristic body configuration of the elderly is a short trunk and long extremities, for the long bones do not undergo significant shortening.[40]

Since the long bones of the upper extremities apparently remain unchanged throughout life, and since for most adults the arm span equals height at maturity, span will be greater than height with advancing years. (However, in one study, the older population had a shorter arm span as well as shorter stature.) Therefore, span has been used to calculate maturity height in the elderly, even for those with marked vertebral osteoporosis or disfigurement of the legs or hips. It appears that loss of height becomes progressively more severe, with the Black population having a greater decrease in height with aging than the white population, especially for the male.[30] One might expect about a 2-inch loss by age 70 and during the eighth and ninth decades a proportionately greater loss.[40] Other postural changes contribute to decreased height. Slight flexion at the knees and hips results when cartilage loses water and joints fuse at the cartilage surfaces. Kyphosis occurs in the thoracic spine which may produce a backward tilting of the head.[52] All of these changes predispose the senior to problems of balance and locomotion. Since the center of gravity has been changed by height alterations and kyphosis has modified posture, the person should be cautioned about reaching, climbing, and walking, especially on slippery or uneven surfaces. Shoes should be well-fitted and have low heels and nonskid heels and soles. An adaptive mechanism for musculoskeletal changes is the wide-based gait with short step and toe pointed out for stability. The cane used by many elderly also gives a wider base for stability and reduces shaking. Postural changes can also affect respiratory, cardiac, and digestive functions as body cavities become compressed.

Osteoporosis is common in the senior. The primary factor in osteoporosis seems to be genetic; the disorder occurs earlier in people with low bone density, especially women and people of Northern European or Asiatic descent. Apparently more osteocytes die in old age so that demineralization is increased. But some researchers feel that this can be prevented somewhat by a daily diet throughout the young years that is adequate in calcium (800 to 1000 mg daily—the equivalent of one quart of milk); vitamin D (400 I.U. daily); phosphorus, protein, and fluoride (1 part per million in drinking water). Vitamin D and fluoride increase absorption and retention of calcium, and thus increase mineralization. Impressive results have been reported in preventing hip fractures in elderly males with osteoporosis through the administration of sodium fluoride. Inorganic phosphate also decreased bone mineral loss.[53] Daily fat intake should be no more than 100 to 125 g because excessive fat intake impairs calcium absorption by forming an insoluble compound. Since calcium intake throughout adulthood is often deficient (200 to 400 mg daily), problems are created in the later years.[4,34]

The osteoporosis can predispose to pathological fractures so that lifting of heavy objects, substantial weight gain, unusual twisting, and jumping should be discouraged. The necessity for maintaining good posture during the early and middle years cannot be stressed enough since the changes of aging will only intensify poor posture, and vice versa. A firm mattress, the use of only a small pillow, and sleeping in a prone position also help preserve better posture.

A reduction in shoulder width and chest size occurs in women. The rib cage is reduced in size by two factors: (1) osteoporosis of the ribs and (2) diminished strength and action of the respiratory muscles.[39] These changes also can be reduced in severity by maintaining good posture and proper lung expansion through slow, deep thoracic respiration.

Weight Changes

Weight has a tendency to plateau between the ages of 65 and 74 and to fall thereafter. The way in which subcutaneous fat is distributed also changes during life. Although weight is usually gained during the fifties and sixties, it may not be distributed the way that it was at an earlier age. For example, fat is lost from the face but there is an increased deposition in the abdomen and hips.[40] Even in the eighties and nineties, fat deposition remains over the hips and abdomen, but the limbs and face lose adipose and subcutaneous tissue and become thin, wrinkled, and lacking in tone. Maintaining optimum weight throughout the early and middle years is the best way to prevent obesity in the later years. A balanced diet and adequate exercise are the two most important elements in weight control.

Other Changes

In women the breasts atrophy with age and may hang at a lower level. Both glandular elements and the fat envelope decrease.

Other contour changes occur in both sexes because of loss of subcutaneous fat. Contours sharpen; hollows become deeper in the eye orbits, axilla, supraclavicular areas, intercostal spaces, and pelvic contour. Bony landmarks—the vertebral tips, scapular angles, xyphoid, ilial spines and crests, patella, foot arch, and metatarsal heads—become increasingly apparent.[40] Muscle bundles and tendonous attachments become distinct, even though muscle substance is lost. Pressure on bony and muscular prominences must be avoided in the bedridden and chairbound patient so that decubitus will not result.

Facial contours also change because of the loss of subcutaneous and adipose tissue. However, additional changes occur as well. The distance between the chin and nose decreases because the lower portion of the face shrinks, which results from reabsorption of bone from the maxilla and mandible. This is caused by the edentulous state. If the senior retains his teeth or wears well-fitted dentures, facial shape changes less. The nose and ears elongate, and the earlobes sag and become wrinkled.[40]

The total weight of all skeletal muscles decreases from 452 g per kilogram of body weight in the third decade, to 339 in the seventh, and to 270 g after 70 years. Aging apparently results in the atrophy of muscle fibers and an increase of intramuscular fat, which results in decreased strength, endurance, and function. Decline in strength occurs in jaw and lip muscles, making it harder for the person to chew and drink liquids, but the decline in strength is most pronounced in the flexor muscles of the forearms and the muscles of the legs and back.[40] Of the two hands, grip in the dominant hand remains stronger. Reduction in muscle strength and endurance predisposes to falls and injuries. Frequent rest periods are necessary when any sustained chore is attempted. Exhausting work, especially hard physical labor, should be eliminated unless it can be broken into work and rest sessions. Perhaps it would be advisable to have a helper to lighten the task. Taking jobs more slowly and allowing more time for completion may permit doing the same jobs as were done in earlier years. According to studies on men aged 70 to 90 years, a regular exercise program, even if started in late life, improves muscle strength, tone, and stamina.[12]

Shakiness and tremors increase, especially of the hands, arms, and head. The degree of tremor amplitude increases with advancing years, especially in relation to hand grip or intention to perform an activity.[54]

Diminished storage of muscle glycogen causes loss of energy reserve for increased activity; muscular activity fatigues the senior more quickly. Work capacity is often better in the afternoon than it is in the morning, perhaps because of food intake.[19,47]

INTEGUMENTARY CHANGES

Skin and Subcutaneous Tissue Changes

Wrinkled skin, particularly of the face, often heralds the signs of aging. The use of the facial muscles in habitual patterns causes these characteristic wrinkles. This should serve as a reminder to all of us to use the muscles for smiling instead of the muscles for frowning. Factors that influence the onset of these wrinkles are skin elasticity, maintenance of subcutaneous fat, solar radiation, and nutrition.

Loss of subcutaneous fat intensifies wrinkle production. Skin becomes lax because of loss of elasticity. Changes also occur because of gravitational pull, such as ptosis of eyelids, ears, and jowls. Often the skin of the neck shrinks, and neck wrinkles may be more marked than facial wrinkling. "Bags" under the eyes result from herniation of fat into the area, often accompanied by some retention of fluid. The bags that develop in the forties and fifties disappear later in life; then the eyes appear sunken because of the loss of fat from the orbit.

The skin of the elderly person's face may present a uniformly pale appearance, which is the result of the loss of capillaries, the decrease in functional melanocytes, and little exposure to sunlight.[40]

Since poor nutritional state, solar radiation, and loss of subcutaneous fat all predispose to wrinkling, precautions should be taken early in life to avoid these factors. Overexposure to the sun during the early and middle years will cause premature wrinkling. Use of sunshades in order to avoid overtanning should be begun early and continued throughout life; the typical sun worshiper will pay a high price for his golden tan in late life. Sudden weight gain and loss cause the skin to become stretched and flabby. Therefore, weight gain during the young and middle years must be avoided, since weight is usually lost in later years. Maintenance of constant optimum weight lessens subcutaneous fat loss and skin stretching. A balanced diet high in protein and vitamins should be followed throughout life, not just for the integrity of the skin but for health maintenance in all body systems.

Skin Lesions

Common skin lesions were investigated in a group of 163 community volunteers 64 years of age and older. Almost all subjects (94 percent) had loss of subcutaneous fat that caused lax skin and loss of skin turgor. *Seborrheic keratosis, a disease of the sebaceous glands, with an increased amount of secretion and formation of a horny or crusty growth on the skin,* occurred in 88 percent and was the most common new growth. The cherry angioma was found in 75 percent. Comedones were apparent in 81 percent. *Dermatophytosis, a fungus infection of the skin of the hands and feet* and *osteatosis, dry, scaly skin,* were seen in 75 percent of the persons. *Nevi (moles)* were present in 63 percent. Lesions found in approximately 50 percent of the subjects included skin tags, *lentigo, freckle-like lesions caused by exposure to the sun and weather,* and varicosities. *Corns, masses of dead skin cells with a sensitive core, are caused by excessive rubbing of shoes on the feet.*[36,46,51]

A longitudinal follow-up study confirmed the above findings. An increased incidence of moderate to severe osteatosis indicates that the skin tends to become less capable of maintaining proper hydration by retaining proper fluid content in epidermal cells. With age, functional capacity of the epidermis alters, especially the skin barrier of the stratum corneum. Furthermore, the sebaceous glands are less active, causing decreased lubrication. Thus, the skin becomes brittle and dry.[47] Use of moisturizing creams and lotions can help. Too frequent bathing or overexposure to cold, dry heat, or water can intensify the condition. Soap should be used sparingly. Because the epidermis is thinner and blood vessels are more fragile, small hemorrhages are often seen under the skin. Trauma such as bumps should be avoided.

Changes in Hair Distribution

Body hair also undergoes aging changes. Hair generally becomes absent or sparse over the entire body except on the face. In both sexes facial hair increases, and hair on other parts of the body thins or disappears entirely. Excessive facial hair can be very disturbing to the woman. Manual removal, depilatories, or electrolysis can help eliminate unwanted hair. Since some products may cause allergic reactions, the person must be cautioned against using products without first seeking medical advice.

Racial, genetic, and sex-linked factors account for the maximum amount of hair a person will have and also the changes that occur with age. Caucasians usually have more hair than persons of Oriental and Negro ancestry. American Indian males have very little facial or body hair.[40]

The hair of men shows the sex-linked characteristic. Male patterns of balding begin in the twenties, with loss of hair on either side of the midline (receding hairline). A patch over the vertex may also bald. Extension and coalescence of these areas occur with age. Many men attempt to use the remaining patch of midline hair to cover balding. This pattern of balding affects men only and is inherited from the mother. In men who do not have this inheritance and in women thinning occurs, but there is no particular pattern. Graying also occurs. Axillary and pubic hair tend to decrease, probably because of decreased hormonal functioning. With aging, axillary hair recedes from periphery to center, the opposite of its development. Thinning of the brows may also occur in normal euthyroid elderly persons. Leg hair is usually scanty or absent in both sexes; arm hair in males may remain but is scanty in women. Abdominal hair sometimes seen in mature menstruating women will abruptly disappear with menopause.[40]

Other Changes

Sweat glands apparently atrophy; they have significance not only for the skin but also for body cooling and temperature control.[48] Since excessive heat cannot be tolerated in later years, the person should be cautioned about overexertion during hot weather and about remaining in the sun.

The toenails become thick and brittle, probably because of decreased peripheral circulation and also because of fungus infections of the nails.[48] These changes, along with reduced ability to stoop or flex knees and hips, may make a regular visit to a podiatrist necessary. Soaking the nails in warm water or warm oil can make cutting easier. However, since peripheral circulation is usually reduced, healing is retarded, and eyesight is impaired, it is probably better for the senior not to attempt nail cutting but to seek assistance in order to avoid injury.

NERVOUS SYSTEM AND SENSORY CHANGES

Central Nervous System Changes

Neurons are lost and brain weight decreases with age. In a study comparing persons 17, 32, and 80 years of age on four cerebral circulatory parameters, no significant difference in mean arterial pressure was found. Progressive reduction in the cerebral blood flow and oxygen consumption and a progressive increase in cerebral vascular resistance were shown. However, there appears to be no direct correlation between the level of oxygen utilization and intellectual deterioration.[17]

Peripheral Nervous System Changes

In the peripheral nervous system, conduction velocity of the nerve impulse decreases with age, particularly after 40 to 50 years. Progressive connective tissue invasion of the actual nerve bundle occurs as well as an increase in the endoperineum. Fibers degenerate and are reduced in number.[17] Reaction time increases; thus, the person in later maturity is usually slower to respond to stimuli and requires more time to complete a task. Patience is needed in working with the elderly. Adjust the pace of your nursing care to the senior's pace: talk to him more slowly; walk with him more slowly; give him time to make a decision or formulate a sentence; do not expect him to finish tasks as quickly as the young person does.

In a study of 256 volunteers aged 60 to 93 who lived in a community environment, certain alterations in neurologic status were found by using reflex hammer, tuning fork, pin, and cotton wisp. The results were as follows:

1. Twenty-two percent showed either above or below average reflex action.
2. Fifteen percent had abnormal gait.
3. Ten percent has loss of arm movements associated with gait.
4. Seven percent had tremors.
5. Twelve percent had reduced or absent vibratory sensibility.
6. Ten percent had reduced two-point discrimination.
7. Five percent had altered tactile sensation or pain.
8. Twenty-six percent had loss of olfactory function.[32]

The number of sensory receptors decreases over body areas because the skin surface is drier, harder, and less vascular.[21] The reduced two-point discrimination and the pain, proprioceptive, and touch alterations are related to reduced sensory receptors. Gait alteration is attributed partially to reduced proprioceptive abilities and fewer sensory receptors in the feet, which can predispose to falls as well as injury to the feet, including burns or frostbite. Additional caution in walking is needed, as is attention to repair of shoes and stockings.

Shoes should be inspected for rough, worn linings and nails coming through the insoles. The feet should be warmed with blankets rather than a hot-water bottle.

Sensory Changes

Older persons are more likely than younger ones to show decrements in at least four of the five senses; a higher threshold of stimulation is required for perception. Apparently the sense receptors become less efficient with age. These impairments contribute to sensory deprivation and social immobility.[25]

Temperature (heat or cold), pressure, pain, and touch sensations are reduced, resulting from skin and vascular changes, which have implications for maintaining comfortable temperature and a safe environment. The patient may not complain of pain and he may not feel the effects of lying too long in one position.

Taste buds decrease with age, which along with altered olfactory sense causes decreased appetite. Extra seasoning often increases food intake, so long as it does not cause gastric irritation. The reduced olfactory sense arises from atrophy of olfactory organs and increased hair in the nostrils.[21] Elderly individuals living alone may not be aware of gas leaks when they occur. Therefore, anyone visiting the home of a senior and noticing the smell of gas must call it to his attention or the visitor must take appropriate action himself.

Visual changes occur with normal aging:

1. Visual acuity is reduced, especially in dim light.
2. Peripheral vision is narrowed.
3. Adaptation to dark areas, low illumination, or flicker is reduced.
4. Sensitivity to glare or bright lights increases because of an altered lens.
5. Accommodation to near objects decreases, beginning between 40 and 50 years. The lens continues to grow, but a nucleus of cells develops that has lost the cell membranes and developed crystallized cytoplasm. Thus, only the portion of the lens near the surface is capable of accommodation.
6. Corneal shape becomes more spherical, causing astigmatism. The spherical cornea and changing lens together may cause a myopic tendency, temporarily causing improved near vision.
7. Reabsorption of intraocular fluid becomes less efficient and may contribute to glaucoma.
8. Pupil size becomes smaller and less responsive to light changes.
9. Color perception changes; bright colors are more easily seen. All colors tend to fade, with a disappearing of boundaries, contours, and depth perception.
10. Color blindness increases, especially among men.
11. Light penetration of lens, cornea, and vitreous humor slows, and the presence of cataract makes the lens opaque.[17,25,42]

Forty percent of men and 60 percent of women over 65 years have vision that is less than 20/70 on testing.[21] In one study, 35 percent of the elderly had low vision (20/100 to 20/70), and 24 percent were legally blind (20/200 or worse).[42]

A longitudinal study of 93 seniors observed over a 10-year period demonstrated increases in glaucoma and cornea guttata (droplike deposits on Descemet's membrane in the posterior endothelial layer of cornea) and a marked decrement in visual acuity. Increases in cataracts and hyalites (yellowish-white vitreous opacities which chemically appear to be deposits of calcium salts) were small. This differed from cross-sectional data; glaucoma and cornea guttata are more likely to be seen in the normal aged who live longer. Conversely, cataracts do not seem to increase as much as the cross-sectional data would suggest.[2] Macular degeneration and resulting blindness increase.[42]

All of these changes point to the necessity of regular vision testing. Tonometry for glaucoma should be done yearly after age 40. Night driving for the elderly should also be carefully appraised. Sunglasses in reduced light and photochromic lenses must be cautiously used by the elderly since visual acuity is already hindered by dim light. Eyeglasses should be worn rather than set on a bedside stand when the person is hospitalized. Eyeglasses that'were appropriate at an earlier age may no longer have the correct lens for the changing eyes. Proper lighting and contrasting colors should be used to avoid glare, prevent accidents, and to maintain participation in various activities. Avoid having the person move abruptly from brightly lit to dark areas. Other ways to enhance vision in the elderly, related to cognitive ability, are discussed in Chapter 10.

Hearing acuity decreases with age as the mean pure-tone threshold at all sound frequencies increases in both sexes. At higher frequencies [above 100 cycles per second (cps)] there is a marked increase in the threshold, especially in men over 60. Most persons over 60 have lost hearing for the higher-pitched frequencies over 4000 cps.[17,25]

Increased rigidity of the ossicles in the middle ear, auditory nerve atrophy, and atrophy of the end organs in the basal turn of the cochlea probably account for hearing loss with age.[21] The importance of protecting hearing at an earlier age cannot be stressed too much. Loud noise damages hearing. The prevalence of loud rock and disco music could create a future generation of deaf elderly individuals.

Although speech frequencies are fairly low, the senior often has difficulty understanding conversation. Apparently discrimination, the ability to identify words, is more severely affected than discrimination of pure-tone thresholds unless the person is in an optimally quiet environment. The change is noted as early as 50 years and increases sharply after 70 years of age.[17,25]

In a longitudinal study with 92 seniors over a 7-year period, hearing acuity was found to diminish with increasing age. Women have better hearing for higher frequencies than do men. However, women in the follow-up study had a greater hearing loss at 3000 cps than did men. Black men had superior hearing compared to white men at both the low and high frequencies.[13]

Consider the elderly person's problem with speech discrimination; stand directly in front of the person and keep your face in the light when you are speaking. Get the person's attention by touch or eye contact. Enunciate distinctly and carefully; do not talk too fast. Rephrase a sentence if necessary. Loud speech does not improve the person's ability to comprehend because the higher pitch is more difficult to hear. Pitch your voice down when you talk to the hearing impaired.

Hearing aids need regular attention to be sure that batteries are functional, fit is adequate, and type is appropriate. Hearing aids must be worn with volume turned up to a level adequate for hearing. The hearing-aid wearer needs regular reexamination by an otologist.

The hearing impaired can be taught the following techniques to enable them to better understand people who are speaking:

1. Combine hearing and seeing to aid understanding. Lipreading is useful, but it involves more than understanding speech from watching mouth movements. It involves reading the whole situation.
2. Watch the total expression and the gestures of the speaker because they provide important clues to what he is saying.
3. Relax because excessive tension interferes with lipreading and hearing.
4. Look for ideas instead of isolated words. Follow along with the speaker. As his speech rhythm becomes familiar to you, key words will emerge that will help you understand him.
5. Avoid facing a bright light and try not to allow the speaker's face to be in the shadow.
6. Try to determine the topic under discussion as quickly as possible; then the conversation can be followed even if a few words or sentences are missed.
7. Put others at ease by assuring them that quiet, natural speech is best for the hearing impaired. Exaggerated lip movements and shouted speech are difficult to understand.
8. Do not be afraid to stare at people while lipreading.
9. Ask the speaker to rephrase his statement if you do not understand what he is saying. If some words are understood, use those words in a question to get the word or words you missed.
10. Pay particular attention to your own speech. A long-term hearing loss, or even a sudden profound loss, may cause a marked deterioration of voice and articulation. This condition must be corrected, for a pleasant, well-modulated voice is a great asset.
11. Do not get into the habit of mouthing the words or the sounds that you are seeing.[51]

ENDOCRINE CHANGES

Closely related to nervous system control is that of chemical regulation by the endocrine glands.

Thyroid Gland Changes

Some researchers feel that the thyroid gland is more important in aging than any other factor (see biologic theories of aging in Chapter 1). Oxygen utilization, and thus basal metabolism rate, decreases with age. However, when oxygen consumption is compared to the actual functioning cell mass, there appears to be no reduction per unit mass of cells. Circulating thyroxine does not appear to decrease with age, but radioactive iodine uptake by the thyroid does. These two factors suggest that the rates of destruction and replacement of thyroid hormone are slowed proportionally. The response of the thyroid to thyroid-stimulating hormone (TSH) appears to be normal, but the turnover rate for thyroxine decreases 50 percent between 20 and 80 years.[17] Because of changed thyroid function, the person may be less alert and active, and he may be more susceptible to cold. Drugs may also be more likely to accumulate and cause side effects or toxicity.

The ability to ward off disease is reduced, apparently because of the reduction in thyrotropic hormone from the pituitary and less thyroid and thymus activity. Yet, the autoimmune response appears to increase, so that cancer cells that are recognized in the earlier years as foreign invaders and eliminated by immune response are permitted to flourish with increasing age. Immune bodies or antibodies, or the cells that produce them, appear defective and often mistakenly destroy healthy tissue.[25,52]

Pancreatic Changes

Studies to date suggest that insulin production or utilization decreases with age. One researcher states that either normal aging decreases glucose tolerance or 70 percent of the 70-year-olds are diabetic. The impaired glucose tolerance test results demonstrated by elderly subjects point to either reduced insulin response or a reduced peripheral sensitivity to released insulin.[17] Researchers believe that the primary disorder in the insulin release mechanism with advancing age is the need for a higher blood glucose level to produce an equivalent insulin level.[27]

Other explanations for glucose intolerance may be decreased peripheral responsiveness to insulin, increased levels of proinsulin (proinsulin has less biologic activity than insulin), and normal or elevated levels of glucagon in aging. Alpha cells that produce glucagon do not appear to be altered by age as do the beta cells that produce insulin. Hyperlipemia may also be acting as an insulin inhibitor. Decreased exercise by the senior is also cited as a possible cause of glucose intolerance, since physical activity seems to increase peripheral utilization of glucose.[27] These latter two factors point to the necessity of weight reduction if overweight and maintenance of an adequate amount of exercise.

Hypothalamic-Pituitary Changes

Deterioration of hypothalamic-pituitary function has not been found in fit elderly people. Disturbed normal circadian pituitary-adrenal rhythm may occur in the elderly, possibly caused by sleep disturbance. Depression is also associated with abnormal sleep and abnormal pituitary-adrenal rhythms.[16]

No systematic studies of blood levels or urinary excretion rates of epinephrine and norepinephrine are available. Reduced epinephrine and norepinephrine release following injection of insulin as a stimulating mechanism (or stressor) does occur. However, these results could be influenced by the reduced response of older persons to insulin. Yet, the less efficient stress response of the older person may be one measure of adrenal gland response to stimulation from pituitary ACTH.[25]

The excretion of aldosterone and secretion of cortisol and conjugated 17-hydroxycorticosteroids decrease with age.[17] With age, testosterone levels and responsiveness to gonadotropin gradually decrease, and the proportionately greater amount of estrogen contributes to receding hairline, hypertrophied prostate, and negative nitrogen balance. Estrogen in women begins to drop between 35 and 40 years, and the proportionately greater amount of androgen contributes to a deepening voice, coarser skin, more facial hair, abdominal fat deposits, and muscular atrophy. Progesterone production and excretion decrease abruptly after the reproductive period. Gonadotrophic hormone in women has a marked postclimacteric increase and then gradually subsides.[17]

The greater decrease in gonadal hormones compared to that of cortisol may result in catabolism, with progressive tissue loss and osteoporosis resulting. Also, apparently androgens enhance and estrogens delay the development of atherosclerosis.[17]

CARDIOPULMONARY CHANGES

Respiratory Changes

With aging, the lungs show a decreased number but increased size of bronchioles and alveoli. Elastin content of the lungs apparently increases while total collagen content remains constant. Despite these latter factors, the aging lung gradually becomes rigid. Vital capacity decreases about 25 percent, although total lung capacity remains fairly constant with aging. Maximum breathing capacity, measured by forced expiratory volume, declines 50 percent between 20 and 80 years.[17] Thus, less air is breathed per unit of time, and less oxygen is available. Less oxygen, combined with a reduction in basal metabolism, means less energy production and synthetic reactions.[25,54]

Carbon dioxide arterial pressure does not normally increase with aging, but oxygen arterial pressure decreases 10 to 15 percent. Ventilation-perfusion mismatching, as well as the increased dead space, probably causes this. Adequate alveolar ventilation must be maintained, since although oxygen consumed under stress is reduced 50 percent, the partial pressure of carbon dioxide does not increase. Apparently, the stressed tissues are either not perfused or they cannot utilize the oxygen.[17]

The aged lung differs from the emphysematous lung; evidence of obstruction, as in emphysema, and the elevated carbon dioxide and bicarbonate blood levels are not seen.[17]

Important clinical considerations in the aged are increased rigidity of the chest wall because of reduced intercostal muscle strength, changes in rib cartilage, and kyphosis; reduced cough efficiency; decreased ciliary activity; and increased lung dead space. Provision should be made for adequate ventilation during bed rest and following surgery. Coughing, deep breathing, intermittent positive pressure breathing (IPPB), and frequent changes of position can all enhance ventilation and should be implemented in the nursing care of the bedridden senior.

Cardiac Changes

The heart in normal aging shows little anatomic change except for the accumulation of the age pigment mentioned earlier. The effect of age pigments on the heart tissue is unknown. Physiologic changes include decreased cardiac output of about 30 to 40 percent between 25 and 65 years. Contraction time is prolonged, especially the isometric phase of contraction, which results in reduced cardiac power and increased energy expended for work achieved. Arterial blood pressure rises during exercise because of the increased cardiac output that results from greater stroke volume, which is the body's attempt to compensate for decreased ability to adequately accelerate the heart rate. Arteriovenous oxygen difference increases at rest but not during exercise when oxygen debt may occur.[17] Because functioning ability decreases, the heart is frequently hypertrophied in late life. Thus, the elderly person must perform strenuous activity more slowly and with interspersed rest periods. Also, he may not be able to perform the same activities as he did in his earlier years. The person must evaluate for himself what his abilities are. If an activity results in pain, exhaustion, or dyspnea, he should probably modify or eliminate it.

Degenerative calcific valve disease is one of the most common pathological changes seen in the aging heart and has been found in up to 37 percent of subjects over 75 years at postmortem.[4]

Vascular Changes

In aging, the blood flow through coronary arteries is reduced, but it appears to be reduced even more to the kidneys and liver than to other organs. Thus, low blood pressure caused by blood loss and shock can be more detrimental to the kidneys of the elderly than to the kidneys of younger persons. The reserve capacity of the kidneys is also reduced. These two combined factors may be sufficient to cause irreversible kidney damage. Therefore, blood pressure readings must be taken frequently (every 15 minutes until stable) following injury and surgery, and prompt action must be taken when a substantial drop occurs in the patient's normal blood pressure.

Because of reduced cardiac output, both systolic and diastolic pressures increase and take longer to return to normal after exercise or stress because of vessel inelasticity and total peripheral resistance from atherosclerosis and arteriosclerosis, despite reduced cardiac output. Peripheral resistance increases because arterial elastic fibers undergo changes, such as straightening, fraying, splitting, fragmenting, and calcification. Collagen in vessels increases and cross-linkages occur, thus producing bundles. Loss of elasticity causes intraaortic systolic pressure to rise abruptly as more blood is forced into the vessel.[17,54] Generally, the upper limit of normal blood pressure for the person over 65 is 160/95 mm mercury.[6]

The blood pressure reading in the aged may vary considerably, depending on the time of day, activity, and stress present. For example, this author has found that the systolic and diastolic pressures are usually lower when the elderly client is assessed in his home than when he is assessed in the doctor's office. The exercise involved in riding a bus or walking to the office, which may include inclines and stairways, the stress of the delayed appointment, the excitement of seeing the doctor all combine to elevate blood pressure. The doctor orders medication based on his office assessment, but the medication causes the person in the home to become hypotensive, fatigued, dizzy, and generally uncomfortable. To feel better, the person does not take his medicine as prescribed, if he takes it at all. It is easy to see why hypertensive patients are difficult to regulate. Calling the patient "noncompliant" does nothing to solve the problem. Experience has shown that in determining drug dosage, consideration of blood pressure readings in the home by a nurse, the patient, or family member promotes better hypertension control. Further, the senior often can adjust the dosage depending on how he feels and by monitoring his own blood pressure. For example, he could take one instead of two tablets. Health professionals should consider the senior as a partner in his treatment.[14] If the blood pressure is reduced by medication to the textbook norm of 120/80, the senior may suffer from hypotension and inadequate perfusion.

Pulse-wave velocity increases with age and is apparently independent of atherosclerosis, although persons with coronary artery disease show greater pulse-wave velocity changes than can be attributed to age alone.[17]

Venous muscle tone and efficiency of venous valves decrease; blood is returned less efficiently to the heart so that venous pooling and dependent edema occur in the lower extremities and abdomen. Capillary permeability is changed, causing poorer nutrition to and waste removal from tissue. Hypoxia of organs and cells and predisposition to thrombus formation also result from poor venous blood flow, which in turn affects arterial flow.

Because of these circulatory changes and the prescription of antihypertensive drugs, the senior is more prone to orthostatic hypotension, dizziness, and faintness when he changes positions or rotates his head. The senior should be cautioned to change position slowly.

DIGESTIVE AND EXCRETORY CHANGES

Digestive Changes

Digestive enzymes, ptyalin, gastric acids and enzymes, and pancreatic enzymes decrease in late life. Senile gastric atrophy causes reduction in the intrinsic factor, which may contribute to anemia.[17]

Absorption is influenced by (1) atrophy of intestinal mucosa and musculature, which slows peristalsis and alters motility through the intestine; (2) altered blood flow; (3) change in adequacy and effectiveness of digestive enzymes; and (4) decreased efficiency of the absorbing surface and transport mechanisms. Fat absorption appears to be delayed with age. Milk and milk products are often poorly tolerated because of a reduction in the enzyme lactase. Some evidence supports reduced absorption of Vitamins B_1 and B_{12} and iron.[17] A change in absorption and utilization of essential minerals—calcium, magnesium, potassium, and sodium—also occurs. Potassium appears reduced in large numbers of elderly people. Changes in dietary calcium intake or absorption may be related to the leaching out of calcium found in osteoporosis. Whether age alone is responsible for nutritional problems or if the difficulty is the result of a lifelong pattern of poor eating habits is unknown.[29] However, the inadequate absorption of a number of nutrients contributes to malnutrition, anemia, and loss of strength and energy, and it indirectly affects many of the body systems as well as the life-style of the senior.

Diverticuli are more common because of decreased muscle tone. Hard food particles and feces become entrapped in the saccular pouches of the intestines, predisposing to infection (diverticulitis) and constipation.[40]

Digestion and absorption are influenced by the number of decayed or missing teeth, which along with a change in the structure of the jaw and mouth, affects the ability to chew. Preventive dental care throughout life is a must if teeth are to be preserved. The necessity for pulling teeth has almost been eliminated by modern dental methods. Dentures may become the antiques of the future.

The person in later maturity is likely to have periodontal disease because of neglect, effects of stress, and aging changes.[21] The person may develop pyorrhea without demonstrating earlier signs of inflammation.[25]

Saliva flow is reduced and the saliva becomes thick and ropy.[35] The dry mouth that results is often a major complaint, especially if the person is also taking antispasmodics, tranquilizers, antihistamines, or other drugs that have the side effect of dry mouth. Holding water in the mouth before swallowing, ice chips, mints, other hard candies, and gum may help relieve the discomfort. Adequate hydration cannot be stressed enough for relief of this problem.

The tongue may become atonic or atrophic, and a burning sensation results from poor blood supply.[35] Chewing and enjoyment of food are interfered with, which effects nutritional status as well as comfort and conversation.

Hyperplastic mucosa in the mouth may occur and should be checked for malignancy; dentures may have to be remade or refitted with a lining as mouth structures change shape. Careful observation of the mouth is necessary; often the condition of the mouth is a sign of other systemic disease.[35]

The gag reflex is less active; the senior is more likely to aspirate food and saliva into the trachea. The Heimlich maneuver to dislodge food from the trachea should be taught to the senior and his family members; it may be lifesaving.

The liver shows decreased weight and cellular change with age. However, tests for liver function, although affected by aging, do not demonstrate abnormal functional capacity.[17] Yet many seniors clinically demonstrate hepatic insufficiency, which contributes to poor absorption of fats and intolerance for fatty foods; deficiency of fat-soluble vitamins; increased flatulence; and decreased detoxification of drugs, causing drug accumulation and toxicity.

Elimination Changes

Studies of large bowel motility are limited, although constipation in the aged is taken for granted. Decreased secretion of intestinal mucosa causes decreased lubrication, which along with loss of intestinal muscle tone contributes to constipation. Lack of bulk in the diet, an irregular meal pattern, dehydration, lack of exercise, and not responding to the urge to defecate also contribute to constipation in the younger as well as in the older person.[40] Teach the person about foods that contribute fiber, the importance of exercise, adequate fluids, and regular mealtimes, and teach him to respond to the gastrocolic reflex. Emphasize the importance of avoiding laxatives and enemas on a regular basis because they contribute to loss of bowel tone. Emphasize also that a daily bowel movement is not essential.

Fecal incontinence increases with age. Confusion and neurologic changes probably are more causative than any other factor. The anal sphincter does appear to have reduced tone; internal sphincter tone is usually maintained, while external sphincter tone is relaxed.[17]

The kidneys also decrease in size, apparently because of loss of nephron units. Glomerular filtration rate decreases 46 percent from 20 to 90 years of age. Renal blood flow decreases 53 percent, which is adaptive, because blood flow is directed to other vital organs initially. Tubular cell function is also reduced; thus, waste elimination eventually decreases. Ability to concentrate urine depends on the integrity of tubular cell function and maintenance of the osmotic gradient. Maximum specific gravity and urinary osmolarity decrease with age.[40] The necessity for avoiding urinary tract infections resulting from reduced blood flow, urine stasis from prostatic hypertrophy or prolapsed uterus, rectum or bladder, and dehydration from inadequate fluid intake cannot be stressed too much. Reduced renal reserve makes infections much more dangerous for the elderly person. Avoidance of catheterization should be a number one nursing goal. Regular toileting and bladder training should be performed to avoid incontinence and retention. Adequate fluid intake, juices and foods that produce an acid ash (prune juice, cranberry juice), and not contaminating the urinary tract will help in avoiding urinary tract infections. Nocturia is frequently present because of decreased bladder capacity; safety precautions must be stressed to avoid falling since the senior sees less well in a darkened room or when the light is suddenly turned off or on. Stress incontinence and frequency and urgency result from poor bladder tone and slowing of the inhibitory neural impulses to the bladder, which cause impaired voluntary control over urination. The resulting embarrassment may cause a curtailment of social roles. Plastic-lined underpants can be worn along with sanitary napkins or extra padding as a precaution against incontinence.

Acid-base balance can still be maintained even though there is a narrowed range of adaptability. As long as acid-base loads do not exceed the excretion capacity, normal balance is possible. However, large acid-base loads in the elderly can more easily overwhelm the regulatory mechanisms than they can in the younger person, and the imbalance remains longer when it does occur. Alkalosis may result because the kidney is unable to excrete excess alkali. During times of reduced fluid intake, loss of fluids from burns, wounds, tubes, diarrhea, vomiting, and fever, and during diuretic therapy observe for signs of fluid and electrolyte imbalance. Diabetes, uremia, and liver disease can also predispose to electrolyte imbalance. The elderly person undergoing fluid replacement must be carefully monitored; fluid overload can cause pulmonary edema to occur more rapidly than in a younger individual since cardiovascular reserves are decreased.

BIOLOGICAL RHYTHMS

Rhythms are an integral part of all biologic life; animals are in a state of continual change, and the seasons and each day have a pattern. Predictable and orderly fluctuations occur internally that cause a person to be different at different periods of the day. These rhythms influence his ability to adapt and affect the regulation and integration of physiological and behavioral responses,[5] and find expression in his physiology, moods, and performance. Apparently, man's mode of life is the synchronizer for his rhythms.

Rhythm periods vary in length. *Circadian rhythms occur approximately every 24 hours. Ultradian rhythms are shorter than the 24-hour cycles. Infradian rhythms are longer than 24 hours.* Physiologic functions that demonstrate circadian rhythms are body temperature, pulse rate, blood pressure, serum and urinary cortisol, electrolyte excretion, and sensory acuity.[49]

Circadian rhythms appear to develop in the first years of life; different rhythms develop at different ages. Rhythms may be developed as the result of inheritance of an internal biological clock or because of neurologic maturation. Or they may be learned through repeated exposure to environment and socialization.[5]

Little is known about how rhythms are affected by aging, if aging is affected by rhythms, or the effect of various physiological or emotional states on rhythms.[5] In one study a sample of 30 institutionalized subjects demonstrated a circadian regularity and synchronization of rhythms,[49] in spite of the elderly person's decreased ability to respond to environmental changes that could affect synchronization (various rhythms occurring in timing with each other).[43] Nursing homes adhere to a routine to facilitate care, which is probably beneficial to the elderly residents in regulating their rhythms.[49]

Rhythms should be assessed prior to therapy. Hall assessed the client's life-style and circadian rhythms of temperature, weight, and vital signs. She planned rehabilitation accordingly and found that the elderly consistently improved performance when the therapy sessions coincided with peak times of the rhythms.[19]

Assess the following patterns to better understand circadian rhythms:

1. Vital signs—when are they at a peak and at the lowest point.
2. Urinary excretion patterns—time and quantity.
3. Behavior patterns in relation to time of day—cheerful, irritable, alert, lethargic, energetic, verbose, quiet.
4. Usual activity pattern—activity-rest cycle, preferred meal times.
5. Environmental stimuli used by the person for time clues—lighting, clock, calendar, radio, television.
6. Subjective feelings—does the person feel best early in the morning or later in the day; physical complaints related to time of day; feelings when schedule is changed.[49]

Use the information for planning care. The schedule imposed by the institution should be compared to the schedule previously followed by the patient. Routine care, some tests, possibly meal schedules, and rest-activity schedules could be modified to reduce the adjustment for the patient. Schedule teaching, counseling, physical exercise, or other therapy at a time of day when the person feels most alert and energetic.

Some medication might be more effective or have side effects reduced or increased, depending on the person's biological rhythms. If sedatives or tranquilizers are given when the person is at lower ebb in energy, metabolism, and feelings, the action of the drugs is increased. Lower dosage may be needed to avoid side effects or toxicity.

Corticosteroid drug effects are related to the circadian rhythms of corticosteroid secretion by the adrenal cortex. Highest corticosteroid levels are found soon after the usual time for awakening, regardless of the time of day. A daily dosage given as several separate administrations throughout the waking hours produces a large amount of adrenal suppression. Administering the total dosage in the morning to day-active people is likely to produce minimal suppression. Research on growth retardation side effects of corticosteroids offers some evidence for giving the drug on alternate days or as a single daily dose around the peak time of adrenocorticol function. Scheduling administration time of corticosteroids has been beneficial for asthmatic patients also. When the drug was given at 7:00 a.m. or 3:00 p.m., it produced greater effects than when given at 3:00 a.m. or 7:00 p.m. Giving unequal doses of two-thirds to three-fourths of the total daily dose on awakening and the remainder at bedtime results in no desynchronization in systemic circadian functions in persons with normal circadian rhythms. These patients respond better to the medication and they feel better.[41]

More research will be appearing relative to rhythms and drug administration. You should stay abreast of developments in rhythm research since you will be held accountable for this knowledge as it is or should be applied to patient care.

CHANGES THAT INFLUENCE SEXUAL FUNCTION

The process of aging plays some part in diminishing sexual function. The manner of sexual expression is influenced to some degree by the senses of touch, smell, taste, hearing, and vision. But the processes of aging are subtle and variable; some men are old at 25 in terms of sexual function, while others are young at 90. Interestingly, some experts on aging believe premature cessation of sexual functioning may accelerate physiological and psychological aging, since disuse of any function usually leads to concomitant changes in other capacities.[37,38]

The menopause which occurs in the middle-aged woman is marked by a changed relationship between production of ovarian estrogen and progesterone and by the secretion of follicle stimulating hormone changes. With anovulation, no progesterone is produced, and estrogen diminishes. Atrophy of the uterus and ovaries and involutional changes in the vagina, labia, and clitoris result. Reduced estrogen results in thinning and drying vaginal epithelium, causing dyspareunia. The urethra and bladder are more mechanically irritated during coitus, and urinary urgency, burning, and incontinence may occur, along with vaginal burning, for as long as 36 hours after coitus. The vaginal barrel decreases in width, length, and expansive ability; the introitus is narrowed, which can also cause dyspareunia. These physiological changes can be treated by estrogen replacement and by engaging in regular intercourse which maintains vaginal lubrication and expansion.[15,23,29]

Yet these changes, which begin in middle age, do not diminish the elderly woman's capacity to achieve orgasm and enjoy sexual relations. Physiological response to sexual stimulation, such as breast engorgement, nipple erection, sexual flush, increased muscle tonus, and clitoral and labial engorgement are slower and reduced in intensity. Duration of orgasm is shorter.[29] But sexual pleasure is more than physiological response.[8,15,23]

Androgen production in the man usually declines steadily until about age 60, after which it remains relatively constant. Some men present 'climacteric symptoms in late middle age. Contrary to popular opinion, sexual response is more likely to weaken with age in men than women; the elderly man is slower to arouse sexually. The size and firmness of testes diminish. The seminiferous tubules thicken and a degenerative process inhibits sperm production. Seminal fluid is thinner and is reduced in amount. The prostate gland enlarges because of excessive androgen production, and its contractions during orgasm weaken. Erection and ejaculation are slower; penile erection may be maintained for extended periods without ejaculation but may not be redeveloped for 12 to 24 hours afterward. Involuntary morning erections decrease in frequency. Ejaculatory force is reduced after age 60; the man does not experience the warning of ejaculatory inevitability. Scrotal vasocongestion, sexual flush, and increased muscle tonus are reduced.[15,23,29]

In spite of these changes, the man maintains erection ability until in the eighties or nineties, although erection takes two to three times longer after age 50. He is less likely to become a father because sperm are fewer and less viable. Regular coitus, along with physical and psychological health, enables the man to maintain sexual function.[8,29]

In conclusion, body systems do not age at the same rate; and the rate of aging varies from person to person. The changes in aging are multiple, complex, and eventually universal throughout all body systems. Causation of aging changes is under investigation by many gerontologists. When causation is found, many of these changes may be preventable. At present, you should focus on carefully assessing and alleviating the effects of these changes and preventing complications that may intensify their disabling characteristics.

REFERENCES

1. American Medical Association Committee on Human Sexuality, *Normal Sexual Development.* Washington, D.C.: American Medical Association, 1972.

2. ANDERSON, BANKS, and ERDMAN PALMORE, "Longitudinal Evaluation of Ocular Function," in *Normal Aging II,* ed. Erdman Palmore. Durham, N.C.: Duke University Press, 1974.

3. ANDERSON, H. C., *Newton's Geriatric Nursing,* 5th ed. St. Louis: The C. V. Mosby Company, 1971.

4. ANDERSON, L., M. DIBBLE, H. MITCHELL, and H. RYNBERGEN, *Nutrition in Nursing.* Philadelphia: J. B. Lippincott Company, 1972.

5. BASSLER, SANDRA, "The Origins and Development of Biological Rhythms," *Nursing Clinics of North America,* 11: No. 4 (1976), 575–82.

6. BATTERMAN, B., M. STEGMAN, and A. FITZ, "Hypertension: Detection, Evaluation, and Treatment," *Nursing Digest,* 4: No. 5 (1976), 55–59.

7. BEESON, P., and W. MCDERMOTT, eds., *Cecil Loeb Textbook of Medicine.* Philadelphia: W. B. Saunders Company, 1971.

8. COMFORT, ALEX, *A Good Age.* New York: Crown Publishers, Inc., 1976.

9. COWDRY, E., and F. STEINBERG, eds., *The Care of the Geriatric Patient.* St. Louis: The C. V. Mosby Company, 1971.

10. DAVENMEUHL, ROBERT, "Aging Versus Illness," in *Normal Aging,* ed. Erdman Palmore. Durham, N.C.: Duke University Press, 1970.

11. DAVENMEUHL, ROBERT, EWALD BUSSE, and GUSTAVE NEWMAN, "Physical Problems of Older People," in *Normal Aging,* ed. Erdman Palmore. Durham, N.C.: Duke University Press, 1970.

12. deVRIES, H., "Physiological Effects of an Exercise Training Regime Upon Men Aged 52–88," *Journal of Gerontology,* 25: No. 4 (1970), 325–36.

13. EISENDORFER, CARL, and FRANCES WILKIE, "Auditory Changes," in *Normal Aging II,* ed. Erdman Palmore. Durham, N.C.: Duke University Press, 1974.

14. GAETA, MICHAEL, and RONALD GAETANO, *The Elderly: Their Health and the Drugs in Their Lives.* Dubuque, Ia.: Kendall/Hunt Publishing Co., 1977.

15. GRIGGS, WINONA, "Staying Well While Growing Old: Sex and the Elderly," *American Journal of Nursing,* 78: No. 8 (1978), 1352–54.

16. GREEN, M. F., "Endocrinology in the Elderly," in *Geriatric Medicine,* eds. W. Ferguson Anderson and T. G. Judge. New York: Academic Press, Inc., 1974.

17. GOLDMAN, RALPH, "Decline in Organ Function with Aging," in *Clinical Geriatrics,* ed. Isadore Rossman. Philadelphia: J. B. Lippincott Company, 1971.

18. GUYTON, ARTHUR, *Basic Human Physiology.* Philadelphia: W. B. Saunders Company, 1971.

19. HALL, LaVONNE, "Circadian Rhythms, Implications for Geriatric Rehabilitation," *Nursing Clinics of North America,* 11: No. 4 (1976), 631–38.

20. HAND, SAMUEL, *A Review of Physiological and Psychological Changes in Aging and Their Implications for Teachers of Adults,* 3rd ed. Tallahassee, Fla: State Department of Education, 1965.

21. HURLOCK, ELIZABETH, *Developmental Psychology,* 4th ed. New York: McGraw-Hill Book Company, 1975.

22. JENNINGS, MURIEL, MARGENE NORDSTROM, and NORINE SHUMAKE, "Physiologic Functioning in the Elderly," *Nursing Clinics of North America,* 7: No. 2 (1972), 237–52.

23. KAAS, MERRIE, "Sexual Expression of the Elderly in Nursing Homes," *The Gerontologist*, 18: No. 4. (1978), 372–78.

24. KENNEDY, R. D., "Recent Advances in Cardiology," in *Geriatric Medicine*, eds. W. Ferguson Anderson and T. G. Judge. New York: Academic Press, Inc., 1974.

25. KIMMEL, DOUGLAS, *Adulthood and Aging*. New York: John Wiley & Sons, Inc., 1974.

26. LEUENBERGER, HANS GEORG W., and INO KUNSTYR, "Gerontological Data of C57 BL/6J Mice II. Changes in the Course of Natural Aging," *Journal of Gerontology*, 31: No. 6 (1976), 648–53.

27. LEVIN, MARVIN E., "Diabetes Mellitus," in *Cowdry's The Care of the Geriatric Patient*, 5th ed., ed. Franz U. Steinberg. St. Louis: The C. V. Mosby Company, 1976.

28. MACKINNEY, ARCHIE, "Effect of Aging on the Blood Lymphocyte Count," *Journal of Gerontology*, 33: No. 2 (1978), 213–16.

29. MASTERS, WILLIAM, and VIRGINIA JOHNSON, *Human Sexual Response*. Boston: Little, Brown & Company, 1965.

30. MCPHERSON, J., D. LANCASTER, and J. CARROLL, "Stature Changes with Aging in Black Americans," *Journal of Gerontology*, 33: No. 1 (1978), 20–25.

31. MILLER, ANNA, and GAIL RIEGLE, "Serum Testosterone and Testicular Response to HCG in Young and Aged Male Rats," *Journal of Gerontology*, 33: No. 2 (1978), 197–203.

32. NEWMAN, GUSTAVE, ROBERT DAVENMUEHL, and EWALD BUSSE, "Alterations in Neurologic Status with Age," in *Normal Aging*, ed. Erdman Palmore. Durham, N.C.: Duke University Press, 1970.

33. NEWMAN, GUSTAVE, and CLAUDE NICHOLS, "Sexual Activities and Attitudes in Older Persons," *Journal of the American Medical Association*, 173: No. 1 (May 7, 1960), 33–35.

34. "Nutrition: Can It Prevent Osteoporosis?" *Geriatric Focus*, 7: No. 12 (1968), 1ff.

35. "Refusal of Dentists to Recognize and Adjust to Physiologic Changes in Aged: A Major Problem," *Geriatric Focus*, 6: No. 4 (1967), 2.

36. ROSSMAN, ISADORE, "The Anatomy of Aging," in *Clinical Geriatrics*, ed. Isadore Rossman. Philadelphia: J. B. Lippincott Company, 1971.

37. RUBIN, ISADORE, *Sexual Life After Sixty*. New York: Basic Books, Inc., 1965.

38. ———, *Sexual Life in the Later Years*. New York: Sex Information and Education Council of the United States Publication Office, 1970.

39. SHOCK, NATHAN, ed., *Aging: Some Social and Biological Aspects*. Washington, D.C.: American Association for the Advancement of Science, 1960.

40. ———, "The Physiology of Aging," *Scientific American*, 206: No. 2 (1962), 100–110.

41. SMOLENSKY, M., and A. REINBERG, "The Chronotherapy of Corticosteroids: Practical Application of Chronobiologic Findings to Nursing," *Nursing Clinics of North America*, 11: No. 4 (1976), 609–20.

42. SNYDER, LORRAINE, JANINE PYRIK, and K. SMITH, "Vision and Mental Function of the Aged," *The Gerontologist*, 16: No. 6 (1976), 491–95.

43. SOLLBERGER, A., *Biological Rhythm Research*. Amsterdam: Elsevier Publishing Company, 1965.

44. STOSKY, B., *The Elderly Patient*. New York: Grune & Stratton, Inc., 1968.

45. STREHLER, BERNARD, "Aging at the Cellular Level," in *Clinical Geriatrics*, ed. Isadore Rossman. Philadelphia: J. B. Lippincott Company, 1971.

46. *Taber's Cyclopedic Medical Dictionary,* 11th ed. Philadelphia: F. A. Davis Company, 1970.

47. TINDALL, JOHN, and ERDMAN PALMORE, "Skin Conditions and Lesions in the Aged: A Longitudinal Study," in *Normal Aging II,* ed. Erdman Palmore. Durham, N.C.: Duke University Press, 1974.

48. TINDALL, JOHN, and J. GRAHAM SMITH, "Skin Lesions in the Aged," in *Normal Aging,* ed. Erdman Palmore. Durham, N.C.: Duke University Press, 1970.

49. TOM, CHERYL, "Nursing Assessment of Biological Rhythms," *Nursing Clinics of North America,* 11: No. 4 (1976), 621–30.

50. "Twelve Ways to Overcome Deafness," *More Years for Your Life,* 7: No. 8 (1968), 3.

51. UHLER, DIANA, "Common Skin Changes in the Elderly," *American Journal of Nursing,* 78: No. 8 (1978), 1342–44.

52. United States Department of Health, Education, and Welfare, Public Health Service, *Working with Older People, Volume II: Biological, Psychological and Sociological Aspects of Aging.* Rockville, Md.: U.S. Department of HEW Public Health Service, 1970.

53. VOSE, GEORGE, *et al,* "Effect of Sodium Fluoride, Inorganic Phosphate, and Oxymetholone Therapies in Osteoporosis: A Six Year Progress Report," *Journal of Gerontology,* 33: No. 2 (1978), 204–12.

54. WEG, RUTH, "Aging and the Aged in Contemporary Society," *Physical Therapy,* 53: No. 7 (1973), 749–56.

55. WESSLER, R., M. RUBIN, and A. SOLLBERGER, "Circadian Rhythm of Activity and Sleep-Wakefulness in Elderly Institutionalized Persons," *Journal of Interdisciplinary Cycle Research,* 7: No. 4 (1976), 333–48.

cognitive characteristics in later maturity

Study of this chapter will enable you to:

1. Describe cognitive changes that normally occur in later maturity.

2. Assess the different components of cognitive function and recognize that certain areas may be limited while the senior functions normally in the remaining areas.

3. Use assessment of normal cognitive changes as a basis for nursing diagnosis, patient care objectives, and a care plan for the senior in various settings.

4. Intervene supportively, using self and environmental and physical aids, to help the senior maintain or regain cognitive competency.

5. Give information as appropriate to the person/family, using the guidelines discussed in this chapter to enhance learning.

6. Counsel the person/family about normal cognitive changes in late life and ways to cope so that function is enhanced.

7. Teach and work with other health team members to provide consistency in care in any health care setting.

8. Evaluate the effectiveness of your care in helping the senior to maintain cognitive competence and in preventing cognitive deterioration.

10

Contrary to the stereotype, the person in later maturity does not automatically degenerate in intellectual function. Assessment and care must be directed toward the healthy characteristics as well as the limitations that may exist.

This chapter will first describe the cognitive functions that have been established to date as normal for the senior. These functions may be assessed by using the method and tools discussed in Chapter 2. Various factors that influence cognitive responses will be explored, since they must be considered during assessment and planning of care. Then intervention measures to maintain or enhance cognitive function will be discussed.

Cognitive functions refer to mental and intellectual processes of drive, perception, interest, motivation, memory, reasoning, thought, learning, problem solving, and judgment. These functions include the ability to examine a situation; take in, process, and recall information; orient self in time and place; organize complex data; and respond appropriately to stimuli in content, emotion, and over time.

INTELLECTUAL ABILITY

Ability Related to Age

Chronological age is rarely a reliable index of the person's mental development. The initial level of ability is crucial; those with high IQ scores as children show progressive gains in general information, comprehension, vocabulary, and arithmetic when retested. A bright 20-year-old, all things being equal, will be a bright 70-year-old, and the bright 70-year-old will function better in certain cognitive skills than the average 20-year-old.[7,14,30,34]

In a study of men aged 65 to 92 years who were medically similar to a group of men whose average age was 21, the older men were significantly superior to the younger ones in verbal intelligence.[5,35] Apparently verbal facility, certain factors of judgment, most areas of learning retention, and well-practiced cognitive skills, such as those used in a profession or occupation, are retained into advanced old age.[2,6,29,30,32]

Intellectual changes in a group of 80-year-old people who were studied over a 25-year period showed less decline in vocabulary skills, comparison ability, and mathematical skills than is popularly believed to be true.[9] Another study extending for 14 years showed negligible changes in elderly persons in verbal meaning, reasoning, and numbers test scores.[48] Test scores on spatial perception and decoding tasks decline, perhaps because of sensory and coordination changes.[29] In one study of men and women ages 64 to 90, 50 percent increased and 50 percent decreased IQ scores. Age, initial endowment, retirement status, health, and other demographic variables were unrelated. Those who decreased scores over the years were isolated and lonely, and they related poorly to people. Those who increased scores were forceful, involved with, and accepted by others.[45]

Jarvik tested 268 pairs of twins ages 68 to 90 years; all of the twins were literate, white, English-speaking, and in satisfactory health. The intelligence performance of the twins equalled or exceeded norms established for persons 50 to 59, despite the younger group's having similar educational background. When the twins were tested one year later, scores had increased, showing continual learning. Mental ability is incremental during adulthood; brighter people show less decline than do normal or below-average people.[8,9] Recent studies also show that intellectual performance is increased with training programs.[44]

Longitudinal studies on the same population are the most useful approach to determining intellectual ability. Past cross-sectional studies that compared intelligence test scores of older persons with younger ones were not valid because older people had not been included in the norms upon which scores were determined. The elderly person typically also has less education, so that he is competing against a better educated younger person who is accustomed to and motivated by testing situations. No wonder the elderly see such testing as irrelevant and often participate in it marginally, if at all.[56]

Considerable time and energy have been spent measuring intellectual decline with increasing age. Perhaps more appropriate would be studies on the increment of wisdom. Listening to the person recall his life experiences could be a measure of his recall and maturity.[41] Verbal, practical, affective, cognitive, and social skills may better describe the senior's mental ability than converted scores on an IQ test.[31]

Problem-Solving Ability

The brain possesses a tremendous reserve capacity. Perhaps this is why the senior may cope very well despite the decrease of functioning nerve cells in the central nervous system, which is influenced by cellular, circulatory, and metabolic changes occurring in the body.[31]

The older person may be able to tolerate extensive degeneration in the central nervous system without serious alteration of behavior or cognitive function if the social environment is supportive. The person often remains relatively unimpaired because he has developed ways to counteract slight memory loss or difficulty in learning. Certain social skills or pleasant responses help the person through a situation, so that others may not notice intellectual deficits. If others' responses remain positive in turn, the senior's self-confidence enables him to use whatever skills he does have. Thus, daily functioning is likely to be unimpaired, and even in unusual situations the person is likely to come up with the best solution for himself.[14,35,42]

The initial level of ability is crucial for continued learning; those with high

IQ scores at a younger age are better able to cope with current stresses, manage new situations, or work more effectively in familiar situations by using a variety of skills that are enhanced by thoughtful experience and maturity.[41]

The elderly person is likely to be superior to the younger person in overall factual knowledge; coordination of facts or ideas, life experience and wisdom; use of authority and power to get things done; and maturity of judgment—all of which can enhance or maintain problem-solving ability and work performance.[16,31] Yet, how the senior uses his skills to do problem solving may differ from that of the younger person. He tends to use redundant information more effectively. Associations between words and events that are logically related and habitual behaviors are strengthened throughout life and are used more by the older than the younger person.[11,14,29,31] The older person performs more accurately when stimuli are logically grouped and sequential, when he is given a larger amount of data to process instead of isolated bits of information, and when he is given a longer time to process the data.[31,46,53] He is likely to work out mentally how to do something before he acts out his solution.

The senior is less likely to take advantage of information that is not directly relevant, and he is unlikely to acquire new ideas or concepts that do not have a definite advantage over currently held ideas or concepts.[11,56]

Tasks that require making analogies, forming new concepts or new classifications, and finding novel or creative answers are more difficult for the senior to perform although he will come up with a workable solution if given time.[11,31,46,53,56]

Creativity

Rigidity and concreteness in thought are considered typical in old age. The older person seems more rigid in his thinking because he is cautious and because he emphasizes accuracy instead of speed. The caution may result from a tendency to avoid risky decisions, perhaps because of fear of failure or because he has learned from past experiences that caution pays. Yet, when a decision cannot be avoided, the elderly are as likely to choose a high risk or innovative solution as are young people. The older person seems more concrete in his thinking because he strives to be functional or practical instead of abstract.[12,14,42]

Reduced use of abstraction skills has other results. Research indicates that appreciation of jokes increases but comprehension of subtle content decreases in old age.[49]

Persons in later maturity usually score lower on tests for creativity, which is in contradiction to the many well-known elderly creative people. Some better known people who were creative in later maturity include the following: (1) Hobbes who wrote productively until age 91; (2) Gladstone who became prime minister for the fourth time at age 84; (3) Jefferson who was inventive until his death at age 83; (4) Franklin who was a member of the Constitutional

Congress at age 81; (5) Sophocles who wrote *Oedipus Tyrannus* at age 80; (6) Goethe who completed *Faust* at age 80; (7) Tennyson who wrote poetry after age 80; (8) Churchill who became prime minister at age 77; (9) Handel, Haydn, and Verdi who created immortal music after age 70; and (10) Michelangelo who completed St. Peter's dome at age 70. You may be able to think of ordinary senior citizens who are also creative in their own way, even if they are not famous.

Past studies on creativity and productivity, measured by publications and discoveries, indicated that people are most creative between 30 and 50 years of age.[7] Actually, there is no age limit for creativity, since creativity is not limited to publications and discoveries. The human is creative in various ways. Current research indicates that the senior is often creative, even if he has not had much education. He uses past experience and insights in new ways to meet current situations. He reintegrates experience on a higher level—absorbing, sifting, and reconstructing reality on his own terms. He treats as hypothesis what most people treat as fact. He recognizes that anything encountered is incomplete, that it is in need of further study and reflection.[7,16,42]

Regardless of how creativity is defined—as superior quality or as total productivity at work—the peaks and declines are the result of more than intellectual changes. Will power, working strength, endurance, and enthusiasm are all part of creativity. With the trends toward longer educational preparation in many fields of work, future studies may reveal that creativity increases with age, since many people will be older before they can become productive.[16]

Reaction Time

Reaction time usually becomes slower as the person ages; although some older people, especially physically active people, react as quickly as some younger people do. The senior needs extra time to perform physical tasks. Performance scores tend to be lower and are used to explain intellectual decline. Yet, by practicing a task the older person can learn to act quickly and improve his reaction time.[14]

The senior performs certain cognitive tasks more slowly for several reasons: (1) decreased visual and auditory acuity, (2) slower motor response to sensory stimulation, (3) loss of recent memory, and (4) changed motivation. He may be less interested in competing in timed intellectual tests. Further, an apparently shorter duration of alpha rhythm in the brain wave affects the timing of response.[53] Reaction time is also slower when the person suffers significant environmental or social losses, when he is unable to engage in social contact, and when he is unable to plan his daily routines. The person who is ill often endures environmental and social losses by virtue of being in the patient role.[6,27,53] Thus, he may be slower responding to your questions or requests.

Yet, some tests have shown that mental reaction time begins to decline after 26 years of age. In one study adults who were 71 were compared with 43-

year-olds. Both sets of subjects were given the same test for vigilance or clock-watching. The seniors were as attentive and vigilant as the young adults for 45 minutes; after that, loss of interest and fatigue reduced their degree of vigilance. However, an attention span of 45 minutes is considered acceptable in young adults, as evidenced by the length of a class hour (50 minutes) in most colleges.[33]

Reaction time is affected by preexisting expectations for stimuli as well as expectations during the experiment. The senior is more likely to expect change rather than repetition in sequences; he had developed a bit of a "gambling" attitude toward life over the years. Thus, he responds faster to stimuli that are not repetitious. Most tests for reaction time involve repetitious stimuli, which may influence test scores.[14,23]

The person over 50 performs less efficiently in tasks requiring speed or when given little advance time to respond to the task. The older person has a longer response initiation time, especially when hand movements are involved. He takes longer to convert verbal stimuli to a mental image.[38,40] Response is slower if action must be carried out without seeing what is being done, when a large quantity of data is presented in illogical order, when a quantity of evidence must be pieced together without using memory aids such as notes, and when abstractions are presented.[14,53] Yet many younger people also have difficulty under such conditions.

The average elderly man performs less accurately in fast-paced than in slow-paced situations; he is less likely to try in fast-paced situations unless he is sure of the accuracy of his response. Performance of the average elderly woman is comparable to that of the younger highly verbal man and woman in fast-paced situations. Throughout life women excel in verbal ability and fluency tests. Older women also tend to respond more readily to cognitive, psychomotor tasks than do elderly men.[14,23,58]

Memory

A progressive loss of *memory, the ability to retain or recall past thoughts, images, ideas, or experiences,* does not necessarily occur in later maturity, although memory loss affects more people as they get older. Loss of *short-term memory, recall for recent events,* is more likely to occur than loss of *remote memory, recall for events that occurred in the past.*

The person's permanent memory is an organized network of concepts interrelated in specific ways. If the relationship between these concepts cannot be used because of loss, decreased retrieval, or slower access, the person loses conceptual richness or spontaneous use of memory links. Such loss is more likely to occur in older people than in younger people and in persons institutionalized than in persons living in the community, apparently because of the number of life crises and less intellectual stimulation for the former group.[39]

Memory loss may occur for various reasons:

1. Interference from other memories that are valued by the person and accumulated with age.
2. Sense of worthlessness or depression, so that less energy is directed toward recall.
3. Loss of interest in current events; past memories are more pleasant.
4. Neurochemical and circulatory changes that may affect cerebral function.
5. Loss of cells in the central nervous system.
6. Difficulty in information acquisition because of deficiency in neural synapses in the storage system.[11]

Short-term memory is central to learning processes that would not otherwise decline with age. Synthesis, analysis, comparison, and ability to organize content are less dependent on short-term memory, and these functions do not decline with age. The problem in learning occurs because the person loses the pieces of immediate information needed to process, code, or synthesize.[35,54] Short-term visual memory appears to be more susceptible to aging than is auditory memory.

The senior has difficulty in ordering the time sequence of more recent events, in rote memory, and in immediate recall of new learning.[7] He uses fewer mental images to enhance verbal phrases he hears and to act as memory mediators, which may account for the poorer performance on memory tests.

Long-term or remote memory, including vocabulary, personal history, past experience, and basic knowledge, is highly resistant to the effects of normal aging.

FACTORS THAT INFLUENCE COGNITIVE RESPONSE

Many factors must be considered when you assess the intellectual level, problem-solving ability, creativity, reaction time, or memory of the older person, including the following:

1. Interest in living and in events about him.
2. Sensory impairments that interfere with integration of sensory input into proper perception.
3. Amount of time since he was in school or in an intellectually demanding position.
4. Educational level, past involvement in informal learning activities, or earlier cognitive incapacities.
5. Amount of deliberate caution, that is, using more time to answer or do a task, which can be interpreted as not knowing.
6. Presence of adaptive mechanisms to conserve energy rather than showing assertion or time-consciousness.

7. Degree of motivation to please those around him or to participate in a testing situation.
8. Presence of ill-health.[24,26,28,30,47,50,57]

Previous life-style, present behavior patterns, and general coping mechanisms all affect cognitive function and must be considered in assessment. Observe behavior in a variety of situations and listen to the person's conversation and reminiscences. Talk with family members or friends. Consider the total, unique individual physically, emotionally, and socially so that you can increase the accuracy of your cognitive assessment.

Too often cognitive impairment of the person in later maturity is considered as irreversible brain damage or chronic brain syndrome. Recent research indicates that mental impairment may be caused by a number of complex and interacting relationships of biological, psychological, social, and environmental factors. Even when brain damage is present, impairment may range from slight to severe.[7]

Emotional Factors

Some of what is called mental impairment results from our approach to older people. Society expects the older person to become deteriorated or "senile." If his self-image is affected by a role expectation of mental dysfunction, his behavior becomes "senile," an example of the self-fulfilling prophecy. Institutional life also limits motivation to behave appropriately because opportunities are not used to draw out functions assumed to be lost in old age. The institution is often devoid of time and environmental cues, and confinement causes disorientation and confusion. Reactions of others markedly affect the person's motivation to stay alert, to learn, to be creative. The person who feels worthless is less likely to try.

The person who suffers marked losses, especially the loss of a significant person, tends to perform less adequately on psychometric and personality tests. Often general behavior and problem-solving abilities are noticeably less effective as well.[46]

The relationship between three cognitive ability factors (ability to process information, manual dexterity in response to stimuli, and ability to analyze patterns) and three personality dimensions (anxiety, extroversion, and openness to experience) were examined in over 900 males aged 25 to 82 years. Persons who were highly anxious scored lower on all three cognitive ability factors. Persons open to experience scored higher on ability to process information and analyze patterns. Introverted persons scored higher on ability to analyze patterns than did extroverts. Older people performed less well than younger ones on manual dexterity and ability to analyze patterns, but they did equally well on ability to process information.[17]

The senior is more apprehensive about new learning situations, especially in a competitive atmosphere. He anticipates difficulty in learning new tasks and asks for more detail and specific directions.[7] Certainly questions should not be interpreted as mental incompetency.

The older person is usually more cautious than the younger adult because of his experience, which accounts in part for the difference in experimental test performance. Whenever possible, tasks are selected that have less risk or at which the person has a higher probability of success, probably to avoid a negative self-evaluation.[7,23,42]

Social Factors

Our culture values a rapid verbal and motor response. The older person has internalized that value, and because he cannot respond rapidly to a question, statement, or task, he may devalue himself. Further, he may have internalized the cultural expectation that school is only for youngsters. Hence, he lacks confidence in pursuing formal or informal learning activities. He may consider himself and other older people too stupid or slow to learn.

The older person should be seen as a productive person who has been learning all of his life. Any decline of mental powers is more likely to result from the brain getting too little rather than too much work. Lack of environmental stimulation, forced isolation, and disengagement hasten mental and physical decline; the person feels less like making the effort to respond intellectually. Those who continue to work have more normal brain function and higher intelligence test scores in later maturity than do those who are idle.[23,24,25,27,29] Society needs the cognitive potential of our senior citizens and should provide opportunities for them to use their skills.

Physical Factors

Sensory impairments that accompany aging, described in Chapter 9, can cause the person to miss certain stimuli and as a result appear intellectually impaired.

In one study of the relationship between visual and mental function, subjects were divided into three groups on the basis of visual acuity: (1) adequate vision—better than 20/70; (2) low vision, 20/70 to 20/100; and (3) legally blind—20/200 or worse. The group with adequate vision scored highest on the mental status questionnaire. Lowest scores were in the legally blind group. That most older people could cooperate with vision and mental testing was also shown.[50]

At this point, whether vision loss causes impaired mental functioning or organic brain disease causes impaired vision is unknown; they are probably interrelated. Also, medications, general physical health, and emotional state can affect both visual and mental function.[50]

A direct relationship also exists between hearing loss and reduced cognitive effectiveness. Hearing loss results in changed speech perception and in reduced ability to define concepts, describe abstract relationships, and even to recall stored information. Thus, hearing loss affects cognitive test scores, reaction time, and personality.[26]

If the person cannot see adequately or hear what you are saying, his response may appear confused, disoriented, or stupid when none of these characteristics is present. The problem is increased if you are speaking English and the elderly person's first language is not English. Inability to differentiate among environmental stimuli and decreased speed of processing information also limit the person's ability to assess the possible constraints and opportunities within the environment, thus limiting his coping strategies.[20]

A serious illness or injury in early life often causes damage to certain brain cells. The person must relearn the functions regulated by these cells; later cognitive impairment can result from incomplete relearning and the illness rather than from the aging process alone.[19]

Numerous illnesses reduce cognitive function and cause disorientation or confusion, as discussed in Units IV and V. Poor health and lower energy levels cause the person to resist becoming involved in planned learning activities and to score poorly on intellectual tests. Even mild disease negatively affects intellectual performance, especially memory, adherence to given tasks, answering appropriately, and ordered sequence of thought. Thus, any ill person will show less mental acuity, which must be considered in planning and giving care.[52,57]

Rapid decline in cognitive function may be a predictor of death if the person has previously been alert and mentally capable. Studies indicate that intellectual functions decline in the aged person primarily one year before natural death.[7,8]

NURSING PROCESS TO PROMOTE AND MAINTAIN COGNITIVE FUNCTIONING

Assessment and Planning Care

Your assessment of a person in later maturity may include the following:

1. Is alert, oriented, and rational, as indicated by speech and behavior.
2. Responds accurately to directions.
3. Recalls data appropriate to the situation.
4. Demonstrates ability to think through situations and make decisions and judgments based upon data.
5. Avoids situations that are unduly hazardous or that will jeopardize self emotionally, socially, financially, or physically.
6. Responds to chosen stimuli with interest and curiosity.

From these and other assessments, your *nursing diagnosis* would be *unimpaired cognitive functioning*. Or an impairment might exist in one of the cognitive areas discussed, but the senior would be functioning normally in all other areas. The nursing diagnosis would be indicative of such an assessment.

Long-term care goals for such a person could include the following:

1. Tasks related to all spheres of daily living are accomplished realistically and with full awareness.
2. Information that is essential to daily living is retained or learned as needed.

Short-term goals could include the following:

1. Reality contact is maintained.
2. Problem-solving activities appropriate to the life situation are accomplished.
3. Creativity is achieved through self-initiated activities.
4. Memory is stimulated through various activities to ensure appropriate responses.
5. New information pertinent to health or self-care is learned.

Additional goals may be appropriate for a patient/client you are caring for with the nursing diagnosis of unimpaired cognition.

Intervention

Because diagnosis usually connotes a pathological state, you may feel that a nursing diagnosis cannot refer to normal functioning. On the contrary, healthy characteristics can be maintained through appropriate planning and intervention. Too often intervention is directed only toward pathology. The following discussion will cover specific measures to maintain or restore cognitive function that can be used by you and other health care workers in any setting.

Supportive Approach

If you personally value cognitive abilities, the occasional memory lapses, slower verbal responses, or apparent lack of interest in learning that you observe in the elderly person may be very threatening. You will need to work through your own attitudes before you can be supportive to the client.

Establishing a trust relationship is supportive and implies that you are available to the person and will not allow anything detrimental to happen to him. Trust implies that you help the person assume whatever responsibility he can for himself, even if his abilities seem marginal. Decision making is left to the client unless his decision will cause hurt or shame to him or others. Work with and respect his assets and limits.

Because you are a nurse, you represent understanding, patience, assistance, encouragement, practical counselor, and teacher to the older person. You can become both guide and companion. Your empathy can support the client so that he maintains present cognitive abilities or regains previous abilities.

Listen to the person talk about the changing cognitive abilities that he perceives. Help him to express frustration and cope with the reality of short-term memory loss, such as forgetting a phone number or the name of someone he just met.

Reinforce that you do not see the person as stupid or less of a person if he makes mistakes. Your kind, sincere approach can lessen the embarrassment caused by poor judgment, slower reaction, or having to struggle to follow the directions on a form.

You will find that the senior responds to your empathy, acceptance, affection, listening, and confidence in his abilities. Often the client demonstrates learning, creativity, and improved recall because he senses that you think he can. The self-fulfilling prophecy works here also.

Equally supportive are the use of touch; clearly stated directions, explanations, or questions; and avoidance of false reassurance or superficially sweet, condescending conversation. The client can better act and think like an adult when you approach him as one.

Interest in the person's activities, however limited, may stimulate further cognition. One 88-year-old lady spent many hours of many lonely days writing down the titles of all the songs she could remember. Each week when the nurse came, the lady would name the song titles; if the nurse knew the songs, they would sing them together. Those unknown to the nurse would be sung alone by the woman, to the obvious pleasure of both. The client often remarked that she did not realize how many songs she knew. The nurse remarked how many songs she had learned. What a lovely way for a bedfast lady to give to another human being.

Creativity can be stimulated in a like manner. When this author was previously writing a book, one of her clients also started writing a story. At each visit, the elderly lady would read a portion of what she had written. Queries about the possibility of having the story published were answered with some encouragement, but when the story was finished, the client said that she would not want to publish it, even if it were acceptable. She stated, "This story is my own creation. It's me. I can't share it with anyone else except you and Chris (her granddaughter). This is for *me* to keep." The worth was in the project and what it had accomplished emotionally for her.

Environmental Support

We all need clocks and calendars to remain oriented; the elderly person is no exception. The face of the clock and the size of the calendar should be large enough to be visible to someone with impaired vision. You may have to wind the clock or watch or remind the person to do so. You can use a large sheet of paper to draw a monthly calendar, adding color and appropriate pictures to add interest. Crossing off each previous day aids orientation if the person needs such assistance.

People in the environment can be supportive and stimulate interest, intellectual ability, and creativity. If the person is institutionalized, membership in one of the groups discussed in Chapter 4 is essential, depending on his needs. If the person lives in the community, you may have to help him secure membership in and transportation to various groups or organizations or arrange for visitors to his home in order to reduce isolation and the resulting impaired cognition.

Sharing your magazines or books can help the client stay abreast of current affairs and think different thoughts. Radio and television are useful in maintaining reality contact if the person lives alone, but the person might enjoy even more the participation in a game or the mental activity involved in a crossword or picture puzzle.

Various objects—pictures, flowers, or knickknacks—can be used to initiate conversation, encourage reminiscing, and stimulate creativity. Often a few basic supplies given to the person will get him started on enjoyable projects.

Sometimes the social environment can provide a reason for staying alert. One lady in the eighties who had always related well with children found a part-time job in her home. She was able to keep several children after school until their parents came home from work. These two hours each afternoon were stimulating to the senior and children alike as she told them stories, engaged them in games, and made a dollhouse with them. Certainly such arrangements could be considered more often by working parents, especially in the one-parent home, if an elderly neighbor is available and willing.

Occupational, physical, and recreational therapy programs are useful to the person who is institutionalized or who can visit the senior citizen center. However, some older people prefer to self-initiate instead of being a part of a structured activity. Their preferences should be respected. Activities should be personally meaningful instead of contrived; otherwise, the person may lose interest and cognitive skills.

Physical Support

Encourage the elderly person to wear prescribed eye glasses or correctly fitted hearing aid if necessary. Then he can receive orienting stimuli and needed information and avoid sensory deprivation and suspicious feelings. Pride about appearance, denial of impairment, or insufficient funds may prevent the person from obtaining the needed prosthesis. Further, the person may be unaware of the sensory loss for a time because he has learned to compensate; your reality input can help him realize his deficit.

In order to enhance cognitive functioning, increased sensory stimuli are necessary to overcome the less efficient sensory receptors.[4,34] However, not all elderly are deaf or visually impaired. Therefore, you do not have to shout or act as if the person were deaf or blind. Use the methods discussed in Chapter 9 to talk with the hearing impaired more effectively.

Avoid excessive stimuli (too much noise or too much visual input) because the aged have more difficulty screening out irrelevant stimuli, which in turn adds to feelings of stress, inability to concentrate, errors, confusion, and disorientation.[52]

Maintain a schedule and routine in your care of the client. If the person lives at home, encourage him to follow a schedule. A schedule for both mental and physical activity provides limits and security; it encourages the person to use his abilities, and it helps the person maintain orientation. Let the person set the pace for his activities and learning so that he feels stimulated but not rushed. Begin and end an activity on time.

Informational Support

Encourage the elderly person to participate in decision making related to his health care and to necessary changes in care or routines. Avoid change in routine whenever possible; if change is unavoidable, the person should be informed as far in advance as practical so that he can get used to the idea. Changes should be discussed with the person; allow time for questions and explanation, and give him a feeling that he is in control. Withholding information about a change in health care causes a loss of sense of control over self and destiny, and it adds to disorientation, confusion, and loss of cognitive ability.[52]

One of your important roles is that of teacher to the client and his family. You will teach both formally and spontaneously. The senior decides to enter the learning activity for various reasons: (1) to find answers to questions, (2) to learn specific cognitive or physical skills or health care measures, (3) to better understand the self, or (4) to further educate the self formally.

You will have to plan and implement experiences for the person in later maturity differently from the way you would for younger adults or children. The senior thinks of self as responsible, self-directing, and mature; an approach that treats him like a child or does not acknowledge his present knowledge or skill is resented. If the elderly person can help plan and conduct the learning activity, he is likely to learn more because he is more involved.[47] Further, the learning activity should be conveniently reached so that he is not too tired to participate. Proper ventilation and temperature are especially important in maintaining alertness and preventing discomfort. The time should be convenient and when the person is at peak functioning. His requests regarding time and place should be considered.

Previously reinforced ways of doing things take precedence over new behavior. The older person seems to learn more easily if essential information is related to previous learning and current needs, interests, and occupation, and he is likely to recall data that can be directly applied or can be seen as relevant.

Because he considers many aspects, he works more slowly and takes longer to make a decision. Thus, his reaction time is longer. He needs time to assimilate new content with past experience and learning.[47]

The person learns better when he is actively involved in discussion and in questions and answers instead of sitting or reading passively. In one study, words at the end of a list were better recalled when the person read the list aloud himself instead of reading the list silently.[3]

Repetition is important for learning at any age. However, sessions do not have to seem repetitious if they are used to reinforce material previously learned and if new and old content is mixed together to maximize understanding. The same general principles can be related to a variety of topics, several motor skills, or tangible experience. Repetition is also facilitated by asking for feedback or a return demonstration.

Demonstration, practice sessions, and written instructions should be provided along with verbal messages to allow for an expansion of ideas and refinement of skills. Content should be divided into units that allow for self-paced learning and that do not overwhelm the person. The real situation should be simulated as much as possible so that the basic steps of the task can be clearly perceived and learned. Focus the person's attention on the task before presenting it so that he will have time to prepare his response. No new verbal stimuli should be given until the person has had time to respond to previous stimuli.[39]

Have a patient, pleasant, and encouraging attitude so that you stimulate the person's desire to learn and prevent discouragement, depression, and a negative self-concept. Help each person to feel that his ideas are important, that his work is successful. Show interest in and appreciation of his efforts.

When you are planning and presenting a learning activity, consider the following points to help the elderly person overcome sensory deficits as you teach:

1. Have illumination that is bright and without glare or flicker.
2. Use visual or other auditory aids to supplement your talk so that the person may use several senses in learning, and place aids or demonstration equipment so that all persons can see and hear.
3. Use sharp contrasts of color against a neutral background when preparing visual aids.
4. Use pictures that are large and colorful.

5. Use large, legible printing or writing on large charts or diagrams.
6. Type duplicated materials in pica type and double space.
7. Speak slowly and distinctly and look directly at the audience. Keep your hands away from your mouth. Use a microphone if there is a possibility that someone cannot hear.
8. Use simple words that are clear and meaningful; avoid jargon or unnecessarily long words.
9. Write unusual or unfamiliar words or names on a blackboard or poster or use an overhead projector.
10. Minimize outside and inside noises or distractions that will interfere with learning.
11. Observe the learner carefully to determine whether or not he is hearing, seeing, and understanding.[39,47]

COMMUNITY SUPPORT FOR EDUCATION

Retirement education is currently attracting much attention among employers, educational institutions, service agencies, and gerontological workers. Traditionally, retirement planning programs were considered the only necessary educational courses. The retired person is now perceived as a continuing learner; the elderly person increasingly enrolls in various academic and non-academic courses. Local school boards may offer formal courses free or at a reduced rate for senior citizens; these courses usually attract many seniors.

Educational opportunities for the senior citizen are directed toward enhancement of self-concept, development of achievement motivation, promotion of creativity, clarification of human values, improvement of human relationships, adaptation to social changes, and acquisition of practical skills. Such education is learner-centered; the teacher serves as facilitator instead of a giver of knowledge. The teacher must be skillful in devoting sufficient time for participation and yet impart sufficient information to help the learner handle his concerns.[11]

Since the older person may not have had contact with a formal learning environment for some years, he will need time to adjust to current teaching methods. The informal democratic participation that younger people take for granted may be enjoyed, but at first the person may consider such behavior inappropriate for "students." Acceptance of the person and appreciation of his individual needs will help him become involved and will help him overcome apprehension and hesitancy.

In conclusion, as a nurse and as a citizen, you have a responsibility to help the person in later maturity maintain normal cognitive function. Accurate assessment and nursing diagnosis, thoughtful planning and intervention, and *evaluation* of your nursing practice are essential. You may evaluate your care as effective if you prevent deterioration, even if the senior has not learned all that you had prepared for him. Additionally, your expertise is useful in guiding community programs that will serve the intellectual needs of the elderly. You should determine which programs are most effective, since they may become a resource for your elderly patient/client/family.

REFERENCES

1. ANDERSON, J. E., ed., *Psychological Aspects of Aging.* Washington, D.C.: American Psychological Association, 1956.

2. ARENBURG, DAVID, "Cognition and Aging: Verbal Learning, Memory, and Problem-Solving," in *The Psychology of Adult Development and Aging,* eds. C. Eisdorfer and M. Lawton. Washington, D.C: American Psychological Association, 1973.

3. ———, "The Effects of Input Condition on Free Recall in Young and Old Adults," *Journal of Gerontology,* 31: No. 5 (1976), 551–55.

4. BERGMAN, M., V. BLUMENFELD, D. CASCARDO, B. DASH, H. LEVITT, and M. MARGULIS, "Age-Related Decrement in Hearing for Speech," *Journal of Gerontology,* 31: No. 5 (1976), 533–38.

5. BIRREN, JAMES, *The Psychology of Aging.* Englewood Cliffs, N.J.: Prentice-Hall, Inc., 1964.

6. ———, "Psychological Aspects of Aging: Intellectual Functioning," *The Gerontologist,* 8: (1968), 16–19.

7. BISCHOFF, LEDFORD, *Adult Psychology.* New York: Harper & Row, Publishers, Inc., 1969.

8. BLUM, J., E. CLARK, and L. JARVIK, "The New York State Psychiatric Institute Study of Aging Twins," in *Intellectual Functioning in Adults,* eds. Lissy Jarvik, C. Eisendorfer, and J. Blum. New York: Springer Publishing Co., Inc., 1973, pp. 13–19.

9. BLUM, JUNE, J. FOSSHAGE, and L. JARVIK, "Intellectual Changes and Sex Differences in Octogenarians: A Twenty-Five Year Longitudinal Study of Aging," *Developmental Psychology,* 7: (1972), 178–87.

10. BOLTON, CHRISTOPHER, "Humanistic-Instructional Strategies and Retirement Education Programming," *The Gerontologist,* 16: No. 6 (1976), 550–55.

11. BOTWINICK, JACK, *Cognitive Processes in Maturity and Old Age.* New York: Springer Publishing Co., Inc., 1967.

12. ———, "Disinclination to Venture Response Versus Cautiousness in Responding: Age Differences," *Journal of Genetic Psychology,* 115: (1969), 55–62.

13. ———, "Geropsychology," *Annual Review of Psychiatry,* 21: (1970), 239–72.

14. ———, *Aging and Behavior.* New York: Springer Publishing Co., Inc., 1973.

15. BOYLE, EDWIN, A. APARICIO, K. JONAS, and M. ACKER, "Auditory and Visual Memory Losses in Aging Populations," *Journal of American Geriatric Society,* 23: (1975), 284–86.

16. BULLOUGH, VERN, BONNIE BULLOUGH, and MADDALENA MANUO, "Age and Achievement: A Dissenting View," *The Gerontologist,* 18: No. 6 (1978), 584–87.

17. BYNUM, J., B. COOPER, and F. ACUFF, "Retirement Reorientation: Senior Adult Education," *Journal of Gerontology,* 33: No. 2 (1978), 253–61.

18. COSTA, PAUL, J. FOZARD, R. McCRAE, and R. BOSSE, "Relations of Age and Personality Dimensions to Cognitive Ability Factors," *Journal of Gerontology,* 31: No. 6 (1976), 663–69.

19. CRAIG, GRACE, *Human Development.* Englewood Cliffs, N.J.: Prentice-Hall, Inc., 1976.

20. DATAN, NANCY, and LEON GINSBERG, eds., *Life-Span Developmental Psychology.* New York: Academic Press, Inc., 1975.

21. EDWARDS, A. E., and G. M. HART, "Hyperbaric Oxygenation and the Cognitive Functioning of the Aged," *Journal of American Geriatric Society,* 22: No. 8 (1974), 376–79.

22. EISENDORFER, C., "Attitudes Toward Old People: A Re-Analysis of the Item-Validity of the Stereotype Scale," *Journal of Gerontology,* 21: (1966), 455–62.

23. FOZARD, J., J. THOMAS, and N. WAUGH, "Effects of Age and Frequency of Stimulus Repetitions on Two-Choice Reaction Time," *Journal of Gerontology,* 31: No. 5 (1976), 556–63.

24. GEIST, HAROLD, *The Psychological Aspects of the Aging Process.* St. Louis: Warren H. Green, Inc., 1968.

25. GRANICK, S., and A. FRIEDMAN, "Educational Experience and Maintenance of Intellectual Function by the Aged: An Overview," in *Intellectual Functioning in Adults,* eds. L. Jarvik, C. Eisendorfer, and J. Blum. New York: Springer Publishing Co., Inc., 1973, pp. 54–69.

26. GRANICK, SAMUEL, M. KLEBAN, and A. WEISS, "Relationships Between Hearing Loss and Cognition in Normally Hearing Aged Persons," *Journal of Gerontology,* 31: No. 4 (1976), 434–40.

27. GRANICK, SAMUEL, and ROBERT PATTERSON, eds., *Human Aging II: An Eleven-Year Follow-up Biomedical and Behavioral Study.* Publication No. (HSM) 71-9037. Washington, D.C.: United States Government Printing Office, 1971.

28. GUTTMAN, DAVID, "Life Events and Decision Making by Older Adults," *The Gerontologist,* 18: No. 5 (1978), 462–67.

29. HAND, SAMUEL, "What It Means to Teach Older Adults," in *A Manual on Planning Education Programs for Older Adults,* ed., Andrew Hendrickson. Tallahassee, Fla.: Florida State University, 1973.

30. HAVIGHURST, ROBERT, W. McDONALD, L. MAEULAN, and J. MAZEL, "Male Social Scientists: Lives After Sixty," *The Gerontologist,* 19: No. 1 (1979), 55–60.

31. Health Services and Mental Health Administration, *Working with Older People: The Practitioner and the Elderly, Volume II.* Rockville, Md.: U.S. Department of Health, Education, and Welfare, May, 1972.

32. HODGKINS, J., "Influence of Age on the Speed of Reaction and Movement in Females," *Journal of Gerontology,* 17: (1962), 385–89.

33. HURLOCK, ELIZABETH, *Developmental Psychology,* 4th ed. New York: McGraw-Hill Book Company, 1975.

34. KIMMEL, DOUGLAS, *Adulthood and Aging.* New York: John Wiley & Sons, Inc., 1974.

35. KIRCHNER, W., "Age Differences in Short-Term Retention of Rapidly Changing Information," *Journal of Experimental Psychology,* 55: (1958), 352–58.

36. LAWSON, J. S., "Changes in Immediate Memory with Age," *British Journal of Psychology,* 56: (1965), 69–75.

37. LEVINE, L. S., *Personal and Social Development.* New York: Holt, Rinehart and Winston, 1963.

38. MISTLER-LACKMAN, JANET, "Spontaneous Shift in Encoding Dimensions Among Elderly Subjects," *Journal of Gerontology,* 32: No. 1 (1977), 68–72.

39. MURRAY, RUTH, and JUDITH ZENTNER, *Nursing Assessment and Health Promotion Through the Life Span,* 2nd ed. Englewood Cliffs, N.J.: Prentice-Hall, Inc., 1979.

40. NEBES, ROBERT, "Verbal-Pictorial Recording in the Elderly," *Journal of Gerontology,* 31: No. 4 (1976), 421–27.

41. NEUGARTEN, BERNICE, "Grow Old Along with Me: The Best Is Yet to Be," *Psychology Today,* 5: No. 7 (1971), 45ff.

42. OKUM, M., and F. DiVESTA, "Cautiousness in Adulthood as a Function of Age and Instruction," *Journal of Gerontology,* 31: No. 5 (1976), 571–76.

43. ———, I. SIEGLER, and L. GEORGE, "Cautiousness and Verbal Learning in Adulthood," *Journal of Gerontology,* 33: No. 1 (1978), 94–97.

44. PLEMONS, J., S. WILLIS, and P. BALTES, "Modifiability of Fluid Intelligence in Aging: A Short-Term Longitudinal Training Approach," *Journal of Gerontology,* 33: No. 2 (1978), 224–31.

45. RHUDICK, P., and C. GORDON, "The Age Center of New England Studies," in *Intellectual Functioning in Adults,* eds. L. Jarvis, C. Eisendorfer, and J. Blum. New York: Springer Publishing Co., Inc., 1973, pp. 7–12.

46. RIEGEL, KLAUS, and RUTH RIEGEL, "Development, Drop, and Death," *Developmental Psychology,* 6: No. 2 (1972), 306–19.

47. ROTROCK, LAWRENCE, and LINDA MILLER, *Active and Alert: Learning Experiences for Older Adults.* Jefferson City, Mo.: Missouri Office of Aging, 1976.

48. SCHAIE, K., G. LABOUVIE, and B. BUECH, "Generational and Cohort—Specific Differences in Adult Cognitive Functioning: A Fourteen Year Study of Independent Samples," *Developmental Psychology,* 9: (1963), 151–61.

49. SCHAIER, ARON, and V. CICERELLI, "Age Differences in Humor Comprehension and Appreciation in Old Age," *Journal of Gerontology,* 31: No. 5 (1976), 577–82.

50. SNYDER, LORRAINE, JANINE PYREK, and K. SMITH, "Vision and Mental Function of the Aged," *The Gerontologist,* 16: No. 6 (1976), 491–95.

51. SPIRDUSO, W., and P. CLIFFORD, "Replication of Age and Physical Activity Effects on Reaction and Movement Time," *Journal of Gerontology,* 33: No. 1 (1978), 26–30.

52. WAHL, PATRICIA, "Psychosocial Implications of Disorientation in the Elderly," *Nursing Clinics of North America,* 11: No. 1 (1976), 145–55.

53. WELFORD, A. T., *Aging and Human Skill.* London: Oxford Publishers, 1958.

54. ———, "Experimental Psychology in the Study of Aging," *British Medical Bulletin,* 20: (1964), 65–69.

55. ———, "Industrial Work Suitable for Older People: Some British Studies," *The Gerontologist,* 6: (1966), 4–9.

56. WETHERICK, N. E., "Changing an Established Concept: A Comparison of the Ability of Young, Middle-Aged, and Old Subjects," *Gerontologia,* 11: (1965), 82–95.

57. WILKE, FRANCES, and CARL EISENDORFER, "Systemic Disease and Behavioral Correlates," in *Intellectual Function in Adults,* eds. L. Jarvik, C. Eisendorfer, and J. Blum. New York: Springer Publishing Co., Inc., 1973, pp. 83–93.

58. ———, "Sex, Verbal Ability, and Pacing Differences in Serial Learning," *Journal of Gerontology,* 32: No. 1 (1977), 63–67.

emotional development in later maturity

Study of this chapter will enable you to:

1. Describe components that contribute to emotional development in later maturity.

2. Discuss factors that influence the senior's emotional health, self-concept/body-image development, personality development, and adaptive capacities.

3. Describe emotional/personality characteristics that may be found in many elderly persons.

4. Assess emotional status, achievement of developmental tasks, and adaptive mechanisms in an elderly person.

5. Use assessment of emotional status as a basis for nursing diagnosis, patient care objectives, and a care plan for the senior in various settings.

6. Discuss various intervention methods that will help the senior maintain emotional health.

7. Use effective communication skills and a trust relationship as a basis for other interventions with the person/family.

8. Work with the senior to help him understand his feelings and how to better meet his emotional needs.

9. Help family members to understand the emotional characteristics and meet the needs of their senior member.

10. Help other health team members to understand the emotional needs and characteristics of the elderly person, and the meaning of his behavior.

11. Work with other team members to promote continued emotional development and prevent psychiatric illness in the senior.

12. Evaluate your feelings in relation to the senior, your care approach, and the effectiveness of your nursing practice.

11

"Old age, to the unlearned, is winter;
to the learned, it is harvest time."

—Yiddish Proverb

In the previous chapters later maturity was discussed as a single life stage; retirement age was used as a marker. Yet some people *feel* that they are middle-aged until 70 or 75 years.[10]

But emotional maturity is different from physical or cognitive maturity. While normal physical or cognitive characteristics for late life may be observed in someone who is 50 or 55 or may not be observed until the person is 80 or 85, emotional maturity is on a continuum. The young-old and the old-old differ in their wisdom and emotional outlook. The clients this author has worked with over many years are not the same people emotionally at 65, 75, 85, and 95.

While normal emotional development will be discussed generally as applicable to all people in later life, some differences between the young-old and old-old will be explored.

EMOTIONAL HEALTH AND MATURITY

What are normal emotional characteristics? What is emotional health? What is maturity? These are difficult questions to answer. The medical and nursing professions have traditionally focused on illness; only recently have they spoken of health promotion. Health is usually defined by the practitioner in a practical way, that is, by the absence of signs and symptoms of disease. Maturity is even more subjective to define. *Maturity may be an attitude, a collection of activities or worthwhile attributes, practical wisdom, stable and socially acceptable behavior, or a ripening and preparation for the next stage of life.*[10] The emotionally healthy, mature senior has satisfying ties with others, does not use any one defense mechanism too frequently, too rigidly in every situation, or for too long a duration after a stressful situation. The person is not a nuisance to himself or to others.[87]

Characteristics of Maturity

The elderly often display in their unique way the characteristics of emotional health and maturity. The following characteristics cited by Jahoda are examples.[50]

Accepting personal strengths and limits and having a firm sense of identity. The senior is firm about what he can and cannot do and may need much encouragement to change behavior or realize a potential talent or skill. He is not easily persuaded from likes and dislikes. He quickly sees through false praise. He usually has a fairly accurate understanding of his positive and negative characteristics, and he accepts and likes himself in spite of his faults. He knows when he needs to be alone and when he needs to be with people. He may say, "I know I seem silly, but this is best for me."

Living to the highest potential; striving for self-actualization. The senior may have difficulty doing all he wants to do because of limitations imposed by declining health or the stressors discussed in Chapter 6. Yet, if given the opportunity and encouragement, he will try new activities, and he usually will enjoy them. Many elderly will push themselves physically as far as they can. Sometimes when the mate dies, the widow says, "In the time I have left I'm going to do what I want to. Let the housework go; there's more to life." And when grief is lessened, she may do volunteer work or travel for the first time. The old-old can do helpful things for others in their own homes, such as making bedpads for use by a home health agency or bandages for the local cancer society.

Resisting stress, conserving energy, attempting to maintain an equilibrium of intrapsychic forces, and developing a philosophy of life. Although he is not likely to seek risky situations, the senior often copes with taxing situations with less overt agitation and anxiety than could be expected in the situation. For example, while an arthritic 84-year-old lady was getting her mail from near the front door of her apartment, the front door slammed. She was locked out and did not have the cane or walker she usually used indoors. Since no one was around, she felt her only recourse was to walk slowly, carefully holding on to the outside of the apartment, and enter her back door which was open. She had not walked alone outdoors for years and had not been outdoors for months. But with determination and caution she walked around the apartment complex, which was about a block in length. Taking her time, she maneuvered down steps, over uneven ground, and up the back steps. She admitted that she had to sit down once she got inside, but her shakiness, weakness, and shortness of breath did not last too long. She did not become overly excited as she was telling about the event, and she said that she had felt that she could make it. God would give her strength, or if she was supposed to die, he would take her, and that was alright too. She did not spend energy or time berating herself or kicking the door.

Showing a sense of autonomy, independence, and ability for self-direction. These characteristics are often valued in the young, but in the old they are called stubbornness. The above situation demonstrates these characteristics. Sometimes the family gets frustrated because the senior will not wait for help or because he attempts tasks that tax him physically. But often while the senior is engaging in challenging physical tasks he is also being very alert mentally and is thinking through his situation from various angles.

Perceiving reality factors accurately, showing social sensitivity, and treating others as worthy of concern. The normal senior is in contact with reality and may, for example, be able to fill you in on local or national events. Often his ideas about how to solve distressful situations are practical. If the person is immobilized, television as well as visitors and phone calls keep him in touch with the world. The person may repeat stories or explain a situation or visit at length in order to show that he is in contact with reality or to reinforce the memory and reality of it for himself. The senior is usually realistic about the demands on his caretakers' time and energy and he will sense and accept when someone truly cannot do as much for him as the other person would like to. If the senior is treated with dignity, his affection, patience, generosity, and interest are returned many times over.

Mastering the environment, working and playing, solving problems, and adapting to life's requirements. The senior does activities appropriate for his stage of life; often we unfavorably compare him to the young active adult as he carries out these activities. Just to manage the stresses discussed in Chapter 6, cope with the negative societal attitudes discussed in Chapter 5, or secure the necessary social, health, or legal services discussed in Chapters 7 and 8 may take considerable problem solving, adaptation, work, and mastery. Play often takes the form of a sense of humor, teasing in conversation, or engaging in the various leisure activities discussed in Chapter 6.

No one ever attains a perfect or ideal state of maturity. No one demonstrates all of the possible characteristics of maturity at one given moment, although they are present most of the time to some degree. If the person has most of the characteristics most of the time, functions adequately in the community, maintains life roles appropriate to his age and situation without being a nuisance to self or others, he is generally considered emotionally healthy or normal. The quality of interaction combined with his functioning is thought of as emotional maturity.

FACTORS THAT INFLUENCE EMOTIONAL HEALTH

Not all seniors believe that old age is harvest time. Various factors influence the senior's emotional status, his feelings about himself, and his ability to cope. In a 30-year study, Larson found that health status, socioeconomic factors, degree of social interaction, marital status, and living situation were strongly related to feelings of well-being and emotional health. Age, sex, race, and employment history showed no consistent relationship.[60]

Health Status

Physical health is one of the major factors that affects emotional status. The person who is generally well can better maintain work, leisure pursuits, and social contacts, and thus he feels worthwhile. Feeling contented emotionally in turn affects physical health positively.

However, the person's perception of his health status may differ from his actual health status. This personal perception of one's health status is a great determinant of the person's emotional status. The person who perceives the self as healthy may actually have considerable chronic health problems. If the person perceives himself as less healthy or less mobile, if he hurts constantly, or if he has chronic illness that needs daily regulation, the natural response is to become more self-preoccupied, less interested in others, and to have less energy available to adapt to other people or life's situations.

The person who does not perceive the self as healthy has often been unhealthy most of his life and now has fewer visitors, spends more time sitting and thinking and less time pursuing activities. Often he feels unhappy and abandoned by others, worries, does not think he has lived a useful life, and wishes that his earlier occupational and social class status could have been higher. The person tends to be depressed and is less emotionally adaptive.[79]

Sociocultural Factors

The sociocultural system influences the emotional status, at least indirectly, as discussed in Chapter 5. American values are antagonistic to old age; status and role are poorly defined for late life. The elderly woman, who has been accustomed traditionally to the expressive role (concerned with the welfare and inner integration of people and the social system and the maintenance of value patterns), adjusts better to retirement than does the man, who changes from the instrumental, task-oriented role to an expressive one, which he considers feminine. If the older person does not stay active in any group and has few or no family contacts, his lack of interaction prevents him from learning new roles, achieving changed status, or validating his own identity and ideas.[56]

The number of social stressors impinging upon the senior (as discussed in Chapter 6), influences emotional status and adaptability. The person who has had a lifetime of disorganization and excessive stress is more likely to decompensate emotionally and neglect the self to an exaggerated degree in late life. Self-neglect may be manifested by domestic and personal filth, hoarding of useless rubbish, persistent refusals of help from community resources, as well as by not eating or taking prescribed medicines. The person may not appear ill, but he is likely to be aloof, shrewd, detached, suspicious, and prone to distort reality.[22] If the person has been able to cope successfully with life stresses, then he becomes like the house built on a firm foundation that is able to withstand the winds and rain beating on it.

Personality Factors

The character structure and personality strengths present in earlier life are crucial to emotional status in later life. If the senior has shown the previously described characteristics of maturity throughout his life, appropriate to his life stage and situation, he will continue to demonstrate them, sometimes even in the face of severe deprivation or stress. This is as true for the person in a residence for the elderly as in home care, barring massive physical or brain deterioration.

The gentle, warm, but assertive, inner-directed senior has often had to adjust to many difficulties and has learned from them. The aggressive, egocentric behavior that we often see in the adults in the 1970's and which is rewarded by our society, may not lay the foundation for flexible, gentle composure that stands firm in the face of hardship.

The sense of **internal locus of control**, *perceiving that his actions control rewards and outcomes in life* (inner-directedness), enhances emotional health and helps the senior feel a higher life satisfaction and self-esteem, maintain stronger ego functioning, and be less prone to mental disorders. Increased sense of inner self-control is related to good health (feeling significant to others, having a sense of hope, and active adherence to a religion). A sense of powerlessness is increased by loss of health, money, spouse, home, or familiar environment.[58] Powerlessness is increased when there are a lack of information, a lack of choice or decision making, intrusions into personal space, a lack of privacy, feelings of isolation and loneliness, or a lack of resources or help.

LATER MATURITY: A DEVELOPMENTAL CRISIS

The person never arrives at a point where he can say with finality, "This is me." Four dimensions relate to the continued state of becoming: The person (1) continues to learn something, no matter how minimal, about himself and the world he lives in; (2) never stops being aware of emotional needs of self, and usually of others, until consciousness leaves; (3) continues to want to direct his own destiny, and (4) never stops trying to find a meaningful and comfortable fit between the self and society. Adult development is not just a process of repair. The truly developmental aspect of the middle and later years is how people transcend their physical limitations to develop different and unique powers instead of adjusting to declining attributes. The mature person never stops growing and changing to meet the changes presented by the self and environment.[67]

Later Maturity: A Crisis? Why?

A *crisis is defined as a turning point, an event in which the usual coping mechanisms of the person are inadequate for the changes encountered.*[35] Living patterns in late life must change in order for the person to remain functional, that is, to cope with the societal, occupational, financial, residential, family, physical, and cognitive changes, described in other chapters, that he will eventually encounter. Change can be threatening. Further, the person's chronological age—65, 75, or 85—conveys a certain meaning to him and society, and he reacts in turn. He strives to maintain a sense of identity, unity, and continuity.

However, emotional reactions and characteristics may reflect his crisis, and emotional maturity will be crucial for surmounting it.

The Social Readjustment Rating Scale assesses the person's perceptions of the adjustment required by 43 life events that involve personal, social, occupational, and family changes.[47] Certain life events are perceived as more stressful by elderly than by younger persons. The extent of readjustment required to accommodate to the changes commonly associated with aging or institutionalization may be beyond the adaptive capacity of the senior. Of all the life events listed in the Social Readjustment Rating Scale, changes in family events were listed as requiring less change than those events of a personal, work, or financial nature. Perhaps the senior has already met and resolved a number of family crises so that he is more adaptive in that area. Or he may no longer have significant family ties; he at least expects the death of spouse and loved ones.[66,73]

Because change is stressful, and stress is a causative factor in disease, a definite relationship exists between the amount of recent change and the onset of illness, which adds another crisis to the senior's life.[47,73]

The crisis of illness is a threat to the senior's self-concept and may contribute to a changed emotional status. Often the ill elderly person seems less mature because of his reactions to illness, treatment, and hospitalization. Illness may mean paralysis, aphasia, possible death, or at best a chronic disease from which he may improve but never recover. If the person was dynamic, vigorous, and successful, recognition of his situation may cause feelings of frustration, anger, depression, hopelessness, confusion, and shame. To cope with these feelings, he may deny his illness and try to do activities that he cannot accomplish in order to prove himself. His adaptive response may be a reaction formation demonstrated by overly cheerful, compliant behavior—his attempt to to avoid rejection or neglect. If the person was always dependent, passive, and uninvolved with others, he may fear that his family will no longer care for him. Life may have no meaning; he feels that he is not worthwhile.

The ill senior often shows emotional lability; he alternates between depression and laughter, anger and calm, inhibition and loss of control. Reduced stress tolerance and inability to respond to the behavior of others are seen. He may feel as frustrated and embarrassed as you do when he is behaving in a pattern at variance for him. Because of his lability, he may cooperate with one nurse but not with another.

Although you may not think so, stubborn or resistive behavior may be a sign of health. He is trying to regain strength, function, and self-control, or he may be telling you that he senses your acceptance, even of his less socially acceptable behavior that he cannot control.

His feelings and behavioral response to the crisis of illness are normal, as discussed in Chapter 13. Do not take personally his lack of response, his lability, or apparent uncooperativeness. Realize that if you work with the senior, you can help him regain earlier behavior patterns and help him to come through the crisis with a higher level of maturity. Helping the person work through his feelings and regain previous personality strengths will also foster the rehabilitation process. Do not label the normal adaptive reactions to crisis as psychiatric illness. Such labeling may cause the person to lose motivation to regain health; he may in turn deteriorate into emotional illness even though he had the potential for greater maturity after the crisis.

Developmental Crisis: Ego Integrity Versus Self-Despair

Erikson, in his Epigenetic Theory describing the eight stages of man, states that the developmental crisis in later maturity is to achieve a sense of ego integrity rather than succumb to a sense of self-despair.[33]

Ego integrity is the coming together of all previous life stages and involves consolidation, protection of, and holding on to the sense of identity or wholeness that the person has accrued over a lifetime. Even in the midst of loss and divestment of usual roles and functions, the person accepts his life as worthwhile. He does not wish that his life would have been different, although he acknowledges that it could have been. He recognizes that he made a contribution to the world and defends the dignity of his life-style. Even if earlier developmental tasks have not been completed, the senior may overcome the handicap through association with younger persons and through helping others to resolve their conflicts. Helping the person retain identities that are important to him, such as parent, spouse, grandparent, sibling, teacher, writer, nurse, or musician is important, because recalling past identities and successes promotes development of ego integrity. The person with ego integrity demonstrates wisdom; he combines knowledge and experience to make a judgment or pursue a course of action.[30,33]

Without resolving the developmental crisis of achieving a sense of ego integrity, the person feels a sense of despair and self-disgust and will be less able to cope with crises related to his changing life. He feels that life has been too short, that it has been futile; he wants another chance to redo his life. If life has not been worth the struggle, death is feared. The person becomes hypercritical of others and projects his own self-disgust, inadequacy, and anger onto others. Such feelings are influenced by society's values, the reactions of others toward him, and his emotional status.[33]

SELF-CONCEPT/BODY-IMAGE DEVELOPMENT

Definitions

Self-concept is defined as the person's total sense of self, feelings about self, awareness of others' reactions toward him and his attitudes, values, and all of life's experiences, some of which may be out of his awareness. Included in self-concept are his body image and sense of self-esteem. *Body image is the mental picture of the body's appearance and function, including internal, external, and postural features of the body as an object in space, attitudes and emotions of the person toward his body, and his reactions to others' responses toward him.* The image is flexible and may not be reflective of actual body structure. *Self-esteem is the evaluation of approval/disapproval given to self; it is based on expectations of self and others, aspirations, and reactions from others.*

Influences on Self-Concept/Body Image

Self-concept and body-image development begin in infancy and are primarily influenced by the reactions of early caretakers toward the person. The early positive or negative feelings about self are hard to change. But a negative self-concept and body image can be modified as the person gains motor, mental, and social skills, receives positive responses from peers and others, and becomes more aware of and develops control over kinesthetic, sensorimotor, sexual, and other internal sensations. Throughout life self-perception is further modified by identification with admired people, the geographical area and home, occupation, education, religion, leisure activities, the many life experiences, and the physical changes of aging. By the time the person enters later maturity, self-concept should be stable. He should like himself and feel accepted by others. All of the physical changes described in Chapter 9 will influence his perception of his body and its competence; he needs time to accept changes in appearance, structure, and function.

Positive self-concept and self-esteem correlate with the following:

1. Having a positive self-concept and self-esteem in earlier life.
2. Perceiving the self as healthy and being physically mobile.
3. Having an adequate income to meet needs.
4. Being married. The widow maintains a more positive self-concept than the widower does, but family life is important to both sexes.
5. Living with spouse or children instead of in an institution.
6. Having a secondary or college education.
7. Having interested children or grandchildren.
8. Maintaining contact with siblings at least monthly.
9. Visiting with friends and belonging to organizations.
10. Having a religious faith and attending church.
11. Being able to vote in the last election.
12. Perceiving the community as a good place in which to live and having an unconfining life space.
13. Anticipating retirement positively.
14. Having a youthful feeling about the self, being independent, and feeling an internal locus of control.[10,38,41,45,62,65,78,79,82,89]

Aging-group-consciousness and becoming a part of the subculture of the later maturity, as discussed in Chapter 5, further enhance positive self-concept. Continued contact with peers helps the person remain realistic about himself and his body as he compares himself to others.[48,54] If the person perceives the self to be doing as well or better in various areas than his peers, he evaluates the self positively. The senior can increase self-esteem by either increasing his successful activities or decreasing his expectations. If he gives up his goals or lowers his expectations, he may feel relief, but he lacks guidelines for self-definition.[62]

The person who is overly concerned about society's negative stereotypes of the aged or its values of youth, beauty, and speed; who feels life has been meaningless; who is without family or friends and is lonely; who is in poor health, dependent, and without basic comforts of life will indeed feel old and will be negative about self, life, and the world in general. If the person's sense of self was tied to work as the one valued activity, retirement will cause him to feel worthless. The subordination of self when living with the children or the reduced interaction with others, depersonalization, and loss of freedom that result from moving into an institution causes a lowering of self-esteem and self-concept. Loss of loved ones further narrows the self. Each death means loss of another role, source of prestige, and social support.[3,23,78] When the person has a negative self-concept, his behavior becomes less sociable and may in turn match the stereotypes and myths discussed in Chapter 5.[5,71,72,91,94]

Comparative Studies of Senior and Younger Populations

In a study comparing self-concept and the ideal self in four age groups, the elderly showed the most positive self-concept and ideal self and highest life satisfaction.[45]

Research comparing self-concepts of people ages 20 to 40 and ages 60 to 80 indicated little differences in ascribed characteristics. Roles and memberships differed between the two groups; the younger persons identified themselves more often in occupational roles, and the older persons identified themselves more often in kinship roles. Over one-half of the younger group described themselves in abstract terms; the seniors did not, possibly because of less education and the practical thinking typical of seniors. The seniors were more spiritual in orientation and described themselves as happy and fortunate more often than did the younger people. The older people were more attuned to current issues, helping others, and feeling affection for others.[20]

In one study comparing college students with older adults, several differences in self-perception were found: (1) college females perceived themselves as higher in affiliation than did college males; (2) college females perceived themselves as more dominating and hostile than did older women, and (3) older men perceived themselves as more cooperative and helpful than did college men. Both generations of women saw themselves as nurturant. College students substantially misperceived older adults, perceiving the seniors as dominant, competitive and very aggressive, contrary to the seniors' self-perceptions. Perhaps these results help to explain the negative stereotypes and inter-generational conflict. The older person who tries to be helpful and cooperative may be misread as being power-oriented and controlling.[36]

In one study of over 4000 persons, the assets most valued in growing old were more leisure, greater independence, and fewer responsibilities. Limitations were identified as poor health, loneliness, financial problems, neglect from others, forced retirement, boredom, and fear of death. In all areas except poor health and forced retirement, people under 65 viewed their problems as more severe than did people over 65. Little difference existed between the seniors and younger adults in basic life satisfaction. Income, race, employment, and education were more likely to influence life satisfaction than age. The seniors were more active and saw themselves as more useful than the younger group perceived them to be.

Thus, the elderly have considerable inner resources. Contrary to stereotypes, seniors do not necessarily have negative feelings about self. The self-concept may be as positive and healthy, or more so, than that of the younger person. Life can be pleasurable, especially if the older person works to maintain a positive attitude. In fact, late life has advantages not found earlier, especially the release from the competitions and anxieties of the middle years.[20] Persons in the young-old years of life, especially women, tend to think of this period as a time of life satisfaction continued from earlier life periods. However, in old-old age, life satisfaction and positive self-image tend to decrease.[21]

PERSONALITY DEVELOPMENT AND CHARACTERISTICS

No specific personality changes occur as a result of aging; values, life orientation, and personality traits remain consistent from at least middle age onward. *The older person becomes more of what he was.* The older person continues to develop emotionally and in personality, but he adds on instead of making drastic changes. If he was physically active and flexible in personality and if he participated in social activities in the young years, he will continue appropriate to his physical status and life situation. If he was hard to live with when he was younger, he will be harder to live with in old age. The garrulous, taciturn person becomes more so, and problems of control and dominance are common. Stereotypes describe the older person as rigid, conservative, opinionated, self-centered, and disagreeable to be with. Such characteristics are not likely to be new but rather are an exaggeration of lifelong traits that cannot be expressed or sublimated in another way.[85]

Influences on Personality Development

Personality, *the distinctive and unique style in which a person behaves or reacts,* is as variable in old age as in youth. Personality development in the senior is affected throughout the years by many variables: health status, integrative processes of the brain, sociocultural background and group membership, social identity and role opportunity, birth order, past and present family interactions, need satisfaction ability, general living situation, changes in habit strengths, and motivation. And all of these variables interact.

Animal studies show that the wider the range and variety of environmental opportunity, the wider the range of behavioral responses and the more flexible the subject. No doubt the same applies to older people. Those who live within a supportive environment that nurtures social and psychological diversity are more likely to have a wider range of behaviors and to be more adaptive. Such elderly will also be less likely to experience personality disturbances or decline.[13]

Because of the continuity of personality, study of the person's past behavior and social competence is a better predictor of personality traits and behavior in later maturity than personality tests or clinical judgments.[29]

Major Personality Types in Later Maturity

Studies of large samples of seniors reaffirm their uniqueness, but researchers have categorized the variety of their behaviors.

Four personality types were described by Neugarten: the integrated, defended, passive dependent, and disintegrated.[67,68]

The *integrated personality* type is characteristic of most elderly. These people function well and have a complex inner life, intact cognitive abilities, and competent ego. They are flexible, open to new stimuli, mellow, and have control over impulses. They adjust to losses and are realistic about the past and present. They have a high sense of life satisfaction. The integrated group is made up of three subtypes: the reorganizers, focused, and disengaged. The *reorganizers* engage in a wide variety of activities; when they lose old roles and related activities they substitute new ones. They are as active after retirement as before. The *focused* are selective in their activities; they devote energy to a few roles that are important to them rather than being involved in many organizations. The *disengaged* are well-integrated persons who have voluntarily moved away from role commitments. Activity level is low, but not because of external losses or physical deficits. They are self-directed, interested in the world, but have chosen the rocking-chair approach to life without guilt. They are calm, aloof, but contented. Thus, Neugarten defines the disengaged person differently from Cummins and Henry.[67,68]

The *defended personality* is seen in ambitious, achievement-oriented persons who have always driven themselves hard and who continue to do so.

They have a number of defenses against anxiety and a tight control over impulses. This "armored" group has medium to high life satisfaction. The defended group is made up of two subtypes: those who hold on and the constricted. The *holding on* persons have a philosophy of, "I'll work until I drop." So long as they can keep busy, they can control their anxieties and feel worthwhile. The *constricted* are preoccupied with their losses and deficits. They have always shut out new experiences and have had minimal social interactions. Their caution continues as they try to defend themselves against aging. Nevertheless, they are satisfied with life, possibly because they know nothing different.[67,68]

The *passive-dependent personality* type is divided into two patterns: the succorance-seeking and the apathetic. The *succorance-seeking* have strong dependency needs and seek help and support from others. They manage fairly well as long as they have one or two people to lean on. They have medium levels of activity and medium life satisfaction. The *apathetic* have an extremely passive personality. They engage in few activities and little social interaction. They have little interest in the world around them. They feel that life has been and continues to be hard and that little can be done about it. They have low satisfaction with life.[67,68]

The *disintegrated or disorganized personality* type is found in a small percentage of elderly who show gross defects in psychological functions and deterioration in thought processes. They may be severely neurotic or psychotic. Yet, these elderly are not necessarily institutionalized. They may manage to live in the community because of the forbearance or protection of others around them.[67,68]

Personality and life-style types were categorized extensively for women and men in one longitudinal study. The four personality types categorized for women were: (1) person-oriented, which comprised over 50 percent of the sample, (2) fearful-ordering, (3) autonomous, and (4) anxiety-asserting. Three personality types were categorized for men: (1) person-oriented, (2) active-competent, and (3) conservative-ordering. Ten life-style categories involved interaction or social behavior, role involvement, satisfaction with environment and others, and perception of change.[64]

Results of the study showed a diversity of behavior in seniors. No correlations existed between personality and life-style, and spouses did not show similar personality types. Health status strongly influenced life-style and personality characteristics; healthy people were more active and involved in life roles. Evidence supports the general hypothesis that personality characteristics in old age are highly correlated with early life characteristics. While early adult life-styles are more likely to continue into old age for men than for women, the early life personality of women is more likely to continue into old age than is the early personality type of men.[64]

Although the popular stereotype is that women cannot cope effectively, this study revealed that *all* women were higher in ability to cope than in ego disorganization, even those who were more rigid in ego defenses, and women were more adaptable than men. Whenever defensiveness or ego disorganization does occur, it is related to general personality predisposition throughout life, outlook on life, and physical health.[64]

Popular beliefs that later maturity means massive decline in psychological functioning or narrowing of life-styles are not supported by this study. On the contrary, most seniors are resourceful and psychologically healthy. Personality problems in old age are related to problems in early life. Even when the younger years are too narrowly lived or painfully overburdened, the later years may offer new opportunities. Different ways of living can be developed as the social environment changes and as the person also changes. Later maturity can provide a second and better chance at life.[64]

The major implications of these personality and life-style studies are the uniqueness of seniors and the need to change public perspectives and attitudes toward the elderly. *Stereotypes have no basis in reality. Further, monolithic planning cannot be done for the elderly.* Choices in housing, retirement plans, health services, and leisure pursuits are essential because of the diversity of interests, capabilities, and needs.[64,67,68]

The old are not necessarily old-fashioned. They have gone through countless changes and have learned a lot from experience, and they store facts, experiences, and feelings within them. They have considerable spunk in spite of aches and ills. If we are going to be stranded on a desert island, at least one person in the group had better be in later maturity because the rest of us have learned little, comparatively, about survival.[28]

Personality Features in the Young-Old and the Old-Old

Authors cite personality trends that are commonly found in the elderly. Some difference is noted between the earlier and later decades of later maturity.

In the *young-old* the personality is frequently flexible, shows characteristics commonly defined as maturity, and is less vulnerable to the harsh reality of aging.

The person manifests self-respect without conceit; tolerates his weakness while using his strength to the fullest; regulates, diverts, or sublimates basic drives and impulses instead of trying to suppress them. He is guided by principles in his behavior but is not a slave to dogma; maintains a steady purpose without pursuing the impossible goal; respects others, even if he does not agree with their behavior; and directs his energies and creativity to master the environment and overcome the vicissitudes of life.[40]

Motivations change; the senior wants different things from life than he did earlier. Concerns about appearance, standards of living, and family change. He needs stronger incentives, support, and encouragement to do what used to be eagerly anticipated. He tends to avoid risks or new challenges. He tends to be increasingly introspective and introverted.[26,68,86]

The elderly are tough; they often endure against great physical and social odds. Experience has taught the senior to be somewhat suspicious, since he is likely to be a victim of "borrowings," a fast-sell job for something he doesn't need, thievery, or physical attacks. Even acquaintances or relatives may try to bilk him out of whatever little money or few treasured possessions he has. As one 78-year-old said, "They (family) think I don't know much, and they are forever suggesting ways for me to invest my money or to put my money into joint accounts—always so they can get to it. I know what they're up to, so I'm careful what I say and do. It's awful to think that way about people, but you can't trust just anyone. And most people won't do even the most simple thing—like mail a letter—unless you pay them." Similar statements have been made by many elderly, and often justifiably.

Yet, generosity is a common trait of the elderly; the person gives of himself fully and shares willingly what little he has with people he cares for and who seem genuinely interested in him.

The elderly person hopes to remain independent and useful as long as possible, to find contentment, and to die without being a burden to others. Increasingly, dependency may undermine self-esteem, especially if the person values independence. Often dependency renews unresolved conflicts from childhood and with his children or caretakers. The dependency-independency conflict is a continuum throughout life, and developmental experiences determine to a large degree success or failure in finding adequate need satisfaction through independent behavior. All of us are dependent to some degree upon others, but in late life dependency may be economic, physical, social, and emotional. The real test of maturity may be how the elderly person deals with his increasing dependency.

Independent behavior has various meanings: (1) strength, (2) denial of weakness and helplessness, (3) youthful feelings or a denial of being old, (4) activity and mobility, (5) being alive and in contact with self and others (while passivity means extinction), (6) a way to combat inferiority and inadequacy, and (7) a way to avoid the risk of rejection or neglect when depending on others.

Independence is also used in other ways by the senior. The senior may be unable to accept help as an unconscious act of hostility, or he may unconsciously punish others by denying them the opportunity to be of help, thus causing them to feel concerned, anxious, and guilty about the senior. If the person cannot accept help, he may be neglected and deprived. Independent behavior (being aloof or assertive instead of close or tender) may be a way of relating to others. Independent behavior may be used to avoid manipulation or exploitation by others, either in relation to receiving services or material goods. If the person is not obligated to or dependent on another, he can come and go as he wishes. Or independent behavior may be a way of controlling others; the senior insists on having his own way or is demanding. The older person may try to remain independent, even when he is not physically or mentally able, to avoid being a burden to another or to live up to others' expectations.[42,84]

Personality characteristics differ for men and women, especially in relation to assertiveness. The man becomes more dependent, passive, and submissive, and more tolerant of his emerging nurturant and affiliative impulses. The woman becomes more dominant and assertive and less guilty about aggressive and egocentric impulses. Perhaps the reversal in overt behavior is caused by hormone changes. Perhaps the man can be more open to his long-unfulfilled emotional needs when he is no longer in the role of chief provider and no longer has to compete in the work world. Perhaps the woman reciprocates in an effort to gratify needs for achievement and worth; she expresses more completely the previously hidden conflicts, abilities, or characteristics.[42,83]

Old-old age is a time for meditation and contemplation, not camaraderie. Camaraderie is for young people who have energy and similarities in background, development, and interest. Old-old people may be friendly and pleasant, but they are also egocentric. Egocentricity is a physiologic necessity, a protective mechanism for survival, not selfishness. Life space shrinks. When old-old people get together, certain factors block camaraderie, even if they want to be sociable: varying stages of deafness and blindness, other faulty sense perceptions, and the fact that they may have little in common other than age and past historical era. Old-old people are even more unique in the life pattern than young-old people because they have lived longer. Further, they have less energy to deal with challenging situations, and relating to a group of oldsters can be challenging.[77,80]

The person in later maturity, especially in old-old age, may be called childish. Rather, the person is childlike; he pays attention to quality in others. He senses when another is not genuine or honest—as a person or in his activities—and he reacts. The old-old person, especially, reacts with sometimes exasperating conduct because he sees clearly through the facade and lacks the emotional energy to be polite, as he would have been earlier. Self-control, will power, and intellectual response are less effective in advanced age. Many of the negative emotional characteristics ascribed to the elderly may be based on this phenomenon. Only the very simple, those who have not grappled with the complexities of life, or the very ill and regressed will be infantile.[77]

The old-old have greater need than ever to hold onto others. They are often perceived as clingy, sticky, demanding, loquacious, and repetitious. This often causes the younger person to want to be rid of the senior, which causes a vicious circle of increased demand and increased rejection.

Preoccupation with the body is a frequent topic of conversation, and other elderly people respond in kind. The behavior is analogous to the collective monologue and parallel play of young children. The talk about the body satisfies narcissistic needs, and it is an attempt to magically relieve anxiety about what is happening. This pattern alienates the young, as well as the young-old, and they tend to avoid or stop conversing with the aged. As one youthful senior said, "I can't stand being around only old folks and listening to their complaints. I'm doing O.K. But soon I'll have to start manufacturing ills, just to compete."

The old-old person knows, like no one else, the importance of the injunctions, "Love thy neighbor," "Be very kind to each other," or "I should have kissed her one more time." They intensely appreciate the richness of the moment, the joys or the sorrows. They realize the transience of life and they are more likely to start each day with a feeling of expectancy, not neutrality or boredom. Their future is today. And as a result, they become more tolerant of others' foibles, more thrilled over minor events, and more aware of their own needs, even if they cannot meet them.[77]

Irritating behavior of the old-old person is frequently related to the frustration of being dependent on others or helpless and the fear that accompanies dependency and helplessness. The tangible issue at hand—coffee too hot or too cold, visitors too early or too late, bowel movement too large or too small—is often not really what is irritating, although the person attaches his complaints to some thing that others can identify. The irritability is with the self, loss of control, lost powers, and present state of being.

While some people in later maturity—young-old or old-old—become more cantankerous, others mellow and become more tolerant. Those who have adequate gratification and have successfully mastered disappointments tend to mellow. Those who have unmet needs and low frustration tolerance become increasingly frustrated and bitter.

ADAPTIVE CAPACITIES

The person in later maturity often continues to be exceedingly adaptive; indeed, he has to be to have survived so long or to manage in today's fast-changing society. Age-linked social trauma, such as retirement or widowhood, rarely leads to mental illness.[1] Yet all the changes that the person encounters, discussed in other chapters, challenge adaptive skills.

Influences on Adaptive Abilities

Past experiences, memories, and relationships are a resource for the senior to draw on; he has a greater amount of self-awareness, which enhances adaptability.[55] The person who has always been active and coped successfully is more likely to be active and cope in later maturity. The person who is healthy, married, better educated, financially secure, has friends, belongs to a church, participates in civic activities, is satisfied with his residence, and is content with himself is more adaptable.[75] Unfortunately, many seniors do not have these advantages, or they lose at least some of them the longer they live. In spite of difficulties, the resiliency of the senior comes through. In one study, ego strength in retired adults was higher in relation to reality, responsibility, and trust than it was in younger adults.[75]

Personality traits that are most useful in remaining adaptive through various stresses and crises include a feeling of hope, introspection, and ability to use information to mobilize inner and outer resources. The older person relies less on a group or on social strengths and turns inward to his own resources. A certain amount of magical thinking, perceiving self as important, being assertive, having a pugnacious stance toward the world, being slightly suspicious, and maintaining a consistent and coherent self-image help the elderly to prevent harm to self and to remain intact in the face of radical environmental change. Passively accepting whatever the other person hands out causes the elderly to be taken advantage of and to fail to cope with many difficulties. The person who cannot find meaningful ways of maintaining the self-image deteriorates in the face of stress and crisis.[29]

Two personality types adjust poorly to the challenges and frustrations of late life. The first is the chronically angry person who is bitter about having failed to achieve earlier goals, blames others for his difficulties, and cannot reconcile himself to growing old. The second is the self-hating person who also feels disappointed about the past, turns his resentment inward, becomes depressed, and feels inadequate and worthless.[75] Both of these personality types manifest the self-despair discussed by Erikson.[33]

Adaptive Mechanisms

The person maintains certain patterns of behavior that were successful earlier in life. But certain mechanisms are developed for successful emotional transition in later maturity.

Peck lists three developmental stages related to adaptation, which show the tasks involved and the mechanisms undergoing change as the person strives to achieve ego integrity. "Ego-differentiation vs. work role preoccupation" is involved in *adaptation to retirement,* and its success depends on the ability to see oneself as worthwhile not just because of a job but because of the basic person one is. "Body transcendence vs. body preoccupation" requires that "happiness" and "comfort" as concepts be redefined to *overcome the changes in body image and the decline of physical strength.* The third task is "ego transcendence vs. ego preoccupation," the task of *accepting inevitable death.* Mechanisms for adapting to the task of facing death will be those that protect against loss of inner contentment and that help to develop a constructive impact on surrounding persons. The development of inner contentment requires the ability to redefine the future.[37, 40]

Certain adaptive or defensive mechanisms are used frequently by the aged in an effort to reduce anxiety, fear, and frustration and to maintain self-esteem.

Rationalization, giving a logical sounding excuse for a situation, is often used to minimize weakness, symptoms, and various difficulties or to build self-esteem. *Compartmentalization, a narrowing of awareness and focusing on one thing at a time,* causes the elderly to seem rigid, repetitive, and resistive. The lower energy level and changing cognitive characteristics contribute to this mechanism. *Denial, blocking of thought or inability to accept a situation,* is used selectively when the person is under great stress. It is an aid in maintaining a higher level of physical or personality integration. For example, the person can deny discomforts and keep ambulating. Or he may live longer and more productively because he denies certain minor symptoms or social stereotypes. *Counterphobia, excessive behavior in an area of life to counter or negate fears about that area of life,* is observed in the person who persists at activities, such as calisthenics or youthful grooming or fashion, to retain a youthful appearance. *Rigidity, resisting change or not being involved in decision making,* is a common defense to help the person feel that he is in control of himself and his life. A stubborn self-assertiveness is compensatory behavior for the person who has been insecure, rigid, and irritable. *Sublimation, channeling aggressive impulses into sociably acceptable activity,* can be an effective defense to meet old age as a challenge and maintain vigor and creativity. Often the elderly desire to live vicariously through the younger generation, and they become involved with the young through mutual activities, listening, or observing their activities. *Regression, returning to earlier patterns of behavior,* may take the form of excessive dependency when the person is capable of self-care. Yet, regression is not negative unless it is massive, since the person gradually needs more help as physical strength declines and as social roles change. Regression may take the form of sexual behavior; the person may be exhibitionistic or behave as if he were in adolescence, the period at which sexual interests and drives are the highest. (However, the elderly are capable of coitus, and revived sexual interests and activity may be a form of self-therapy to recapture a sense of capability and self-esteem.) *Somatization, complaints about physical symptoms and preoccupation with the body,* may become an outlet for free-floating anxiety. The person can cope with vague insecurities and rapid life changes by having a tangible physical problem to deal with, especially since others seem more interested and concerned about disease symptoms than feelings about self. *Isolation, repressing the emotion associated with a situation or idea,* enables the person to cope with very threatening ideas and situations, such as his own and loved ones' disease, aging, and death. Thus, the elderly may appear relatively calm in the face of crisis. The elderly person may control his life through intellectual processes. *Withdrawal, becoming excessively distant, quiet, isolated from others, or sleeping a great deal,* is a way to cope with decreased energy, health problems, or perceived lack of interest from others. However, withdrawal tends to interfere with optimal meeting of needs.

Often to maintain self-identity and to meet needs in a manner resembling the former life pattern, the senior has to change his standards, goals, and behavioral strategies. He experiences the futility of dreams; swallows pride; accepts reduced life satisfaction, activity, and productivity; and sometimes avoids group responsibilities. The senior has to cope with life stresses while he is experiencing changed social environments, physical coordination and sensations, and greater fatigue. Imperfect results and dependency must be accepted.[77] Further, others expect the senior to be less energetic, autonomous, creative, or effective, all of which influence the will to cope.[44]

DEVELOPMENTAL TASKS

Later maturity is called the Examination Stage by Havighurst, a time characterized by reflection, purposefully dropping some activities while pursuing others (often with a new vigor); becoming an observer and mentor to others; facing new and unresolved problems, and continuing to learn.[44]

The pattern of achieving developmental tasks varies greatly from one senior to another; the assumption with children and adolescents is that all are working on basically the same set of developmental tasks. However, certain tasks must be accomplished in late life although the chronological time and outward manifestation vary. These tasks are to:

1. Decide where and how to live out the remaining years.
2. Continue a supportive, close, warm relationship with the spouse or significant other, including a satisfactory sexual relationship whenever possible.
3. Find a satisfactory home or living arrangement and establish a safe, comfortable household routine to fit health and economic status.
4. Adjust living standards to retirement income; supplement retirement income if possible with remunerative activity.
5. Maintain maximum level of health: care for the self physically and emotionally by getting regular health examinations, needed medical or dental care, eating an adequate diet, and maintaining personal hygiene.
6. Maintain contact with children, grandchildren, and other living relatives, finding emotional satisfaction with them.
7. Maintain interest in people outside the family and in social, civic, and political responsibility.
8. Pursue new interests and maintain former activities in order to gain status, recognition, and a feeling of being needed.
9. Find meaning in life after retirement and in facing inevitable illness and death of self and spouse as well as other loved ones.
10. Work out a significant philosophy of life, finding comfort in a philosophy or religion.
11. Adjust to the death of spouse and other loved ones.[30, 33, 44]

One elderly person considers three developmental tasks to be crucial in old age: (1) attending to spiritual matters, (2) gaining new self-insight, and (3) realizing life's ephemerality and trying to impart that wisdom to younger people, for the senior wishes that he had done so sooner.[77]

NURSING PROCESS TO PROMOTE AND MAINTAIN EMOTIONAL HEALTH

Assessment, Nursing Diagnosis, and Planning Care

The *assessment tool* in Chapter 2 may be helpful in determining emotional status. Your assessment of the person in later maturity may include any of the following behaviors:

1. States acceptance of himself, his life stage, and his past life.
2. Demonstrates behaviors and characteristics correlated with positive self-concept and adequate self-esteem.
3. Demonstrates a variety of personality characteristics that are appropriate to the situation, even if they are unique to him.
4. Adapts to stress and crisis by using appropriate, effective adaptive mechanisms and available resources.
5. Gives evidence of working through or achieving at least most of the developmental tasks of this era.

From these and other assessments your *nursing diagnosis* would be *unimpaired emotional functioning*.

However, the senior may be healthier or more competent in some aspects of emotional life than in others. Fluctuations in mood or lack of knowledge of the person's pattern make assessment more difficult. Just as few young adults reach complete maturity, few older persons attain an ideal state of personality or ego integration. What is considered normal behavior in the elderly should be stretched to the limit. Emphasize strengths and recognize various life-styles and coping mechanisms which the person has used successfully through many historical and social changes.[43]

Long-term care goals for such a person could include the following:

1. Statements and behavior indicative of integrated identity, positive self-concept, adequate self-esteem, and life satisfaction are expressed.
2. Ability to cope with late life stresses is demonstrated.
3. Ability to use help from others as well as own inner resources is apparent in working through life crises.
4. Life review is done.
5. Symptoms of psychiatric illness are not apparent.

Short-term care goals could include the following:

1. A sense of security is felt and expressed in most situations.'
2. A range of behaviors and emotional responses are demonstrated in a variety of situations.
3. Social relationships are maintained.
4. Adequate attention, without preoccupation, is given to physical needs and personal hygiene.
5. Reminiscing is done in relation to life review.
6. Satisfaction with the life situation is expressed.

You may think of other care goals for your patient/client.

General Intervention

Use the insights gained from Chapter 3; use of communication principles and of yourself as a therapeutic tool are essential. The senior is often very candid; he reveals intimacies more directly and quickly than a younger person might do. The senior is open as he reminisces. You may also involve the senior in a group; the information presented in Chapter 4 will help you select an appropriate group. Because intellectual function is closely related to how the person feels about himself, and therefore his emotional status, using the information presented in Chapter 10 will promote a positive self-concept and enhance the person's emotional response.

You will also need to work with family members, sometimes using the same principles of care you use with the senior to help them better understand the emotional life and needs of their loved one. Share practical ideas that you have found effective that will help them to live more harmoniously with the elderly person. Help them determine how they can work with the senior to better meet his needs.

In any health care setting you will also be involved in teaching other staff members so that they can better understand and care for the elderly person. Consistency of approach by all members of the health team is essential to enhance the senior's sense of security and positive self-concept and to help the senior to meet his needs.

Meeting Basic Needs

You need to make a strong commitment to assist the elderly person in remaining as healthy and adaptive as possible. All humans are incapable of remaining emotionally healthy without adequate feedback on their behavior, without adequate input either psychologically or physically.

The senior needs to have physiological needs met so that energy is available for continued emotional development. He needs to feel safe and secure in his environment and with other people; to receive and give affection, love, esteem, and approval. He needs to be able to use his skills, talents, and potential (to self-actualize) as long as he is able, to maintain social relationships, spend leisure time happily, and maintain spiritual values and practices.

Needs of the elderly depend on earlier life-style. If the person was married, had strong family ties, lived actively involved with others, and had affectionate, diffuse social relationships, he will continue to have a significant need to give and receive love from family, friends, and others. If he was involved with things, with work, special interests, or hobbies while he eased himself through life with minimal involvement with people, he will have a strong need for similar environmental stimuli, hobbies, and involvement in activities and with things in order to feel satisfied.

The elderly person also has other needs that you can assist him with: privacy from unwarranted verbal or physical intrusions; space or territory for himself and treasured possessions and respectful handling of his possessions; hope which is honestly instilled to overcome insecure and helpless feelings and dependency. You do not create dependency. All people have dependency needs that must be met if exploitative, clinging, resentful, hostile behavior is to be avoided. Meeting dependency needs releases psychic energy so that independence can emerge. The senior can be self-sufficient only when he is assured that someone cares if his needs are met.

Cross-cultural studies reveal certain universal needs of the elderly. These needs are to: (1) *live as long as possible* or until life's satisfactions no longer compensate for its privations and pain; (2) get some *release from wearisome exertion* of doing humdrum tasks and protection from exposure to physical hazards; (3) safeguard and even *strengthen skills,* possessions, rights, authority, and prestige acquired earlier; (4) *remain an active participant* in the affairs of life and share group interests; and (5) *withdraw from life as comfortably* and honorably as possible when it is time.[8] Be mindful of these needs as you administer care in any setting.

One elderly author says that the basic requirements in order for old age to be reasonably secure include the following: (1) sufficient income to provide an adequate diet, comfortable housing, and proper medical care and the individual's creativity and will to make that income provide the essentials; (2) an active mind and some genuine interests; (3) a feeling of being needed and useful; (4) a basic life-living attitude; and (5) some kind of physical contact with others, such as touch, caresses, or sexual intimacy.[20] You have a responsibility to help the person meet these needs; the last need can be met as you touch the person during routine care or an affectionate encounter.

As you care for persons in later maturity, you will not be able to meet all of their needs, but your concern, attention, knowledge, and labors can help to meet some of them. The more you can direct your practice toward that of the geriatric nurse practitioner described in Chapter 7, the more you will be instrumental in meeting basic needs and thus promoting emotional health. Helping the person to stay in control of himself and master his environment, to the degree possible, increases his sense of dignity, self-esteem, and positive self-concept.

The person in later maturity frequently seems more self-assertive, possibly to compensate for his insecurity. Perhaps he also has firmly established his beliefs for himself. If you assess that the person has a high need for independence, provide opportunities for self-assertive behavior. Let the person make decisions about his own life and defend his roles. Channel his energy into constructive involvement and activity in daily care, occupational or recreational therapy, or in assuming responsibility for another, if possible.

Supportive Approach

Preserve the individuality of the senior, even if some psychopathology is present. Alleviate troublesome symptoms or life problems so that you can help the person return as quickly as possible to previous equilibrium, even if that equilibrium seems eccentric. If the person has a pattern of behaving that meets his needs, we should be loathe to change it.[43]

Accept the personality traits that help the person remain adaptive, even if they are bothersome to you. Do nothing to break the person's spirit. Inspire hope by your attitude. Encourage him to use his inner resources and to stand up for his rights by your acknowledging the worth of his unique personality and life-style characteristics. Help him to accept help from you or from others whenever necessary. Help him modify goals and expectations when the situation requires it without losing sense of integrity or worth.

To be supportive, you must receive support from others. Share your frustrations and accomplishments with your colleagues. Work together as a team to arrive at solutions. Also accept the affection and support the senior and his family give to you as you care for them in any setting. Let the senior be active in helping find solutions to his problems. He and his family are part of the team.

Becoming a Confidant

The presence of a *confidant*, *someone whom the senior can confide in about feelings and problems,* is essential in maintaining a sense of reality, identity, positive self-concept, and self-worth. The confidant also buffers against loss, role changes, or reduced social interactions. The confidant is a supportive person, especially if a long-term relationship ensues.

Women are more likely than men to have a confidant; married persons more likely than widows; widows more likely than single persons. The confidant may be the spouse, a child, a friend, or yourself, if you are in the maintenance phase of the helping relationship described in Chapter 3. The sex difference in having a confidant may be related to the greater longevity of women and their lower rate of suicide, the lower rate of mental illness following widowhood among women as compared to men, and to the fact that women are more expressive of feelings throughout life.

Loss of a confidant has a more negative effect on morale than other social losses unless the senior has a long-term relationship with another person. This has implications for how you handle the termination phase of your relationship.

Promoting the Consultative Role

Help the elderly person remain mentally alert and emotionally gratified by placing him in a *consultative role*, *seeking his advice on matters which he is qualified to speak to.* You do not bring him your personal problems (unless the person is a beloved friend or relative); you seek his ideas on matters related to his care or life situation.

The consultative role is a part of achieving ego integrity. It implies that the senior is able to help others objectively because he has survived a full life and has profited in experience, training, discrimination, judgment, and wisdom. Whether the advice given is good or bad is not the point. The important thing is that an answer was asked for and given, which fulfills the senior's role of consultant. The senior often talks at length about how he would correct certain problems or improve the world situation. Listen to and acknowledge his comments.

Society honors certain people by formally placing them in the consultative role: elderly grandparents, judges, scientists, educators, physicians, and nurses. The consultative role is a continuation of the generative stage, but it does not have the accompanying responsibility. When the consultative role can be filled reasonably, the person experiences successful aging. When the role cannot be fulfilled, self-esteem falls and depression results.

Encouraging Reminiscing and Life Review

Reminiscing and life review are adaptive processes that promote a psychological reorganization in the senior. *Reminiscing, or talking about a past event,* is a general response to any crisis, including the developmental crisis of aging. Looking back over a lifetime, recalling pleasurable memories and past achievements, and ignoring or selecting certain memories in the search for meaning strengthen identity and the sense of what has been lived.[17,18] It is a central part in achieving ego integrity.

Reminiscing is not just idle talk, escape from reality, childish regressing, seeking attention, being unable to control thoughts, or filling up empty time.[17,18] It involves patching together all of the life's experiences to construct a meaningful existence, an integrated, unique whole never to be repeated.[32] Reminiscing helps you to learn about the client, and it is essential for him to do life review.

People have a habitual pattern of reminiscing; they talk about the good old days or their mistakes, or they tell "tall tales." The person who talks about the good old days is fairly well-adjusted to his lot in life. Those who regale others feel adequate self-worth and they feel that they have something to share. The reminiscing person is a perpetual learner and will incorporate present situations into their memory and adaptive patterns.[32]

Life review is a naturally occurring, universal mental process characterized by looking back over the life lived and recalling either pleasurable memories or unresolved conflicts which can be surveyed and integrated. Life review is the creative process of appraising self, reconstructing reality, and reintegrating experience, which involves seeking consistency between the past, present, and future selves. Life review is manifested in thoughts, dreams, mirror gazing, and story telling, but the artistic senior may also engage in life review through paintings, poetry, literature, and music. Using others as a sounding board and receiving their feedback help to accomplish life review. Thus, the person gains greater wisdom and new insights into his life experiences, reaffirms his identity, and retires from life with an acceptable image and dignity.[17,18]

Life review is stimulated by the anticipation of death; it occurs not only in the elderly but in terminally ill adults, those preoccupied with death, regardless of health status, and in people facing crisis. Thinking about the past is not limited to the elderly. One study found that teen-agers thought more about the past than did any other age group. (The teen-age years are a time of defining identity and self and seeking a sense of integration; the senior, however, goes through this process on a different level.)

Most people of any age think primarily about the present as well as the past and future. Although people over 65 think slightly less about the future, their thoughts are not dominated by the past.[19,25,39] Do not think of life review and reminiscing as garrulous behavior. Instead, take time to listen, even if you have heard the story before or if the story seems without purpose. Ask related questions; you will not interfere with reality contact by talking about the past. Do not interrupt or distract when the senior talks about how things were (it is your chance to learn about history), what he used to hope for and do. Acknowledge his past achievements. Listen (and gain philosophical insights) when the senior rehashes old conflicts, relives old pleasures and pains, reviews the meaning and importance of his existence, and considers what death and judgment might be like. Often he feels nostalgic for past activities and an acceptance of the past and present as he talks.

The person may avoid life review; the less he looks, the fewer problems he finds. He may die before he has done much life review, or life review may cause feelings of discontent, self-despair, deep terror, or rarely, pathology. As the person reminisces about his life, he may feel angry about events, berate himself for committed or omitted acts, feel guilt or regret; depression may result. The most tragic life review situations involve increasing, but *partial,* insight, which causes a sense of a wasted life without a chance to redo.[17,18] Such unhappy feelings and partial insight are less likely to result if the senior can share his life review with a professional as well as with peers and family. The professional who listens and gives constructive feedback, acknowledging the bad times but pointing out the positive features of the person's life, can help the person gain more complete insight and a sense of satisfaction. Peers and relatives are not necessarily good listeners. Peers will try to compete with his story and will interrupt the reminiscing. Family members often tell the senior to stop talking about the past because they have probably heard the story so many times. Or the listener may walk away or pretend not to hear. These reactions are likely to increase the senior's anger and despair; his life must not have been worth much if no one wants to hear about it.

The person's emotional status also determines the direction of life review. The depressed senior castigates himself and ruminates about the unpleasant. He feels ashamed. The person can be helped to reminisce by externalizing anger and dissatisfaction about how the young people have botched up the world. Appreciate his global anger at a world that has used the lifeblood of elders to shape a society of affluence and comfort for us. Acknowledge the pain of elders who are not reaping the fruits of their labor.[32]

The confused person reminisces in a repetitive, annoying manner as he ineffectively tries to focus his thoughts. Assist him to select and elaborate a particular memory and explore it with him to stimulate reality orientation.[32]

The helpless, demanding person insists that he is inept; you may become irritated with him but do not accept his self-image. Engage him in active exploration of past and present strengths.[32]

The frightened person cowers in submissiveness, feeling that if he is quiet and good, he will be ignored and none of his horrendous fantasies will come to pass. Explore the source of his fears and past supports.[32]

Spontaneous memories often reflect current situations. If the aged person remembers only the extreme helplessness of being a small child, he may be saying that he feels helpless in his present situation. Spontaneous memories can be used to assess present perceptions.[32]

Thus, your role in listening, accepting, and being interested in the senior's reminiscences and life review is crucial in promoting further personality growth. Although listening takes time, often it can be done during the bath or other care procedures. Having the same nurse assigned to the senior over a period of time also helps because the senior can continue sequentially instead of having to start at the beginning with each caretaker.

If you find the person gazing at himself in the mirror, either do not interrupt or else talk to him about what he's thinking and feeling. Do not chastise or tease him because the senior seldom looks in the mirror to admire his beauty. Later on you may want to follow up on whatever comments about himself he has directed to the mirror and encourage him to look at himself in the mirror. Mirror gazing aids not only life review but also reintegration of the changed physical self.

You may stimulate reminiscing and life review by talking about present objects or events—food, pictures, weather, seasons, music, or whatever. Almost everything you mention can trigger memories in the senior, which he often pursues for only a few minutes before returning to present thoughts. If you work in a residence or institution for the elderly, you can encourage reminiscing through informal group discussion and activities. Encourage the seniors to form friendships and talk to each other. Power and cohesiveness grow from sharing memories with peers.[32] You may form one of the groups discussed in Chapter 4.

Some people in later maturity, especially in the young-old (sixties and seventies) may not want to reminisce to any great extent. Present reality and future plans should be the subjects of their conversation.[31] Offer new activities and opportunities to learn.

Environmental Support

The physical environment affects behavior. For example, slippery waxed floors, few chairs, formal furniture arrangement, and lack of elevators discourage walking, general mobility, and socialization in a nursing home or residence for seniors. The elderly person remains more mobile and sociable if he can help decide about environmental characteristics. The living environment should be functional and comfortable. Often new buildings present a sterility and force loss of familiar objects.

The environment that offers the senior opportunities to participate voluntarily in interesting activities promotes emotional health. You can initiate constructive use of leisure by having supplies available and encouraging the senior's participation and creativity. Leisure pursuits enjoyed by the elderly were discussed in Chapter 6. Community services, such as senior citizen centers, telephone services, geriatric day care, and various organizations, all discussed in Chapter 6, can also be used to keep the senior involved.

In one study a photography course was used to teach new skills, increase the sense of competence, encourage social interaction, and provide feedback to increase positive feelings about self.[4]

In another program each senior became responsible for an adult mentally retarded person; each senior acted like a foster grandparent. In the process both the senior and the retardate benefited.[52]

Behavior Modification Approach

Certainly the elderly person's behavior should not be modified for the caretaker's benefit. But often the senior's social environment is reinforcement deficient; staff, family, or friends gradually withdraw their attention, respect, and love. Then the person becomes less sociable and adaptable.

Reinforcing the senior's social behavior and giving positive feedback to his efforts to relate and behave appropriately are essential for him to maintain reality contact and sense of identity. Reminding him of past coping mechanisms will help him reawaken a sense of mastery. Formal behavior modification programs can be useful, but they should not be used without also developing and maintaining a nurse-patient relationship. More information about behavior modification programs can be found in several references.[6,62]

The senior can also be taught to strengthen, maintain, or weaken certain behavior or ideas by controlling his own reinforcement and the consequences of such behavior. For example, the person can be taught to use more positive than negative statements about himself when he is talking with others; more than likely the person will get a more positive response in return. Such feedback is reinforcing, and as the person makes more positive statements which are true, he comes to believe them and grows to feel more positive about himself. However, anytime the elderly person is asked to give up certain behavior in favor of other behavior, he loses the satisfaction that accompanied other behaviors related to the original behavior. For example, if he received more attention when he complained about his aches, asking him to talk about subjects other than his physical symptoms will not be satisfying unless he gets an equal amount of or more attention. Or giving up a "rigid" response or a ritual means losing the security of knowing how something will turn out; he will need much positive reinforcement for trying a different behavior before he can feel good about the change.[73]

Evaluation

Evaluation of your nursing practice relates to your care objectives, your relationship with the person, and whether or not the person continues to cope with his situation and function realistically.

Recognize the emotional effects that intervening emotionally with the elderly have on you. Do you perceive and relate to the senior as if he were a parent, grandparent, or other relative? If you are in the child role, you may manifest fear or ambivalence instead of the firmness needed to help them. Can you face your own aging process? Do you think about what you may be like emotionally when you are old? Can you accept your limits in helping the elderly? Are your emotional needs met elsewhere or are you accepting the warmth and interest of the elderly person/family for your own benefit? As you care for the senior, you will have to continually rework your feelings about life, death, age, parental relationships (especially if your own experiences with parents were unhappy) and chronic illness/disability if you are to remain objective and yet be able to give of yourself to the elderly person.

Emotional status and function do not automatically deteriorate with age. Disease, major social losses, and long-standing personality characteristics have more to do with mental illness than age.[67] Avoid labeling the old, ill, bereft senior as mentally ill just because his behavior is different or makes you uncomfortable. Although Unit V explores in-depth various psychiatric illnesses of later maturity, only a small percentage of the elderly will ever be diagnosed as emotionally ill.

REFERENCES

1. "Age-linked Social Trauma Rarely Leads to Mental Ills," *Geriatric Focus,* 6: No. 13 (1967), 1ff.

2. ALLPORT, GORDON, *Pattern and Growth in Personality.* New York: Holt, Rinehart and Winston, 1961.

3. ANDERSON, NANCY, "Institutionalization, Interaction, and Self-Conception in Aging," in *Older People and Their Social World,* eds. Arnold Rose and Warren Petersen. Philadelphia: F. A. Davis Company, 1965, pp. 245–57.

4. ARONSON, DAVID, and A. GRAZIANO, "Improving Elderly Clients' Attitudes Through Photography," *The Gerontologist,* 16: No. 4 (1976), 363–67.

5. ATCHLEY, R. C., *The Social Forces in Later Life.* Belmont, Calif.: Wadsworth Publishing Co., Inc., 1972.

6. BERNI, ROSEMARIAN, and WILBERT FORDYCE, *Behavior Modification and the Nursing Process.* St. Louis: The C. V. Mosby Company, 1973.

7. BEVERLEY, E., "The Beginnings of Wisdom About Aging," *Geriatrics,* 30: (July, 1975), 17–28.

8. BIRREN, JAMES, ed., *Handbook on Aging and the Individual: Psychological and Biological Aspects.* Chicago: The University of Chicago Press, 1959.

9. ———, *The Psychology of Aging.* Englewood Cliffs, N.J.: Prentice-Hall, Inc., 1964.

10. BISCHOFF, LEDFORD, *Adult Psychology.* New York: Harper & Row, Publishers, Inc., 1969.

11. BLOOM, K., "Age and the Self-Concept," *American Journal of Psychiatry,* 118: (1961), 534–38.

12. BOTWINICK, JACK, *Aging and Behavior.* New York: Springer Publishing Company, Inc., 1973.

13. BRITTON, J., and O. BRITTON, *Personality Changes in Aging.* New York: Springer Publishing Co., Inc., 1972.

14. BRUBAKER, TIMOTHY, and EDWARD POWERS, "The Stereotype of 'Old'—A Review and Alternative Approach," *Journal of Gerontology,* 31: No. 4 (1976), 441–47.

15. BUHLER, C., "Meaningful Living in the Mature Years," in *Aging and Leisure,* ed. R. Kleemeier. New York: Oxford University Press, 1961.

16. BULTENA, G., and E. POWERS, "Effects of Age-Grade Comparisons on Adjustment in Later Life," in *Late Life: Time, Roles, and Self in Old Age,* ed. J. Gubrium. New York: Behavioral Public, 1976.

17. BUTLER, ROBERT, "The Life Review: An Interpretation of Reminiscence in the Aged," *Psychiatry,* 26: No. 1 (1963), 65–76.

18. ———, "Age: The Life Review," *Psychology Today,* 5: No. 7 (1971), 49ff.

19. CAMERON, PAUL, "The Generation Gap: Time Orientation," *The Gerontologist,* 12: No. 2 (1972), 117–19.

20. CARLSON, AVIS, *In the Fullness of Time: The Pleasures and Inconveniences of Growing Old.* Chicago: Henry Regnery Company, 1977.

21. CHIRIBOGA, DAVID, "Evaluated Time: A Life Course Perspective," *Journal of Gerontology,* 33: No. 3 (1978), 388–93.

22. CLARK, A. *et al.,* "Diogenes Syndrome," *Lancet,* 1: (February 15, 1975), 366–68.

23. CLOSURDO, JANETTE, "Behavior Modification and the Nursing Process," *Perspectives in Psychiatric Care,* 13: No. 1 (1975), 25–35.

24. COE, RODNEY, "Self-Concept and Institutionalization," in *Older People and Their Social World,* eds., Arnold Rose and Warren Petersen. Philadelphia: F. A. Davis Company, 1965, pp. 225–43.

25. COLEMAN, P., "Measuring Reminiscence Characteristics from Conversation as Adaptive Features of Old Age," *International Journal of Aging and Human Development,* 5: (1974), 281–94.

26. COSTA, P., and R. McCRAE, "Age Differences in Personality Structure: A Cluster Analytic Approach," *Journal of Gerontology,* 31: No. 5 (1976), 564–70.

27. CRAIG, GRACE, *Human Development.* Englewood Cliffs, N.J.: Prentice-Hall, Inc., 1976.

28. CURTIN, SHARON, *Nobody Ever Died of Old Age.* Boston: Little, Brown & Company, 1972.

29. DATUM, NANCY, and LEON GINSBURG, eds., *Life Span Developmental Psychology.* New York: Academic Press, Inc., 1975.

30. DRESEN, SHEILA, "Staying Well While Growing Old: Autonomy—A Continuing Development Task," *American Journal of Nursing,* 78: No. 8 (1978), 1344–46.

31. DUVALL, EVELYN, *Family Development,* 5th ed. Philadelphia, J. B. Lippincott Company, 1977.

32. EBERSOLE, PRISCILLA, "Reminiscing," *American Journal of Nursing,* 76: No. 8 (1976), 1304–05.

33. ERIKSON, ERIK, *Childhood and Society,* 2nd ed. New York: W. W. Norton & Co., Inc., 1963.

34. FILLENBAUM, G. and G. MADDOX, "Work After Retirement: An Investigation into Some Psychologically Relevant Variables," *The Gerontologist,* 14: (1974), 418–24.

35. FINK, STEPHEN, "Crisis and Motivation: A Theoretical Model," *Archives of Physical Medicine and Rehabilitation,* 48: No. 11 (1967), 592–97.

36. FITZGERALD, J., "Actual and Perceived Sex and Generational Differences in Interpersonal Style: Structural and Quantitative Issues," *Journal of Gerontology,* 33: No. 3 (1978), 394–401.

37. FORD, CAROLINE, "Ego Adaptive Mechanisms of Older Persons," in *Human Life Cycle,* ed. Wm. Sze. New York: Jason Aronson, Inc., 1975, pp. 599–608.

38. GEORGE, LINDA, and GEORGE MADDOX, "Subjective Adaptation to Loss of Work Role: A Longitudinal Study," *Journal of Gerontology,* 32: No. 4 (1977), 456–62.

39. GIAMBRO, LEONARD, "Daydreaming About the Past—The Time Setting of Spontaneous Thought Intrusions," *The Gerontologist,* 17: No. 1 (1977), 35–38.

40. GITELSON, MAXWELL, "The Emotional Problems of Elderly People," in *Human Life Cycle,* ed. Wm. Sze. New York: Jason Aronson, Inc., 1975, pp. 575–87.

41. GRIGGS, WINONA, "Staying Well While Growing Old: Sex and the Elderly," *American Journal of Nursing,* 78: No. 8 (1978), 1352–54.

42. GUTMAN, DAVID, "Aging Among the Highland Maya: A Comparative Study," *Journal of Personality and Social Psychology,* 7: No. 1 (1967), 28–35.

43. HALL, JOANNE, and BARBARA WEAVER, *Nursing of Families in Crisis.* Philadelphia: J. B. Lippincott Company, 1974.

44. HAVIGHURST, ROBERT, "A Social-Psychological Perspective on Aging," in *Human Life Cycle,* ed. Wm. Sze. New York: Jason Aronson, Inc., 1975, pp. 627–35.

45. HESS, ANNE, and H. BRADSHAW, "Positiveness of Self-Concept and Ideal Self as a Function of Old Age," *Journal of Genetic Psychology,* 117: (1970), 57ff.

46. HIRSCHFELD, MIRIAM, "The Aging Holocaust Survivor," *American Journal of Nursing,* 77: No. 7 (1977), 1187–89.

47. HOLMES, T. and R. RAHE, "The Social Readjustment Rating Scale," *Journal of Psychosomatic Research,* 11: No. 8 (1967), 213–17.

48. HYMAN, H., "The Psychology of Status," *Archives of Psychology,* 38: (1942), 1–94.

49. "Is Aging Just for the Old?" *Modern Maturity,* August–September, 1974, p. 6.

50. JAHODA, MARIE, *Current Concepts of Positive Mental Health.* New York: Basic Books, Inc., 1958.

51. JEFFERS, FRANCIS, and ADRIAN VERVOERDT, "How the Old Face Death," in *Behavior and Adaptation in Late Life,* eds. Ewald Busse and Eric Pfeiffer. Boston: Little, Brown & Company, 1969, pp. 163–81.

52. KALSON, LEON, "MASH: A Program of Social Interaction Between Institutionalized Aged and Adult Mentally Retarded Persons," *The Gerontologist,* 16: No. 4 (1976), 340–48.

53. KARP, S., "Field Dependence and Occupational Activity in the Aged," *Perceptual and Motor Skills,* 24: (1967), 603–9.

54. KELLY, H., "The Two Functions of Reference Groups," in *Readings in Social Psychology,* eds. G. Swanson, T. Newcomb, and E. Hartley. New York: Holt, Rinehart and Winston, 1962.

55. KENT, D., and M. MATSON, "The Impact of Health on the Aged Family," *Family Coordinator,* 21: (1972), 29–36.

56. KENT, DONALD, "Social and Cultural Factors Influencing Mental Health of the Aged," in *Human Life Cycle,* ed. Wm. Sze. New York: Jason Aronson, Inc., 1975, pp. 643–49.

57. KIMMEL, DOUGLAS, *Adulthood and Aging.* New York: John Wiley & Sons, Inc., 1974.

58. KIVETT, VERA, ALLEN WATSON, and J. BUSCH, "The Relative Importance of Physical, Psychological, and Social Variables to Locus of Control Orientation in Middle Age," *Journal of Gerontology,* 32: No. 2 (1977), 203–10.

59. KOIS, DENNIS, "How You Live Called Key to How Long You Live," *St. Louis Globe-Democrat,* January 17–18, 1976, Sec. A, p. 15.

60. LARSON, REED, "Thirty Years of Research on the Subjective Well-Being of Older Americans," *Journal of Gerontology,* 33: No. 1 (1978), 109–25.

61. LEBOW, MICHAEL, *Behavior Modification.* Englewood Cliffs, N.J.: Prentice-Hall, Inc., 1973.

62. LEE, ROBERTA, "Self-Images of the Elderly," *Nursing Clinics of North America,* 11: No. 1 (1976), 119–24.

63. LOWENTHAL, MARJORIE, and CLAYTON HAVEN, "Interaction and Adaptation: Intimacy as a Critical Variable," *American Sociological Review*, 33: No. 1 (1968), 20–30.

64. MAAS, HENRY, and JOSEPH KUYPERS, *From Thirty to Seventy*. San Francisco: Jossey-Bass, Inc., Publishers, 1974.

65. MEDLEY, MORRIS, "Satisfaction with Life Among Persons Sixty-Five Years and Older," *Journal of Gerontology*, 31: No. 4 (1976), 448–55.

66. MUHLENKAMP, ANN, LUCILLE GRESS, and MAY FLOOD, "Perception of Life Change Events by the Elderly," *Nursing Research*, 24: No. 2 (1975), 109–13.

67. NEUGARTEN, B., "Grow Old Along With Me! The Best Is Yet to Be," *Psychology Today*, 5: No. 7 (1971), 45ff.

68. ———, "Adult Personality: A Developmental View," in *Readings in Psychological Development Through Life*, eds. D. Charles and W. Looft. New York: Holt, Rinehart and Winston, 1973, pp. 356–66.

69. O'CONNELL, V., and A. O'CONNELL. *Choice and Change: An Introduction to the Psychology of Growth*. Englewood Cliffs, N.J.: Prentice-Hall, Inc., 1974.

70. PALMORE, ERDMAN, and VERA KIVETT, "Change in Life Satisfaction: A Longitudinal Study of Persons Aged 41–70," *Journal of Gerontology*, 32: No. 3 (1977), 311–16.

71. PRESTON, C., "Subjectively Perceived Agedness and Retirement," *Journal of Gerontology*, 23: (1968), 201–4.

72. ———, and K. GUDIKSEN, "A Measure of Self-Perception Among Older People," *Journal of Gerontology*, 21: (1966), 63–71.

73. RAHE, R. and R. ARTHUR, "Life-Change Patterns Surrounding Illness Perception, *Journal of Psychosomatic Research*, 11: No. 3 (1968), 341–45.

74. REBOK, GEORGE, and WM. HOZER, "The Functional Context of Elderly Behavior," *The Gerontologist*, 17: No. 1 (1977), 27–34.

75. REICHARD, SUZANNE, FLORENCE LIVSON, and PAUL PETERSON. *Aging and Personality*. New York: John Wiley & Sons, Inc., 1962.

76. REID, DAVID, GWEN HAAS, and DOUGLAS HAWKINGS, "Locus of Desired Control and Positive Self-Concept of the Elderly," *Journal of Gerontology*, 32: No. 4 (1977), 441–50.

77. RENDER, HELENA, "My Old Age," *Nursing Outlook*, 12: No. 11 (1964), 31–33.

78. ROSE, ARNOLD, "Mental Health of Older Persons," in *Older People and Their Social World*, eds. Arnold Rose and Warren Petersen. Philadelphia: F. A. Davis Company, 1965, pp. 193–99.

79. ———, "Physical Health and Mental Outlook Among the Aging," in *Older People and Their Social World*, eds. Arnold Rose and Warren Petersen. Philadelphia: F. A. Davis Company, 1965, pp. 201–9.

80. ROSEN, J., and B. NEUGARTEN, "Ego Functions in Middle and Later Years: A Thematic Apperception Study," in *Personality in Middle and Late Life: Empirical Studies*, ed. Bernice Neugarten. New York: Atherton Press, 1964.

81. ROWE, ALAN, "Retired Academics and Research Activity," *Journal of Gerontology*, 31: No. 4 (1976), 456–61.

82. SAUER, WILLIAM, "Morale of the Urban Aged: A Regression Analysis by Race," *Journal of Gerontology*, 32: No. 5 (1977), 600–608.

83. SCHWARTZ, D., and S. KARP, "Field Dependence in a Geriatric Population," *Perceptual and Motor Skills,* 24: No. 4 (1967), 495–504.

84. SHUKIN, A., and B. NEUGARTEN, "Personality and Social Interaction," in *Personality in Middle and Late Life,* ed. Bernice Neugarten. New York: Atherton Press, 1964.

85. SLATER, P., and H. SCARR, "Personality in Old Age," *Genetic Psychological Monographs,* 70: (1964), 229–69.

86. STINNETT, N., and J. MONTGOMERY, "Youth's Perceptions of Marriages of Older Persons," *Journal of Marriage and the Family,* 30: (1968), 392–96.

87. SULLIVAN, HARRY S., *The Interpersonal Theory of Psychiatry.* New York: W. W. Norton & Co., Inc., 1953.

88. THOMPSON, W., *Correlates of the Self-Concept.* Nashville: Counselor Recordings and Tests, 1972.

89. TOSELAND, RON, and JAMES SYKES, "Senior Citizen Center Participation and Other Correlates of Life Satisfaction," *The Gerontologist,* 17: No. 3 (1977), 235–41.

90. TUCKMAN, J., and I. LORGE, "Attitude Toward Aging of Individuals with Experiences with the Aged," *Journal of Genetic Psychology,* 92: (1958), 199–204.

91. WEG, RUTH, "Aging and the Aged in Contemporary Society," *Physical Therapy,* 53: No. 7 (1973), 749–56.

92. WEINBERGER, L., and J. MILLHAN, "A Multi-Dimensional, Multiple Method Analysis of Attitudes Toward the Elderly," *Journal of Gerontology,* 30: (1975), 343–48.

93. YOUMANS, E., and M. YARROW, "Aging and Social Adaptation: A Longitudinal Study of Healthy Old Men," in *Human Aging,* Vol. II, eds., S. Granick and R. Patterson. Washington D.C.: U.S. Department of Health, Education and Welfare, (1971), pp. 95ff.

94. ZOLA, I., "Feelings About Age Among Older People," *Journal of Gerontology,* 17: (1962), 65–68.

family relationships in later maturity

Study of this chapter will enable you to:

1. Discuss how the elderly family differs in composition and functions from young adult and middle-aged families.

2. Identify cultural factors and norms and other variables that affect the elderly family unit.

3. Observe the variety and adequacy of living arrangements for elderly families in your community.

4. Describe the relationships that may develop within the elderly family: between partners, between siblings, as well as between parent, child, grandchild, and greatgrandchild.

5. Discuss the myths and stereotypes related to sexuality in late life and how they can be overcome.

6. Identify manifestations of sexuality in elderly persons whom you observe or care for.

7. Formulate an assessment tool and assess a family unit, considering the information presented in this chapter.

8. Formulate a nursing diagnosis and family care objectives appropriate to an elderly family.

9. Intervene with a family unit through purposeful communication, a helping relationship, teaching, counseling, referral, or doing special health care measures as indicated.

10. Work with other health care professionals or agencies to give comprehensive, coordinated care to a family.

11. Discuss how intervention with a family unit differs from intervention with an individual.

12. Evaluate the effectiveness of your care and ability to simultaneously care for several people who comprise one unit.

12

INTRODUCTION

Definitions

Many people may not consider the elderly couple or elderly siblings who live together to be a family. Traditional definitions of family refer to husband, wife, and child, as well as the extended family, and refer to functions of reproduction.

However, in the eight-stage family life cycle the *aging family stage exists from retirement to death of both spouses.* The *aging family* may be defined as *a primary group and a social subsystem that consists of two or more persons related by marriage, blood, or adoption who reside together, characterized by face-to-face association, role and economic cooperation, and a sharing of values, responsibilities, and rewards.*[15]

The elderly family may consist of husband and wife, several siblings or cousins, very old parents with an elderly offspring who is single or widowed, a widower living with an elderly relative, or a man and woman who live together by mutual consent without getting married so that they will not lose their Social Security benefits. Same-sexed friends who are as close as siblings may perceive themselves as a family unit; the relationship may be companionable and not necessarily homosexual.

The *extended family*, consisting of the nuclear family (*husband, wife, children*), *parents, aunts, uncles, cousins, and grandparents,* was more prominent in the past but seldom lived under one roof in the United States to the extent that extended families lived together in other parts of the world. Yet, in the past, relatives lived and worked closely together, had great impact on each other, and contributed to childrearing. Today geographic mobility related to occupation and life-style may preclude such close contact. Yet, the extended family does exist. The *psychologically extended family is one in which there is supportive interaction between several generations of relatives although they do not live in the same household.*[19,40]

Functions of the Family

While the functions of the family typically include sexual regulation, reproduction, physical and emotional maintenance, division of labor, socialization of young, placement of members into the larger society, and maintenance of order,[15] functions of the aging family differ to some extent. The primary functions of the aging family include companionship between its members, providing physical necessities, maintaining motivation and morale, and continuing communication and patterns of interaction.

Sexual intimacy may or may not be a function; division of labor may be minimal if only one member is healthy enough to do most of the work. Instead of releasing members into society and recruiting members into the family, which occurs in the younger years, the aging family gets smaller as members are lost to death, and ties with the community may be tenuous.[15]

Family ties are important to the senior because of their emotional, supportive, and sometimes economic functions. As the person ages, he becomes more involved in family than he does in non-kin relations if family exist. The problem is the lack of cultural norms for intergenerational relations, which cause the senior to expect different contacts from what are sometimes provided by the younger family members.

Changing Cultural Norms

As society becomes increasingly mechanized and depersonalized, the family remains one of the few groups that has a primary, or close, relationship; yet the family is different for today's senior.[40]

The person in later maturity grew up in an extended family, with discipline from and responsibility to grandparents, aunts, uncles, and parents. The family was typically patriarchal; father was chief decision maker. Thus, the senior has difficulty understanding his offspring's nuclear family who lives in a democratic pattern and has less contact with other relatives. Norms regarding mate selection, marriage, reproduction, childrearing, sex roles, mate relations, divorce, care of parents, and family and social roles for the elderly have changed. What the senior considers his offspring's responsibility the offspring may consider an obligation or a task to be done by a social agency. Having children no longer automatically offers a residence, economic advantage, or care.

As society emphasized productivity, upward socioeconomic mobility, individuality, geographic mobility, and anonymity of urban life, the older person had more difficulty maintaining family ties. Our open society offers many choices, but it also contributes to isolation of the person.[4] Two kinds of isolation may occur with the elderly: (1) a lower degree of involvement with near or distant relatives, children, or former friends, so that the senior feels that he must rely on himself and (2) divergence from cultural values, interests, and activities that are important to younger people, causing conflict between generations and the senior's feelings of being obsolete.[17]

Yet, the elderly family is like the young adult family in that the main reason to live together is for affection and companionship. However, the elderly are not as likely to divorce if the members are not having a harmonious relationship. To live alone may seem worse to some seniors than to be unhappy; or at least, they cannot visualize their life pattern differently.

In the future, extension of healthful vigor to age 85 to 90 may lead to more second marriages, changing sexual norms such as polygamy or several women sharing a husband, and more divorces in late life.[9,33]

Living Arrangements

Most young-old do not live alone. They live in a family unit, maintaining a household with spouse, children, or a relative. The senior may invite another elderly relative to live with him because of singlehood or widowhood. The senior may be invited to join a family unit because he can give financial assistance or help with young children.[7,40]

Most old-old persons live alone, especially the woman who frequently outlives the man. When family ties are few or distant, the old-old is likely to be institutionalized when he cannot perform self-care tasks.[7]

The senior prefers his own residence but wants to live near offspring and to maintain ties. About one-half of the elderly live in close proximity (within one-half hour's drive) to at least one child or relative. Parents may live with a married or widowed child if a housing shortage exists, if the adult child needs help, or if the senior is ill.[39,40,41,46]

Proximity of children compensates for loss of mate; the extended family compensates for having no children. Friends or neighbors may play a supportive role.[41]

SIBLING RELATIONSHIPS

Bonds between siblings extend throughout life and are often second only to mother-child ties. In childhood siblings fulfill a number of functions: parent substitute, teacher, role model, challenger, or stimulator.[10] During young adulthood and the childrearing years siblings tend to drift apart and often communicate indirectly through the parents, or ties may be maintained through infrequent letters, visits, or phone calls. But when parents die or their own children leave home, sibling ties are usually renewed.[21]

The elderly feel closer to their siblings than to other relatives (except the children), especially if the senior never married, is widowed or divorced, or had no children. The sister-sister tie is the closest sibling tie, and it may be closer than the husband-wife tie. Past sibling rivalries may be reactivated, but they are usually suppressed for the sake of companionship.[20] Contact with an older sibling can provide anticipatory socialization as the aging person learns about coping with retirement, illness, disability, and loss of spouse. Siblings provide emotional support, encouragement, morale lifting, and counseling during crises, and they act as confidant and teacher. Siblings are often expected to help each other financially if necessary. Older sisters may assume a maternal role with the entire family, especially with brothers, and help keep the extended family together after the parents' death.[11]

Influence of Retirement

For the reasons discussed in Chapter 6, retirement causes both partners to redefine marital roles and may increase conflicts for both. The independent breadwinner loses status upon retirement. The dependent wife gains status or power and increases decision making.[41]

The couple interacts more. Conflicts that were suppressed when children were in the home or the man (or woman) was preoccupied with a job may arise and increase in intensity because of role reversals and decreasing adaptability.[41] The conflicts may cause the man to join his buddies at the local bar or in leisure pursuits and the woman to pursue volunteer work or interests with female friends. If the couple live in a rural area or has a home with a yard and garden, the extra space and related tasks may diffuse the conflict.

Yet, this can be a happy time for the couple. Their lives are calmer. Problems with dominating in-laws may be over. They have new freedom to do as they please. Adjustment is smoother if they have previously enjoyed each other, worked together in the house, shared common interests, and if neither has to bolster the ego by projecting inadequacies or displacing anger onto the mate.[43]

Interdependence of the Elderly Couple

In spite of frictions that result from more closeness, the elderly couple at the end of a long life together have established a symbiotic relationship. Each is extremely dependent on the other and they identify with each other, even if their life together looks less than ideal. They provide a familiar landmark for each other in a drastically changed environment. They give each other support and security; each is predictable. Often the senior's grumbling or seemingly sarcastic remarks are the habitual way of showing love to a spouse who is known very well and who knows what the remarks mean.

Husband and wife often become more alike in behavior patterns over the years from imitative learning. Certain personality traits also become more dominant in family interaction as energy for defense mechanisms diminishes. The patterns of living may be either healthy or neurotic, but they are not likely to be changed very much. The dominant pattern will also have been learned by the children and will often be continued in the offspring's family. The closer the family ties between generations, the more the pattern will be strengthened. If the elderly parents' living pattern has been unhealthy, involving domination, submission, scapegoating, rumination, manipulation, or other patterns, the offspring either contribute toward the elderly couple's behavior or break away from it by keeping an emotional and geographical distance.[16]

SEXUALITY IN LATER MATURITY

Sexuality is defined as the deep, pervasive aspect of the person, the sum total of attitudes, feelings, and behavior as a male or female, the expression of which goes beyond genital response.[24]

Myths and Stereotypes About Sexuality

The elderly are seen as sexually unattractive and neuter beings, without sexual interests or activities, by relatives, researchers, physicians, social scientists, and the elderly themselves. Until recently, sexual activity was procreative instead of recreative. Repression of ideas about sexual behavior in seniors may also be related to the Oedipal conflict; at some time in childhood the direct sexual wishes and fantasies connected to parents are repressed, and even adult offspring often fail to see their parents as sexual beings.[52] Taboos about sexual activity in later maturity may be partly an extension of the incest taboo. By fostering the stereotype of the asexual senior, the elderly are not viewed as sexual competitors or sexual objects.[11]

A number of myths about sexual behavior in the elderly may still prevail, in spite of attempts at sex education. Myths include:

1. Too much sexual activity in young life hastens old age and death; semen emission is weakening and causes coital inability in old age.
2. Menopause and hysterectomy decrease sexual satisfaction and mark the end of sex life for the woman.
3. Certain foods have aphrodisiac qualities and improve potency.
4. Masturbation is annoying if practiced by children but sick if practiced by older persons.
5. Older men are especially prone to exhibitionism, child molesting, and other deviations.
6. Older people are too fragile to make love if they want to.[13,36,50]

Myths and stereotypes are harmful; the senior adopts the societal views and develops a negative self-image as a sexual being. The myth becomes a self-fulfilling prophecy. The widowed are forced to live alone and forego companionship of a partner because of offspring's attitudes. Celibacy between married couples is enforced in institutions for the aged. Administrative justice is harsh on the older man accused of sexual offenses. And medical and psychologic diagnoses may be incorrect because sexuality is denied.[13,34,36,50]

Expressions of Sexuality

The meaning and value of intercourse are not strictly organic. They are also psychological and sociocultural. Sexual behavior and satisfaction vary considerably among the elderly, depending on earlier sexual activity.

Sexuality refers to more than coitus. Sexuality includes the close hug, kiss, and companionship shared when frailties do not permit genital intimacy; the alert and practiced eye of the elderly male and his comments about a lady's pretty legs; and the feeble hand reaching out to receive the warmth of a touch and affection. Sexuality is expressed in intellectual interest in romance or eroticism.[8,13,34,35]

Coitus or general sexual behavior serves many functions: making love; showing affection, trust, companionship, or respect; releasing tension; giving of self to another; reaffirming self-concept; conveying that another is attractive or valued; increasing self-esteem, bolstered by the knowledge that one is desired or valued by another. Aggression, dominance, or submission can also be expressed by sexual behavior.[13,50]

Influences upon Expressions of Sexuality

Sexual desire and ability do not normally diminish in later maturity. Various factors influence the type and frequency of the senior's sexual behavior. Cultural taboos and restraints imposed by rigid moral or religious principles inhibit psychologically. Normal physical aging changes discussed in Chapter 9 have a minimal effect upon function or enjoyment as long as the person regularly engages in coitus. Negative self-concept, behavioral effects of values related to youth and beauty, fatigue, illness, surgery, medications, and overindulgence in food and drink result in reduced sexual function. Secondary impotence in the male is more directly associated with excessive alcohol consumption than any other factor, although fear of unsatisfactory performance, boredom with partner, and preoccupation with economic problems are other factors. The degree of marriage harmony also influences sexual activity.[11,22,34,35]

Abstinence causes difficulty in resuming coitus; after illness or surgery, coitus should be resumed as quickly as possible. If the partners are compatible, coitus necessitates less energy expenditure than commonly thought, although heroic feats should not be attempted. Sexual frustration may consume as much energy, especially if sexual activity is a major part of the self-concept. Only if the heart has been severely damaged or if other severe impairment is present should sexual activity be adjusted or contraindicated.[6,12,34,35]

Certain illnesses are more likely to cause impotency, such as diabetes, because of neuropathy of the sacral parasympathetic fibers that supply the penis, and vascular disease, because of the effect on the increased blood supply that is needed to distend vascular spaces of the erectile penile tissue. Effects of arthritis on sexuality are discussed in Chapter 15. Prostatectomy may cause impotency. Senile vaginitis, cystocele, and rectocele may inhibit the woman's enjoyment, but these conditions are treatable. Often the fear of impotency resulting from a disease is more likely to cause impotency than the disease itself.[22,34,35,50]

The older male may temporarily experience impotence; if he and the partner accept this as normal, the male can function the next time. The closeness of each other can be very gratifying without penetration or orgasm. If the self-concept and marriage are shaky, an episode of impotency may be shattering and result in more impotency. The man may seek correction in sex pills or foods, penile splints, or other devices, all of which are generally a waste of money. The solution to impotency is found in the communication and closeness between the partners, which may be enhanced by knowledgeable, thoughtful counseling.[11]

The woman's sexual desire and capacity for function are frequently greater after menopause. Most cessation of coitus is attributed, by both men and women, to the male partner. The partners may subtly or silently agree to stop intercourse if this has been viewed as a chore or as unpleasant; usually this happens long before old age. If the partners have a positive self-concept and love for each other, sexual function may improve. They have more time for experimentation; neither is bothered by young children, fear of pregnancy, or job pressures. Companionship from other sources may be reduced; if the marital relationship is happy, the partners may turn more to each other for companionship. Research studies show a variety of percentages of seniors who regularly engage in coitus; the percentages will probably rise as our more sexually oriented younger population becomes older. Oral, manual, and digital manipulations between partners are also becoming more common, can be an outlet for present seniors, and will surely be used more by future elderly. Sexual satisfaction does not depend on coitus.[10,11,12,13,21,22,34,48,50]

The older person who is single, widowed, or divorced is not expected by society to have any sexual needs or activity, and this group has the lowest incidence of sexual activity. Although the strength of their sexual drive may cause tension and anxiety, it is not usually great enough to cause them to overcome the social disapproval and personal difficulties involved. The older person living alone may find release in masturbation and can be counseled accordingly. However, the attitude that masturbation is evil and a childish form of behavior is hard to erase.

Although the frequency and intensity of coitus may be reduced, not until old-old age does the person normally lose capacity for coitus. Sexual interests and activity may remain until death.[11]

RELATIONSHIPS WITH ADULT CHILDREN

Parenthood as a psychobiological process ends only with the parent's loss of memory or death. Being a parent remains central to the self-concept and in late life it normally bolsters self-esteem. The senior clings to adult children; he seeks in them the psychic image of what they were and always will be—his children.[4]

Relating to the Offspring

Marriage of offspring, which usually occurs when the parents are in middle age, is likely to be a critical period in the parent's life. Henceforth, parents are no longer the closest of kin legally. The new in-law is the closest kin, regardless of how short a time the offspring has been married.[4] Confusion exists about even the role of parents to adult offspring in our society.[17]

Formerly in our culture when young adult children married someone nearby, both sets of parents lived close to the young couple. Conflicts between in-laws often resulted. Now, geographically and socially, marriage of offspring may entail quite a separation from parents. Yet, ties between parents and offspring, especially same-sexed, can remain close.

In cultures in which the young wife goes to live in the husband's home the marriage of a daughter means complete separation between parents and daughter. The mother cannot help the daughter adjust or cannot remain involved in the daughter's life, as is commonly done in our culture.[4]

The elderly man may feel jealous of his offspring, especially of the son who is virile and active in the work area. At times the senior may take credit for the success or he may depreciate the efforts of his son. If the son understands the feelings of his once powerful father, who is now emotionally dependent on the son's love, respect, and admiration to maintain his self-esteem, the son can help keep the relationship smooth. If the elderly person is also economically dependent on the son, the senior's already diminished self-esteem increases the need for respect and sensitivity to his real and imagined offenses.[4]

The elderly woman may try to remain involved with her daughter, and the mother's increasingly dominant personality conflicts with her daughter's desire to be independent and establish her identity and role. Conflicts ensue unless the daughter and her husband can listen objectively and avoid arguing with the mother. Further, the mother may have helpful ideas at times.

Father usually remains more distant from the married daughter. Perhaps Oedipal feelings and jealousy are revived by the son-in-law.[4]

Both parents are likely to give more advice, ask more questions, or visit more frequently than is desired by the offspring. Parents mean to be helpful but may be perceived as intruding. Some of the senior's need to give advice may result from a desire to continue the ties that were present when the child was dependent, to act in the consultative role, and to help them prevent mistakes as they observe the marital and parenting behavior of the child.[4] If the separation of generations cannot be accepted, the desired close bonds may actually be broken.

Parents are more heavily invested in their children than the children are in the parents, although mutually maintaining emotional ties and giving aid are culturally expected. Parents prefer offspring to keep in touch through visits rather than letters or phone calls, although all three are desired. The elderly also feel that the children are willing to support them financially but are unable to, which may be a denial of the weak intergenerational ties, since most children do not support their parents.[17]

However, the more harmonious the parent-child relationship in the past, the more the parents were able to meet the child's developing needs, the more companionable the offspring will be to the parents in late life.

Role Reversal

Sometimes in later maturity role reversal occurs. The senior becomes dependent on his child for assistance, which can be psychologically threatening to both generations and intensify role conflicts.[41] The senior may cast family members into parental roles, expecting them to supply needs, guard his status, or make decisions. But many elderly are unwilling to relinquish authority over the offspring even when they are dependent on them for financial support as well as care and companionship. Further, the offspring may resent the obligation and take out long-suppressed hostilities on the parent.[17,41,52]

Sense of duty varies with the offspring's sex, birth order, experiences during childhood, and present life situation. But care of the sick elderly parent is also more difficult in today's society in which most women work; usually there is no unmarried, unemployed daughter in the home. If the aged parents live with the adult children and cause a downward adjustment in living standards, problems result. Often the parent is placed in a home when much care is needed or when the middle-aged children can no longer cope with the three-generational family.[17,41]

Most seniors are satisfied with ties to their offspring, regardless of geographic proximity. Mutual affection, continued communication, reciprocal giving, and the senior's feeling of financial security, regardless of objective level of income, contribute to positive feelings. Harmony is greater when the senior keeps busy with various interests. Normally, the offspring contribute directly and indirectly to the well-being of the senior.[16,44]

THE THREE- AND FOUR-GENERATIONAL FAMILY

The senior is usually part of a series of separate but interrelated families. His middle-aged offspring are helping their adolescent and young adult children to become emancipated from home while simultaneously caring for the increasingly dependent, elderly parent(s), and sometimes up to four even older grandparents. Elderly aunts and uncles may also need some care.

Sociocultural Influences

The norms held by most elderly persons are that (1) adult children should live without parental interference but parents should help when necessary, excluding financially; (2) seniors should enjoy their children and grandchildren; and (3) seniors are responsible for themselves until deteriorated, disabled, or in financial distress, at which time adult children are expected to help.[17]

Four variables appear to affect the quality of intergenerational ties: (1) health, (2) living environment for the elderly and their children, (3) finances, and (4) values on and attitudes toward aging. As the population becomes more urban and secular and as living standards rise, offspring are more reluctant to support aged parents. Adult children are torn between the needs of their parents and their children.

Housing patterns in urban areas mitigate against three generations under one roof, although the practice is more common in working class and low-income families and in certain ethnic groups. When the senior lives with the offspring and grandchildren, certain problems must be resolved. Who remains head of the house is usually determined by who owns or rents the house, income of family members, and who assumes the dominant role. Since the elderly person is not likely to be head of the house, feelings of rejection and being a burden may ensue. In times of great need, the offspring and family may move in with the elderly parent if necessary.[41]

Aged parents who have higher incomes are more likely to have an active role in the family because of increased power in the interaction, but conflict is reduced when the elderly parent can yield authority to the woman of the house, especially in relation to childrearing and household routines. The grandmother has a more secure place in the culture and is perceived as more useful than the grandfather since most family roles for the elderly are traditionally female roles.

Kinship ties vary with race, social class, occupation, and education, and in one study they were measured by the high school seniors' knowledge of the grandparent's occupation. The extent of knowledge of grandfather's occupation correlated with higher social class, occupational, and educational achievement of parent; homogeneity and higher denominational status (Episcopalian, Congregational, Presbyterian) of parents' religion; residence with both parents; and student's higher academic aptitude, educational achievement, and occupational aspiration. However, children of blue-collar workers are better able to name collateral relatives of the extended family than are children of white-collar workers. Apparently, blue-collar families do much visiting and share mutual aid and support with distant aunts, uncles, and cousins.[31]

Advantages of the Three-Generational Family

Benefits of the three-generational family are mutual. The elderly receives a place to live, economic help, protection, affection, and sometimes nursing care. The offspring receives help with childrearing and household tasks and has someone to turn to for help and support during crises.

The grandparent can also support grandchildren in times of stress and provide the extra affection that busy parents may not show.

GRANDPARENTHOOD

Not all seniors become grandparents. But even with the current lower birth rate, the late phase of parenthood usually begins with grandparenthood and continues until death. Grandparenthood can provide a new lease on life and may foster more harmonious relations between the senior and the offspring. For the offspring, independence is declared with parenthood; the child is now bestowing status on the parent. For the elderly parent, grandchildren are a new love object with which to identify, a kind of immortality, a way to relive parenthood.[4]

The Age Factor

Although the parent can become a grandparent in the late thirties, forties, or fifties, the older person is more likely to enjoy and benefit from the status of grandparenthood. Having a grandchild while children are still at home may be more of a problem than a joy. The grandchild may be perceived as another child and reared by the grandmother instead of the young mother. The grandchild may be resented because his coming may have interfered with plans for or aspirations of the parent or grandparent. Even if the grandchild is wanted, involvement is usually less for the younger grandparent because of life-style and emotional needs.

Relieved by the immediate stresses and responsibilities of parenthood, the elderly grandparent typically enjoys the grandchildren more than the children, at least for relatively short periods of time. Extended contacts can be fatiguing.

Grandparent-Grandchild Relationships

Indulgence in a relationship that is harmonious between the elderly parent and offspring does not involve only candy, toys, or time spent in playing with the grandchild. The grandparent's love and pride give the child a sense of security in being loved without doing anything to deserve it. The undemanding love of a grandparent gives the child a sense of omnipotence. In turn, the grandparent receives a loving glance, a trusting hand, an appeal for help, a message of being needed, wanted, and loved. That gives a new lease on life!

The interaction between grandparents and grandchildren typically involves short and long visits; exchange of gifts, letters, and phone calls; sharing of the youngster's adventures and the senior's wisdom. Grandparents provide a validation of life and death and an example of the aging process. Grandparents also serve as the middleman or arbiter in conflicts between the adult children and grandchildren, mitigating the parents' anger at the child while getting some of that anger directed at them. Grandparents are allowed (at least overtly it is accepted) to interfere in parent-child relationships to a degree. Since roles of the mother-in-law and father-in-law frequently conflict with grandparent roles in the extended family, they may therefore contribute to conflict between the generations.

The grandparent role for both sexes in the extended family is really that of the grandmother's role—babysitting, child care, companionship, and household tasks. The role of authority and responsibility formerly associated with the grandfather has been diminished by social changes. Further, the grandfather usually does not live as long as the grandmother does. The child's father usually provides financial support and authority, although situations exist when grandparents have to financially support the offspring and grandchildren.[5] Although the grandfather is not necessarily as close as the grandmother is to the grandchildren, he may be affectionate and proud of the young ones, whereas grandmother may view the young ones negatively because she has been more closely involved with their care.[19]

The feelings of grandparents toward their children and grandchildren and what is expected of the grandparents depend on cultural and socioeconomic status; past relationships with offspring and with their own parents and grandparents; and current social changes.[4]

Grandchildren often grow away from the elderly grandparents. The ambivalence and rebellion of adolescence are directed more toward parents than toward grandparents, since parents are the main objects of their conflicting instinctual drives, unless the grandparents live in the same house. The grandparents become the recipient of considerate, indulging behavior; the youth sees the weakness of the grandparent, often earlier than justified. But the grandparent responds to the protective, if condescending, love of the grandchildren as a balm for wounds inflicted by old age.[4] However, as the grandchild matures emotionally and becomes settled into job, home, and family, the young adult grandchild may reestablish a close bond with the old-old grandparent, which will now be different but can be equally rewarding for both.

Emotional reserves of the aged are maintained by contact with the young and by rekindling memories of past gratifications.[4] But self-preoccupied ruminating about the past is irritating to both children and grandchildren and is a sure way to alienate both generations. Yet, the more frustrated the senior, the greater the need to hang onto the gratifying past and to make inconsiderate demands.

In old-old age the senior has less emotional reserve to empathize with the grandchild or his children. The aged parent expects from the child and grandchild what they expected from him as a parent or grandparent—the removing of all hurts and pains, which is impossible. The solace offered by the younger generations may not gratify demands and it cannot remove the weakness and burdens. The children and grandchildren can become as frustrated as the elderly parent.[4]

Not all elderly people will be grandparents, certainly not the childless couple and usually not the single person. But even the couple with a child(ren) may have no grandchildren. Yet, the grandparent role is one of the few status roles for the elderly in our country. Thus, the Foster Grandparent Program, described in Chapters 7 and 8, exists to help seniors remain involved in the community and contribute their love and talents toward the well-being of a child, and therefore toward the next generation.

Great-Grandparenthood

Because of increasing longevity, many old-old people are becoming great-grandparents and the heads of four-generational families. The grandparents may be in the position of dividing their time and energy between caring for their aging parents and providing attention to adult offspring and their grandchildren.

The relationships discussed under grandparenthood may be applicable to the great-grandparent, depending on age, health status, and closeness of family ties. Since the great-grandparent will not usually be capable of doing as much with the great-grandchild for as long as he did with the grandchild, who is now the parent generation, the tie is more tenuous. Then too, because of geographical mobility in the United States, the older person may have grandchildren and great-grandchildren living throughout the country; contact may be at holidays or even less frequently. For many young children, the main tie to great-grandparents may be in the genealogical record.

CHANGING MARITAL STATUS

The elderly couple may be in a second or third marriage because of death of a former spouse, or less commonly, divorce. However, often the couple have celebrated their fortieth or fiftieth anniversary. The longer the marriage, the less likelihood of divorce.

Death of Spouse

But eventually marriage ends. The surviving spouse takes on the new legal and social role of widow(er). Widowhood may last a few years for the old-old; it may last 10, 20, or 30 years for the young-old. The loss of spouse is probably more difficult to handle at this time because the senior has usually suffered multiple losses—friends, family, roles, finances and perhaps residence. Because of the time spent together, the widow(er) feels that part of self-identity is gone forever. Especially for the woman, whose identity and status are closely related to being married and to her husband's position, the loss of social status is considerable. Then, too, the senior may be less resilient, have less effective coping mechanisms, and fewer supportive persons to help him regain coping skills. The senior also has fewer other roles that can be used as distractions to fill the lonely hours.

Often the surviving spouse feels great guilt and worthlessness, depending on the circumstances of the partner's death. If the survivor cared for the deceased, the person is likely to berate the self for not having done more or for times of less effective care. With the partner dead, the survivor may perceive the self as having no other role. The more active the senior was in caring for the ill partner, the more personal interests and social activities had to be given up. After the partner's death, the survivor may feel very lonely and isolated in a couple-oriented society. Previous friendships may have been dropped if the mate was ill a long time; the bereaved person may not have the psychic or physical energy to renew those friendships. All of the manifestations of grief discussed in Chapter 13 are evident. Suicidal thoughts are common; suicide is often successful and is contemplated as a way to join the dead partner. The survivor needs much support, affection, and interest. As one elderly lady said, "Everybody's bringing me things—things I don't want or need. All I want is for someone to come sit with me, so that I don't have to listen to the shouting silence of empty rooms."

Death of spouse is probably equally difficult for the man and woman. Although the man is more likely to remarry, he often has been very dependent on his wife for personal attention and homemaking skills. He may be unable to fend well for himself and may regress quickly unless he is given help. The woman is usually able to manage household duties but has more difficulty taking on financial responsibility; often the older woman has been completely uninvolved in the business transactions of the family. She often has to learn quickly and painfully how to manage, sometimes suffering additional losses in the process. The elderly widow also suffers a more restricted social role; certain activities are less acceptable for the woman than for the man to do alone. Usually the survivor has to establish friendships with other widows or singles.

Widowhood is always an ego-shattering, lonely experience if the marital relationship was close, but today's middle-aged women may be able to cope better in widowhood with the business and legal aspects because many of them have had careers and experience in handling business, money, and property affairs. Further, the women's liberation movement is slowly affecting social roles of both men and women.

Remarriage

In the first marriage, the person has no other marriage experience with which to compare the spouse; in remarriage after widowhood the survivor may feel dissatisfaction when comparing the first and second mate. If the widowed person felt close to the first mate, guilt or uncertainty about loving another arises. Often the second marriage is rationalized by saying that it is different, that it is more mature, that it is for companionship, or that it is to share economic resources or live more reasonably. The widow(er) may idealize the first partner and marriage so that he cannot find a second mate who lives up to the first mate's image. In a successful and happy remarriage the recollections of the first spouse are favorable or neutral.[3]

Certain areas of potential difficulty exist for the couple when one partner in a remarriage is a widow(er). First is the idealization of the deceased mate, which causes an unrealistic comparison of the new spouse. Second, the first marriage was not terminated voluntarily, which implies that the second mate is second choice, which may cause anxiety for the new spouse. Third, the second spouse is moving into established relationships and may be treated like an intruder or compared to the first spouse by relatives and friends. Fourth, remarriage expands family relationships; another set of in-laws has to be adjusted to and former in-laws have to be appeased. The family of the deceased spouse may consider remarriage disrespectful to the person's memory. Finally, numerous problems exist when children are involved. The former in-laws may fear that their relationship to the offspring and grandchildren will be replaced by the new in-laws. The children must also adjust to a new stepparent while retaining memory of the first parent. The widow(er) must adjust to someone new in the counter-parent role, which is more difficult if the widow(er) combined parental roles before remarriage. The influence of the deceased parent may remain strong for the offspring, especially if the surviving parent reminds them of the deceased parent's expectations. What the surviving parent attributes to the deceased may be neither true nor appropriate, which causes conflict in the children, and possibly resentment in the new spouse.[3]

Remarriages are usually successful; the partners are usually older and have fewer romantic expectations. Older persons may have less exacting standards and be more understanding and patient than when they were younger. The contrast of loneliness without a spouse and companionship and security of marriage causes both partners to work harder at making the marriage harmonious.[3] Adjustment is easier if the age difference between the remarried spouses is not too great; values, education, and social background are similar; income is adequate; both are sexually active; family and friends show approval, and both are in good health initially.[3,18]

THE SINGLE SENIOR

A sizable number of people in later maturity never married or were divorced or widowed many years earlier, so that they perceive themselves as single especially if they had no children. The single senior is not necessarily lonely and unhappy in old age. The single person has learned how to develop interests and has become involved with other people and organizations in order to compensate for lack of family. Thus, the single person may be less lonely than if all of life was centered around job, home, family, and spouse. Usually the single person has worked in a career or profession throughout life. Foresight about financial needs in old age may have caused the person to invest in more than a pension or Social Security plan.[18]

Yet, more single seniors are women than men because of the imbalance in the number of each sex in the United States. Traditionally, the woman held low-paying jobs, perhaps not covered by either a pension or Social Security. Thus, the elderly single person may live in poverty because of the effects of inflation upon whatever savings were accumulated.

The problem for the single elderly person becomes more acute when health fails, since friends and kin may already be dead and no one can assist with care or business matters. The single person has probably been independent throughout life and will have difficulty giving up that independence. Some may move willingly to a residence for senior citizens in order to gain companionship and convenience. But the move to a nursing home may be seen as a declaration of dependency emotionally, physically, and economically, or as incompetence. Often the single senior struggles to remain in the same housing situation for as long as possible, but many suffer neglect and deprivation in the process. Some may eventually move to low-rent hotels or apartments which may be dirty or without hot water or cooking facilities. In every city a small percentage of the elderly live mostly in abandoned buildings or on the streets and carry their few possessions with them. They may feel very lonely, abused by society, and necessarily suspicious of others in the environment, and they may suffer great health problems as well.

NURSING PROCESS WITH THE FAMILY

Assessment, Nursing Diagnosis, and Family Care Goals

As you care for the elderly couple, you need to observe how they relate to each other as well as observe the individual's physical and emotional status. Each couple/family will be as unique as an individual person is. You may construct a family assessment tool by using some of the questions from the sociocultural and psychological tools in Chapter 2 or by utilizing other resources.

As you assess the family to determine how you can be of assistance, avoid assumptions or judgments. An interaction pattern that may appear to be an unhappy or destructive one on casual observation may not be. Usually the behavioral pattern is of long standing; each spouse knows what to expect from the other. Neither is likely to want to give up the familiar. Even when one partner tells you how frustrating certain habits of the mate are, do not assume that the senior has any intervention in mind other than your listening to the catharsis of tensions and validation of realistic ideas. Remember, every family has its squabbles.

One area of importance to assess is how the physical, cognitive, and emotional characteristics—normal or ill—of each member of the elderly family affect the entire family unit. Does the wife's deafness interfere with communication to the point that the husband never talks because he cannot shout loud enough for her to hear? Do they use nonverbal methods, or does the wife wonder why he is so distant and quiet? Does she think that something is wrong with him because he does not talk? Is she completely unaware of her hearing impairment?

Questions should be asked and observations should be made in relation to all major physical functions, social roles and activities, emotional responses and behaviors, and their effects on the family function. For example, since retirement the husband's main activity has been to sit in front of the television; he refuses to go with his wife for a walk around the block or shopping. He previously had been gregarious and enjoyed many hobbies. His wife feels concerned, angry, and rejected. After further assessment, your nursing diagnosis, patient-care goals, and intervention may be directed toward his depression following retirement and to helping his wife understand and cope with his behavior, express her feelings, and maintain healthy responses.

If the family's interaction is grossly disturbed, so that all or several members are functioning inadequately, assess the family together as a unit for a period of time before formulating your nursing diagnosis and care goals. Consider the many aspects discussed in previous chapters as you adapt assessment from one person to several people simultaneously, formulate nursing diagnoses and family-care goals, and plan care.

Based on your assessment, your *nursing diagnoses* may include:

1. *Open communication and harmonious family relationships.*
2. *Impaired family communication.*
3. *Impaired ability to cope with family crisis because of social stresses.*
4. *Disharmonious or destructive emotional reactions between family members.*
5. *Unresolved grief because of loss of spouse.*

Formulation of *goals* may include the following:

1. Family members will continue to be supportive.
2. Family members will relate more harmoniously to each other.
3. Family members will improve in ability to talk about personal feelings with each other.
4. Family members will work together to cope with their problems or social stresses or to secure help as necessary.
5. The widow(er) will resolve loss of spouse and establish another close relationship.

General Intervention

Your role is not to be a family therapist unless you have the proper education and competency. If you are working with a troubled elderly family, use the communication methods and information on helping relationships described in Chapter 3 as a basis for intervention. As you listen to family members, establish trust, and work with them over time, you will use and share information presented in any of the chapters of this text appropriate to their physical, emotional, cognitive, social, spiritual, and health status. This information will help the members be more understanding of themselves and other family members and will help them be better able to cope with changes that occur in the family. You may tell them about helpful community resources or general legal considerations so that they can determine whether or not an agency or organization should be contacted as a source of help or whether or not they need legal assistance. You may teach one family member how to care for and rehabilitate another or how to carry on a reality orientation program begun in the hospital. You may use principles of crisis intervention to help the family resolve a situation or a survivor work through grief.[25]

You will be promoting health and adaptability as you show acceptance, listen, teach, present alternatives, encourage self-help, or refer to a community agency. Now you will be working with more than one person; therefore, you must direct your attention to the whole unit while you remain open to each individual. You must divide your time between members competing for your attention so that no one is overlooked. At times you will need assistance from health care workers in other disciplines.

Intervention Related to Sexuality

You have an important role with the elderly person in relation to sexuality. First, you must work through your stereotyped attitudes and unlearn the myths. Then you can use the results of research to present information that can help the senior recognize the validity of his present sexual activity or overcome inhibitions. If you assume that sexual behavior is normal in late life, you will be more likely to include questions about sexuality in your assessment and nursing history. However, you need to ask the questions diplomatically; some elderly people consider sexuality a very private matter and will not answer unless they see a reason for your questions. Yet, your asking conveys that sexual behavior is normal. Your questioning is done to learn of the senior's need for information and to impart information *as needed* about how the medical, surgical, or psychiatric condition affects his sexual practices. It is essential to convey that your questions are not based on nosiness, jest, ridicule, or condemnation. Counseling with the senior and his partner can be done in a casual and indirect manner as well as in a more formal manner. The counseling may relate not only to information about physical changes or coital capacity, but also to how the condition or medication affects desire and capacity. Even more important may be discussions about the senior's feelings about self and partner and their relationship, about release of tension without a partner, or the joys and problems related to remarriage. You may also counsel the adult offspring to correct their misperceptions and to help them understand their parents' needs.

Sexual expression is highly individual. The couple may prefer kissing, hugging, touching, and lying next to each other instead of intercourse. However, you can share some practical information. Estrogen-progesterone creams or water-soluble jelly may alleviate vaginal discomfort for the woman; estrogen products are usually prescribed with care because of the carcinogenic possibilities. A vaginal pessary or surgery corrects a cystocele or prolapsed uterus. *Kegal exercises, alternately contracting and releasing the vaginal area,* strengthen perineal muscles. The person with a chronic or disabling illness may assume a more passive role in coitus. Timing coitus to the period of the day when biological rhythms are at a peak or the partners are least fatigued enhances enjoyment. Weight reduction may aid performance. More direct stimulation is also needed to produce erection.

The most important attitude that you can convey is the normality of sexual activity in late life; the commonest cause of sexual nonfunction in all ages is anxiety about performance. Premature cessation of sexual function may accelerate physiologic and psychologic aging. The enjoyment of intimacy is worth the time and emotional and physical investment. When intercourse is impaired, other sexual needs persist, including closeness, sensuality, and being valued as a person. Further, assume that more people in later maturity have sex than talk about it. Giving information can help the senior avoid being exploited by those who rely on personal insecurities to sell sex products.[11]

You also have a role in helping to change administrative attitudes and policies that segregate sexes in residences or nursing homes for seniors. Physicians and people in charge often lack information about sexuality and establish rules based on social stereotypes or their own personal problems about sexuality. Married couples in any residential setting for the elderly should stay living together. Imagine being married for 50 years and then being separated to live on different floors upon admission to a nursing home! The added crisis is inexcusable!

The elderly have a right to privacy and to establish relationships as they wish. They should not be demeaned by being treated like naughty children if interest is shown in the opposite sex—whether the person is married or unmarried. They know their own minds and do not need their morals policed by busybodies who regard sexual interests or activities as a sign of dementia.[11]

Residential or nursing homes that follow the sexual mores of the outside world have happier, less deteriorated residents who consume fewer tranquilizers.[11] It is to the advantage of the elderly as well as his caretakers to provide for an outlet for sexual drives. When overt libidinal expression is inhibited, the energy is likely to be channeled into aggressive drives so that the person becomes more irritable and harder to live with. Reactions of frustration and anger from the elderly are not uncommon; they are tolerated and justified by society. In addition, as sexual interests diminish, the person becomes increasingly preoccupied with his body functioning, especially the bowels and stomach. The gastrointestinal tract becomes libidinized. A regular physical exam, including rectal and vaginal exam, may be interpreted as a sexual attack. In fact, the health care workers as well as the aged person often divert attention to various body functions in order to handle apparent sexual feelings of the aged.[52]

Evaluation

The accuracy and thoroughness of your assessment, the effectiveness of your care planning, nursing approach, and general or specific intervention measures can be evaluated as you observe the family unit change. The family members may increase harmony, gain new coping skills, talk more freely with each other and their children, reach a higher level of health, correct some long-term problems, or become more involved in the community. Perhaps with your assistance the family will be utilizing services of one or two agencies in town instead of four or five, as sometimes happens when no one is coordinating care. You may see a change in the interaction pattern, or perhaps the members express a more positive self-concept and greater self-esteem. Has the family unit reestablished ties with other relatives? Have members resolved grief from death of another member?

Try to be objective as you look at yourself. Do you have sufficient emotional energy to be concerned for and involved with several needy people simultaneously? Can you be impartial? Can you avoid a show of favoritism to the same- or opposite-sexed family member or to any one member? Can you encourage others to be actively involved in their care? Can you persist and be creative in finding assistance when needs are present and community resources seem lacking? Do you feel a sense of reward from watching the change in a total unit, in several persons, over time? Can you work with another professional in intervention or step aside when you are no longer needed and let the other professional continue specialized intervention? Can you let the family solve its problems without your assistance when they are able?

REFERENCES

1. American Medical Association Committee on Human Sexuality, *Normal Sexual Development.* Washington, D.C.: American Medical Association, 1972.

2. BARFIELD, R. and J. MORGAN, "Trends in Satisfaction with Retirement," *The Gerontologist,* 18: No. 1 (1978), 19–23.

3. BELL, ROBERT, *Marriage and Family Interaction.* Homewood, Ill.: Dorsey Press, 1963.

4. BENEDEK, THERESE, "Parenthood During the Life Cycle," in *Parenthood: Its Psychology and Psychopathology,* eds. E. J. Anthony and T. Benedek. Boston: Little, Brown & Company, 1970, pp. 185–206.

5. BISCHOFF, LEDFORD, *Adult Psychology.* New York: Harper & Row, Publishers, Inc., 1969.

6. BOTWINICK, JACK, *Aging and Behavior.* New York: Springer Publishing Co., Inc., 1973.

7. BRODY, STANLEY, WALTER POULSHOCK, and CARLA MASCIOCCHI, "The Family Caring Unit: A Major Consideration in the Long-Term Support System," *The Gerontologist,* 18: No. 6 (1978), 556–61.

8. BURNSIDE, IRENE, "Listen to the Aged," *American Journal of Nursing,* 75: No. 10 (1975), 1800–1803.

9. "Change in Family Structure Important Trend for Future," *Geriatric Focus,* 9: No. 7 (1970), 3ff.

10. CICIRELLI, V., "Family Structure and Interaction: Sibling Effects on Socialization," in *Child Psychiatry: Treatment and Research,* eds. M. McMillan and H. Sergio. New York: Brunner/Mazel Publishers, 1977.

11. ———, "Relationships of Siblings to the Elderly Person's Feelings and Concerns," *Journal of Gerontology,* 32: No. 3 (1977), 317–22.

12. COMFORT, ALEX, *A Good Age.* New York: Crown Publishers, Inc., 1976.

13. COSTELLO, MARILYN, "Sex, Intimacy, and Aging," *American Journal of Nursing,* 75: No. 8 (1975), 1330–32.

14. CUMMINGS, ELAINE, and D. SCHNEIDER, "Sibling Solidarity: A Property of American Kinship," *American Anthropologist,* 63 (1961), 498–507.

15. DUVALL, EVELYN, *Family Development,* 4th ed. Philadelphia: J. B. Lippincott Company, 1971.

16. FISHER, SEYMOUR, and DAVID MENDELL, "The Communication of Neurotic Patterns over Two and Three Generations," in *A Modern Introduction to the Family,* eds. Norman Bell and Ezra Vogel. New York: The Free Press, 1960, pp. 616–22.

17. HAWKINSON, WM., "Wish, Expectancy, and Practice in the Interaction of Generations," in *Older People and Their Social World,* eds. Arnold Rose and Warren Peterson. Philadelphia: F. A. Davis Company, 1965, pp. 181–90.

18. HURLOCK, ELIZABETH, *Developmental Psychology,* 4th ed. New York: McGraw-Hill Book Company, 1975.

19. JOHNSON, ELIZABETH, "Good Relationships Between Older Mothers and Their Daughters: A Causal Model," *The Gerontologist,* 18: No. 3 (1978), 301–6.

20. LAVERTY, R., "Reactivation of Sibling Rivalry in Older People," *Social Work* 7: (1962), 23–30.

21. MANNEY, J. D., *Aging in American Society.* Ann Arbor, Mich.: Institute of Gerontology, 1975.

22. MASTERS, WILLIAM, and VIRGINIA JOHNSON, *Human Sexual Response.* Boston: Little, Brown & Company, 1966.

23. MORGAN, LESLIE, "A Re-Examination of Widowhood and Morale," *Journal of Gerontology,* 31: No. 6 (1976), 687–95.

24. MURRAY, RUTH, and JUDITH ZENTNER, *Nursing Assessment and Health Promotion Through the Life Span,* 2nd ed. Englewood Cliffs, N. J.: Prentice-Hall, Inc., 1979.

25. ———, *Nursing Concepts for Health Promotion,* 2nd ed. Englewood Cliffs, N.J.: Prentice-Hall, Inc., 1979.

26. NEWMAN, G., and C. NICHOLS, "Sexual Activities and Attitudes in Older Persons," in *Normal Aging,* ed. E. Palmore. Durham, N.C.: Duke University Press, 1970, pp. 277–81.

27. ———, "Sexual Activities and Attitudes in Older Persons," in *Human Life Cycle,* ed. Wm. Sze. New York: Jason Aronson, Inc., 1975, pp. 637–42.

28. PFEIFFER, ERIC, "Sexual Behavior in Old Age," in *Behavior and Adaptation in Later Life,* eds. Ewald Busse and Eric Pfeiffer. Boston: Little, Brown & Company, 1969, pp. 151–62.

29. ———, ADRIAAN VERWOERDT, and HSIOH-SHAN WANG, "The Natural History of Sexual Behavior in Aged Men and Women: Observations on 154 Community Volunteers," *Archives of General Psychiatry,* 19: No. 12 (1968), 753–58.

30. ———, "Sexual Behavior in Aged Men and Women," in *Normal Aging,* ed. E. Palmore. Durham, N.C.: Duke University Press, 1970, pp. 299–303.

31. PHILBLAD, C. TERENCE, and ROBERT HABERSTEIN, "Social Factors in Grandparent Orientation of High School Youth," in *Older People and Their Social World,* eds. Arnold Rose and Warren Peterson. Philadelphia: F. A. Davis Company, 1965, pp. 163–80.

32. ———, and ROBERT MCNAMARA, "Social Adjustment of Elderly People in Three Small Towns," in *Older People and Their Social World,* eds. Arnold Rose and Warren Peterson. Philadelphia: F. A. Davis Company, 1965, pp. 49–73.

33. "Polygamy Is Projected for American Elderly," *St. Louis Post-Dispatch,* February 17, 1974, Sec. F, p. 7.

34. RUBIN, I., *Sexual Life After Sixty.* New York: Basic Books, 1965.

35. ———, *Sexual Life in the Later Years.* New York: Sex Information and Education Council of the United States, Publication Office, 1970.

36. ———, "The Sexless Older Years: A Social Harmful Stereotype," in *Readings in Psychological Development Through Life,* eds. D. Charles and W. Looft. New York: Holt, Rinehart and Winston, 1973, pp. 367–79.

37. RUNER, M., *To the Good Long Life: What We Know About Growing Old.* New York: Universe Books, 1974.

38. SEELBACH, W., and W. SAUER, "Filial Responsibility, Expectations, and Morale Among Aged Parents," *The Gerontologist,* 17: No. 6 (1977), 492–99.

39. SHANAS, E., *et al., Old People in Three Industrial Societies.* New York: Atherton Press, 1968.

40. "Social Myth as Hypothesis: The Case of the Family Relations of Old People," *The Gerontologist,* 19: No. 1 (1979), 3–9.

41. SMITH, HAROLD, "Family Interaction Patterns of the Aged: A Review," in *Older People and Their Social World,* eds., Arnold Rose and Warren Peterson. Philadelphia: F. A. Davis Company, 1965, pp. 143–62.

42. STANFORD, DENNYSE, "All About Sex . . . After Middle Age," *American Journal of Nursing,* 77: No. 4 (1977), 608–10.

43. STINNETT, N., L. CARTER, and J. MONTGOMERY, "Older Persons' Perceptions of Their Marriage," *Journal of Marriage and Family,* 34: (1972), 665–70.

44. SUSSMAN, M., and L. BURCHIVAL, "Parental Aid to Married Children: Implications for Family Functioning," *Marriage and Family Living,* 24: (1962), 320–32.

45. TREAS, JUDITH, "Family Support Systems for the Aged," *The Gerontologist,* 17: No. 6 (1977), 486–91.

46. TROLL, L., "The Family of Later Life: A Decade Review," *Marriage and Family Living,* 33: (1971), 263–90.

47. VERWOERDT, ADRIAAN, *Clinical Geropsychiatry.* Baltimore: The Williams & Wilkins Company, 1976.

48. VIDEBICK, R., and ALAN KNOX, "Alternative Participatory Responses to Aging," in *Older People and Their Social World,* eds. Arnold Rose and Warren Peterson. Philadelphia: F. A. Davis Company, 1965, pp. 37–48.

49. WOLPE, JOSEPH, and ARNOLD LAZURUS, *Behavior Therapy Techniques.* London: Pergamon Press, 1966, pp. 105–106.

50. YEAWORTH, ROSALIE, and JOYCE FRIEDEMAN, "Sexuality in Later Life," *Nursing Clinics of North America,* 10: No. 3 (1975), 565–74.

51. YORK, J., and R. CALSYN, "Family Involvement in Nursing Homes," *The Gerontologist,* 17: No. 6 (1977), 500–505.

52. ZINBERG, NORMAN, and IRVING KAUFMAN, *Normal Psychology of the Aging Process.* New York: International Universities Press, Inc., 1963.

53. ZOLAR, M., "Human Sexuality: A Component of Total Patient Care," *Nursing Digest,* 3: No. 6 (1975), 40–43.

crisis in later maturity: loss and death

13

The person in late life has encountered daily stress and any number of crises for many years. Later maturity as a developmental crisis is described in Chapter 11. Some of the events that can be stressful or actually overwhelm the senior and become a crisis are described in Chapters 5 and 6: the impact of cultural attitudes upon the self, retirement, income reduction, relocation of living quarters, lack of transportation, excessive leisure time or inability to pursue leisure interests, and the problems of being a consumer in today's society. Any of the illnesses described in Units IV and V and the necessary adjustments to various health care or social agencies, described in Chapter 7, are also crises. All of these events involve loss, as does the ultimate crisis, death of loved ones, friends, pets, and self, which will be described later in this chapter.

THE CONCEPT OF CRISIS

Various changes in late life are perceived as *crises when the situation is a threat to the senior's self-esteem, cannot be handled with the usual coping mechanisms, and disrupts his life-style.* How soon and how completely the senior is overwhelmed by the event depends on his management of past stressors and crises, present personality and character structure, energy and health status, symbolism of the event, his support system, and economic status. What is a stressor for one senior may result in disequilibrium, a crisis, for another. What may be a minor crisis for a young person may be extremely difficult for the senior to handle, or vice versa. Various mechanisms to cope with stress are discussed in Chapter 11 and are initially used to confront a crisis until they are found to be ineffective.

Eventually the senior goes through a series of phases in the course of crisis: (1) shock and disbelief, when the stress level is very high; (2) defensive retreat, in which denial and the usual adaptive patterns are used but become ineffective; (3) gradual awareness of the real situation, accompanied by mourning, depression, bitterness, and suicidal thoughts; and (4) resolution, the acceptance of or adaptation to the event, which usually takes 6 weeks to 6 months or a year. The time needed to progress through these *normal* phases depends on the person and the crisis event. Further basic information about crises can be obtained from various sources.[26,29,64,69]

LOSS, GRIEF, AND MOURNING

Definitions

Crisis means that the self must change. Hence, it involves loss, grief, and mourning.

Loss refers to giving up a valued internal or external support that is required to meet basic needs, such as a person, thing, relationship, situation, status, role, ritual, health, or independence. The person feels deprived of something significant.[26]

Grief is a sequence of subjective emotional and physical states, including intense sorrow, caused by loss. Grief is the emotion involved in the work of mourning.[26]

Mourning is a broad range of physical and emotional reactions that follows a loss or accompanies an anticipated one. It is the process whereby the person seeks to disengage from an emotionally demanding relationship and reinvest in a new, satisfying one.[26]

Every change faced by the senior involves loss; something is given up even if something desirable is gained. Normally the senior has developed adequate coping abilities, but the cumulative effect of loss in late life may be devastating.

Anticipatory grief is the reaction to possible or inevitable loss; the person goes through some of the grief syndrome and mourning process prior to the loss. Premature mourning can exhaust emotional resources, so that when the loss, such as death, does occur, the survivor feels nothing and may act inappropriately to the occasion. However, anticipatory grief work can also help the senior prepare for the inevitable and may prevent him from being overwhelmed at the time of the actual loss. He considers ahead of time how he will cope when the valued object or person is gone; thus, he remains more flexible and coping is enhanced.[26]

Manifestations of the Phases of Crisis, Including Grief and Mourning

A review of the grief syndrome described by Lindeman and the stages of grief and mourning described by Engel helps us to understand what the senior experiences as he works through the various phases of crisis associated with loss.[26,29,42,58]

Shock and disbelief are the initial response when the senior becomes aware of loss. The grief syndrome is manifested initially by physical symptoms and altered sensorium which last from 20 minutes to several days. Symptoms include muscular weakness, tremors, tightness in the throat, choking, shortness of breath, sighing, hyperventilation, palpitations, pallor, chills, parasthesias, tightness in the chest or abdomen, anorexia, and fatigue. Altered sensorium includes feelings of disbelief or unreality, helplessness, threatened self-esteem, and a high level of anxiety or panic. The person cannot think or plan logically; judgment is impaired. He may strike at or be sarcastic with someone who is trying to help. He may act automatically but not perceive his inadequacy. He may wander aimlessly. The senior may act as if nothing happened, or he may be intensely preoccupied with the loss. He may ignore or focus on physical symptoms. Socially, he is unable to function appropriately, being either very withdrawn and docile or hyperactive and chaotic. The implications of the loss are not fully comprehended in spite of verbal acceptance of the loss. The senior needs help in meeting basic needs because of feelings of worthlessness and lack of energy, organization, and initiative in carrying out daily tasks. Initially, there may be no tears, but the impact of loss occurs sooner or later, and the deep anguish and despair are expressed by crying, either silently and covertly or loudly and uncontrollably, depending on cultural norms.

As the senior perceives for himself or is told what has happened, he copes with the discontinuity in his life and the threat to self through defensive retreat.

Defensive retreat may last for a few hours, days, or longer. Habitual behavior and previously successful ways of solving problems are tried, but tension and discomfort are not reduced. The senior withdraws or retreats into himself to preserve self-esteem and a sense of reality. He may deny, fantasize that the lost object or person is still present, or give unrealistic suggestions about how to manage the situation. He may express **emotional isolation**, *talking about the loss without showing any affect.* He may be apathetic, euphoric, overly calm, or disoriented. He may curl up in fetal position on the bed. He may continue with tasks that are unnecessary or unrelated to the loss, such as cleaning, and neglect necessary tasks. Resistance to ideas suggested by others and repeating the same ideas are common. Physical symptoms may be minimal, but behavioral disorganization seen during the shock stage may continue.

Denial is a *normal* mechanism for this period and acts to buffer against extreme anxiety and the overwhelming sense of helplessness. Denial gives the person time to "collect" himself and to begin to use more effective, realistic behaviors. The more sudden or unexpected the loss, the greater may be the denial and defensive retreat. But even if the loss, such as death of a loved one, was expected, some denial and defensive retreat are seen briefly. Perhaps the person continues with a task already started, says he cannot believe the event happened, or retreats to the privacy of a little used area of the home to be alone for a time.

Denial varies in degree and involves the use of three other mental mechanisms: (1) rationalization or excuses about what is happening or felt by the person, (2) displacement of dangerous, disquieting, uncomfortable information onto others, often in the form of demands or complaints, and (3) projection of personal feelings of inadequacy onto others, saying how inept or neglectful others are. Thus, the person maintains an intact sense of self during defensive retreat, regardless of his behavior.

Isolation of affect, denial, or excessive motor activity are temporary and necessary defenses, but they cannot maintain effective adjustment. Eventually the senior must confront the loss and continue grief and mourning. Few people can avoid this confrontation because the loss of the loved one is obvious and others around them continue to talk about the loss and change activity or routines accordingly.

Acknowledgment of reality begins slowly and may alternate at first with the behaviors of defensive retreat, but it is the result of the facts being perceived. The mourner feels empty, insecure, and alone as he becomes aware of the innumerable ways in which he was dependent on that which is lost for gratification, a feeling of well-being, effective functioning, and sense of self. Characteristics of the grief syndrome are apparent, for as the mourner slowly redefines the loss and attempts to do problem solving to overcome it, anxiety and tension again increase. Physical symptoms previously experienced may last for months, especially those of the cardiovascular, respiratory, and gastrointestinal systems. Symptoms such as cardiac arrhythmias, tachycardia, hypertension, tachypnea, dyspnea, dysphagia, anorexia, indigestion, diarrhea, or constipation may be present off and on during the mourning process, are a normal response, and are not imaginary. The person should consult a physician because he may need treatment.

In addition to the symptoms that are a normal part of grieving, the senior may develop symptoms similar to those suffered by the deceased loved one. This identification process maintains a tie with and appeases some of the guilt feelings for having earlier aggressive or angry feelings toward the deceased. How the symptoms are expressed depends on the senior's constitutional factors as well as on past learning about what symptoms are most likely to get attention or be defined as illness by self and others.

Reality may seem harsh; depression, agitation, apathy, self-hate, and low self-esteem are felt. The senior may state that he does not feel worthy of your help; yet, he may complain that you are neglecting him if you fail to do something important for him. Coping abilities and self-concept may disintegrate to some degree before the senior can constructively direct his energies. Thinking may at first be disorganized, but with your help, gradually he can begin to make appropriate plans. Certain unrealistic ideas or goals will be given up as unattainable.

The senior is preoccupied with the loss; he wishes to have a continuing experience. He may start to talk to the deceased many times a day or cook for two people instead of one. He may feel the presence of the deceased spouse in a ghostlike form. He may return to the site of his old job after retirement; look for an object taken by a burglar when he knows it won't be recovered; or visit the grave of the loved one repeatedly. He wants to talk about the loss, although others may not want to listen. He searches for evidence of failure on his part "to do right" or to prevent the loss, verbally accuses self or others of wrongdoing, and expresses ambivalence toward the lost object or person.

The greater the ambivalence felt, the greater the sense of guilt and shame experienced. In any love relationship the person will at times feel frustration, anger, or dislike. The senior often has lived with the loved person or has had the beloved object or position for a long time; therefore, many opportunities for ambivalence to creep in would have occurred. The grieving person may feel angry at the deceased for having left him, but he may also feel glad to still be alive. Guilt and anger feelings, a normal part of grieving, are frequently displaced onto others: doctor, nurse, employer, relative, friend, or God. If guilt is not resolved, self-blame for the loss and preoccupation with past, present, and future losses, as well as with personal death, will occur.

The senior may go to the funeral of a stranger or watch a movie and weep intensely. He is grieving for the lost person but also for his own inevitable death, especially if there is no one close to help the senior proceed through grief and mourning.

Talking about the loss, its meaning, and associated pleasant memories is one way of reinforcing reality as well as expiating guilt. The senior becomes assured that he did everything possible in the situation to prevent loss or undo earlier unkind acts toward the loved one. Reminiscing promotes *idealization,* so that only positive characteristics remain in the senior's memory about the lost object or person. Idealization follows the difficult and painful experience of guilt, fear, and regret for real or fantasized past hostile acts, neglect, lack of appreciation, or personal responsibility for the death or loss.

Identification follows idealization; the mourner consciously adopts some of the behavior, goals, or admired qualities of the deceased. If an object was lost, the person tries to obtain a replacement that is very similar. Lost roles, status, or activities are replaced with something similar whenever possible. A memorial may be established in an effort to shed guilt and as a tangible identification object. As identification is accomplished, preoccupation with the loss, ambivalence, guilt, and sadness decrease. Thoughts return to life and daily routines. The senior wants to be useful; he realizes that he has been a social burden and makes plans to resume former roles to the degree possible.

If strong guilt is present, the senior may identify with negative characteristics, including the last disease symptoms, of the deceased. This negative identity could later lead to psychopathology. Or the negative identity may be manifested by antisocial behaviors, self-neglect, or suicidal gestures.

Resolution of mourning may take a short time if anticipatory grieving was done, or it may take from 6 to 12 months. The mourning of an older person for spouse may take longer. Crisis resolution occurs when the person perceives the situation without hostility, guilt, or bitterness, when the painful loss can be integrated into self. The senior may wish that things had been different, but he accepts that they cannot. He will cope, slowly conquering the cluster of adjustments, apprehensions, and uncertainties that mark loss and deprivation crises. Slowly he reorganizes and redirects his energy to life. The person becomes interested first in other mourners, because it is easier to feel close to someone who has had a similar experience. Then the senior becomes reinterested in friends, relatives, and activities and will seek new relationships or activities if he is still active enough to do so. The senior who has loved ones who stand by him will get through the crisis better. Finally, the person remembers the lost object or person realistically—both the pleasures and disappointments—and feels less lonely and insecure than immediately after the loss.

Gradually the senior feels a new sense of worth; now he can see a reason to continue to live whereas earlier he may have wanted to die, especially if his loss was a loved one. He feels satisfied with his ability to have mastered the loss situation and to come through mourning with an intact identity and as mentally, emotionally, and socially competent. The person has added to his maturity and wisdom and has firmed his sense of ego integrity.

Few seniors resolve the crisis of loss by permanent repression and denial, chronic physical disability, or major personality disorganization, such as neurosis and psychosis. However, if the senior has suffered too many losses in too short a time, he endures an overload of negative thoughts and feelings. When grief cannot be handled, an outlet is found in physical symptoms or pathologic behavior. Thus, helping the senior resolve each crisis is paramount.

The mourning process, as it fits into the stages of crisis, will probably not proceed in a sharply delineated manner. One stage will merge with another. The person may be effective in one sphere of life but less so in another.

You can teach the senior about ways of coping with grief, which include to:

1. Recognize that the physical and emotional reactions are normal responses to loss and that loss and death are a part of life.
2. Develop new interests, acquaintances, and relationships.
3. Treasure memories but not to live only with memories.
4. Allow time to resolve the loss.
5. Use ceremonies and rituals to help resolve loss if they are meaningful and not excessive or inappropriate.
6. Try to face the full reality of what has happened.[42]

The ultimate goals of grief work and mourning are to remember without emotional pain; to reinvest emotional energy; and to know defeat, suffering, struggle, and loss and to find a way out of these depths, in turn enriching life and gaining a stronger sense of compassion.[65]

Influences on the Outcome of Mourning

How well the senior accomplishes mourning depends on his ability to cope with crisis, as previously discussed. Other factors must also be considered. The more dependent the senior was on the lost person or object, the more difficult the emancipation. The greater the ambivalence and guilt, the longer the mourning. If the loss was anticipated and prepared for, resolution will be smoother and often sooner. The more supportive people he has to help fill the void, enhance self-esteem, and create new roles or replace the loss, the more readily he can reestablish ties and move through mourning. Societal, religious, and cultural roles for the mourner can help; unfortunately, in the United States the mourner is expected to resume a cheery face and former activities soon after the funeral. The Orthodox Jewish religion probably has the most supportive prescribed ritual to assist the mourner over a period of time. Most people have to struggle by themselves. Society makes little provision for loss replacement or discharge of normal hostility and guilt.

Ineffective Resolution of Loss

The senior experiences grief more intensely because his emotional involvements are concentrated on fewer people, since he gradually loses contact with friends or relatives through geographical moves or death. Further, any loss of material possessions is very threatening, for often he has so few material goods or financial reserves and he has no way to make up the loss.

Morbidity and mortality are increased among the bereaved, especially if denial and isolation are used excessively and if the survivor cannot talk about his loss, anger, and grief.[59] The elderly survivor is likely to have a harder time working through grief and mourning, especially from death of spouse, because of a sense of hopelessness and lack of significant persons who can listen and promote reality. Adjustment to death of a loved one is related to conflicts that existed in the relationship and feelings of uncertainty about decisions made regarding the dying person.[22]

Medical office consultations for psychiatric symptoms and chronic somatic conditions, such as arthritis, increase for the first 6 months after loss of spouse.[70] Relatives of the deceased have a higher mortality rate within the first year of mourning, especially elderly widow(ers). Apparently the emotional stress of a loved one's death, compounded by deterioration of physical condition during care of the deceased, lowers body resistance to disease, affects organs through the sympathetic nervous system response, and affects the person's "will to live." The survivor suffers the "giving up—given up" complex, feeling helpless and hopeless, which also contributes to a higher suicide rate among elderly survivors. Symptoms such as insomnia, trembling, nightmares, general nervousness, cognitive impairment, and depression occur more frequently in mourners than in nonmourners. Other psychosomatic symptoms of headache, vomiting, indigestion, anorexia with weight loss, chest pain, frequent infection, and general aching also occur. The senior who is unable to express his feelings or seek help with his grief work will have more physical problems.[20,26,37,71]

The anniversary syndrome may also occur; here the survivor becomes ill a year after the loss, often to the day, and often with the same symptoms as the deceased suffered.[17,38,70]

Various other abnormal reactions occur when grief is not adequately resolved. Abnormal grief is manifested by prolonged, excessive sadness or extreme apathy; lack of initiative; excessive withdrawal from, anger at, or suspicions of others; or inappropriate euphoria or depression.[42] Extreme denial may cause the person to act as if the deceased was still alive. Everything in the house is kept as it was prior to the loved one's death; daily activities are planned to include the deceased, or business affairs previously handled by the deceased are neglected. Denial and repression may be prolonged, but a delayed mourning reaction often occurs later when another loss is experienced. Studies show increased incidence of affective disorders, especially reactive and neurotic depression, in the bereaved.[17,33,39,70,72] The more socially isolated the mourner, the more likely he will suffer an abnormal emotion reaction.[33] Suicide after recent death of a loved one or major object loss occurs all too frequently.

Maladaptation may include expressing hostility toward authority figures who were uninvolved in the death or acting out socially in a way to be apprehended by the police. The person may become overgenerous and give away money or possessions of value. Often such acts are a desperate attempt to gain attention and make contact with another. The person may also become compulsively busy or ritualistic, or indulge excessively in alcohol, food, or drugs as a crutch or an escape from feelings.

Unfortunately, all of these reactions interfere further with grief work and add to the senior's burden when he encounters future crises.

THE CRISIS OF DEATH

Sociocultural Perspectives in Attitudes Toward Death

In the Middle Ages, the person was very aware of natural signs or premonitions that he was dying and was active in doing the rituals that prepared for death. Loved ones quietly kept the vigil with him. Death was familiar and near; it evoked no great sorrow, awe, or fear. About the eighteenth century, death became romanticized, intertwined with love; concern about another's death became of greater concern than personal death. Gradually, death was viewed as a disruption; sorrow was openly and intensely expressed.[2]

In the twentieth century, death has become frightening, taboo, and unfamiliar. Care of the dying has been moved from the home to the hospital. Although death is frequently presented in the mass media and movies and many disasters are publicized, few people have direct contact with death. Mourning has been suppressed. The language of our culture avoids death with phrases like: "He passed on." "He grew weak." "He is sinking." "He is gone." Humor may be used to refer to dying, express fears of death, predict death, or convey doubts about staff competence.[2,25,48] Medical care technology further depersonalizes and denies death. The person is no longer in charge of his dying, even if he is aware of his status.

The senior has lived through some of this evolution. He may have helped care for sick and dying parents at home and is perplexed, perhaps angry, when he is sent to a nursing home or hospital instead of remaining part of the family unit.

Although considerable literature and mass media coverage is devoted to death and dying, people in the United States still seem uncomfortable with the topic of death. In spite of increased efforts at professional education about dying and death, care of the dying elderly population continues to be neglectful in many institutions.

Some cultures believe that life and death can be controlled by the person. Voodoo deaths or spontaneous deaths are well documented; the person is either a victim of the enemy or wills himself to death when he has broken a taboo and dies shortly thereafter. The medicine man is important in many cultures to organize the community's attitude toward the dying person; if support is withdrawn, the person gives up and soon dies. If the medicine man conveys that the person is curable, the community becomes supportive and the person survives. The situation for our elderly may not be too much different. Being hospitalized—cut off from the community—may hasten death, something Native Americans, Orientals, Chicanos, as well as the elderly have "known" as they were subjected to impersonal treatment.[62] However, since hospitals are at times necessary, efforts should be made to create a warm, supportive environment.

Among Alaskan Indians, the elderly person has a strong premonition about when he will die, can accurately predict his death, and gathers his loved ones for final rituals and farewells prior to his death. The person exhibits a willfullness and choice about the timing of his death.[79]

Premonitions of death are apparently present in many seniors, although they may be reluctant to say so. Sometimes the senior will predict when he will die. The elderly may exert more control over their longevity and time of death than is commonly realized. Often it appears that the person will not give up life until he has said farewell to a certain loved one. Longevity is increased when the senior has the following characteristics: useful, satisfying role; positive view of life; assertive attitude; competent physical and mental functioning; willingness to adjust and change; lifetime habits of moderation; interest in others and the future; and creative and expansive thinking.[11,40,47,68] Interestingly, one study found that the patient who survived longer than predicted was angry about his illness, fearful of death, and determined to live instead of being resigned to death.[12]

Attitudes about death differ in various cultures. Mortality occurs at an earlier age in lower socioeconomic groups and among racial minorities in the United States. Therefore, death may be perceived differently by different groups. In a study comparing Black, Mexican, and White Americans, fears of death were related more to age than to racial group. Middle-agers expressed more fear than the elderly, and women were more expressive of their feelings than men but they did not think about death as frequently. Whites were less preoccupied with death than the other minorities. Elderly Mexican Americans expressed the least fear of death; young Mexican Americans expressed the most.[5]

In the United States, death is expected to come to the elderly, to people no longer in the work force. Thus, society overall is not concerned with death unless it occurs to the young or occurs violently. Even if death comes early, little disruption occurs because work is organized so that major institutions are relatively independent of the persons who carry out work roles within them.[9]

Fear of death is apparently more common in the young than in the elderly, although the elderly express fear of death when a crisis in the social environment is disrupting prior life-style and acceptance. For example, those who are moved to or live in a nursing home are more fearful than the elderly who live in the community and are not experiencing relocation.[28,56] The elderly suffering psychiatric illness may also express fear of death.[83] The elderly in a stable situation feel more peace and equanimity about death.

Meaning of Death

Results of many studies done on feelings about, attitudes toward, or meaning of death are contradictory. Some researchers report death anxiety; others report death acceptance. Actually, the results could vary within the same sample, depending on when the subjects were surveyed. Most studies have not clearly differentiated reactions to eventual death for the combined variables of sex, age, race, socioeconomic status, cultural background, past occupation, religious or philosophical outlook, self-image, sense of hope, health status, and past and current life situations. Dying and death affect the *total* person—mind, body, feelings, spirit, and life experience. All of the self—what was, is, and will be—is involved.

To the elderly, death may have many meanings: a friend who brings an end to pain and suffering; a teacher of transcendental truths uncomprehended during life; an adventure into the unknown; reunion with loved ones; a reward for life well-lived. Death may mean the great destroyer; the cessation of life with eternal nothingness; punishment and separation; or a way to force others to give more affection than they were willing to give in the past.[27,43] Suicide may be seen as a way to gain control over dying, join loved ones, or end an apparently hopeless situation.

The mature person recognizes that dying and death are phases of living and life. The decreased energy level, religious beliefs, and loss of most significant people also facilitate a philosophical attitude toward closure. Children and grandchildren also bestow on the older person the reminder of continuity of life and tangible evidence of his own ongoing contribution to mankind.[43] The person who has left issues unsettled, dreams unfulfilled, hopes shattered, or let meaningful things pass him by is reluctant to die. Knowing of one's mortality allows the person to start preparing early for the last developmental stage—to live life instead of passing through it.

Preparation for Death

Most people admit to thinking about death at some time; usually these thoughts are triggered by external events, such as an accident or near-accident, a serious illness, or death of someone close. Yet, some older people do not make plans for death, as if planning will hasten death. In one study, about 70 percent had life insurance, 25 percent had made a will and some kind of funeral or burial arrangements, and about 50 percent had talked to close relatives about death.[43,74] The elderly are more concerned about the dying process—the pain, being a burden, loss of bodily and mental functions, dependence on others, rejection, isolation and separation from loved ones, inability to take care of personal business, and loss of social roles.[8,38,43,74,75,78] The more relationships that are important to the senior, the more ties he has to undo, the greater his grief.[61] Although most seniors do not wish to have life prolonged by a machine, there are times that such treatment is warranted. The life-support machine gives the senior, if he is aware, and the family extra time to prepare for inevitable death.[34]

Some seniors feel that the best way to avoid prolonged suffering and dying and to prepare for death is to express their desires to family and physician through the Living Will, discussed in Chapter 8.

Death can be planned for in different ways. For example, a prominent Protestant theologian and his wife put all of their affairs in order, said their farewells, wrote a short note to their children and grandchildren explaining the reason for their behavior, and then committed suicide. They wrote that their health was quickly failing; they required almost constant medical treatment. Soon they would be too dependent to live with dignity. They did not want to take up space in a world in which there were too many mouths and too little food. They felt that it was a misuse of medical science to keep them technically alive. They had thought carefully, believed that they had the right to decide when to die, and felt that the decision was not turning against life as the highest value. They clearly were not acting out of depression, despair, pain, or mental incompetence. They knew they risked condemnation from others; their religion does not sanction suicide. But they felt that their action was logical and will become more usual and acceptable in the future.[21]

Charles Lindbergh also planned his death, but in a different way. When he knew he was terminally ill, he selected his grave site on the tropical island of Maui and made all of the necessary legal and business arrangements. Eight days before his death, when the doctors told him he had little time left to live, he flew from New York City to Maui, and with his family, physician, and two nurses spent the last days looking at the place he loved and reminiscing. He received the necessary care but no measures to prolong life. His death was like his life: simple, well-planned, considerate, and humble.

Most seniors do not have the means to fulfill their dreams as Lindbergh did. Many are taken to the institution; endure a variety of tests, drugs, and procedures; and have minimal control over their living or dying. Preoccupation with symptoms, pain, and the rigors of treatment preclude quiet contemplation, meaningful life review, or serene acceptance of death. Medical staff may resist death more vigorously than the patient and often do not credit the senior with enough maturity to understand or accept the finality of his condition.

Although a few seniors maintain denial, most desire to plan for their demise. You may be of assistance to them as they validate ideas or need specific tasks to be done. Or you may assist them by letting the doctor know that the senior can accept his condition and wants to settle his affairs. The doctor can state the diagnosis and prognosis honestly without conferring hopelessness. If the person insists that he does not want to be told anything, his request should be honored. Often that person is aware of the truth but wants to avoid talking about it.

Preparation for death is more important for some elderly than for others. Some need to make provisions for their heirs and finalize business and legal affairs.

If the senior or his family have delayed or seem uncertain how to prepare for death, you may want to suggest two books that cover the many details very well. They are *Concerning Death: A Practical Guide for the Living,* edited by Earl Grollman,[35] and *How to Prepare for Death: A Practical Guide,* by Yaffe Drazmin.[23] Grief and mourning can be facilitated by careful preplanning.

To others a spiritual preparation for death is of greater importance. Premonition of impending death may give opportunity for long-deferred self-examination and for gaining new meaning in life and death. A reconciliation of conflicts in one's religious faith can be accomplished. Personal hurts can be amended and tenuous relationships can be strengthened. Each day becomes precious and meaningful.[38]

People die as they live. Those who found meaning in life are unafraid of its end. If success in life has been measured by material standards, death may be approached with bitterness and anguish. Religious faith is not necessarily a factor; an agnostic or atheist may accept death with as much tranquillity as a religious believer.[38]

Certain developmental changes occur in the last year prior to death that are unrelated to age and illness and appear to be predictors of death. Characteristics of approaching death which are often monitored by the ill elderly include poorer performance of various tasks, lower energy level, slower reaction time, decline in cognitive functioning, shortened memory, decreased planning ability, reduced emotional complexity, decreased ability to cope with stress, a more negative self-image, less capacity for learning, less assertiveness and flexibility, and increased introspection. The senior expresses more anxiety, hopelessness, and less expectation about the future. He feels that his body is no longer functioning as well as it did, even before overt signs and specific symptoms appear. The person may say, "I feel like I'm slipping. I don't think I'll be here next year at this time." The senior may show increased interest in his social and material environment; it is a disservice to isolate the senior at this time.[43,54,56,73]

Awareness of Dying

People today are better educated generally by the mass media about the manifestations of the main killers, cardiovascular disease and cancer, than they were in the past. Further, the legal aspects of informed consent are rigorous; many procedures cannot be performed without giving the senior an honest explanation. Thus, most people are likely to know intellectually even if they do not emotionally accept their terminal illness. Yet, some doctors and families persist in wanting to keep the diagnosis and prognosis from the patient; they feel that the elderly person will be unable to accept the news. Glaser and Strauss describe the stages the terminally ill patient may experience.[32]

Closed awareness exists when the person has not been informed and has not discovered the severity of his condition, when he may not be knowledgeable about signs of terminal illness, or when he may be in denial. Maintaining closed awareness is easier in the hospital than at home. You are in the middle in such a situation, for it is hard to communicate openly when a secret must be kept. Family members are robbed of an opportunity to be honest, share their grief with their loved one, or plan together for the future. The patient has no opportunity to work through his doubts or fears or make plans for his loved ones. No one ever learns of the resilience or maturity of the senior, who may be more able to cope than anyone realizes. Keeping the patient uninformed is a travesty of care in most cases. However silent the patient might be about his condition, he may have a premonition about his status. The senior watches his caretakers and family closely for clues about himself. He may come to the conclusion that he is very sick and dying as he overhears snatches of conversation or sees teary eyes.[32]

Isolation is experienced when family and friends relate differently to the patient after they learn that he is dying from a terminal illness. They no longer share with the patient; conversation becomes superficial, stilted, and lacks spontaneity as they try to keep the patient from learning his diagnosis.[32]

Suspicious awareness exists when the person believes that he is dying but says nothing to confirm his idea. Usually his deteriorating physical status, others' silence or their brusque answers to his queries, a move closer to the nurses' station, extra attention from relatives rarely seen, or shorter and fewer contacts with the health team confirm his suspicions. The senior now knows that he is dying but realizes that others around him do not know that he knows.[32]

Mutual pretense occurs when the patient, family, and staff enter into a game. All realize that the patient knows that he is dying, and all continue to pretend otherwise. The patient can plan to a degree for his remaining life, but he cannot share this with anyone close. No one can be honest; no one benefits from the patient's awareness. Even the patient cannot do anticipatory grieving or legal and business planning very well.[32]

Open awareness exists when the patient and family are fully aware of the terminal condition and can talk about it, although the nearness of death may not be established. Now the senior can reminisce and conduct life review. He can give treasured possessions to the right person. He can be in control of his situation to a greater degree as he finishes important work and makes plans for and says farewells to the family. He learns how family members perceive their coming loss—his death. He can share his feelings of loss as he anticipates death. The anguish is not reduced, but it can be faced together. The staff will also be more involved with the senior as he talks to them about his death. The staff may find it more difficult to care for the person who knows. Staff cannot hide behind clichés; they have to involve something of the self and see him as a person, not a thing. The senior or family may request extra privileges, which the rule-bound nurse finds difficult to fulfill. The senior may wish to die at home, and the family and staff may work together to set up a care routine at home and secure the help of a home health agency. The senior who knows may quietly but firmly convey that he wishes to be granted privacy and dignity, both of which may be difficult to obtain.[32]

Sequence of Reactions to Approaching Death

Kubler-Ross describes a series of reactions that the person and family go through as death approaches.

Denial and isolation are the initial and natural reactions when the senior becomes ill or learns of a terminal diagnosis: "It can't be true; I don't believe it." Denial is more likely in the person who is told too quickly or abruptly by the doctor. Denial may be manifested by minimizing or refusing to acknowledge his illness or diagnosis or that the diagnosis may change his life-style. The senior may make overly optimistic comments about his condition, refuse to follow doctor's orders, seek other doctors' opinions, try home remedies, or delay hospital admission. He may even begin unrealistic plans or projects that will be finished in the distant future. However, denial does not usually last when pain, fatigue, or weakness interfere with activity.[52]

As the senior becomes aware of his condition, either because of the extent of his symptoms or because he is repeatedly told by others, he may use emotional isolation as a defense. He talks about his illness and even the possibility of death intellectually, without emotion, as if the topic referred to someone else. Isolation enables the person to carry on practical activities of life that are necessary in order to prepare for hospitalization, prolonged illness, or eventual death.[52]

Anger is the second reaction and occurs with acknowledgment of the reality of the prognosis. As denial and isolation decrease, anger, envy, and resentment of the living are felt. In America direct expressions of anger are unacceptable; therefore, angry feelings are likely to be displaced onto the doctor, nurse, family, or even the food. Angry demands are a way to avoid neglect and to feel a sense of control over an uncontrollable event. The person feels that he does not deserve to be sick, let alone to die. He is bitter and hard to manage as he thinks, "Why me?"[52]

Bargaining, the third reaction, may be difficult to observe unless you care for the person regularly. The person tries to enter into some kind of agreement which may postpone death. He tries to be on his best behavior in order to be granted the special wish of longer life, preferably without pain. Bargaining may be life-promoting; the person is hopeful and he expresses faith in God and the future. The body's physical defenses may be enhanced by mental or emotional processes yet unknown, and a bargaining attitude may account for the not-so-uncommon cases in which the person has a prolonged, unexpected remission from a disease process. The senior who has a negative self-concept or is alone and isolated lacks a sense of hope and is not likely to bargain; he feels that he has nothing to bargain for.[52]

During this stage the senior vacillates between doubt and hope. Sources of doubt include new and unexpected symptoms, any additional or unexpected stressor related to treatment, financial concerns, or the temporary absence of the doctor or primary nurse. When the source of stress is relieved, so is the doubt. Hope arises when the senior hears the medical personnel say, "We can help you"; by being encouraged to be actively involved in treatment and aligned with doctors and nurses against the disease, by being treated at a leading medical center, and from overtly hopeful attitudes of the staff.[14]

Depression, the fourth reaction to his condition, occurs when the person gets weaker, needs more treatment or pain medication, and worries about realistic mounting medical costs and even obtaining necessities. Role reversal and related problems add to the depression.[52] The senior feels shame about his condition and guilt about being a burden on others. He may feel that he is being punished for past misdeeds. He thinks about past losses and his present condition, and he worries about his future. He feels hopeless. He fears being left alone, losing independence, being disfigured, having pain, or losing his sanity.[18] The mild depression that is frequently present in the senior is worsened as he anticipates death. The senior may lie with his face to the wall; answer slowly, if at all; speak with an expressionless voice; talk in short and muddled sentences; or stare out of the window.[86]

Preparatory depression differs from reactive depression. He now grieves for the impending losses he will endure. Not only will his loved ones lose him, but he is losing all significant relationships and things. He will not be able to do some of the things that he wanted to do. The person begins to separate himself from the world. He reviews the meaning of his life, tries to share his insights with others, and gradually withdraws from involvement in life around him. If others continue to convey that they expect him to want to live, he may feel misunderstood and more depression, turmoil, and grief. This depression is difficult for family and staff, but he needs to be allowed to emotionally prepare for death.[52]

The quality of life that is being left behind is defined differently by each person, depending on (1) present life situation, (2) family relationships, (3) work abilities, (4) religious beliefs, (5) past ability to cope with stresses, (6) amount of pain, (7) feelings of despair and dependency, (8) amount of body mutilation and related feelings of repugnance from the disease or its treatment, (9) feelings of loneliness and isolation, (10) loss of freedom imposed by the medical care system, (11) ability to carry on regular routines, and (12) sense of mastery over oneself and one's life.[50]

Acceptance, the final reaction, comes when the person has time to prepare for death, is given help in working through previous reactions, and remains alert long enough to emotionally resolve his death. Now he is resigned to his fate. He is withdrawn, neither angry, depressed, envious, nor resentful of the living.[52] The person is emotionally and socially bankrupt; nothing of obvious importance can be added to his life and nothing can be regained. Apathy rather than serenity or acceptance may be seen. The senior cannot or will not further accommodate to the indignities of his disease. He has lived his life and does not wish to relive it. He says his good-byes.[52] Only the senior who continues to add to the spiritual dimensions of his life will be able to use this time for growth emotionally and spiritually, and feel that he is adding something to himself as he is dying. He may feel an inner peace and self-possession. He lives with the certainty of a limited future.[50] He plans his inheritance and assigns his treasures to others.[43]

Unless he is unconscious, the senior who is dying continues to feel, think, and respond to the present and limited future, to his illness, and to those around him. He does not just lie passively and await death. He may strive to control and manipulate others; to prevent their leaving him or withdrawing their love. He may pretend to avoid feelings of loss and despair.[75]

The person may not proceed to acceptance. He may refuse to admit he is dying and show anger, bitterness, and self-pity. He may retaliate against others, demand, cling, or berate himself.[75]

The person who is dying often fluctuates between avoidance, denial, anxious hope, rejection, uneasy resignation, and calm acceptance. The person tries to maintain ties with those closest to him while he wrestles with impending extinction.[28]

The Kubler-Ross framework is analogous to Fink's framework of four phases of crisis and can be used for assessing dying persons, but *all dying seniors do not move through those stages or in the designated sequence. Do not expect the person to be in any specific stage.* Do not behave in a way that conveys to him that he must act a certain way at a certain time. *Be open to his unique behavior.*

Another author describes a slightly different sequence of stages that the dying person encounters. His framework was used with 400 terminally ill patients and their families.[66]

The Stage of Shock and Denial versus Panic begins with news of the fatal diagnosis, causing the person to feel stunned and overwhelmed. Denial, the defense that helps the person pretend that he did not hear what he cannot emotionally accept, follows shortly. Without the use of denial, the person is in panic and resorts to impulsive, uncontrolled, and unrealistic behavior. Fright and terror may make the situation seem so overwhelming that the senior sees no way out except to escape reality through suicide or psychosis.[66]

The Stage of Emotion: Catharsis versus Depression occurs next. Shock is shortlived, and reality is perceived slowly as denial lifts. The flood of emotion that follows either finds expression in catharsis or is turned inward against the self in depression. Anger at having a fatal disease may also be directed at a loved one, the doctor, or God. Frequently the senior is not allowed to experience catharsis; external controls may be applied by family, friends, medical staff, and even the minister. Most professional workers will try to keep the patient happy, pleasant, and cooperative and will not encourage catharsis. The person may also have strong internal controls against expressing negative feelings; he may feel that it is wrong or unchristian to express anger. When anger is turned inward, the realistic guilt and shame achieve neurotic proportions, and depression results.[66]

The Stage of Negotiation: Bargaining versus Selling Out is the third stage. The guilt, shame, and depression often result in a selling out instead of attempting to live to the fullest. The badness and unworthiness that the person feels convince him that he is getting what he deserves. Or his depressive withdrawal causes him to feel so alienated from others that he feels it is no use living. Hopefully the senior moves into bargaining; he will do his share and cooperate if the medical team will do its best. The patient feels hope that there is yet a way out.[66]

The Stage of Cognition: Realistic Hope versus Despair is the fourth stage. Negotiation does not last long. The progress of illness and treatment procedures remind the patient of reality. The senior increasingly realizes his situation and faces the meaning of it. If he is left alone without support, awareness of dying simply confirms that there is no meaning and no hope. Bitterness, gloom, despair, and depression result. He may be helped to experience realistic hope by discovering some sense of meaning and purpose through personal fulfillment. Since medical personnel tend to associate hope with getting well, they may have difficulty offering hope. However, hope can relate to the present concerns of the person regarding comfort and to the concern of being alone at the time of death. The availability of a caring person can give a sense of hope.[66]

Now the senior tries to work through the questions of "Why me?" "Why now?" "What is the meaning of life?" "What is in the future?" "Is there an afterlife?"[66]

The person who is in despair is rarely helped unless he can go back and relive earlier stages of his terminal illness and emotional struggle constructively. The person can be helped to find a relevant life perspective through which he can reassess his life pilgrimage past, present, and future and can come to a new awareness of himself and his destiny.[66]

The Stage of Commitment: Acceptance versus Resignation is the fifth stage. It is difficult to distinguish between when realistic hope becomes acceptance and when despair turns to resignation. The shift is experienced as movement from the intellectual response to emotional response. Acceptance is affirmed in the confidence and assurance that meaning will be experienced. Acceptance means emotionally realizing that death is the natural fulfillment of life and the completion of its meaning and purpose. Resignation is the emotional confirmation of deep despair, of the feeling of a meaningless end to existence. You can become the one who helps the senior to experience internalized trust in the goodness of life, its meaning and purpose, and the ultimate fulfillment in death. You can help the patient resolve remaining bitterness, grief, and previous hurts that interfere with developing faith and to develop a congruence between what he believes about life and death.[66]

The Stage of Completion: Fulfillment versus Forlornness is the last stage. As death becomes an inevitable reality, the senior ends the pilgrimage of life with either a sense of forlornness, withdrawal, depression, and being forsaken or abandoned or with a sense of fulfillment. If the patient was not helped through these various stages, then indeed his resulting forlornness might be the result of our abandonment.[66]

Reactions of the Family to the Dying Relative

The senior's family may go through the stages previously described, either at the same pace, more quickly, or more slowly. Various conflicts may arise in the family.

If the senior was in a pivotal position as leader in the family or if he was the main scapegoat for their problems, the balance of the family system is threatened. Change in role behavior affects work, leisure, interactions, and self-gratification now and in the future. If one family member is dying, some other family members may have to give up their sick role behavior. Dependency needs are threatened because the emotional or financial support given by the dying person to the family is no longer available. The family may identify with the patient. Or they may resent having to directly care for him and the many emotional, physical, financial, and family stresses related to his illness. The patient's immobility, care needs, and his personality characteristics may evoke hostility and aggressive behavior. If the senior was hard to live with, the family may be eager for him to die, feel a sense of triumph about his helplessness, or even be abusive verbally or physically. If the senior does not cooperate, fails to adhere to treatment, was accustomed to and continues to demand indulgence, or constantly complains about neglect or unfulfilled ambitions, his family may refuse to care for him at home or visit him in the institution. Or aggressive reactions may be redirected into the mechanism of reaction formation in which the family shows excessive concern for the senior since aggressive reactions may cause guilt. As family members care for the senior, they may show emotional isolation; the lack of emotional expression helps them do necessary tasks for the senior.

While the patient may prefer to die at home, the family may not be willing or able to handle this. Hospitalization may be a function of family needs. The extended family may provide a wider network of support and may be willing to help, but the nuclear family may perceive them as unsupportive. Often the members of the nuclear family feel very alone because they feel that they have little community support.[60]

To Maintain Life or to Hasten Death

The "right to die with dignity" is currently a frequently heard phrase. To some people it means a conscious control or decision about ending life peacefully; to others it means murder. The issue is not simple. The following discussion will attempt to present pertinent questions and a variety of ideas on the subject.

Chapter 8 defines euthanasia and discusses the right to die from a strictly legal framework. Opponents to the person's right to choose when and how he wishes to die use both religious and secular arguments. The commandment, "Thou shalt not kill," refers to any act of euthanasia except voluntary and direct, that is, when the person commits suicide. Secular objections are based on concerns about the danger of abuse and difficulty in obtaining consent, the risk of incorrect diagnosis, and the possibility of new medical discoveries or spontaneous recovery by the patient. The *wedge argument* is also used; the argument is that the door will be opened for various undesirable practices, such as active involuntary euthanasia, socially condoned murder, or genocide as practiced by the Nazis. Further, use of drugs negates the need for mercy killing since pain can be controlled. Not all chronically ill or dying patients have severe pain. Many resources are available to help those in need.[4,24]

Think about your responsibility of routinely using life-prolonging or heroic measures and the difference between life-preserving and life-prolonging treatments, as defined in Chapter 8. For example, a 75-year-old woman is resuscitated after a myocardial infarction and continues to live a full life. A 75-year-old severe diabetic is resuscitated after cardiac arrest preoperatively to an above-knee amputation. A 75-year-old patient with inoperable cancer of the colon is resuscitated. Which of these three people received life-preserving or life-prolonging treatment? How far can you go to honor the Living Will signed by the senior? What is meant by "incapacitated"? When would the person consider himself incapacitated? Is incapacity defined as a vegetative state, inability to walk, inability to speak, or disfigurement by surgery?

To arrive at your own answer, you will want to review the definitions and legal implications. You may want to study a variety of references: theological, ethical, psychological, and sociological. Whether you like it or not, you will not be able to escape the issue. As you assume more independence in practice, you will have to make decisions about life-preserving services. You will be accountable for the decision. The answer will not be easy and it will not be an answer for all time.

The senior may talk freely about death, say that he wants to die because he feels that he is a burden or wants to be released from suffering, or say that he does not fear death and is looking forward to eternal life. Yet, he may dread the thought of personal extinction and the loss of life's pleasures and he may fear the unknown future.[28]

Thus, when the older person says that he wants to be allowed to die, his wish may be a temporary one because of pain or stress. He does not necessarily mean permanent extinction. Those who talk of active or passive euthanasia in response to the person's wishes to die need to listen to the covert message, to the nonverbal or subtle clues that indicate otherwise. Perhaps the best way to assess his wish to live is to hear the statements about enjoyment of life that come after pain control and anxiety release, such as, "It's good to be alive," or "I'm feeling much better."

As a health professional, you must look at personal attitudes and values about life and death and you must be committed to helping the terminally ill person live as comfortably and with as much meaning as possible until he dies. Some authors feel that the elderly and the chronically and terminally ill are taking space, food, oxygen, and money that could be used for technological advances to help those who are well or at least curable. It would be easy to assume that we are helping the chronically or terminally ill and the dying person by ending their misery—putting them to sleep, with their consent, of course. (They would not dare to refuse their consent with social attitudes and pressures threatening them.) Each of us must work vigorously to prevent such an ethic from taking hold. Do so by clearly knowing inside yourself that every person is valuable, including the dying person. Suffering can be comforted, although a vegetative state need not be artificially prolonged. The patient can refuse treatment. Know clearly that unless you work to humanize care of the chronically or terminally ill person, you can predict what you will receive when you are in that situation yourself. For selfish reasons, if not for altruistic reasons, it is essential to assert your values, knowledge, and skills on the side of those most vulnerable and least able to speak for themselves. A look into yourself, an increased awareness about your values and attitudes, is the first step in the right direction.

Yet, the modern methods of resuscitation that are used when lives can be saved are out of place when disease or accident has nearly ended the senior's life, especially if resuscitation renews his suffering and he is prepared for and desirous of death. The dying ought to be allowed to depart in peace, and after death, the body should not be immediately disturbed. Disturbance of the dead body may have no effect on the deceased, but it robs bereaved bystanders of their peace and consolation.[85]

NURSING DIAGNOSES AND FORMULATION OF PATIENT CARE GOALS

Nursing Diagnoses

Although dying is related to a medical diagnosis, the elderly person may also demonstrate behaviors that indicate any one of a number of *nursing diagnoses.* Based on your assessments, your nursing diagnosis may be: (1) *pain,* (2) *self-despair,* (3) *unresolved previous crises,* (4) *lack of awareness of diagnosis,* (5) *denial,* (6) *negative self-concept, feeling worthless or a burden,* (7) *inadequate emotional response for the situation,* (8) *grief and mourning,* (9) *concern about family integrity,* (10) *alterations in faith or sense of hopelessness,* (11) *impaired ability to communicate, or* (12) *immobility.* Any of the nursing diagnoses described in Units IV and V are also applicable. If you are working with the family, some of the above diagnoses could also apply to members of the family unit.

Formulating Patient Care Goals

Your care plan and long- and short-term goals must always be individualized for the patient and family unit. Because the dying person can have a number of conditions needing care, any of the following *patient care goals* may guide your intervention:

1. Pain is controlled to maintain comfort and to prevent interference with daily living to the degree possible.
2. Reminiscence and life review are done to gain a sense of ego integrity or resolve past crises.
3. Information about condition and prognosis is obtained to the extent that it is desired or needed.
4. A sense of self-acceptance and having lived a meaningful life is demonstrated verbally or through behavior.
5. Adaptation to approaching death and the current life situation is demonstrated verbally, emotionally, or behaviorally.
6. A sense of hope, trust, and faith is maintained or strengthened.

7. Verbal or nonverbal communication skills are maintained to the extent possible or strengthened.
8. Communication is maintained or strengthened with family members.

Any of the care goals given in Units IV and V are also applicable. Formulate goals pertinent to your individual patient.

ASSESSMENT

Self-Assessment

Being aware of and coping with your personal feelings about death are difficult, but it is essential in order to care for the dying person and his family members.

You may find yourself going through the same crisis stages as the senior while you work closely with him. Or "professional" behavior, which may be a combination of denial and emotional isolation, may be your way of keeping a distance between patient and self, of coping with frustration, ambivalence, helplessness, or guilt, or the secret wish that the patient would die.

What are your feelings and attitudes about death? You will continue to rework your feelings and attitudes as you continue to care for dying persons.

You are a product of your culture. If you are 20, your perception of any loss, the crises of illness and death, the necessary care, and worth of the dying old person may be different from that of the 50-year-old nurse. Religious, educational, and family experiences also affect your ability to cope with all kinds of crises, including death.

You may identify with the dying person either unconsciously or consciously. You may see yourself in the dying person. The more believable the identification, the more difficulty you may have in giving care, since you are reminded of personal mortality. Or you may be reminded of a family member or friend as you care for the dying patient, and react to him as you would to a family member or friend. Such a reaction or me-you pattern will not be helpful for the patient who may sense that you are distressed and avoid asking for necessary care. If the senior is badly disfigured or in great pain, you may want to avoid rather than face his condition. You may enter his room brusquely, remain only the minimum amount of time, show your repulsion nonverbally, or unnecessarily delay answering the call-bell.

You will encounter frustrations as you work with the person in crisis or care for the dying person. Solutions may be difficult to find; since pain may be constant and difficult to relieve, you may feel incompetent. You may find it difficult to talk with the senior or listen to his concerns. You may resent his demands or lack of conforming to the patient role. You may be repulsed by his appearance, smell, or behavior. The family may make what seems to be unreasonable demands or accusations about neglect. Thus, in spite of good intentions, moral and religious convictions, and educational programs, you may avoid the senior and his family, who may then be left to face the crisis of loss and death alone.

As you repeatedly rework feelings about crisis, dying, and death and become more comfortable with distressing reactions from others, you will be able to serve more spontaneously and openly in situations previously avoided. You will be able to admit, without guilt, that you have certain limitations and cannot care for every senior—dying or otherwise. You will be able to admit the unrealistic fears of contributing to the person's death and work through your sense of inadequacy in the face of death. You will be able to utilize and support other team members, yet do as much as possible for the patient/family without showing shock, repugnance, or disapproval.

All of these reactions are normal. Face them, and then seek help from other professional colleagues (nurses, chaplains, counselors) to admit, talk about, and diminish such feelings and behavior. Or you may realize that you prefer working in an age specialty other than with the elderly. To come to grips with yourself takes courage, but it is essential for your personal as well as professional growth.

Think of death as the last developmental stage and as a fulfillment. Think of the dying person as a teacher. The meaning of death can serve as an important organizing principle in conducting your life. You will also realize how very important you are to the dying person.

As you care for elderly dying patients and their families, you will need to repeatedly study your attitudes and feelings about aging and life extinction. You will not arrive at any final answer, for as you continue to grow, to deepen your insights about life, you will continue to rework the meaning of life and death. Listen to the dying person and read a variety of literature to help you to rework your feelings and ideas. You will not work through your feelings once and for all. Each dying patient whom you care for is a unique person and will arouse feelings in you specific to his situation.

Assessment of Patient and Family

Use information about crisis, loss, and death to help you determine the feelings and needs of the dying elderly person and his family. Portions of the psychological assessment tool in Chapter 2 will also be helpful in assessing the person in crisis. Determine the senior's feelings and anxiety level, the extent of his loss or change, how he usually copes with problems and has tried to cope with this problem, his overall adaptive abilities, and his support system. Often the senior in crisis is bereft of a support system; his loss may have been the one person upon whom he depended. Determine the phase of crisis he is in.

If he is terminally ill, assess his stage of awareness and reaction to the diagnosis. Consider the wholeness of both patient and family members—the physical, emotional, cognitive, social, and spiritual needs and strengths. Learn what the patient and family know about the senior's condition and what they have been told by the doctor and others.

Listen to the topics of conversation the senior discusses to determine his feelings and needs. Determine what is important to him in care and conversation; observe for daily rituals. Learn about his special preferences. Be perceptive to the patient's and family's feelings, their fears of loneliness and abandonment, their response to suffering, or the presence of pathological depression.

Because the dying patient may have any of the conditions described in Units IV and V and may have aspects of normality discussed in Chapters 9, 10, 11, and 12, use the information presented in those chapters to help you assess specific needs and care problems.

The Dying Process

The dying person has four developmental tasks: (1) to manage reactions to symptoms of the terminal state and pathophysiology, (2) to prepare for impending separation from loved ones, (3) to react to the prospect of going into an unknown state, and (4) to adjust his perception of how he lived in relation to how he wanted to live.[7]

Most dying persons know that death is near and will say so to those able to listen. Often discomfort and suffering are great earlier in the illness and in the early stages of dying. But dying is often relatively easy right at the last, regardless of how great the earlier suffering. A brief interval of peace comes before death, and the senior may die smiling. Apparently most people do not suffer pain or agony at the end, as many persons who have remained conscious to the end testify to the persons sitting with them.[85]

Physical changes during the last hours before death include mottled skin and cyanotic lips and nailbeds from hypoxia; a thready, weak, or absent pulse; hypotension, and either a subnormal or elevated temperature. Shortness of breath and Cheyne-Stokes respirations, which occur when death is imminent, occasionally cause a patient to become panic-stricken, but most deaths are a quiet "slipping away" with only a few seconds of struggle or restlessness at the time of death.[81]

The mental condition of the senior near death varies from deep coma to full alertness. The patient may appear comatose when he is really able to be aroused. Occasionally just before death the person recovers consciousness and is able to speak a few sentences. Regardless of state of consciousness, he is able to hear. Usually in the process of dying, consciousness is gradually lost, as is the person's ability to communicate his thoughts. But the person may be able to signify assent or dissent by slight movements of the head, hand, or eyes. Only the acute observer notices that often the mind is active until the end, although the person appears stuporous.[85]

As the person nears death, he may have visions and talk to loved ones, either living but absent or deceased. Such visions and premonitions occur even in people who are not religiously inclined or who do not believe in an afterlife. Whatever may be the explanation of such visions, they are apparently comforting to the dying, for these visions are evidence of the reality and nearness of those who have gone before.[85] Do not regard this phenomenon as the hallucination of a sick mind.

INTERVENTION

To care for the dying patient, you may use any of the interventions described in other chapters, depending on his physical, emotional, cognitive, and spiritual status and on his social situation. Specific care measures may have to be adapted, depending on whether care is given in the person's home, hospital, or nursing home.

Major components of nursing care of terminally ill persons include the following: (1) giving thorough physical care, (2) maintaining a dignified self-image, (3) giving emotional support, (4) preserving a rewarding relationship, (5) carrying out prescribed treatments, (6) teaching and counseling, (7) coordinating the health team so that the comfort and dignity of patient and family are maintained, (8) referring to or using community services, and (9) facilitating a peaceful death.[10,83] The following discussion will cover guidelines that are useful for the dying senior and his family.

Principles of Crisis Intervention

General principles of crisis intervention are based on effective communication techniques and guidelines for a relationship described in Chapter 3. Since the person in crisis is at a turning point and is ripe for help, a little help at the right time does considerable good. The distress felt by the senior motivates him to change, to adjust behavior. In crisis work, help the person talk about his feelings and the related event. Focus on the present event. Catharsis lowers tension, clarifies the problem, promotes comprehension of reality and consequences of the situation, and mobilizes energy for constructive action. Have the senior repeat his story as often as he feels a need to. Ask related questions to encourage him to tell about the event in the sequence of its happening, if possible, in order to clarify what happened and what he has done about it. Help the senior confront the crisis in manageable doses. Accept the person's denial, but help him to gradually recognize reality by careful questioning. Help him dispel fantasies and find facts. Avoid false reassurance, but recognize his strengths and encourage him appropriately. Do not encourage him to blame others for what has happened, but help him not to focus on self-blame either. Instead, encourage the senior to discuss possible solutions and show faith in his ability to manage the crises. Your warmth, patience, and support will enable the senior to work through the loss rather than be emotionally crippled by it.

Intervention with the Family

You may work with other health team members to assist the family to care for the terminally ill senior. Many patients prefer to die at home, and if the family is willing and able to assume that care, help from various community and home health care agencies, other relatives, and neighbors should be sought. Equipment can be obtained from a medical supply house or pharmacy. Families often have considerable resources, coping abilities, and motivation which should be supported by the institutional staff. The family and patient can be taught to do the essential care at home. The community nurse can act as an advocate and support for the patient and family.[49]

While the senior may be cared for at home in the initial stages of the terminal illness, most people die in an institution. Your compassionate, gentle, but thorough physical care to the senior helps the family feel more comfortable. Good grooming, hygiene measures, and an orderly environment are the external signs of emotional care, along with prompt pain relief and allowing the patient to be as independent as possible.[31,36] The family perceives your attitude to and interest in the patient.

The family is important for the patient's sense of identity and emotional health; avoid being rigid about visiting hours. The family may help with feeding, grooming, fluffing the pillow, wiping the brow, holding the arm with the intravenous tubing in it, or other nontechnical aspects of care as a way to show their love or compensate for frustration, helplessness, or guilt. Often family members can get the patient to eat when no one else can, because they go slowly, they talk during the meal, or they may bring in favorite foods. Sometimes what the family says to or does with the senior seems strange and nontherapeutic to the staff, but it may be a comforting family pattern to the patient. Do not interfere unless the family is doing something unsafe or is annoying the patient. Sometimes you need to help the family regulate their visits so that they do not interfere with care or tire the senior.

Explore with the family some ways to talk with and support the patient, such as not to whisper in his presence but instead to talk to him as if he can hear, even though he is comatose. He may be able to understand them. Hearing is the last sense to be lost, but you and the family may need to speak close to his ear and distinctly in order for him to hear as death nears.

Recognize when family members are fatigued or anxious. Relieve them from care duties at that point and encourage them to rest and meet their needs. A lounge where they can rest and yet be near the patient is helpful. Out-of-town visitors may need special consideration or help in finding meals and lodging.

Show acceptance of and help family members understand the mourning process and express their grief. In some cultures the dying person is comforted by the family's expression of grief directly to him. For other families, privacy is sought for grieving; provide privacy if necessary, give support, and help them understand what they are going through. Help the family understand the member who is not overtly grieving. Defenses are useful and normal. Grief may come later.

Keep the family informed of daily progress. Prepare family members for sudden changes in the senior's condition or appearance so that they will be less shocked or overwhelmed when they walk into the senior's room.

The crisis of the senior's death may result in other life crises for the family. Living routines and arrangements may be difficult to change. Role reversal and assuming extra responsibilities, fatigue from caring for a loved one for a long time, working with other family members without the guidance or support of the senior, change in responsibilities and leisure activities, or meeting financial obligations can seem overwhelming. Failure of relatives and friends to help or their insistence upon helping or giving unneeded advice are equally burdensome. You can help by being a listener, exploring with them how to cope with new demands, or encouraging them to seek help from other persons or agencies. Your listening and acceptance of their feelings and statements may be enough to help the family mobilize their strengths to work together and cope with remaining problems.[36]

During the time when the senior is disengaging himself from them and the world, be prepared to explain the process to the family and to give extra support. Help the family remain in touch with the dying senior through short visits, touch, and caring silence. If the senior has always been head of the family, help family members to direct their views, questions, or concerns to someone else. Help them realize that the senior has found his peace and cannot hold on to former relationships if he accepts the inevitability of death or if he is physically and mentally near death.

News of impending or actual death is best conveyed to the family unit instead of to a lone individual in order to allow the people involved to give each other mutual support. The message must always be given in a private area so that they may express grief appropriate to them. Stay with them as long as necessary. Sometimes the senior has only one other close person who survives him—sibling, spouse, child, niece, or friend. Have someone (yourself, a unit secretary, aide, volunteer, or chaplain) remain with that person for as long as necessary.

You may also have to give considerable help with decision making, make initial plans with the mortician, or even arrange for transportation of the family members to the home of a neighbor or friend. Even when death is expected, the aging or lone family member may feel overwhelmed, be confused, or be unable to think logically when the death actually occurs. The most beneficial aid that can be given to the bereaved is help with immediate plans. Advise that major decisions on life-style of the survivor be delayed for about a month after death of the family member to allow for a more realistic solution.[20]

Sometimes the elderly person has no surviving family members or friends, or if he has, they do not come to visit. You may become the family surrogate to the senior, doing the little extras for him that the family would ordinarily do. Your relationship may be the only meaningful thing remaining to him. Or you may be able to engage a volunteer or someone else to do extra tasks for the senior. You may have to assume extra responsibility at the time of the senior's death with funeral arrangements and business/legal concerns, unless the senior has appointed a person/agency to carry out arrangements.[20]

Follow-up care with the family should be an integral part of service, but it is usually lacking. Follow-up visits to the bereaved family would enable you to observe their coping abilities, enhance catharsis, and promote mourning and return to normal routines. An unresolved grief reaction could be prevented, especially in the elderly spouse of the deceased. Even a condolence call by the professional involved in the senior's care before death expresses concern and makes the mourner feel that he is not alone, and it can contribute to effective grief work through attentive listening.[30] Explore with the family about how they will manage. Encourage them to participate in religious or family ceremonies or rituals. A later follow-up telephone call or home visit gradually terminates the relationship and gives support during their grief. Also, such a visit could also help evaluate the effectiveness of your previous care to patient and family.

Intervention with the Dying Person

You have major responsibility for the dying senior's care even if you do not do all of the care. You have the opportunity for a close relationship to the senior. Try to see him as the person, not the disease. The positive transference discussed in Chapters 3 and 4 can be an asset and give meaning to the senior's life. Use insights about the meaning of death and the dying process to help the senior work through his grief and to understand and accept his condition. Recognize the value of a caring attitude and of compassionate service with your hands during intervention. Protect the vulnerable senior from some of the distress or concerns felt by loved ones. Help him maintain the role that is important to him. Help the patient bring his life to a satisfactory close, to be as comfortable as possible, to truly live until he dies.

Physical care of the dying person includes providing for pain relief, nutrition, hygiene, rest, position, elimination, and other basic needs. Meticulous physical care provides emotional and physical rest. Pace your care slowly enough and at intervals in order to lessen fatigue. Many comfort measures that are essential for effective care are described in Unit IV and other basic nursing texts.

Control of pain in the terminally ill patient is essential. Medication should be given before pain becomes too severe. Concern about addiction is unwarranted. Promote comfort through the time-honored nursing measures of positioning, a backrub, creating a quiet environment, and letting the senior decide what will work best to alleviate his pain and promote his comfort. Your close relationship also soothes his physical pain as well as his anxiety and depression, especially when analgesics have lost their effect. Letting the patient know that he is a valued person instead of a helpless case gives him strength to endure the pain.

Mouth care is often neglected, but it is as essential as skin and hair care, and it is often more challenging. As total bodily deterioration progresses, the mouth increasingly becomes the most convenient, and later the only, mode of communication as hands lose coordination and the person loses the will and strength for writing. The mouth remains the last area for gratification and satisfaction with which he is able to indulge himself or can be indulged, such as through desired foods, talking to loved ones, and requesting desired satisfactions.[53]

The mouth can be a significant source of discomfort or pain in people dying from oral cancer, cancer of other body parts, or chronic diseases. The mouth often becomes dry and sore. Moniliasis or other infections, taste disturbances, halitosis, drooling, and disturbances of chewing, swallowing, and speech are often present. Further, the drugs that the patient receives may also cause side effects or toxicity symptoms in the mouth. Inability to eat or talk is perceived as deprivation, a hopeless prognosis, and loss of relationships. Emotional reactions of others to the condition of the senior's mouth are a source of embarrassment and shame.

The mouth should be allowed to remain a prized body area. It should be as comfortable, usable, and attractive as possible to the patient and others. The lips, oral cavity, and teeth should be kept in as optimum a condition as possible. The dentist is an important member of the health team to include in the care of the chronically or terminally ill patient.[53]

Maintaining nutrition and hydration is also a challenge, since dysphagia, anorexia, nausea, and vomiting are symptoms common to most terminal illnesses. The diet should be modified as necessary for as long as possible. If the senior desires a meal of bread, butter, jelly, and beer and can retain it, let him have it. Do not be overly concerned about the Basic Four in the terminally ill person. Do not deprive him of the joy of eating something he really wants, even if the combination sounds strange to you. Gastric tube feedings and intravenous fluids are given as the person's condition deteriorates, and the special care measures for each of these procedures (described in medical-surgical nursing texts) should be followed.

Maintaining elimination is often a problem. The patient often alternately has constipation, impaction, and diarrhea. Bulk foods, fluids, stool softeners, and enemas, or an antidiarrheal medication should be given as indicated. Urinary retention or oliguria may be present, especially if the person is dehydrated.

***Palliative care**, measures to reduce discomfort,* is a major intervention, since the terminally ill senior may present a variety of symptoms, depending on the physical disease process. A variety of medications are frequently given. Observe for side effects. Carry out nursing measures as indicated for the specific drug.

As the person nears death, physical care takes an increasing amount of time. The process of dying is progressive, from the lower limbs upward, rather than a simultaneous failure of vital functions. Sphincters relax; the person is incontinent of stool and mucus. Unless a catheter is in place, urinary incontinence occurs. Continuous and thorough skin cleansing and bed linen changes are essential.

Peristalsis gradually ceases; food and fluids are not tolerated. Dysphagia may cause aspiration. Thus, medication should be given intravenously if possible, or intramuscularly.

The jaws drop and the mouth hangs open; the tongue becomes edematous and the mouth condition deteriorates. Offer sips of water, if tolerated. Or provide a small amount of moisture by placing ice chips wrapped in gauze between the gums and cheek, or place a water-soaked gauze between the lips for the person to suck on. A *light* layer of Vaseline on the lips and tongue will prevent cracking; avoid an excessive amount to prevent aspiration. If there is drooling of saliva, place a gauze wick between the cheek and gums and extend it between the lips to afford relief from choking. Turning the person on his side also prevents aspiration.

Diaphoresis often occurs. The person may feel hot inside although his skin feels cold to the touch. Keeping the skin dry and using a light cover and fan or air conditioner help to keep the person more comfortable.

The body should be maintained in normal alignment as much as possible. Near the end of life extra pillows under the head, arms, and legs often add to comfort. Place the person in whatever position he desires, although he may be too restless to maintain any position for very long.

Many terminally ill patients die in a tangle of plastic bags or glass jars; tubes in the vein, mouth, nostrils, and bladder; monitor wires; and often bars and pulleys. The person may feel like a machine, especially if staff members focus on the objects surrounding him instead of on him. Family members can scarcely reach him to comfort him because of all the equipment. Technology can make dying an undignified ordeal for patient and family. You should do everything possible to minimize the machine. Instead, you should focus on the dignity and uniqueness of the patient and on helping the family stay in touch with him.

Although physical care is essential and time-consuming, do not focus exclusively on physical symptoms or physical care measures. Physical complaints may be a cover for anxiety, depression, or other feelings, and they may indicate a desire to talk about feelings.

Psychological care includes showing interest, acceptance, and concern; promoting a sense of trust, self-esteem, positive self-concept, and realistic body image; providing for privacy, sensory stimulation, and independence; and encouraging participation in decision making.

Communication with the terminally ill senior is recognized as an essential nursing intervention, but it is frequently neglected. Health workers seem afraid to talk, especially about death. Actually, the patient is not as interested in your answers as he is in your listening ear.

What can you talk about with the terminally ill senior? *Let him take the lead in conversation.* Ask about his family; talk about the pictures or floral arrangements at his bedside; refer to his past work, interests, hobbies, or special talents. Talk about whatever will help you better know and appreciate him as a person. Talk about the things that affect him now. No topic should be avoided that the person is willing to talk about. Nonverbal communication (a shake or squeeze of the hand, a hug, a tear, silence, acts of thoughtfulness) is as important as verbalizing our concerns. Touch is a way to learn more about another—his feelings, his dependency, or his aversion to touch.[18]

If the patient introduces the subject of dying, it means that he wants to talk about it and hopes that you will listen. He is more likely to confide in some people than in others, depending on how he feels about the person and the person's apparent ability to listen without uttering pseudo-reassuring clichés. Often he will test the listener first with some obtuse statement; the patient often does not come right out with what is on his mind.[18]

If he needs to talk, he will give some kind of signal. Ambiguities, ambivalences, trailing sentences, discrepancy between verbal and nonverbal communication are cues to a listening ear. If signals are picked up gently, he may talk. When he gives such signals and then does not talk, it may mean that the listener failed to pick up on cues or else responded too strongly.

Respond to questions as simply, honestly, and positively as possible. Avoid false reassurance. Invite the patient to talk about himself and his feelings through open-ended questions that are related to his initial remarks and/or concerns. If he talks about death, listen. You are not expected to have any answers or to expound your philosophy or beliefs. You are not likely to say anything wrong if you answer with a feeling of concern and interest. Focus your attention on the patient instead of on yourself. Your listening will convey that the patient has meaning to you; in turn, he will feel a sense of esteem and hope and that his life has had meaning. If he cannot talk about his feelings, help him reduce tension and depression through other means, for example, crying, physical activity, or sublimative activities, such as in occupational therapy.

Spend sufficient time with the senior to preserve his self-esteem and convey that you care and are available. You do not necessarily have to spend 30 or 60 minutes. Ten minutes of time focused completely on the senior and his concerns may actually be better. The senior will feel less fatigued physically after your interaction. But your frequent, short visits emphasize your availability and concern and that he and his approaching death are important. And you permit him the opportunity to say as little or as much as he can for that time. You permit privacy. Intense feelings cannot always come forth all at once. However, when the senior has much to say all at once, be prepared to spend more time in one sitting. Often you can combine helpful listening while you are giving physical care. Planned, attentive listening helps the senior clarify feelings and usually reduces his demands or manipulative, angry behavior.[86]

If you realistically cannot stay with the patient more than 10 minutes because of the needs of other patients, you may do one of several things. Be honest; tell him why you cannot stay. Offer to return later; tell him that you want to hear what he has to say if he can wait. Offer to call another team member to whom he also feels close. Offer to bring a tape recorder, so that you may later listen and respond. The more verbal person or someone who is interested in machines may not feel intimidated by talking into a machine and may appreciate your interest in having his thoughts and feelings saved. He may find the catharsis on tape and the relistening to be very therapeutic for himself. Sometimes saying things aloud is enough to release tension, promote problem solving, encourage decision making, or foster self-acceptance. If you are very important to the senior, he may choose to wait until you can return.

You may also help the senior feel that his reminiscing, words of counsel, or life review are important enough to save, not only for your response, but also for loved ones to keep. What better way for grandchildren or greatgrandchildren to remember the grandparent's voice and listen to his wisdom when they are old enough to understand. The senior who fears what his future may hold, who is concerned about what will happen to certain family members, who wants a memory of him to remain, or who does not believe in immortality may feel reassured by having the opportunity to say what is important and by knowing that if some members of the family did not really understand the first time, they can hear it again. Some elderly people may prefer writing or art work as the medium instead of the tape recorder.

If you observe the patient in the various phases of approaching death described earlier, you may wonder how to respond. The following are possible responses that you can use.

If the senior *denies* his condition, at first listen and accept his denial as necessary for him. Help him to feel secure with you. You may then gradually encourage him to face reality, but do not probe or repeatedly talk about his condition.

If he is *angry*, listen to him talk about when he became ill, who was involved, and details about the present situation. Blame for his feelings, defense of the medical team or treatment, return arguments, or statements about how well off he is should be avoided. Remain open and calm; repeatedly listen to the same story.[18] Suggestions on how to help a senior resolve his anger are made in Chapter 22.

If he is *bargaining,* let him talk about the good deeds he will do if he is allowed to live. Do not contradict his plans; instead, promote a sense of hope. Help him achieve desired goals if possible; help him modify goals if necessary.

The *depressed* person can be helped by staying with him through tears, listening to his sorrow, sitting with him in silence and avoiding cheery phrases.[18] The depression accompanying terminal illness can be reduced by helping the senior realize that family members and professional staff feel more useful and at ease when they can help take care of him. People measure their worth on their ability to help others, especially in a love relationship. To be the constant recipient of care, attention, and kindness, as happens to the patient, is intolerable for some people. But if the helping efforts of family, friends, and staff can be interpreted as an expression of love to the patient, as the patient helping them to be useful, then hopefully the patient feels less useless and dependent. Review with him the many times he has been helpful to others; he now deserves to be helped. To be lovingly cared for can be comforting. To be taken care of routinely as an obligation can be demeaning.[50]

The dying patient who is in *suspicious awareness, mutual pretense, or open awareness* presents a special challenge. Often the person appears very cooperative, cheerful, friendly, and well-adjusted. You would think that if patient, family, and nurse were all aware of the terminal illness, open communication would be easy. That is not necessarily true. The patient with these behaviors may be so gentle, well-educated, or soft-spoken that he remains very much in control of the conversation. No one would dare mention anything that would distress him. He may, because of personality characteristics, be liked very much, but you may be unable to bring yourself to spend much time with him. You may talk on a superficial level to avoid showing feelings of sadness. You may engage in physical care primarily to make up for lack of communication. You may rationalize that the family, who appear to be devoted to the patient, are adequately meeting the patient's emotional needs. Recognize personal feelings and behavior and consider the amount of energy it may be costing the patient to retain constant composure, to be a "good patient," and to protect himself from the nurse's avoidance.[52]

The senior may have worked through his grief and have no need to talk. Primary concerns may be comfort, easing pain, little pleasures the day may bring, making final arrangements in business, setting old wrongs right, and bidding farewells. Perhaps such behavior merely represents a deeper level of denial. How far acceptance can go is relative. Maybe it is best to have a cover for deep denial. How far can a person go toward accepting his own nonbeing? If some degree of repose is achieved, it is unlikely that the patient will say much about dying, or if he does, it will be to one or two people to whom he feels closest or most comfortable.[72]

When the patient becomes comatose, talk to him as if he can understand. Tell him what you are doing, that you are interested in his well-being, that his family loves him (if they seem to). Do not talk over him to others in the room as if he did not exist.

Inform the senior as fully as possible about his care routine and the expectations of the institution. Convey that you want his suggestions about how to carry out procedures or treatment measures so that he is most comfortable.

Encourage him to be active in making decisions about his care as long as he is able. However, he needs honest information and your flexibility and willingness in order to enter into his care planning and be a member of the health team. Giving information, teaching, or counseling do not mean that you tell him everything you know or everything that is known about his condition or prognosis. Lengthy explanations of pathophysiology are inappropriate and usually not understood. You cannot predict when he will die. What he needs is basic information clearly presented so that he can decide what is best for him to do: to begin or refuse a new therapy; to omit routine measures such as a bath; to take more of the prescribed analgesic; to use nursing measures such as positioning and backrub instead of medication to relieve discomfort; to sleep without sedation if he can; to eat something contraindicated on his diet. Avoid too strict a routine; then the senior will be willing to state preferences, give suggestions, and enter into decision making. If he senses that you can change your plans to meet his needs, he will be more willing to follow your schedule when there is no choice. And then he suffers neither loss of self-esteem nor sense of integrity. The senior should be assisted in maintaining roles of spouse, parent, or whatever, if possible and as long as he desires, so that he can be commended for his role behavior as a person. He needs to be told that he is doing well in the personal sense. He can take pride in performing cooperatively with his own treatment and care. A comment such as the following should be directed to patient (and family) to encourage and support them: "You are coping well in a difficult situation. I admire your strength in dealing with a hard problem."[50]

Spiritual care of the patient includes any of the interventions discussed in Chapter 14. Assist in meeting the person's spiritual needs if you feel comfortable. If you do not, contact the clergy. If the patient indicates no desire for such care, avoid proselyting. It is important for the religious professional not to discuss his own religious convictions or insights with the dying person unless the dying person wants to hear them. Instead, let the dying person share his religious history and convictions. Listen carefully, even if what the person says is contradictory to your own beliefs. The task of the professional *is not* to convert the dying person to his religion or to any religion. If the person says that he is an atheist, the above statements also apply. Undoubtedly, his contact with religion in the past made him an atheist or agnostic. Find out how this came about if he is willing to tell you, and respect his convictions.[18]

Social needs must be considered until the patient wishes to be left alone or is comatose. Welcome his visitors; keep visiting hours flexible whenever possible. Help him get dressed and groomed appropriately to receive visitors, leave his room, or meet other patients.

Monitor the environment surrounding the dying patient. Avoid a factory-like atmosphere. Surroundings should be attractive, orderly, clean, cheerful, and well-lit to offset the failing vision instead of dark and depressing. Exclude extraneous noise. If possible, provide familiar, comforting objects around him, for example, pictures, flowers, and personal clothing. Soothing music may be enjoyed. The patient may want to visit his home; this may be arranged if the family is willing, the patient's condition warrants it, and modifications in care can be made. Often the senior can accept life's closure after he has had a chance to say farewell not only to important people but also to treasured objects and his home.

Provide continuity of care. Exchange information with the whole medical team, including patient and family, in order to maintain consistency in carrying out procedures or care routines and to reduce feelings of uncertainty and neglect.

Encourage communication between the patient and health team. Encourage the patient to ask his own questions and state his needs and problems, but if he cannot, be his advocate. Realize that the senior may choose to talk with team members other than yourself about his feelings or that he may choose not to talk at all. Time, place, and identity of the person limit open expression.

Privacy must be respected, but you can offer help and availability to the patient. The feelings of the patient can be recognized verbally and generally, so that the patient can choose how much of himself to reveal and how much help to respond to. Intervals of silence are necessary to give the patient time to sort out his thoughts and feelings.[86]

Personalized care is a goal for the dying patient and means that he has (1) continuity of contact with at least one person who is interested in him as a human being, (2) opportunity for active involvement in living and in his care to the extent he is able, (3) confidence and trust in those who are providing his care, and (4) benefit of administrative priorities, policies, and practices that motivate staff members to give individualized care.

EVALUATION

Continually consider whether or not your care is holistic, appropriate, and effective for the dying patient and his family. Look at your own feelings and your resulting behavior. Distinguish between your fears of death generally, of another's dying, and of personal expectations.

Look at the overall care given to the patient. Is he kept sedated so that staff can avoid having to handle personal feelings as well as the feelings of the patient and family? What is the effect of the institution on the dying person and his family?

Psychological care is often more difficult to give and evaluate than physical care for several reasons: (1) lack of one primary caretaker for the patient, (2) lack of any system of reward for the nurse who spends time listening to and talking with the patient and family, (3) lack of perceived authority to provide the emotional care deemed necessary or to secure someone who can, and

(4) lack of accountability for psychological care. Thus, there is little incentive for some nurses to extend themselves in that direction. If psychological care is given low priority, it will be done infrequently. Yet, such information obtained through evaluation of care could provide the impetus for more effort and competency directed toward giving emotional care to the patient and family.[6]

Personalized care in institutions is given when staff members are given an opportunity to talk about their problems in being with and caring for dying patients; when professionals are interested in, available to, and willing to support patients and each other; and when the psychological and social needs, as well as the physical needs, of patients are recognized.[6]

Psychosocial supports for staff members who work with people in crises or who are terminally ill or dying need to be built into the system. Long-term care of the elderly or dying offers little excitement; much nursing care is closely intertwined with ordinary and usual activities of daily living—eating, bathing, going for a walk, or playing a quiet game. The challenge is to make work that is mundane into a meaningful experience. The staff need authority to go with responsibility of care.

REFERENCES

1. ANDERSON, W., "The Elderly at the End of Life," in *The Hour of Our Death,* eds. Sylvia Lack and Richard Lamerton. London: Geoffrey Chapman, 1974, pp. 8–17.

2. ARIES, PHILIPPE, *Western Attitudes Toward Death.* Baltimore: The Johns Hopkins University Press, 1974.

3. BARRACLOUGH, B., "Suicide in the Elderly," in *Recent Developments in Psycho-Geriatrics,* eds. D. Kay and A. Walk. London: Royal Medico-Psychological Association, 1968, pp. 87–98.

4. BEAUCHAMP, JOYCE, "Euthanasia and the Nurse Practitioner," *Nursing Digest,* 4: No. 5 (1976), 83–85.

5. BENGSTON, VERN, J. CUELLAR, and P. KAGAN, "Stratum Contrasts and Similarities in Attitudes Toward Death," *Journal of Gerontology,* 23: No. 1 (1977), 76–88.

6. BENOLIEL, JEANNE QUINT, "Talking to Patients About Death," *Nursing Forum,* 9: No. 3 (1970), 254–68.

7. BIRRIN, JAMES, *The Psychology of Aging.* Englewood Cliffs, N.J.: Prentice-Hall, Inc., 1964.

8. BISCHOFF, LEDFORD, *Adult Psychology.* New York: Harper & Row, Publishers, Inc., 1969.

9. BLAUMER, R., "Death and Social Structure," *Psychiatry,* 29: (1966), 378ff.

10. BLUMBERG, JEANNE, and ELEANOR DRUMMOND, *Nursing Care of the Long-Term Patient.* New York: Springer Publishing Co., Inc., 1963.

11. BOTWINICK, JACK, *Aging and Behavior.* New York: Springer Publishing Co., Inc., 1973.

12. BRADEN, WILLIAM, "Long-Livers Find Death Frightening," *St. Louis Post-Dispatch,* December 14, 1975, Sec. H, p. 9.

13. BRODEN, ALEXANDER, "Reactions to Loss in the Aged," in *Loss and Grief: Psychological Management in Medical Practice,* eds. B. Schoenberg, A. Carr, D. Peretz, and A. Kutscher. New York: Columbia University Press, 1970, pp. 199–217.

14. BUEHLER, JANICE, "What Contributes to Hope in the Cancer Patient?" *American Journal of Nursing,* 75: No. 8 (1975), 1353–56.

15. BURNSIDE, IRENE, "Listen to the Aged," *American Journal of Nursing,* 75: No. 10 (1975), 1800–1803.

16. CAREY, RAYMOND, "Living Until Death: A Program of Service and Research for the Terminally Ill," in *Death, The Final Stage of Growth,* ed. Elisabeth Kubler-Ross. Englewood Cliffs, N.J.: Prentice-Hall, Inc., 1975, pp. 75–86.

17. CARR, A., and B. SCHOENBERG, "Object Loss and Somatic Symptom Formation," in *Loss and Grief: Psychological Management in Medical Practice,* eds. B. Schoenberg, A. Carr, D. Peretz, and A. Kutscher. New York: Columbia University Press, 1970, pp. 36–48.

18. CASSINI, N., "Care of the Dying Person," in *Concerning Death: A Practical Guide for the Living,* ed. Earl Grollman. Boston: Beacon Press, 1974, pp. 13–48.

19. CAUGHILL, RITA, ed., *The Dying Patient: A Supportive Approach.* Boston: Little, Brown & Company, 1976.

20. CLAYTON, PAULA, JAMES HALIKES, and WILLIAM MAURICE, "The Bereavement of the Widowed," *Diseases of the Nervous System,* 32: No. 9 (1971), 597–604.

21. COUSINS, NORMAN, "The Right to Die," *Saturday Review,* June 14, 1975, p. 4.

22. CRANE, DIANE, "Dying and Its Dilemmas as a Field of Research," *The Dying Person,* eds. O. Brien, H. Freeman, S. Levine, and N. Scotch. New York: Russell Sage Foundation, 1970, pp. 303–25.

23. DRAZMIN, YAFFE, *How to Prepare for Death: A Practical Guide.* New York: Hawthorn Books, Inc., 1976.

24. ELLIOTT, NEIL, *The Gods of Life.* New York: Macmillan Publishing Co., Inc., 1974.

25. EMERSON, JOAN, "Social Functions of Humor in a Hospital Setting," Ph.D. Dissertation, University of California, Berkeley, 1963.

26. ENGEL, GEORGE, *Psychological Development in Health and Disease.* Philadelphia: W. B. Saunders Company, 1962.

27. FEIFEL, H., ed., *The Meaning of Death.* New York: McGraw-Hill Book Company, 1959.

28. ――――, "Attitudes of Critically Ill Toward Death and Dying," *Geriatric Focus,* 6: No. 5 (1967), 1ff.

29. FINK, STEPHEN, "Crisis and Motivation: A Theoretical Model," *Archives of Physical Medicine and Rehabilitation,* 48: No. 11 (1967), 592–97.

30. FLESCH, REGINA, "The Condolence or Sympathy Call," in *Concerning Death: A Practical Guide for the Living,* ed. Earl Grollman. Boston: Beacon Press, 1974, pp. 265–79.

31. FREIHOFER, PATRICIA, and GERALDINE FELTON, "Nursing Behaviors in Bereavement," *Nursing Research,* 25: No. 5 (1976), 332–37.

32. GLASER, B., and A. STRAUSS, *Awareness of Dying.* Chicago: Aldine Publishing Company, 1965.

33. GORE, GEOFFREY, *Death, Grief and Mourning.* Garden City, N.Y.: Anchor Books, 1967.

34. GRIFFIN, JERRY, "Family Decision," *American Journal of Nursing,* 75: No. 5 (1975), 795–96.

35. GROLLMAN, EARL, ed., *Concerning Death: A Practical Guide for the Living.* Boston: Beacon Press, 1974.

36. HAMPE, SANDRA, "Needs of the Grieving Spouse in a Hospital Setting," *Nursing Research,* 24: No. 2 (1975), 113–20.

37. HENDIN, DAVID, *Death as a Fact of Life.* New York: Warner Paperback Library Edition, 1973.

38. HERTER, FREDERIC, "The Right to Die in Dignity," *Archives of the Foundation of Thanatology,* 1: No. 3 (1969), 93–97.

39. HINKLE, L., *et al.,* "An Investigation of the Relation Between Life Experience, Personality Characteristics, and General Susceptibility to Illness," *Psychosomatic Medicine,* 20: No. 4 (1958), 278–95.

40. HORNER, ELEANOR, "Creativity and Fear of Death," *St. Louis Globe-Democrat,* September 25, 1975, Sec. A, p. 54.

41. HURLOCK, ELIZABETH, *Developmental Psychology,* 4th ed. New York: McGraw-Hill Book Company, 1975.

42. JACKSON, EDGAR, "Grief," in *Concerning Death: A Practical Guide for the Living,* ed. Earl Grollman. Boston: Beacon Press, 1974, pp. 1–12.

43. JEFFERS, FRANCES, and ADRIANN VERWOERDT, "How the Old Face Death," in *Behavior and Adaptation in Late Life,* eds. Ewald Busse and Eric Pfeiffer. Boston: Little, Brown & Company, 1969, pp. 163–81.

44. JORDAN, MERLE, "The Protestant Way in Death and Mourning," in *Concerning Death: A Practical Guide for the Living,* ed. Earl Grollman. Boston: Beacon Press, 1974, pp. 81–100.

45. KALISH, RICHARD, "Life and Death: Dividing the Indivisible," *Social Service and Medicine,* 2: (1968), 249–59.

46. KASTENBAUM, ROBERT, "Pathologic Behavior in Old Age May Be Result of Bereavement Overload, Psychologist Says," *Geriatric Focus,* 8: No. 12 (1969), 2–3.

47. KIMMEL, DOUGLAS, *Adulthood and Aging.* New York: John Wiley & Sons, Inc., 1974.

48. KNUTSON, ANDIE, "Cultural Beliefs on Life and Death," in *The Dying Patient,* eds. O. Brien, H. Freeman, S. Levine, and N. Scotch. New York: Russell Sage Foundation, 1970, pp. 42–64.

49. KOBRZYCKI, PAULA, "Dying with Dignity at Home," *American Journal of Nursing,* 75: No. 8 (1975), 1312–13.

50. KOENIG, RONALD, "Dying vs. Well-Being," *OMEGA,* 4: No. 3 (1973), 181–94.

51. KOIS, DENNIS, "How You Live Called Key to How Long You Live," *St. Louis Globe-Democrat,* January 17–18, 1976, Sec. A, p. 15.

52. KUBLER-ROSS, ELISABETH, *On Death and Dying.* London: Collier-Macmillan, Ltd., 1969.

53. KUTSCHER, AUSTIN, "The Psychosocial Aspects of the Oral Care of the Dying Patient," in *Psychosocial Aspects of Terminal Care,* eds. B. Schoenberg, A. Carr, D. Peretz, and A. Kutscher. New York: Columbia University Press, 1972, pp. 126–40.

54. LIEBERMAN, M., "Psychological Correlates of Impending Death: Some Preliminary Observations," *Journal of Gerontology,* 20: No. 2 (1965), 181–90.

55. ———, "Social Setting Determines Attitudes of Aged to Death," *Geriatric Focus,* 6: No. 16 (1967), 1ff.

56. ———, and COPLAN, ANNIE, "Distance from Death as a Variable in the Study of Aging," *Developmental Psychology,* 2: No. 1 (1969), 71–84.

57. "Lindbergh Chose a Planned Death," *St. Louis Post-Dispatch,* May 22, 1977, Sec. I, p. 19.

58. LINDEMANN, ERIC, "Symptomology and Management of Acute Grief," *American Journal of Psychiatry,* 101: (1944), 141–48.

59. MADDISON, DAVID, "Death Denial. A Question as to Its Significance," *Archives of the Foundation of Thanatology,* 2: No. 1 (1970), 11–12.

60. ———, and BEVERLY RAPHAEL, "The Family of the Dying Patient," in *Psychosocial Aspects of Terminal Care,* eds. B. Schoenberg, A. Carr, D. Peretz, and A. Kutscher. New York: Columbia University Press, 1972, pp. 185–200.

61. MEYEROWITZ, JOSEPH, "Dying: Dromenon Versus Drama," in *Anticipatory Grief,* eds. B. Schoenberg, A. Carr, A. Kutscher, D. Peretz, and I. Goldberg. New York: Columbia University Press, 1974, pp. 79–93.

62. MORGENSON, DONALD, "Death and Interpersonal Failure," *Canada's Mental Health,* 21: No. 3–4 (1973), 10–12.

63. MUEHLENKAMP, ANN, LUCILLE GRESS, and MAY FLOOD, "Perception of Life Change Events by the Elderly," *Nursing Research,* 24: No. 2 (1975), 109–13.

64. MURRAY, RUTH, and JUDITH ZENTNER, *Nursing Concepts for Health Promotion,* 2nd ed. Englewood Cliffs, N.J.: Prentice-Hall, Inc., 1979.

65. NICHOLS, RAY, and JANE NICHOLS, "Funerals: A Time for Grief and Growth," in *Death, The Final Stage of Growth,* ed. Elisabeth Kubler-Ross. Englewood Cliffs, N.J.: Prentice-Hall, Inc., 1975, pp. 87–96.

66. NIGHSWONGER, CARL, "Ministry to the Dying as a Learning Encounter," *Journal of Thanatology,* 1: No. 2 (1971), 101–108.

67. "Older Person's Unconscious Attitudes to Dying May Be Determined by the Proximity of Death," *Geriatric Focus,* 7: No. 17 (1968), 2ff.

68. PALMORE, E., ed., *Normal Aging.* Durham, N.C.: Duke University Press, 1970.

69. PARAD, H., ed., *Crisis Intervention: Selected Readings.* New York: Family Service Association of America, 1965.

70. PERETZ, DAVID, "Reaction to Loss," in *Loss and Grief: Psychological Management in Medical Practice,* eds. B. Schoenberg, A. Carr, D. Peretz, and A. Kutscher. New York: Columbia University Press, 1970, pp. 20–35.

71. REES, W., and S. LUTKINS, "Mortality of Bereavement," *British Medical Journal,* 4: (1967), 13–16.

72. REEVES, ROBERT, "Reflections on Two False Expectations," in *Anticipatory Grief,* eds. B. Schoenberg, A. Carr, A. Kutscher, D. Peretz, and I. Goldberg. New York: Columbia University Press, 1974, pp. 280–84.

73. REIMANIS, G., and R. GREEN, "Imminence of Death and Intellectual Decrement in Aging," *Developmental Psychology,* 5: (1971), 270–72.

74. RILEY, JOHN, "What People Think About Death," in *The Dying Patient,* eds. O. Brien, H. Freeman, S. Levine, and N. Scotch. New York: Russell Sage Foundation, 1970, pp. 30–41.

75. SOBEL, DAVID, "Death and Dying," *American Journal of Nursing,* 74: No. 1 (1974), 98–99.

76. SUDNOW, DAVID, *Passing On: The Social Organization of Dying.* Englewood Cliffs, N.J.: Prentice-Hall, Inc., 1967.

77. SULLIVAN, HARRY S., *The Interpersonal Theory of Psychiatry.* New York: W. W. Norton and Co., Inc., 1953.

78. SWENSON, W., "Attitudes Toward Death Among the Aged," *Minnesota Medicine,* 42: (1959), 399.

79. TRELEASE, MURRAY, "Dying Among Alaskan Indians: A Matter of Choice," in *Death, The Final Stage of Growth,* ed. Elisabeth Kubler-Ross. Englewood Cliffs, N.J.: Prentice-Hall, Inc., 1975, pp. 33–37.

80. VAILLOT, SR. MADELINE, "Hope: The Restoration of Being," *American Journal of Nursing,* 70: No. 2 (1970), 268–73.

81. WALKER, MARGARET, "The Last Hour Before Death," *American Journal of Nursing,* 73: No. 9 (1973), 1592–93.

82. WEBER, LEONARD, "Ethics and Euthanasia: Another View," *American Journal of Nursing,* 73: No. 7 (1973), 1228–31.

83. WEISMAN, AVERY, and ROBERT KASTENBAUM, "The Psychological Autopsy: A Study of the Terminal Phase of Life," *Community Mental Health Journal, Monograph No. 4.* New York: Behavioral Publications, Inc., 1968.

84. WESTHOFF, MARY, "Listening to Relieve the Fear of Death," *Supervisor Nurse,* 3: No. 3 (1972), 80ff.

85. WORCHESTER, ALFRED, *The Care of the Aged, the Dying, and the Dead,* 2nd ed. Springfield, Ill.: Charles C Thomas, Publisher, 1961, pp. 33–66.

86. WYZANT, W., "Dying, But Not Alone," *American Journal of Nursing,* 67: No. 3 (1967), 547–77.

moral and spiritual development in later maturity

Study of this chapter will enable you to:

---

1. Differentiate moral development from spiritual development.

2. Consider the spiritual dimensions of the senior as an important aspect of his life.

3. Explore how your moral development and spiritual beliefs influence your care of the elderly person.

4. Contrast specific beliefs of the major religions in the United States and discuss the implications of these beliefs for nursing practice.

5. Assess spiritual needs of the senior, using information from this and previous chapters.

6. Work with the senior in formulating goals related to his spiritual care.

7. Foster spiritual development, indirectly or through specific measures, as is appropriate to the senior's beliefs, needs, and wishes.

8. Explore with the senior to evaluate the effectiveness of your spiritual care.

14

Today's generation of seniors was reared in an era in which right actions, religious belief, and going to church were emphasized. Church-related activities were often the main social affairs. Many seniors still hold those earlier values. The church membership is a reference group that gives support and security to the religious person. For some elderly, the church congregation is perceived as a family constellation.

The senior is at a unique time in his life in that spiritual matters—concerns about mortality and immortality, pain and suffering, loss, weakness and strength, and rights and responsibilities of self and others—take on new meaning as death approaches. Further, he has time to think about his life; he cannot run away from himself in work or other activities. Just as the senior continues to develop and change physically, socially, emotionally, and in his family life, so he continues to develop morally and spiritually. Formulating a philosophy of life or a spiritual outlook on life remains a developmental task into later maturity.[16] The senior's ultimate philosophical or spiritual belief is uniquely his own, and such an abstract part of the person is very difficult to write about.

MORAL DEVELOPMENT

Morality refers to behavior that is considered good or bad. The senior may be in the *Post-Conventional level* of moral development, in which he follows the principles that he has defined as appropriate for his life. He no longer behaves a certain way just because the majority of other people do. In *Stage 1* of this level, he adheres to the legal viewpoint of society but believes that laws can be changed as people's needs change, and he lives by the universal principles of justice, equality, and human rights. Such universal principles take precedence over the man-made rules of a locale. In *Stage 2,* he still lives by Stage 1, but he is able to incorporate injustice, pain, and death as an integral part of existence.[25]

However, most seniors stay at the Conventional level, and some will still be at the Pre-Conventional level. In the *Conventional level,* the person follows the social rules of conduct and law and order in response to others' expectations. He values conformity, loyalty, and social order. In *Stage 1* he considers an action good if it pleases others. In *Stage 2* he values law and order; he wants established rules from authority. He obeys the law just because it is the law. In the *Pre-Conventional level,* he obeys rules to avoid pain and obtain pleasure. He defers to the person in power. In *Stage 1* he defines good and bad in terms of himself. In *Stage 2* he sometimes does acts to meet another's needs as well as his own.[25]

Although religious and moral development are progressive, there is no link between religious affiliation or education and moral development. Moral

development is linked positively with empathy and the ability to act reciprocally with another while maintaining personal values and principles.[25]

The senior who adheres to the Post-Conventional level of moral development may have to forsake his principles if he is institutionalized; if he continues
to speak and practice his beliefs, he may be considered a nuisance. He may
question rituals, rules, and policies that have been established for the institution's efficiency or profit rather than for the patient's benefit. His behavior may
receive such disapproval that he learns to keep quiet in order to get his minimum needs cared for. He learns that it is easier to live at the Pre-Conventional
level. For example, an alert 80-year-old male in one nursing home who tried to
report to the public the physical and emotional abuse that occurred in the
home was himself beaten with a Coke bottle by an attendant. He said no more
in defense of himself or others; the institution's staff hardly gave a thought to
his death a few weeks later.

An area of research yet untouched is what happens physically and emotionally to the senior when he feels that he is forced to give up his principles.
Perhaps the "senility" of institutionalization can be related to the inability to
adhere to moral, philosophical, or spiritual principles and beliefs.

SPIRITUAL DEVELOPMENT

All people have a spiritual dimension to the self, whether or not they follow a
formal religion. *Spiritual refers to the transcendental relationship between the
person and a Higher Being, a quality that goes beyond a specific religious affiliation, that strives for reverence, awe, and inspiration, and that gives answers about
the infinite.* *Religion is a ritualized form of expressing belief in a Higher Being
and is a means of expressing and meeting spiritual needs.*

Most studies of people in late life indicate that the senior who has a religious faith goes to church if he possibly can.[5,11,21] (Many churches have more
oldsters than young people in the congregation.) In addition to meeting spiritual needs, church attendance is important as a social event, to reaffirm the self
as a person, to add structure to the week, and to feel needed and responsible
through participation in church activities. Further, the person who attends
church regularly feels more assured that people will look after him if he becomes ill or is in need, especially if he lives alone. And finally, he feels that he
will be remembered after death and at least a few people will attend his funeral
and see him to his grave. Thus, the person may not have been an active church
member during the young and middle adult years, but if he was reared with
any church connection at all, he is likely to reestablish church ties as he gets
older. Church attendance drops only when the senior becomes ill or infirm,
feels embarrassed about lack of money or appropriate clothes for attending

church, feels unwanted by younger members, or lacks transportation. Sometimes the senior becomes displeased because the church members are not more helpful to him, especially if he was always active as a member.[21]

However, there is much more to the spiritual dimension of the senior than attending church.

GENERAL ASSESSMENT

In order to understand the spiritual depth of the senior, you must do an astute assessment over a period of time. Contributing to his spiritual understanding are his physical, emotional, and cognitive status; socioeconomic level; cultural, racial, or ethnic background; urban or rural residence; religious affiliation; and life stresses. Information presented in the previous chapters will assist you in your spiritual assessment.

Certain qualities are likely to be found in the senior who has wrestled with some of the questions of life and who has transcended some of the mundane answers. If he is emotionally mature, the senior shows a spiritual integrity much as he shows ego integrity.[17]

He has an acceptance, patience, and tolerance for others who are different or who practice their religious faith differently. He sees the commonalities in all religions and is less likely to insist that only one way is right, although he may devotedly practice his religion in the same way that he always has. He listens attentively as others explore their own beliefs.

He shows characteristics that are similar to those of ego integrity discussed in Chapter 12. He trusts and has faith in a Higher Being, a Creative Force, Fate, God. He has a sense of autonomy, of being a unique, valued person—valued because he is a child of God or a child of the Universe. He has a sense of spiritual identity, with Christ, God, Allah, his ancestors, or whomever or whatever his belief dictates. He feels an intimacy, a closeness and commitment to something other than just himself and his immediate loved ones. His spiritual integrity shows in other ways as well. He speaks of and shows love for others, a love that is selfless and forgiving. He can be kind, loving, and gracious, even to those who act maliciously toward him. He transcends the basic meanness of life; he no longer puts energy into revengeful feelings as the younger person might. He is tranquil in the face of adversity because of his strong belief that in the end he will be cared for, that the force of God is with him.

He continues to search for meaning and to refine his philosophy about life, the small time spent on earth, and the whole of eternity.

Even if the senior is disoriented, confused, delirious, cognitively impaired, or emotionally ill, he is still a spiritual person. His apparent ramblings may be an effort to resolve spiritual conflicts, or they may be an expression of spiritual insights phrased in a way we do not understand. Regardless of his condition, he is still a spiritual being and assessment should include that component.

Not all seniors will openly demonstrate the characteristics of spiritual maturity just described. Their life, conversation, and actions may appear to be spiritually void. Yet, if you talk about spiritual matters with them, you will learn that their inner thoughts and private rituals include spiritual convictions and practices. Other seniors will feel a spiritual void; abandoned by God; unloved by anyone, including a spiritual being; worthless; and fearful of death. They may frantically "try on" different religions in an effort to quiet their longings and to find meaning in life. They will be demonstrating the characteristics described in Chapter 12 for self-despair and self-disgust.

However, even the atheistic or agnostic senior, as well as the despairing, will often develop spiritually in times of crisis, as shown by the following case study:

Mrs. V., aged 88, openly and frequently condemned organized religion for how ineffective it was, including the Greek Orthodox Church to which Mr. V. belonged. He had attended church when he was younger; she had never attended any church. Her excuses included, "All they want is my money." "The priests think they are so much better than anyone else. They'd step on you if you were lying in the streets." She did not speak of any belief in a God or in immortality.

But she slowly began to change as she cared for Mr. V. in their home for the year of his terminal illness. One of her friends who called daily was a devout Baptist who would always say that she had included Mr. and Mrs. V. in her morning prayers. As Mrs. V. began to get more fatigued from the burden of doing Mr. V.'s physical care, the friend would say things like: "Have faith. God will give you strength to care for him and to keep him at home. He is watching over you. He will keep you." And gradually Mrs. V. took these words into herself. As she cared for Mr. V., struggling to turn him or change the bed, she would say, "But I can do it. God will give me strength." Later, she would say, "I'm managing. God is giving me the strength or I know I could never do it."

She began to change in other ways too. She no longer condemned the church, and she called the nearby Greek Orthodox priest to see Mr. V. She spoke of life hereafter and of how when Mr. V. died, she'd soon go to join him.

After his death, she clung to any statements from others that were spiritual in nature. She continued to say, "God gave me the strength to take care of my husband. Now I am at God's mercy. I am in His hands. I am so lonely. I have so little. I can't make it without Him."

Although she never expressed the profound beliefs of someone who had always been spiritually bound to a Higher Being or God, in her simple, childlike way she had shown spiritual development.

In assessing the senior, whether he is spiritually profound or has a very childlike, simple faith, do not make assumptions. Do not assume that the spiritually simple person receives any less comfort from his beliefs than does the profound person. Further, do not project your spiritual values, belief, or development onto the senior.

SPECIFIC ASSESSMENT RELATED TO SPECIFIC RELIGIOUS BELIEFS

A knowledge of the major religious faiths is essential if you are to make a meaningful assessment and to individualize intervention. Since most older people tend to be more orthodox or traditional in their religious beliefs, the following discussion about some of the major religions and sects in the United States covers the traditional beliefs related to the needs or concerns of the senior. Recognize, however, that the beliefs and practices of a senior may not follow exactly the tenets of the religion, and that some denominations and sects have several branches, for example, the Lutherans, Baptists, and Pentecostals. Thus, the spiritual needs of the people belonging to Northern or Southern Baptist churches, urban or rural Methodist churches, or Missouri or American Synod Lutheran churches may vary considerably, even if their religious faith is listed as Baptist, Methodist, or Lutheran.

Yet, there are commonalities between religions. Christianity, Judaism, and Islam all adhere to a monotheistic God, have a historical fixed scripture for public use, make covenants with God or Allah for protection, obey God's or Allah's commandments, and often proselytize. The believers are "doers." Believers of Taoism and Confucianism believe that everything is in the being of God or that there is no Godhead. These people try to be in harmony with the world around them as well as with others. Buddhism and Hinduism have their roots in India and teach that everything is in the being of God. These believers are interested in "being" instead of "doing." They have a collective literature for private devotion. Control of the mind and body is desired and achieved through some of the yoga practices. They look inside of the self for answers about spiritual matters, as do believers of Taoism, Confucianism, and Shintoism. Common sense rather than doctrine determines behavior and good acts. Members of the Native American tribes may belong to Christian denominations or sects, but they may also practice tribal religions, which include folklore and herbal medicine, and they may rely on a superhuman power. Mind and body are seen as closely interrelated; to be in harmony with nature and others is essential for the spirit and for health.

Christianity

Christianity consists of many denominations and sects. Although Christianity was divided into Eastern Orthodox and Roman Catholic in 1054 A.D. and the Protestant Reformation in the sixteenth century created a third division, Christians share the basic belief that Jesus Christ as described in the New Testament is God's Son. His birth marks the beginning of the time A.D. His short life and works are described in the New Testament. According to the belief, Jesus was fully man and God at the same time. The main symbol is the cross, the structure on which Christ was crucified for the sins of mankind. The cross also symbolizes the finished redemption: Christ arising from the dead and ascending to God, his Father, in order to rule with Him, continuously influencing the lives of His followers. God is perceived as three persons—the Father, the Son, and the Holy Ghost (Holy Spirit); the Holy Ghost provides a spirit of love and truth. No one comes to God the Father except through belief in Jesus Christ the Son. Christians differ in their beliefs and practices but all regard themselves as children of God, created in His image, protected by Him, yet responsible for their own souls. Christians try to live so that they have eternal life after death with God and Jesus Christ.

Roman Catholicism emphasizes the authority of the church through the Scriptures. Jesus chose apostles as God, the Father's, representatives to preach, teach, and guide other people, and establish the Church. Jesus appointed Saint Peter as the head of the Church to preserve unity and to have authority over the apostles. This same mission continues through the Pope, his Cardinals, and his Bishops.

The Catholic believes that the Sacraments are grace-giving rites that help the person share in Christ's life and that sustain him in following Christ's example. The Sacraments received once in life are Baptism, Confirmation, Holy Orders, and Matrimony. Baptism, for the infant or the adult who joins the church, incorporates the soul into the life of Christ to share His divinity. Through Confirmation the Holy Spirit is imparted in a fuller measure to help strengthen the person in his spiritual life. Matrimony acknowledges the love and lifelong commitment between a man and woman. Holy Orders ordains priests and deacons.

Sacraments which may be received more than once are Penance (Confession), Holy Eucharist (Holy Communion), and the Anointing of the Sick (Sacrament of the Sick). Penance, required once a year by Church law, involves acknowledgment and forgiveness of the person's sins in the presence of a priest and is usually received according to individual need. The Mass, often called the Eucharist, is the liturgical celebration which has the Sacrament of the Holy Eucharist as its central portion: Bread and wine are consecrated and become the body and blood of Christ, which are received in Holy Communion. Catholics are required to attend Mass on Sunday or late Saturday and on specified holy days, which in the United States are January 1, Ascension Thursday (40 days after Easter), August 15, November 1, December 8, and December 25, unless they are prevented by illness or another serious reason. Many older Catholics desire daily Communion. Anointing of the Sick, formerly known as Extreme Unction or last rites, is symbolic of Christ's healing love and the concern of the Christian community. Anointing of the Sick provides spiritual strength to those who are ill; the elderly person may still consider this Sacrament as indicative of approaching death. Explanation may be necessary to offset fears. This Sacrament should be administered to those approaching death, and it should also be given if the patient or family request it. If the person is dead when the priest arrives, the body is not anointed, but the priest leads the family in prayers for the dead person.

Because the Catholic reveres life, the amputated limb should be offered to the family for burial in consecrated ground. There is no blanket mandate, but burial may be required by the diocese.

The Catholic believes that suffering and illness are allowed by God because of man's disobedience (his original sin), but that they are not necessarily willed by God or given as punishment for personal sins. Yet many Catholics perceive illness as a test of their spiritual strength and of their relationship with God.

Friday abstinence and Lenten fasting have been relaxed in recent years. Today, many dioceses observe Friday abstinence only during Lent and fasting on Ash Wednesday and Good Friday.

Since the *Eastern Orthodox Church* is divided by nationality, slight differences in beliefs and practices may occur from group to group. Eastern Orthodoxy is common to those of Turkish, Egyptian, Syrian, Rumanian, Bulgarian, Albanian, Cypriot, Polish, and Czechoslovakian ethnic descent. The Russian Orthodox Church and the Greek Orthodox Church are autonomous branches of the Eastern Orthodox Church. The Eastern Orthodox Church has no Pope, but otherwise it is similar to the Roman Catholic Church. There are seven Sacraments, including Anointing of the Sick, administered by the priest. The Divine Liturgy, the Eucharistic service, is presented in the native language and sometimes in English. Confession at least once a year is prerequisite to participation in the Eucharist, which is required at least four times a year: at Christmas, Easter, on the Feast Day of St. Peter and St. Paul (June 30), and on the day celebrating the sleeping of the Virgin Mary (August 15).

Fasting (avoiding meat, dairy products, and olive oil) is done for spiritual betterment. The fasting period is from the last meal in the evening until after Communion and on other traditional fast days: each Wednesday (representing the seizure of Jesus), each Friday (representing His death), 40 days before Christmas and before Easter.

For the Greek Orthodox, last rites consist of Holy Communion. Last rites are obligatory if death is impending to the Russian Orthodox; to the Eastern Orthodox the Anointment of the Sick is a blessing, not a last rite. Cremation is discouraged by the Eastern, Greek, and Russian Orthodox churches. The Greek and Russian Orthodox churches also forbid autopsies and embalming.

Protestantism is divided into many denominations and sects, which in turn often have numerous branches that vary slightly in their beliefs and practices. Protestants employ a freedom of spiritual searching and reinterpretation; thus, new groups form as certain persons and their followers believe that they see

Christ's teachings in a new and better light. Most Protestants read the Bible for guidance; a few groups, those that emphasize individual freedom, allow no written creed and expect members to follow an unwritten code of behavior. Protestants believe that the person's spiritual relationship is between himself and God and Jesus; no Pope or saints are needed to intervene for them. No one person or group of persons has sole authority to interpret His truth to others. They believe that they should follow Christ's teachings, are responsible for their actions and following God's will, and should be able to worship freely. The minister represents friendship, love, acceptance, understanding, and forgiveness. Some sects, such as Friends (Quakers), do not have a minister but rely upon inspired persons within the group for guidance and interpretation of God's word.

Some of the major Protestant churches in the United States, beginning with the most formal in liturgy and sacraments, are the Episcopal and Lutheran Churches; in between are the Presbyterians, United Church of Christ, United Methodists, and Disciples of Christ (Christian Church). The freest liturgically and least sacramental are the Baptists, Pentecostals, and other fundamentalist sects. The Friends and Mennonites are not sacramental or liturgical sects.

Some of the opposing doctrines and practices are as follows: living in versus living above sin; predestination versus free will; infant versus believer's baptism, and loose versus tightly knit church organization. Some believe that the Scriptures are infallible; others believe that the Scriptures are a guide and are to be interpreted for today's living. Some Protestants view death as penalty and punishment for sins; others see death as a transition when the soul leaves the body for eternal reward. Most believe that science can be used to relieve suffering but techniques should not be used unjustly, in contradiction to Christian theology, or in conflict with the individual's personality and will.

Certain Christian groups have specific beliefs that must be considered in nursing intervention. They are discussed in the following paragraphs.

Seventh-Day Adventists rely on Old Testament laws more than other Christian churches do. They accept the Bible literally and believe that following the commandments is evidence of salvation. Members believe they must warn mankind to prepare for the Second Coming of Christ. Some sects regard the Sabbath from sundown Friday to sundown Saturday, during which time they do minimum work and avoid study or outside influences. Because Adventists view the body as the "temple of God," health care is given high priority.

The Church of Jesus Christ of Latter-Day Saints (commonly called the Mormon Church) takes inspiration from the Book of Mormon, translated from the golden tablets found by the young prophet Joseph Smith. The Mormons believe that this Book of Mormon and two other books supplement the Bible. Every Mormon serves several years as a missionary; there is no official congregational leader but a seventy and high priest to represent authority. The Mormon Church believes in taking care of the whole person, and it provides education, recreation, and financial aid for its members. Mormons believe that disease comes from failing to obey the laws of health and God's commandments, although the righteous may become ill because of microorganisms.

The Church of Christ, Scientist (Christian Scientist) uses Mary Baker Eddy's book, Science and Health with Key to the Scriptures, and the Bible as spiritual guides. Science and Health emphasizes wholeness, and those who follow it think of God as Divine Mind, of spirit as real and eternal, of matter as unreal illusion. Sin, sickness, and death are unrealities or errors of the human mind and can be eliminated by altering thoughts, not by using medicine, psychotherapy, or hypnotism. The elderly Christian Scientist is usually cared for either at home or in nursing homes or sanitariums established by the Church and recognized under the federal Medicare program and in insurance regulations. The facilities are operated by trained Christian Scientist nurses who provide basic hygiene measures, first aid, and spiritual assistance. Medication, intravenous fluids, or blood transfusions are not given. The Christian Scientist practitioner devotes his time to healing and helping people apply natural spiritual law. If the Christian Scientist is in a regular hospital, he has probably tried Christian Science healing first and may have been placed in the hospital by a non-Scientist relative. He will prefer to have minimum medical treatment and to have a practitioner called to continue treatment through prayer.

The Friends (Quakers) differ from most Protestants in that the Bible is not their ultimate authority; the final authority resides in the person's direct experience of God within himself. The Friend obeys the inner light or divine inspiration; this spiritual quality causes the Friend to esteem himself and listen to inner direction. The Friends have no minister, no symbols, and no religious decor; all Friends are spiritual equals. Unprogrammed corporate worship consists of silent meditation with each person seeking divine guidance and sharing his inspiration if he is so moved.

The Unity School of Christianity blends concepts from Christian Science, Quakerism, and Hinduism. The school emphasizes positive thoughts, reason, knowledge, and prayer. Each person has the right to approach God individually; each person has a responsibility to live in a spiritual, positive manner. Health is considered natural; sickness is considered unnatural. Illness is real, but it can be overcome by concentrating on spiritual goals. The Unity Village in Missouri publishes inspirational periodicals and has a staff available on a 24-hour basis to answer calls from people seeking spiritual help, prayer, and counseling.

Judaism

Many elderly Jews will be Orthodox, although they may belong to Reform or Conservative congregations. The Orthodox Jew believes that God gave the law exactly as it is written in the Torah, the first five books of the Old Testament, and in the Talmud, a commentary on the Torah and a collection of civil and religious laws. The law should be followed precisely. The *Reform Jew* believes that the law was written by inspired men at various times and thus is subject to reinterpretation. *Conservative Jews* are in the middle; they take some practices from both groups. The Jewish spiritual leader is a rabbi; the spiritual symbol is a menorah, a seven-branched candelabrum. The fundamental Jewish concept is expressed in the prayer, "Hear, O Israel, the Lord our God, the Lord is One." God is One; He loves His creation, wants his people to live justly, and wants to bless their food, drink, and celebration. Judaism's theme might be, "Enjoy life now, and share it with God." Thus, belief in an afterlife is not emphasized, although some Jewish people do believe in one. Jews believe in observance of the Law, in their historical role as God's chosen people, and in their hope for better days. Their beliefs have helped them to survive seemingly insurmountable persecution and suffering. However, suffering or illness are not inherently valued.

Important holy days are Rosh Hashana, the Jewish New Year; Yom Kippur, the day of atonement; Tishah b'Ab, the day of lamentation; and Passover. The New Year is a time to be with the family, give thanks for good health, and renew traditions. Yom Kippur is a time to ask forgiveness of family members for wrong doing. The Jew fasts for 24 hours on Yom Kippur as a symbolic act of self-denial, mourning, and petition. Tishah b'Ab, which commemorates the destruction of the First and Second Temples of Jerusalem, is another 24-hour fast period. Passover celebrates the ancient Jews' deliverance from bondage in Egypt; unleavened bread, matzo, is eaten instead of leavened bread during this 8-day period.

The Jewish person values his religion, but he also values his loved ones, family life, health, and education. He is future oriented; thus, he wants to know the implications of the diagnosis and treatment. He may seek several medical opinions before agreeing to a treatment plan.

Islam

This monotheistic religion has an Arabic history; members are called Muslims. Allah is the true God; Mohammed is his prophet, and this belief must be said at least once but is usually said many times during the Muslim's lifetime. The Koran (Quran) is the scripture written by Mohammed, and the Hadith, the collective body of traditions relating to Mohammed and his companions, offer guidelines for thinking, devotional life, and social obligations. The Muslim has a direct relationship with God; he believes himself to be an unique individual with an eternal soul. He believes in heaven and hell and in living a good life. He does not worship an image or picture of Mohammed, since the prophet is not deified.

The Muslim prays five times a day: on arising, at midday, in the afternoon, in the early evening, and before retiring. He performs a ritual washing before each prayer because the Koran emphasizes cleanliness. Then he kneels on a prayer rug, faces Mecca, goes through prescribed body motions, and says various passages in supplication and praise. All Muslims aspire to make a pilgrimage to Mecca at least once in a lifetime to renew spiritual faith.

Ramadan (Ramayan) is a fast month, during which time the Muslim eats or drinks nothing from sunrise to sunset as an act of discipline to understand those who have little food. After sunset he takes nourishment only in moderation. At the end of Ramadan, he enters a festive period with feelings of good will and gift exchanges.

The Koran teaches that the follower shall be responsible to society, avoid gambling, and give a portion of his money to the poor.

The *Black Muslims* (*Nation of Islam*) in the United States have used part of the basic Islam faith in forming their religion. The sect has stringent rules, for example, members may not indulge in any activity (even sleeping) more than is necessary for health.

NURSING DIAGNOSIS, FORMULATION OF PATIENT CARE GOALS, AND INTERVENTION

Your *nursing diagnosis* may be any of the following: *belief in a specific religion, alterations in faith, agnostic, or atheist.* Usually the senior will be best able to tell you where he is spiritually. He will make the nursing diagnosis, so to speak.

Long-term nursing goals may be as follows:

1. The direction of spiritual development that the senior has begun will be continued.
2. Meaning in life will be related to the person's spiritual and philosophical beliefs.
3. The level of moral development will be maintained.

Short-term nursing goals may include the following:

1. Spiritual practices that are not detrimental to health will be continued during the period of health care.
2. Assistance to meet spiritual needs will be given according to the indications of the senior.
3. Health care interventions or policies will not intimidate the spiritual or moral integrity of the senior.

Regardless of the spiritual level of the person, your goal will not be to convert the patient to a religion (including your own) and not to preach your beliefs and values.

General Intervention

You cannot give what you do not have. You cannot practice what you do not know. You may decide that you cannot or do not wish to involve yourself with the spiritual life of the senior you care for. But you cannot avoid the spiritual dimension. You have a spiritual dimension, regardless of your religious beliefs. The senior also has a spiritual dimension that is manifested through his behavior and that you cannot avoid. Both you and the senior are continuing to develop in every sphere, including the spiritual.

If you believe the following words by Robert Browning, you will be better able to care for the senior, including his spiritual self:

> Grow old along with me!
> The best is yet to be,
> The last of life, for which the first was made:
> Our times are in His hands
> Who saith, "A whole I planned,
> Youth shows but half; Trust God, see all, nor be afraid."

Intervention in the spiritual dimension involves intangible aspects as well as overt measures. You will not be able to state a theoretical or scientific base as you would for intervention related to conditions described in Units IV and V. Hopefully, you will be willing to try to integrate spiritual aspects of care into the scientific aspects.

Basic to caring for the spiritual side of the senior is an acceptance of your own and his spirituality, of the sacredness of yourself and the senior as human beings. If you can convey to the senior that you believe he is valuable, worthy of your trust and care, then you will help his spirit to come alive, and you will help him to believe in himself and in something outside himself.[29]

Awareness of your own developmental progression, including the spiritual, is also essential if you are to be aware of or to assess the senior accurately. Self-awareness should also help you to be more attuned to the senior's needs, for you will be able to sort out his beliefs, needs, and wishes because you are aware of your own.

Meeting the spiritual needs of the elderly is probably the greatest challenge you will face because it requires that you accept your own spirituality, finiteness, need for others, and need for a belief system. As you develop spiritual maturity, you may experience a sense of your greatest vulnerability and your greatest strength, your deepest degree of uniqueness and your deepest degree of universality, your deepest joys and most frightening fears. Vulnerability comes from knowledge of finiteness. Acceptance of finiteness means that you must learn how to live. As you learn how to live, you can help another live to the fullest.

Intervention to foster spiritual development will often involve measures that overtly appear to have nothing to do with religion or spirituality. For example, you can help the senior maintain his sense of autonomy by developing a relationship and using communication skills described in Chapter 3. You foster his spiritual development and avoid regression by treating him like the adult that he is instead of like an infant. (Geriatrics is not pediatrics.) The more dependent or impaired the senior, the more devastating the approach which makes him feel like an infant, a burden, even more dependent. It is equally important that you avoid labels like failing, slipping, debilitated, decrepit, or worse, senile. Your label is likely to be self-fulfilling. If you use a label, you foster what you think is present. The senior is still living and developing; he is succeeding in meeting his life tasks.

You foster spiritual development as you give conscientious physical care, relieve pain, reorient him, use touch, help him maintain an intact body image, help him to reminisce and do life review, or make his environment more pleasant and esthetic. You care for the whole person.

You foster spiritual development as you try to maintain his lifelong patterns, as you include family and friends in assessment and intervention, and as you let family and friends assist in the senior's care, if they wish to assist. Often the presence of children, either relatives or friends, will spark the senior's spirit, rekindle his interest in life, give him a reason to live, and help him find meaning in life.

Talk with the senior so that you can learn his philosophy of life. Understanding his cultural background, religious beliefs and specific practices, and philosophy of life can help you determine and foster his acceptance of aging and body image changes and of the losses incurred in old age. Refer to the references at the end of Chapter 6 to understand special needs of people from different cultures.

Carrying out the specific practices described in the following section can also help the senior feel that he is unique and worthy as a person. For example, the senior who has attended Mass daily all of his life but is now physically too weak to go to chapel in the hospital will appreciate a short, simple prayer said by yourself or someone who feels comfortable praying with him. Or refer him to the minister of his faith. Helping him to maintain hope will be a way of touching his spiritual dimension.

Specific Intervention Measures

The understanding gained from reading the previous brief section on people's religions and from reading the references at the end of this chapter can help you to individualize spiritual care.

You can assist the *Roman Catholic* patient in meeting his spiritual needs by calling a priest, taking him to Mass, and providing for an hour's fast and a quiet environment before he receives the Eucharist. He will appreciate being able to keep the rosary, Bible, prayerbook, crucifix, and various medals at the bedside. Holy water and lighted candles are also meaningful symbols.

When he is ill, he and the family may want the priest to administer the Sacrament for Anointing of the Sick; certainly this Sacrament is wanted when the senior is approaching death. Some older Catholics adhere devotedly to fast days and to the former rule of abstaining from meat on Fridays and during Lent. The ill person is exempt from fasting but may need assurance from his priest.

The *Orthodox* patient will also want to talk with a priest who speaks his language, attend church service, and keep religious symbols, such as the Bible, prayerbook, and icons (pictures of Jesus, Mary, or revered saints) at his bedside. He will also appreciate holy water and lighted candles. The ill person desires Holy Communion; fasting is from the last meal the evening before Communion. The ill senior may need assurance from the priest that he does not have to keep other fast days; or fasting may be allowed if it does not interfere with medical procedures. The Orthodox patient generally, but especially the *Greek Orthodox,* opposes euthanasia and believes that every reasonable effort should be made to preserve life until it is terminated by God. The *Russian Orthodox* senior male should not be shaved except in preparation for surgery. The cross necklace is worn at all times and should be replaced immediately after surgery. After death, the arms are crossed. Clothing worn at death must be of natural fiber so that the body will change to ashes sooner.

The *Protestant* wants to have the Bible or special devotional or prayer books with him. He appreciates someone saying grace before feeding him, calling his minister, reading or quoting Scripture, and taking him to chapel. For most Protestants, there are no dietary restrictions. Most Protestants desire Holy Communion but do not believe in last rites. Ill members read the Scriptures and pray.

Certain denominations and sects have specific beliefs that must be followed. *Episcopalians* may abstain from meat on Friday and fast before receiving Holy Communion. Generally, Protestants do not fast prior to Holy Communion. For both *Episcopalians* and *Lutherans,* last rites are optional. The *Mormon* wears a white garment under his clothing which was received after a special ceremony in the temple and has priesthood marks at the navel and knee. This garment is considered protection against danger and you should not remove it.

Dietary restrictions are followed by some denominations and sects. The *Seventh-Day Adventist* does not eat pork or fish that has both scales and fins. Some Adventists are strict vegetarians. Others are lacto-ovo-vegetarians; they drink milk and eat eggs, but they do not eat meat. The *Pentecostal* refrains from eating pork or any strangled animal or food to which blood has been added. The *Jehovah's Witness* does not eat anything to which blood has been added, but he can eat animal flesh that has been drained. The *Mormon* believes in eating healthful foods and sparingly of meat.

Avoidance of coffee and tea, which contain a stimulant, is followed by devout *Seventh-Day Adventists, Christian Scientists, Mormons,* and some *Baptists.*

The *Adventists* and *Christian Scientists,* some *Mormons,* and *Friends* also avoid narcotics and other drugs, if possible.

Many elderly people smoke and like an appetizer of wine or whiskey in eggnog before sleep. However, these practices would not be followed by the following believers: *Church of Christ, Church of God, Seventh-Day Adventist, Grace Brethren, Friends, Nazarene, Pentecostal, Mormon,* and some *Baptists* and *Methodists.* The *Mennonite* and many members of fundamental sects refrain only from alcoholic beverages.

Some Protestants believe in laying on of the hands for healing: some *Baptists,* followers of the *Church of Christ, Nazarene, Pentecostal,* and *Mormon* religions. Anointing with oil is practiced by the *Seventh-Day Adventist, Church of Christ, Grace Brethren,* and *Pentecostal.*

The *Seventh-Day Adventist* may refuse medical treatment and the use of secular items, such as television, on the Sabbath, preferring instead to read the Scriptures.

The beliefs of most Protestants do not conflict with modern medical practices, but there are exceptions. The *Mennonite* values individual dignity and self-determination; thus, he will probably oppose shock treatment, drugs, and any treatment that affects the personality or exercise of the will. *Jehovah's Witnesses* refuse to accept blood transfusions. This belief is based on a Levitical Commandment given by God to Moses that states that no one in the House of David should eat blood or he will be cut off from his people and on a New Testament reference (in Acts) that prohibits the tasting of blood. Intravenous fluids that are like the body's fluid composition are acceptable. The *Christian Scientist* does not seek biopsies or medical treatment, except that of an orthopedist to set a fractured bone, and opposes use of drugs and blood transfusions. Most Fundamentalists do not dance or play cards; thus, certain recreational therapies are avoided. *Jewish* law may be suspended for the ill patient, but the elderly Jewish person will be more comfortable following as many practices as possible.

Sabbath is observed from sundown on Friday to shortly after sundown on Saturday. The Orthodox Jew prepares for the Sabbath by cleaning the home, cooking enough food for the Sabbath day, bathing, and thinking about the spiritual refreshment that the Sabbath brings. Thus, during the Sabbath the Orthodox Jew may refuse freshly cooked food, medicine, treatment, surgery, and the use of radio, television, and writing equipment in order to avoid having thoughts diverted from this special day.

The Orthodox elderly male usually wears a yarmulke or skullcap continuously; he will also want to wear socks in bed because he believes that neither head nor feet should be uncovered. He may refuse to use a razor because of the Levitical ban on shaving. He will probably avoid direct eye contact with the nurse or any other woman except his wife in order to avoid behaving in a way that might be interpreted as seductive. He will want to use the Siddur, a prayerbook, and phylacteries, which are leather boxes containing slips inscribed with Scriptures passages, at weekday morning prayer.

The Orthodox Jew follows certain dietary rules because God has so commanded; and he believes in eating in moderation as a health measure. Food that is ritually correct is called *kosher;* unfit food is called *treyfe* (or treyfah). Forbidden foods include pig, horse, shrimp, lobster, crab, oyster, and fowl that are birds of prey. Animals that are ruminants and have divided hooves, such as cows, sheep, or goats, may be eaten. Fish must have both fins and scales in order to be eaten. Kosher animals must be healthy and slaughtered in a prescribed manner. Because of the Biblical passage that forbids soaking a young goat in its mother's milk, the Jew does not eat meat and milk products together. The utensils used to cook these products or the dishes from which to eat these foods are never intermixed. Kosher products are marked with *U* or *pareve.* Other dietary guidelines for the Orthodox Jew are:

1. Serve milk before meat products. Meat may be eaten a few minutes after milk, but milk cannot be eaten for 6 hours after meat.
2. If the person refuses meat because of incorrect slaughter, encourage a vegetarian diet with protein supplements, such as fish and eggs, which are considered neutral unless they are prepared with milk or meat shortening.
3. Obtain frozen kosher products, heat, and serve in the original container and use disposable utensils.

The Jewish person respects the elderly and feels responsible to visit with and care for them. Jewish tradition demands that someone remain with the dying person; the soul should leave in the presence of people, just as life is with people. The bedside vigil shields the mourner from guilt and serves as a time to encourage a personal confession by the dying. Confession on the deathbed acknowledges the ending of one cycle and the beginning of another unknown cycle. The confession and the recitation of the shame in the last moments help the dying to affirm faith in God and focus on familiar rituals of life.

After death, the body is ritually washed by members of the Ritual Burial Society, and burial should occur within 24 hours. If a Jew dies on the Sabbath, he cannot be moved, except by a Gentile, until sundown. Jewish law does not allow autopsy and cremation.

The Jewish religion provides for survivors to work through the crisis of loss and mourning for a year. For the first 3 days deep grief is expressed by crying and the tearing of clothes to symbolize the tearing of a life from others. Seven days of lesser mourning follow; then 30 days are allowed for gradual readjustment. The remainder of the year is devoted to remembrance and healing. The dead are remembered by the Jewish community annually on the anniversary of the death.

The *Islam* religion excuses ill persons from religious rules, but many elderly Muslims will want to follow them as closely as possible. The person will want to go through his prayers at least symbolically if he is bedfast. Dietary beliefs should be respected. The Muslim does not drink alcoholic beverages, and pork is forbidden. The older, more conservative Muslim may have a fatalistic attitude that interferes with compliance to medical treatment; whatever happens is considered God's will. The family should be with the dying person. The dying person must confess his sins and beg forgiveness. After death, the family washes the body, folds the hands, and then faces the body toward Mecca. Only relatives and friends may touch the dead body; autopsy is forbidden.

EVALUATION

No known laboratory results or vital sign measures correlate with effective spiritual care, although as the person gains a feeling of peace and serenity, his disease condition may improve or he may be more active and alert than he was previously.

Spirituality cuts across all cultural and denominational lines and makes us all more alike than different. Genuine respect and love can break through barriers of confusion, loneliness, alienation, and social, cultural, and denominational differences.

REFERENCES

1. ABBOTT, WALTER, and JOSEPH GALLAGER, eds., *The Documents of Vatican II.* New York: The American Press, 1966.

2. ABERNETHY, GEORGE, and THOMAS LANGFORD, eds., *Philosophy of Religion: A Book of Readings.* London: Macmillan Co., 1968.

3. ALLPORT, GORDON, *The Individual and His Religion.* New York: Macmillan Publishing Co., Inc., 1961.

4. BERKOWITZ, PHILIP, and NANCY BERKOWITZ, "The Jewish Patient in the Hospital," *American Journal of Nursing,* 67: No. 11 (1967), 2335–37.

5. BISCHOFF, LEDFORD, *Adult Psychology.* New York: Harper & Row, Publishers, Inc., 1969.

6. BOROS, LADISLAUS, *Pain and Providence,* trans. Edward Quinn. Baltimore: Helicon Press, 1965.

7. BROWN, ROBERT, *The Spirit of Protestantism.* New York: Oxford University Press, 1961.

8. BUTLER, RICHARD, "The Roman Catholic Way in Death and Mourning," in *Concerning Death: A Practical Guide for the Living,* ed. Earl Grollman. Boston: Beacon Press, 1974, pp. 101–18.

9. CAMPBELL, TERESA, and BETTY CHANG, "Health Care of the Chinese in America," *Nursing Outlook,* 21: No. 4 (1973), 245–49.

10. CRAIG, GRACE, *Human Development.* Englewood Cliffs, N.J.: Prentice-Hall, Inc., 1976.

11. CROONENBURG, ENGELBERT, *Gateway to Reality: An Introduction to Philosophy.* Pittsburgh: Duquesne University, 1967.

12. deSAINT EXUPERY, ANTOINE, *The Little Prince.* New York: Harcourt, Brace and World, Inc., 1943.

13. DEVOL, THOMAS, "Ecstatic Pentecostal Prayer and Meditation," *Journal of Religion and Health,* 13: No. 4 (1974), 285–88.

14. DIXON, DOROTHY, *World Religions for the Classroom.* West Mystic, Conn.: Twenty-Third Publications, 1975.

15. DUSKA, RONALD, and MARIELLEN WHELAN, *Moral Development: A Guide to Piaget and Kohlberg.* New York: Paulist Press, 1975.

16. DUVALL, EVELYN, *Family Devlopment,* 5th ed. Philadelphia: J. B. Lippincott Company, 1977.

17. ERIKSON, ERIK, *Childhood and Society,* 2nd ed. New York: W. W. Norton and Co., Inc., 1963.

18. GOLDBRUNNER, JOSEF, *Holiness Is Wholeness: and Other Essays.* Notre Dame, Ind.: University of Notre Dame Press, 1964.

19. GORDON, AUDREY, "The Jewish View of Death: Guidelines for Mourning," in *Death, The Final Stage of Growth,* ed. Elisabeth Kubler-Ross. Englewood Cliffs, N.J.: Prentice-Hall, Inc., 1975, pp. 44–51.

20. HAMMOND, GUYTON, *Paul Tillich and Erich Fromm Compared: Man in Estrangement.* Nashville, Tenn.: Vanderbilt University Press, 1965.

21. HURLOCK, ELIZABETH, *Developmental Psychology,* 4th ed. New York: McGraw-Hill Book Company, 1975.

22. JORDON, MERLE, "The Protestant Way in Death and Mourning," in *Concerning Death: A Practical Guide for the Living,* ed. Earl Grollman. Boston: Beacon Press, 1974, pp. 81–100.

23. JUNG, CARL, *Man and His Symbols.* Garden City, N.Y.: Doubleday and Co., Inc., 1964.

24. ———, *Analytical Psychology: Its Theory and Practice.* New York: Random House, Inc., 1968.

25. KOHLBERG, LAWRENCE, *Recent Research in Moral Development.* New York: Holt, Rinehart and Winston, 1971.

26. LANG, BRUCE, "The Death That Ends Death in Hinduism and Buddhism," in *Death, the Final Stage of Growth,* ed. Elisabeth Kubler-Ross. Englewood Cliffs, N.J.: Prentice-Hall, Inc., 1975, pp. 52–57.

27. MAY, ROLLO, *Man's Search for Himself.* New York: W. W. Norton and Co., Inc., 1953.

28. McCONKIE, BRUCE, *Mormon Doctrine.* Salt Lake City, Utah: Bookcraft, 1966.

29. McMAHON, EDWIN, and PETER CAMPBELL. *Please Touch.* Mission, Kansas: Sheed & Ward, Inc., 1969.

30. MEAD, FRANK, *Handbook of Denominations in the United States,* 4th ed. New York: Abingdon Press, 1965.

31. MORRIS, K., and J. FOERSTER, "Team Work: Nurse and Chaplain," *American Journal of Nursing,* 72: No. 12 (1972), 2197–99.

32. MURRAY, RUTH, and JUDITH ZENTNER, *Nursing Concepts for Health Promotion*, 2nd ed. Englewood Cliffs, N.J.: Prentice-Hall, Inc., 1979.

33. NAIMAN, H., "Nursing in Jewish Law," *American Journal of Nursing*, 70: No. 11 (1970), 2378–79.

34. NOUWEN, HENRI, *Intimacy: Pastoral Psychological Essays.* Notre Dame, Ind.: Fides Publishers, Inc., 1969.

35. ———, *The Wounded Healer.* Garden City, N.Y.: Doubleday and Co., Inc., 1972.

36. ———, *Reaching Out: The Three Movements of the Spiritual Life.* Garden City, N.Y.: Doubleday and Co., Inc., 1975.

37. ———, "Coping with the Seven O'Clock News: Compassion in a Calloused World," *Sojourners,* September, 1977, 15–18.

38. PADAVANO, ANTHONY, *Dawn Without Darkness.* New Jersey: Paulist Press, 1971.

39. PAULUS, TRINA, *Hope for the Flowers.* New York: Newman Press, 1972.

40. PIEPGRAS, RUTH, "The Other Dimension: Spiritual Help," *American Journal of Nursing,* 68: No. 12 (1968), 2610–13.

41. PILL, ROBERT, "The Christian Science Practitioner," *Journal of Pastoral Counseling,* 4: No. 1 (1969), 39–42.

42. PORATH, THOMAS, "Humanizing the Sacrament of the Sick," *Hospital Progress,* 53: No. 7 (1972), 45–47.

43. POWELL, JOHN, *Why Am I Afraid to Tell You Who I Am?* Niles, Ill.: Argus Communications, 1969.

44. ———, *Fully Human, Fully Alive.* Niles, Ill.: Argus Communications, 1976.

45. "Recognizing Your Patient's Spiritual Needs," *Nursing '77,* 7: No. 12 (1977), 64–70.

46. SAUNDERS, E. DALE, *Buddhism in Japan.* Philadelphia: University of Philadelphia Press, 1964, 265–86.

47. SMITH, HUSTON, *The Religions of Man.* New York: Harper & Row, Publishers, Inc., 1965.

48. TILLICH, PAUL, *The Courage to Be.* New Haven, Conn.: Yale University Press, 1952.

49. TINNEY, JAMES, "Black Muslims," *Christianity Today,* 20: (March 12, 1976), 51–52.

50. TOURNIER, PAUL, *The Meaning of Persons.* New York: Harper & Row, Publishers, Inc., 1957.

51. ———, *The Adventure of Living.* New York: Harper & Row, Publishers, Inc., 1957.

52. ———, *Learn to Grow Old.* New York: Harper & Row, Publishers, Inc., 1972.

53. *Unity School of Christianity.* Unity Village, Mo.: Unity School of Christianity, n.d.

54. UTT, RICHARD, *The Builders: A Photo Story of Seventh Day Adventists at Work Around the World.* Mountain View, Calif.: Pacific Press Publishing Association, 1970.

55. VAN KAAM, ADRIAN, *Religion and Personality.* Englewood Cliffs, N.J.: Prentice Hall, Inc., 1964.

56. ———, *Spirituality and the Gentle Life.* Denville, N.J.: Bimention Books, Inc., 1974.

PHYSICAL ILLNESS IN LATER MATURITY:
Related Nursing Process

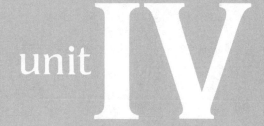

unit **IV**

problems of mobility in later maturity

15

Many persons in later maturity experience problems in transporting themselves within their environment as a result of aging changes, disease, and social or psychological factors. This chapter will deal primarily with changes within the musculoskeletal system that make walking and other movements difficult.

Chapter 9 presents physical aging changes caused by passage of time rather than those resulting from disease process or injury. This chapter applies the nursing process to the person with the nursing diagnosis of *limited mobility*, regardless of underlying pathogenesis. The steps of assessment, formulation of goals and planning, implementation, and evaluation will be identified and discussed for specific nursing diagnoses.

IMMOBILITY: A CONCEPT

Definitions

Although this chapter focuses on limitations of physical mobility, the concept of immobility must first be explored. *Immobility, unavoidable or prescribed restriction of movement in any sphere of a person's life,* must be viewed in a broad context.[30] Immobility may be physical, emotional, social, or intellectual in nature. *Physical immobility* refers not only to arthritis, casts, or traction, but also to being unable to shop because there are too many stairs or insufficient energy to carry the packages. *Emotional immobility* refers to excessively rigid thinking that prevents trying new activities or to emotional illness such as depression that prevents expression of feelings and interchange with others. *Social immobility* refers to disengagement, apathy, or even widowhood which causes the person to curtail or avoid social relationships. *Intellectual immobility* refers to loss or disuse of memory and problem-solving skills so that the person does not continue to learn information that is essential to living. Physical impairments have emotional and social ramifications. In turn, being emotionally upset or socially isolated has physiological consequences. Such interrelationships in immobility are especially apparent in later maturity.[10,30]

Hazards of Immobility

Major effects of physical immobility on the body are summarized in the following charts.[31]

Cardiovascular

1. Vasomotor control is affected; orthostatic hypotension, venous stasis, and decreased neurovascular reflex control of blood vessels with vasodilation occur.
2. Cardiac workload is increased in the supine position because of altered dis-

tribution of blood throughout the body and increased circulating blood volume.
3. Thrombus formation is increased because of venous stasis, increased blood viscosity associated with dehydration, and increased blood calcium level, producing blood hypercoagulability.
4. Intima of blood vessels are damaged by maintaining one position for a prolonged time, inhibiting circulation and predisposing to thrombus.

Respiratory
1. Respiratory rate decreases and oxygen-carbon dioxide balance is altered because of reduced basal metabolism, less oxygen requirement by cells, and less carbon dioxide production in cell metabolism.
2. Chest expansion is reduced because of position, posture, rigid rib cage, and reduced strength of pectoral muscles.
3. Secretions pool because of reduced respiratory movement.
4. Respiratory acidosis may occur because of adaptational response to accumulation of carbon dioxide from lack of respiratory movement and pooled secretions. Temporary stimulation of the respiratory center causes the aortic and carotid bodies to react against the stimulus, in turn depressing respiratory centers.

Nutrition and Elimination
1. Nitrogen balance is reversed, increasing catabolism and protein loss.
2. Anorexia occurs first as an adaptive response to decreased metabolic requirements but then contributes to undernutrition.
3. Gastrointestinal function and metabolic processes are impaired, affecting food ingestion and waste elimination.
4. Constipation or fecal impaction results from decreased peristalsis, weakened abdominal muscles, unnatural position for defecation, ignoring of gastrocolic reflex, and nutritional factors such as dehydration and lack of bulk food intake.

Skeletal Muscular
1. Osteoporosis and resulting bone compression or fracture from demineralization occur because osteoblasts stop forming new bone when the stimulus of movement is gone while osteoclasts continue their destructive process.
2. Muscular strength is reduced because of atony and disuse atrophy.
3. Muscular contracture results from disuse atrophy and pull of the flexor muscle.
4. Joint range of motion is reduced; contractures may result.
5. Circulatory exchange to soft tissue decreases with muscle disuse.

Integumentary
1. Skin breakdown occurs because of impaired circulation and localized ischemia from pressure, with lack of oxygen and nutrition to the cells, and resulting from negative nitrogen balance that causes malnourishment.

2. Heat loss is increased because of vasodilation caused by the supine position and pressure on body surfaces, resulting in perspiration.

Urinary Excretion
1. Urinary stasis occurs in the renal pelvis because urine must leave the kidney against an upward gradient when the person is supine.
2. Urine volume decreases because of altered circulation.
3. Urine composition changes because of protein breakdown, bone demineralization, circulatory changes, and often the presence of dehydration.
4. Renal calculi form and infections occur because of urine stasis, alkaline urine, decreased urine volume, and increased mineral salts in the urine.

Psychosocial
1. Ego identity is distorted because movement is restricted and socialization is reduced.
2. Emotional responses of withdrawal, apathy, regression, or aggressivity occur because of perceived loss of control.
3. Drives and expectations are reduced; body rhythms and life-style are tied to inactivity.
4. Sensory diminution or deprivation may occur, causing changes in time, space, and reality perception, suspicion, hallucinations, illusions, and delusions.
5. Ability to concentrate and do problem solving are reduced, causing impaired learning and motivation.
6. Social roles are reversed, changed, or eliminated, causing low self-esteem and changed reactions from others.
7. Values and ideals concerning motion or movement are threatened, causing further regression and disorganization of personality.

ASSESSMENT

Your assessment must always consider the presence of the various hazards of immobility as well as the more specific points discussed in the following pages. Comprehensive assessment contributes to individualized care.

Range of Motion

Mobility assessment begins with determination of range of motion in all joints. The normal range of motion of the major joints in the body is summarized below.[3,13]

Upper Extremity

Wrists: Flexion, 90°   Extension, 70°
         Radial deviation, 20°   Ulnar deviation, 55°

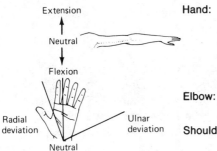

Hand: Metacarpophalangeal:
            Flexion, 90°   Hyperextension, 30°
       Proximal interphalangeal:
            Flexion, 120°   Extension, 0°
       Distal interphalangeal:
            Flexion, 80°

Elbow: Flexion, 160°   Extension, 0°
        Supination, 90°   Pronation, 90°

Shoulder: Forward flexion, 180°   Extension, 50°
           External rotation, 90°   Internal rotation, 90°
           Abduction   Adduction
             (away from body), 180°   (toward body), 50°

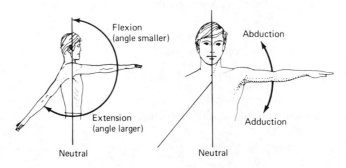

Lower Extremity

Ankle: Dorsiflexion, 20°   Plantar flexion, 45°
        Inversion, 30°   Eversion, 20°

Knee: Flexion, 130°   Hyperextension, 15°

Hip: With knee straight
            Flexion, 90°   Hyperextension, 15°
        With knee flexed—   Flexion, 120°
            Abduction, 45°   Adduction, 30°
            Internal rotation, 40°   External rotation, 45°

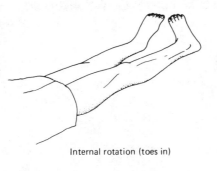

Internal rotation (toes in)

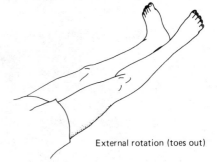

External rotation (toes out)

Spine

Neck: Chin to chest, 45°; Occiput to spine, 55°
        Lateral bending, 40° to right and left
        Rotation, 70° to right and left

Back: Flexion—forward bending, 75–90°
        Extension—backward bending, 30°
        Lateral bending, 35° to right and left
        Rotation, 30° to right and left

When checking range of motion of joints, also note swelling, heat, redness, pain, crepitation, masses, and deformity.

Muscle Strength

Muscle strength contributes to mobility and must be assessed. Grading muscles of extremities and neck from zero to 5 is subjective, but it does provide some frame of reference for reporting.[10]

5 – Strength at 100%   – Normal – Complete range of motion against gravity with full resistance.

4 – Strength at 75%   – Good – Complete range of motion against gravity with some resistance.

3 – Strength at 50%   – Fair – Complete range of motion against gravity.

2 – Strength at 25%   – Poor – Complete range of motion without gravity.

1 – Strength at 10%   – Trace – Evidence of slight contractility. No joint motion.

0 – Strength at 0%   – Zero – No evidence of contractility.[13,25]

Muscle tone is decreased in diseases of the anterior brain cell, peripheral nerves, and cerebellum. A spastic tone is found in pyramidal tract diseases and varies from normal to marked increase as the extremity is flexed and extended. If there is continued pressure, the tone gradually decreases. Rigidity characterizes extrapyramidal disease, and increased tone is present throughout the full range of motion.[3,13]

Reflexes

Nerve innervation at the reflex level is assessed with range of motion and muscle strength. A deep tendon reflex is dependent on intactness of sensory nerves, functioning synapse in the spinal cord, intactness of the motor nerves and neuromuscular junction, and a competent muscle. Reflexes of this type are not dependent on higher levels of motor function in the cord and brain. Higher motor pathways can affect reflex activity and are required for smooth, coordinated, voluntary movements.[3,13]

These higher motor pathways are summarized in Table 15.1.[3,25]

TABLE 15.1   Summary of Higher Motor Pathways That Affect Reflex Action

Structure	Origin	Pathway	Function
Pyramidal tract	Motor cortex of brain	Between brain stem, cord, anterior horn cell.	Maintains fine, discrete, conscious, voluntary movement.
Extrapyramidal tracts	Cortex	Between cortex, basal ganglia, brainstem, and cord but outside pyramidal tract.	Maintain muscle tone; control gross automatic muscular movements.
Cerebellar system	Cerebellum	Receives both sensory and motor input.	Coordinates muscular activity; maintains equilibrium; controls posture.

All three of these motor pathways ultimately are dependent on the anterior horn cell. A lesion in any of these tracts or areas will affect reflex and other movement. The type and location of the motor deficit help to localize the lesion.[3]

The deep tendon reflexes localize the segmental level of the cord if pathology exists there. The reflex and segmental level being tested are listed below:[3,13,25]

Reflex	Segmental level
Biceps	Cervical 5, 6
Brachioradialis	Cervical 5, 6
Triceps	Cervical 7, 8
Knee—patellar	Lumbar 2, 3, 4
Ankle—Achilles	Lumbar 5 to Sacral 2

A book on physical diagnosis should be consulted on how to test these reflexes.[3,24] A grading system similar to that for muscle strength is used for reporting reflexes.[13,25]

0	Absent
1+	Decreased
2+	Normal
3+	Hyperactive
4+	Hyperactive with clonus (a sustained spastic flexing of a joint after quickly extending or flexing it and maintaining tension on the tendon).

Hypoactive reflexes occur in any disease that interferes with the anterior horn cell or the sensory or motor muscle. Hyperactive reflexes almost invariably represent disease of the upper motor neuron or pyramidal tract.[25]

Gait and Posture

Gait and posture are assessed immediately upon meeting the patient (review posture changes described in Chapter 9). A normal person should be able to walk a fairly straight line for 10 to 20 feet with eyes open or closed.[25]

Since cerebellar functioning (such as gait and balance) is important to mobility, it is tested. The **Romberg test**, *in which the person is asked to stand with eyes closed and feet together,* tests standing balance. A positive Romberg is the inability to maintain balance with eyes closed but ability to do so with eyes open. Coordination and ability to perform rapid alternating movements test cerebellar status. The person can be asked to pronate and supinate the hands rapidly and may be directed to tap each foot rapidly on the floor. Running the heel of one foot down the opposite shin from knee to ankle is another cerebellar test.[13,25]

Characteristic gaits that indicate pathology are summarized in Table 15.2.[3,13,25]

TABLE 15.2.   Summary of Gaits Indicating Pathology

Gait	Definition	Pathology
Spastic hemiparesis	One arm flexed, close to side and immobile. Leg circled stiffly outward and forward; toe dragging.	Unilateral upper motor neuron disease.
Scissors	Legs advanced slowly and thighs crossed forward on each other.	Bilateral spastic paresis of the legs.
Steppage	Feet lifted high, knees flexed and then brought down with slap.	Associated with footdrop secondary to lower motor neuron disease.
Sensory ataxia	Unsteady with feet wide apart, lifted high, and brought down with slap. Watches his feet; cannot stand with eyes closed.	Loss of position sense in legs. Posterior column disease, as seen in tabes dorsalis.
Cerebellar ataxia	Staggering, wide-based, and exaggeration on turns. Cannot stand steadily with feet together with eyes open or closed.	Disease of cerebellum. Staggering is toward affected side.
Parkinsonian	Stooped posture with hip and knees flexed. Short, shuffling steps. Decreased arm swings. Turns stiffly as a whole.	Basal ganglia defect of Parkinson's Disease.
Trendelenburg	Fall of pelvis on side opposite the involved hip when it is weight bearing.	Weakness of the abductor muscles due to muscle disease, lack of innervation of the muscle or unstable hip joint.

TABLE 15.2. *Continued*

Gait	Definition	Pathology
Antalgic	Leans over the involved hip as weight is borne on it.	Patient's attempts to minimize the force borne through to hip to decrease pain or arthritis or other hip joint pathology.

Peripheral Sensation

The senses of vibration, motion, position, pain, temperature, and touch are assessed because peripheral sensation is fundamental to mobility. At the same time the skin and peripheral vasculature should be noted for intactness and adequacy of function. Color, temperature, presence of hair, lesions, condition of nails, and presence of calluses, corns, rashes, and injuries should all be noted in the extremities. A corn can inhibit mobility considerably.

Extraneous Movements

Abnormal movements will interfere with mobility and should be assessed. The more common ones that appear are described below:[13,25]

Resting, nonintention tremor (Parkinsonism)	Evident in both hands, arms, head, tongue, and legs. Associated with increased muscle tone and cogwheeling of joints (rhythmical increase and decrease in tone superimposed on passive movements produced by examiner).
Essential (familial or senile) tremor	Absent or minimal at rest but more pronounced with sustained posture or movement. More likely to involve the head. No alteration in muscle tone.
Intention tremor (Multiple Sclerosis)	Evident when purposeful movement is called for.
Choreic movements	Purposeless, irregular, involuntary, spontaneous movements of one or more joints, face, mouth, or tongue. Increased tone present.
Athetoid movements	Slow, writhing movements of proximal parts of the extremities, trunk, and face. Seen in cerebral palsy.

Activities of Daily Living

Activities of daily living are assessed relative to mobility. Mobility must be present to some degree if the person is to be an independent, contributing member of a community. The ability to carry out activities of daily living is based not only on being able to perform the task manually but also on having the motivation, opportunity, and resources to perform it safely and effectively. Thus, activities of daily living are best assessed in the individual's own environment whenever possible, preferably when he is not aware that he is being tested. The community health nurse may be the one best equipped to assess this.

Activities that should be assessed are:

1. *Walking*—distance without discomfort; number of stairs without discomfort; usual amount each day; assistive devices needed, such as walker, cane, crutches.
2. *Wheelchair*—ability to transfer from bed to chair and back; from chair to auto and back; from chair to toilet and back; from chair to tub or shower and back.
3. *Bedridden*—ability to change position.
4. *Stooping, bending, kneeling, reaching,* and *climbing.*
5. *Hygiene*—ability to toilet or manipulate bedpan, urinal, toilet tissue; bathe, shave, use makeup, comb and shampoo hair; and perform oral hygiene.
6. *Eating*—ability to shop for groceries; prepare meals; eat meals, cut food, and use utensils; drink from glass or cup.
7. *Dressing*—ability to get into underpants, bra, undershirt; dress, shirt, trousers; socks, stockings, shoes; corset, girdle, brace, sling; and fasten buttons, zippers, belts, and snaps.
8. *Other*—ability to speak, hear, and see; dial, answer, talk, and hear on phone; read and write; straighten and clean environment; leave immediate environment and travel to another place by walking, driving, or using public transportation; and care for financial and other affairs.

Assessment of the person in his home includes considering his role in the home, the presence or absence of others, and the extent to which the home is an asset or detriment. Assessment of safety and hygiene factors are important, but comfort and security factors are equally important. We can become so concerned about the elderly eating enough or hurting themselves that the solutions for protection we offer may cut off opportunities for enjoyment of life, freedom of choice, or contact with things that are an extension of self or a source of productivity or amusement.[1]

Emotional and Social Response

Chronicity and grief are aspects of limited mobility, since most persons in later maturity can move less freely than earlier in life. Normal biological changes, upon which is superimposed any of the conditions to be discussed in this chapter, limit motion to some degree, even if the person can manage self-care and normal household tasks. For some elderly people, the bed or wheelchair constitutes their world. Regardless of the degree of limited mobility, the person perceives himself becoming less mobile instead of more active in the future. He is gradually or suddenly losing something highly valued, depending on the situation, which usually is never fully regained. As a result, self-concept and personality changes may occur. He is likely to feel restricted or damaged, less worthwhile, more fearful, and suspicious of and angry at people who move fast. Irritability at self and others is common. He grieves over the loss of the former active self; depression results unless the person is able to mourn his loss and then recognize his remaining strengths.

Body image, the mental picture of the body as an object in space and attitudes about the body, changes. Often deformity, pain, decreased strength and endurance, incoordination, or extraneous movements combine with the reduced range of motion to cause the person to feel unattractive, inefficient, and rejected by others. The ability to maintain an intact and realistic body image depends on the opportunity to maneuver the body physically in the environment. The more physically active person has a better defined body boundary and a more precise mental picture of what his body can do and how much space he needs to do a task. The wheelchair-bound person tends to have a distorted body image, and until the wheelchair becomes a part of his body image he frequently bumps into objects and has difficulty pushing himself. Even the ambulatory person can no longer depend on his body to carry out tasks automatically and effectively. He feels vulnerable to intrusion as he receives stares from others, is accidentally bumped or deliberately shoved, and is overwhelmed by bombardment from environmental stimuli. He feels less able to protect himself from ordinary or unusual hazards: uneven sidewalks; narrow, steep stairways; strong gusts of wind; fast-moving vehicles; running children; purse snatchings; or fire in a building. The discussion about body image and self-concept in Chapter 11 is relevant to the person with limited mobility.

Sexuality, how the person sees self as man or woman and ability to maintain a physical and emotional relationship, is threatened by actual physical as well as body image changes. The person may be too uncomfortable or tired for intercourse; the partner may fear hurting the person or feel repulsed by the person's appearance. This mutual avoidance may result in the spouses not touching, kissing, or fondling each other, even though each may desire being close to the other. Often conflicts over physical sexuality spill over into other areas of life; they cause arguments or resentful silence, interfere with social and leisure activities, or cause the partner to spend less time at home.[19] The discussion about sexuality in Chapter 11 is pertinent to the person with the nursing diagnosis of limited mobility.

Interactions with family members and others are often affected by limited mobility. The more limited the mobility, the more dependent is the person. The more dependent, the more he feels like a burden and of no value. Thus, the person may strive to remain independent and may overcompensate, attempting tasks he cannot manage, which exasperates the family because of the hazards involved. The person who cannot accept help causes the family to feel rejected, helpless, guilty, and angry. Alternately, the person may demand to be cared for; the person who in the past was pushed into excessive responsibility and was forced to be independent may feel that it is his turn to be waited on. Or family members may smother the person with care and attention, simultaneously expressing nonverbally their feelings of anger at his inability to care for himself. The elderly person is left with feelings of confusion, bewilderment, and ultimately feelings of worthlessness. Most families try hard to be as helpful as possible, but, there is usually a limit to the dependency they can tolerate. Health workers and family may convey to the person that his dependency is unacceptable. Thus, the person must work through dependency and independency conflicts, feelings of infantilization, and desires to be self-sufficient. The discussion about family relationships in Chapter 12 is pertinent to this situation.

Many of these emotional and social responses can be assessed in contacts with the person, that is, through observing what he says and does and how he appears. Tactful questions can also provide some of the answers. However, what the patient or family says is not always indicative of actual or potential abilities or emotional and social responses.

After assessing mobility, an accurate recording should be made so that others may be aware of this person's uniqueness. Documentation is necessary for planning and evaluating care; documentation is also the foundation for accountability for the level, amount, and quality of care given the patient.

NURSING DIAGNOSIS AND FORMULATION OF PATIENT CARE GOALS

Nursing Diagnosis

When your assessment indicates impairment in the areas just described, the *nursing diagnosis is limited or impaired mobility,* which relates to several medical diagnoses, as follows:

1. Limited mobility of a muscular origin.
2. Limited mobility arising from joint pathology.
3. Limited mobility resulting from fractures and orthopedic surgery.
4. Limited mobility caused by paralysis (CVA).
5. Limited mobility of a extrapyramidal origin (Parkinsonism).
6. Limited mobility of a cerebellar origin.

In this chapter discussion of the first three diagnoses will relate nursing diagnosis, patient care goals, and nursing intervention to pathology. The last three diagnoses will be discussed in Chapter 16 on neuroregulatory mechanisms because of the interrelationship of those nursing diagnoses and pathologies.

Patient Care Goals

Long-term care goals for any person with limited mobility include:

1. Full range of motion is present in all joints.
2. Joints with limitation in motion are stabilized or improved.
3. Pain is not present or is controlled.
4. Activities of daily living are performed independently or with minimal assistance.
5. Ambulation and self-care are resumed as soon after injury or surgery as possible.
6. Complications such as pneumonia, atelectasis, decubiti, wound infections, and impaction are not experienced.

These goals are optimal and may not be applicable to all patients/clients. However, they are a guide to help you to formulate specific, individualized goals.

Short-term goals are written pertinent to the specific symptoms, needs, and condition of the individual person and relate to each long-term goal. What short-term goals can you formulate that are specific to the person you are caring for?

NURSING INTERVENTION

Nursing Interventions Applicable to All Persons with Limited Mobility

Since most elderly persons with limited mobility are living at home, health promotion measures are as important in your repertoire of nursing interventions as are measures related to the hospital or nursing home.

This chapter will first discuss general nursing interventions that are useful in achieving the patient care goals listed above. Then specific nursing intervention will be discussed in relation to limited mobility of muscular origin, arising from joint pathology, and resulting from fractures and orthopedic surgery.

Emotional care may be the most essential, for if the senior has a negative attitude or upset feelings, safety factors and rehabilitation measures are likely to be disregarded.

Help the person work through his situation of being less active and to resolve feelings related to chronicity and grief. Listen to him complain about what he cannot do, reminisce about his past active life, and express bitterness about future plans that he will not be able to realize. Listening and emotional support is time-consuming; the topic is not pleasant, and response to your support may be slow. Yet, unless the senior can ventilate his feelings, your teaching, positive reinforcement, and efforts at rehabilitation will not be utilized. Becoming less mobile is an aspect of the crisis of getting old, which then becomes part of a chronic problem. Crisis, grief, and chronicity are often best resolved by having the person express his feelings verbally. Then he can begin to perceive what he can still do, which is more effective than being told how well off he is. Ventilating anger, sadness, and fears also frees him to begin to hope, to problem solve, and to think about how to modify his environment, life routines, and leisure activities to meet his needs to the best of his ability for the remaining years. Use principles related to resolution of grief and mourning from Chapter 13 as you work with this person and family.

Reintegration of body image can be promoted in several ways. Your acceptance of the person's appearance and disability is essential to his eventual self-acceptance. Give him every possible opportunity to practice using various positions, exercises, or devices to help him better maneuver himself and manage activities of daily living. Verbal explanation of what he is practicing and use of visual cues, such as looking in a mirror or at a videotape or photograph, also help him better visualize mentally his body as it functions. Recognize his personality strengths and accomplishments toward self-care and independent living. Other principles of care that apply to this person are found in Chapter 11.

Explore obvious coping mechanisms with the senior. Often the person with limited mobility uses the adaptive mechanisms of normalization and renormalization. *Normalization includes doing everything possible to keep up with others and putting on a facade or giving excuses when he cannot stay apace.* for example, he may blame slower movements and deformity on an accident rather than arthritis because he perceives his disease as a stigma. *Renormalizing means to adjust to physical changes by decreasing activity, justifying inactivity, working through fears of dependency, eliciting help when necessary, and balancing the effect of drugs taken for symptom relief against the side effects* these drugs sometimes produce.[43]

Exploration of coping mechanisms does not mean a deep interpretation of all behavior and thoughts. Such exploration would be threatening, and the person who is ill or in pain has little energy to be introspective or to stand back and observe all of his reactions. At times the senior is so involved with maintaining his sense of self that he has reduced self-awareness. Exploration of behavior and feelings must always be done in the context of a relationship and with empathy and concern. At times, instead of exploring you will be supportive to his behavior. Yet, helping the person understand the normalization and renormalization mechanisms can help him become more accepting of his situation and of his need for help.

Encourage communication between partners about personal and each other's feelings, desires, and reactions so that sexuality can remain an integrated part of self-concept and life. Explore with the couple the importance of maintaining masculinity or femininity in various ways and expressing affection in ways other than coitus. Various social activities as well as intercourse can be planned for when the person is less uncomfortable or tired. Rest, heat, and medications can be used prior to activities. The couple can also explore the use of different positions during intercourse so that the person can participate more fully and with more enjoyment. Certainly, you must feel comfortable about the topic of sexuality, in its broadest sense, to discuss it with anyone.[19]

Work with family members as necessary: listen to their feelings; help them find solutions to their problems; encourage family members to talk honestly with each other, and refer them to other services if necessary.

Promote independence by teaching the senior how to maintain a balance between rest and activity. Include family members in your teaching so that they will allow the senior to do as much as he is able. They can also help to motivate the person to maintain a job or social activities by expressing their encouragement and interest. Encourage the person to accept help with tasks that are beyond his functional abilities.

Encourage adequate nutrition first by determining daily eating patterns, food preferences, and nutritional intake. Then appropriate instruction can be given. The person who lives alone or is homebound is more likely to use processed, packaged foods. Some of these have questionable nutritional value and may be high in calories. Instruction in the Basic 4 foods or referral to meals-on-wheels may be needed. If there is no meals-on-wheels program available, a neighbor or family member should be approached to do grocery shopping and possibly to prepare meals. If the person can do his own shopping, he should be taught which foods are less expensive and of higher nutritional value. For example, a person living alone may find it difficult to finish a whole can of vegetables before spoilage occurs. Frozen vegetables and fruits or small cans may be more economical. Potato flakes, instant rice, dry onion flakes, dry cereals, frozen orange juice, powdered milk, and instant tea and coffee can all be kept for a considerable time with proper storage. Meat can also be kept frozen for long periods of time. Individual servings, wrapped and frozen, can be prepared rapidly and with minimal effort. Bread can also be frozen and individual portions used as needed. If the patient does not have a freezer or refrigerator, more of a problem is presented. Then dry and canned foods must be relied on.

Cooking becomes increasingly hazardous as the person ages and loses mobility. Some TV dinners or ready-to-heat-and-serve-foods are tasty and adequate nutritionally. Family members or friends can prepare such packages for later use if the person has a freezer. A small countertop electric oven can be purchased and used to heat most foods. Standing at the stove to cook is fatiguing; bending over to transfer food in and out of the oven can result in fainting, falls, or burns.

Promoting a safe environment is a challenge for the person and family. Your responsibility as a nurse begins well before the accident occurs. Much orthopedic surgery, especially that precipitated by fractures, can be prevented by appropriate safety measures.[12] Through your home assessment and instruction you can help the elderly person understand the importance of the following safety measures:

1. Dark halls and stairwells must be adequately illuminated and free of clutter.
2. Night lights should be used.
3. Rugs, floors, and steps should be kept in good repair. Floors and steps should be kept unwaxed and clean of litter and spillage. Floor coverings should be free from holes, wrinkles, and rough spots, and firmly anchored.
4. Handrails should be installed on stairs, in bathrooms and hallways.
5. A tub seat and a tub handgrasp, or a chair alongside the tub and a chair or stool in the shower, as well as nonskid treads in the tub or on the shower floor should be used.
6. Electrical cords should not be stretched across heavily traveled areas in the room.
7. Electrical cords and outlets should be in good condition.
8. Pot handles should not extend over the edge of the stove; heavy pots should not be used for cooking.
9. Utensils, food, or other articles frequently used should be in an easily reached place.
10. Standing on ladders or chairs or reaching by standing on tiptoe should be discouraged since balance is reduced and tremor or ischemic attacks make this activity extremely hazardous.
11. Heavy objects should not be lifted since this may result in compression fractures due to osteoporosis.
12. Eyes should be examined frequently; failing sight and inadequate glasses are the cause of many accidents.
13. Low-heeled, well-fitted walking shoes in good repair should be worn instead of scuffs or slippers.

A very thorough safety checklist can be obtained from the National Society for Crippled Children and Adults.[35]

Constantly be alert for hazards that could result in accidents. The elderly driver should be aware that night driving may be more hazardous than in earlier life because his reaction time, recovery time from glare, and dark adaptation time all take longer.

The elderly must be discouraged from going out in icy and snowy weather. Even short trips can have tragic results. For example, Mrs. J. Z., 66 years old, walked from her porch to the garage to take out the trash. She slipped on a small icy patch; a fractured neck of the femur required a prosthesis. An ounce of prevention is truly worth a pound of cure.

The local fire and police departments should be notified where every elderly person with limited mobility lives in their districts. They can be very helpful in observing the person and his external environment and they are often called to help in nonemergency but stressful situations.

Limited Mobility of a Muscular Origin: Pathology and Nursing Intervention

Muscular weakness, wasting of skeletal muscles, and decrease in muscular strength and endurance are common in later maturity and can be caused by the aging process. The number of muscle fibers decreases and regeneration does not occur. These changes first become obvious in the hands. Then arm and leg muscles become thin and flabby. The degree of weakness does not increase proportionally with the apparent wasting, but mobility is limited to some extent.

Muscle cramps may occur in later maturity because of peripheral vascular insufficiency, lowered sodium or calcium plasma levels, or peripheral nerve disease. In many situations the cause cannot be determined.

Muscle weakness can also arise from pathology of nervous innervation; weakness is a symptom in almost all disorders of the neuromuscular system. Muscle wasting accompanies weakness in diseases of the motor cortex, pyramidal tract, or extrapyramidal system. Weakness is accompanied by pain or tenderness of the muscles in spinal cord tumors and disc disorders. Abnormal movements such as fasciculations accompany weakness in progressive muscular atrophy, and grosser abnormal movements occur in some extrapyramidal diseases.

Disorders at the neuromuscular junction, such as in myasthenia gravis, also cause weakness. The muscles innervated by the cranial nerves are particularly involved (neck, trunk, and extremities). Initial symptoms are most common in the extraocular muscles. Muscles of respiration are affected in severe disease.

Electrolyte imbalance, especially insufficient potassium, will cause muscle weakness. Since so many persons in later maturity receive diuretics, loss of potassium occurs and is a common cause of weakness. Substantial losses also occur in vomitus and diarrhea. Weakness is characteristically demonstrated in the muscles of one or more extremity, trunk, neck, and sometimes respiratory muscles. Tendon reflexes are decreased.

Hyperkalemia caused by renal disease; too rapid intravenous administration of potassium; hemolysis; acute acidosis; burns; and crush injuries can also cause impairment of skeletal, cardiac, and smooth muscle. Weakness occurs, but electromyographic and electrocardiographic findings vary from those found in hypokalemia.

Endocrine disorders also cause muscle weakness. Both hypofunction and hyperfunction of the thyroid, adrenals, and pituitary will cause muscle weakness.

Other causes of muscular weakness and fatigue are diabetes, artherosclerosis of the large vessels of the lower extremities, chronic malnutrition, disuse, and emotional problems.[38]

Medical treatment will be determined by the cause of the weakness. Thorough assessment, including physical examination, careful history, laboratory tests, and X-rays are required for diagnosis.

Nursing intervention depends on the cause. However, the nursing diagnosis of limited mobility of a muscular weakness origin should result in formulating goals and planning initial care to assure safety. Being available for assistance in ambulating, turning, and personal care are required.

Prevention of weakness may also be possible through health teaching about use of exercise, diet, and drugs. For example, the retired person often cuts exercise dramatically, limiting it to that necessary for daily living and little else. However, the sedentary person can maintain muscle tone and joint mobility. A booklet of exercises, *Exercises While You Watch TV,* can be obtained from Sickroom Supplies, Inc., 2534 S. Kinnickinnic Avenue, Milwaukee, Wisconsin 53207. The booklet has been endorsed by the National Council on Aging, *Aging* magazine (a publication of the HEW Office of Aging), and the National Institute of Health.

The elderly person living alone seldom takes time to get a balanced diet. If diuretics of the thiazide type are ordered without potassium supplement, encourage the person to eat a dietary supplement, such as orange juice, bananas, strawberries, prunes, Coca Cola (not Pepsi), apricots, asparagus, carrots, peaches, plums, spinach, milk, coffee, tea, cocoa and dried fruit. Good food sources are meat, fish, fowl, cereals, fruits, and vegetables. A diet adequate in protein, calcium, and iron contains enough potassium for ordinary requirements.[34]

Limited Mobility Resulting from Joint Pathology and Nursing Intervention

Osteoarthritis (*degenerative joint disease*) *is characterized by deterioration of the articular cartilage and formation of new bone at joint surfaces.* This pathology is common in later maturity and is a more common cause of disability than gout and rheumatoid arthritis combined.[5] Apparent contributing factors are age, trauma, mechanical stress, and genetic predisposition.

Early signs of the disease include joint tenderness upon pressure, pain on motion, and mild heat. Crepitation on motion is often present. Later changes include bony hypertrophy in the involved joints. The weight-bearing joints (hips, knees, lumbar, and cervical spine) are usually involved. The distal interphalangeal and proximal interphalangeal joints of the hands and the first metatarsophalangeal joints of the feet may also show changes. *Heberden nodes, enlargement of the terminal interphalangeal joint,* often occur in postmenopausal women.[7] Advanced changes may include deformities such as *subluxation* (*dislocation*), *genu varum* (*bowleg*) or *valgum* (*knock-knee*), and *coxa vera* (*decreased angle at head of femur with shaft*).[21]

Diagnosis can be made with X-rays that show narrowing of the joint space, which is caused by loss of cartilage, sclerosis of subchondrial bone, bony hypertrophy at joint margins, bone cysts, and deformities. Other laboratory tests are negative and help to differentiate osteoarthritis from other systemic arthropathy.[21]

Rheumatoid Arthritis is a systemic disease of the connective tissue, which is characterized by inflammation in the synovial membranes lining the joints and tendons. The cause is unknown, but it appears to be related to the body's immune system. This inflamed synovium hypertrophies and invades surrounding cartilage, bone, and tendons. The onset may be insidious or sudden. The polyarthritis is characterized by pain, swelling, heat, low-grade fever, malaise, and increased fatigability. Symmetrical joints are usually involved.[7] Joints of the hands and feet (proximal interphalangeal, metacarpaphalangeal, metatarsal phalangeal joints), wrists, knees, elbows, ankles, shoulders, hips, and temporomandibular are most frequently involved. The cervical spine is less frequently involved. The most characteristic lesion is the rheumatoid nodule found in connective tissue of almost any organ, but especially in synovial or periarticular tissue. Ulnar subluxation and deviation of the phalanges and flexion contractures may occur. These contractures are major causes of disability.[21] Early morning stiffness that subsides with exercise, known as the *gel phenomenon,* helps to distinguish rheumatoid from osteoarthritis. Osteoarthritis usually interferes with activity.

Laboratory findings include the presence of the rheumatoid factor (RA factor) in the serum of 80 to 90 percent of patients[7], elevated erythrocyte sedimentation rates, mild anemia, and positive antinuclear antibodies and/or lupus erythematosis cells in 10 to 20 percent of patients. X-rays show periarticular demineralization and soft-tissue swelling. Later, erosions of marginal bone and loss of cartilage appear. Deformities are apparent in advanced disease because of fibrous ankylosis and flexion contractures.[21]

Gout is an inflammatory arthropathy caused by the formation of microcrystals of monosodium urate or calcium pyrophosphate dehydrate in joints and surrounding tissues. The joints rapidly become swollen, red, hot, and painful. The joints most commonly involved are the great toe, instep, ankle, knee, elbow, and wrist. The attack, in which fever and leukocytosis are present, subsides after several days and a remission follows. As time passes, attacks become more frequent and joint involvement increases. Continual inflammation of multiple joints results and deformities occur. Tophaceous deposits are present in the chronic form of the illness and are found in ears, elbows, and tendons of the fingers and ankles.[21]

X-ray changes show soft-tissue swelling around the involved joints and punched-out lesions in the surrounding bone. Hyperuricemia occurs in acute attacks in most patients. Urate crystals in synovial fluid is diagnostic.[21]

Nursing intervention is directed toward maintaining a balance between rest and activity as well as meeting the patient care goals stated earlier. The person needs motivation to remain active in the presence of pain, especially if the demands of maintaining a job, keeping a house, or raising a family no longer exist. The drive to remain independent can be destroyed by the disability and pain of an arthropathy. One of your major objectives of nursing care is to assist the patient and his family in motivation, preservation of independence, and prevention of complications and added disability.

Any elderly person with an arthropathy in the hospital or long-term care facility needs a planned activity program as part of the rehabilitation plan. This program needs to be continued at home. Having the person do his own care is essential, even though he has pain or if it would be faster and easier for you to do it. Keep him up and mobile most of the day and maintain a normal schedule of sleeping and rising. Use of heat, massage, range of motion exercises, and proper alignment also help relieve stiffness and preserve joint function and muscular strength.

If an acute attack of rheumatoid arthritis or gout occurs, the patient may need to be on bedrest, but bedrest must be for as brief a time as possible. Even during bedrest the joints should be put through full range of motion exercises, if tolerated, and position should be changed every hour or two to prevent contracture formation. Bedrest should be avoided whenever possible because of the resulting hazards to the body, as described earlier, and indicated by the following case study.

Mr. J. H., a 63-year-old diabetic and arthritic, was confined to bed with diabetic acidosis for several weeks. When he could finally be ambulatory again, his hip was found to be ankylosed and partially flexed so that he could no longer assume a sitting or standing position. This extremely disabling and painful condition was finally corrected about one year later by a total hip replacement. Before surgery Mr. H.'s only wish was to be dead.

Teach the patient how to be independent in activities of daily living. Clothing with front closures, zippers instead of buttons, and elastic shoe strings make dressing easier. Back scratchers, long-handled graspers (e.g., fireplace log tongs), and built-up handles on silverware can assist with reaching and holding objects. Rearrangement of furniture and household goods in cabinets, closets, and refrigerator can make objects more accessible. Include the family in your teaching about maintaining and promoting self-care and independence; a well-meaning family can undo rehabilitation if they are not aware of the goals and approaches of care.

Referral of the homebound person to a home nursing agency, assistance from nursing, physical therapy, home health aid, and homemaker services, and sometimes meals-on-wheels, may result in the person maintaining some independence. Canes, crutches, walkers, and wheelchairs, as well as commodes, hospital beds, and other aids can often be obtained through the home health agency. However, one admonition is necessary. Assistive devices should not be initiated prematurely; for example, a person who is ambulatory should not be given a wheelchair to use routinely.

Other agencies that may exist in your community and that can be of assistance are the Council for the Aging; Health Department Nursing Services; Veterans' Administration Home Care Program; church-related nursing services, such as Cardinal Ritter Institute in St. Louis; or home care programs conducted by private hospitals, such as the one operated by Jewish Hospital in St. Louis. Nurses in occupational health, doctors' offices, hospitals, or nursing homes can make such referrals, depending on the person's needs and preference.

Surveillance of drug therapy is one of your important responsibilities. Many drugs have side effects that need to be observed and reported immediately.[27] Side effects, precautions, and contraindications have been summarized in Table 15.3.[6,21]

TABLE 15.3   Nursing Responsibilities for Drug Therapy in Arthropathy

Drug	Side Effects	Precautions	Contraindications
Salicylates (usually given in large doses)	Dyspepsia, gastrointestinal bleeding, peptic ulcer. Tinnitus, hearing impairment. Headaches. Vertigo. Irritability.	Patients with allergies, especially asthma, may have a severe allergic reaction to salicylates. Give with food. Observe for symptoms.	Potentiates warfarin (Coumadin). Should not be given to patients on Coumadin therapy or with peptic ulcer disease.
Ibuprofen (Motrin)	Less gastrointestinal toxicity than salicylates. Dyspepsia. Allergic reactions. Headache.	Observe for side effects.	
Indomethacin (Indocin) (initial dose low, not to exceed 100 mg)	Allergic reactions. Dyspepsia, gastrointestinal bleeding, peptic ulcer. Severe headaches, confusion, and mental disorders.	Give with food or an antacid. Observe for side effects.	Should be used with great caution in the elderly. May potentiate warfarin.
Phenylbutazone (Butazolidin); Oxyphenylbutazone (Tandearil)	Less toxic than Indomethacin. Bone marrow suppression (agranulocytosis). Salt and fluid retention. Dyspepsia, gastrointestinal bleeding or ul-	Give with antacid or meals. Blood cell counts should be checked every 1 to 2 weeks for 6 weeks and then every 1 to 2 months. Thorough mouth care.	Should be used cautiously in patients with congestive heart failure (a diuretic may be prescribed along with the drug). Potentiates warfarin.

TABLE 15.3   *Continued*

Drug	Side Effects	Precautions	Contraindications
	ceration. Allergic reactions. Oral ulceration.	Observe for side effects.	
Gold Salts gold sodium thromalate (Myochrysine); Aurothioglucose (Salganal) (usually used for rheumatoid arthritis)	Dermatitis. Bone marrow suppression (platelets, neutrophils or erythrocytes). Mouth ulceration. Nephritis. Vasomotor reactions.	Complete blood counts and urinalyses every week. Platelet counts every 2 weeks. Can be reduced to once a month and eventually every 3 months if no toxicity. Mouth care. Observe for side effects.	Any decrease in blood cell counts or proteinuria is cause for discontinuing drug at least temporarily.
Corticosteroids	Capillary fragility and easy bruising. Osteoporosis, aseptic necrosis of the bone. Gastrointestinal bleeding, peptic ulcer. Cushingoid habitus, hirsutism, moon face, acne, hyperglycemia, salt retention, increased susceptibility to infections, cataracts, glaucoma, adrenal suppression.	Reserve therapy for patients who fail to improve with more conservative treatment. Must be discontinued gradually over a period of weeks. Increased steroid doses will be required during stress (e.g. surgery, injuries). Safety and dietary precautions. Observe for side effects. Frequent weights.	Peptic ulcer disease. Hypertension. Diabetes.
Penicillamine	Abnormalities in taste. Allergic reactions. Glomerulonephritis. Optic neuritis. Bleeding into the skin, thrombocytopenia. Leukopenia. Aplastic anemia.	Complete blood cell counts during therapy. Safety measures. Observe for evidence of bleeding and infection.	Patients with penicillin allergies should not receive.
Azathioprine (Imuran)	Bone marrow suppression of any or all blood cells. Nausea, diarrhea. Hepatocellular damage. Increased inci-	Complete blood cell counts and serum transaminases during therapy. Observe for bleeding, infections, and jaun-	Liver disease. Highly toxic and should only be used when less conservative therapy fails.

TABLE 15.3 *Continued*

Drug	Side Effects	Precautions	Contraindications
	dence of lymphomas.	dice. Safety and dietary measures.	
Cyclophospha-mide (Cytoxan)	Suppression of bone marrow, especially granu-locytes. Alopecia. Sterility. Nausea, diarrhea. Hemor-rhagic cystitis and fibrosing cystitis. Increased inci-dence of lymphomas.	Complete blood counts during therapy. Observe for bleeding and infections. Safety measures. Ade-quate diet. Avoid contact with crowds or situa-tions in which in-fection may be acquired.	Preexisting bladder disease. Since sterility may be ir-reversible, con-traindicated in child-bearing age. Highly toxic and should only be used when less conservative ther-apy fails.
Colchicine	Dyspepsia, diar-rhea. Anaphylaxis when intraveous route is used.	Dose reduction if weakness, an-orexia develop. Treat diarrhea and vomiting.	Caution when ad-ministered to el-derly and debilitated, espe-cially those with renal, GI, and heart disease.
Allopurinal (Zyloprim)	Allergic dermatitis. Hepatitis. Leuko-penia. (The latter two are rare.)	Liver function tests. Do not use iron salts. Fluid intake of 2,000 ml. daily.	Preexisting liver dis-ease is a contrain-dication. Patients with renal disease need close observation.
Probenecid (Benemid); Sulfinypyra-zone (Anturan)	Formation of urate stones in the uri-nary tract. Aller-gic dermatitis. Gastrointestinal irritation and pep-tic ulceration.	Salicylates block their activity and should not be used simultaneously.	Contraindicated in patients with sig-nificant renal dis-ease and peptic ulcer.

Teach the person and family about drug dosage and side effects; suggest-ability should be considered when side effects are detailed, since the person may imagine the side effects he has been taught. Emphasize the importance of medical checkups when drugs requiring blood and urine surveillance are being used. Since memory may be affected by advancing years, the senior should be assisted in remembering when drugs are to be taken. On arising, a day's supply of medication can be placed in small pill boxes, plastic cups, or the cups of an egg carton and marked to be taken during the day at specific times, for exam-ple, before meals, after meals, after putting on pajamas at bedtime, before shaving in the morning, or in conjunction with a regular television program. Then he will be less likely to repeat or skip a dose. For the person confined to home, prescription drugs can be reordered by telephone with either direct or mail delivery.

Failure to take medication correctly, as prescribed by the physician, may occur in 25 to 50 percent of outpatients.[26] Health history should include a report on all medications taken over a 24-hour period, when and how much taken, what the medication is taken for, and whether it is prescribed or obtained over the counter.[36] A medication history for prescribed and over-the-counter drugs organizes the data; an example has been prepared by Parker.[32]

In all medication studies, the types of errors seem to follow a pattern: (1) errors of omission, (2) inappropriate self-medication, (3) incorrect dosage, (4) improper timing, and (5) inaccurate knowledge of purpose.[36]

Many elderly persons have conditions that are controlled by regular drug therapy so that they remain symptomless and may feel that they are cured. When they feel good, they do not take their medications. Further, many people take many different medications for a variety of ills—perhaps several hundred weekly. Taking pills becomes a full-time occupation, one that is tiring, irritating, cumbersome, and a constant reminder of infirmity. Resistance to the routine is easy to understand. If the person is not mentally alert or if side effects from the drugs reduce cognitive abilities, underdosing or overdosing is easy to understand.[36]

Errors are fewer when the person is included in the planning of a schedule for taking medication. Instructions on the bottle label should be specific. Encourage the person to return unused medications when he returns for follow-up visits. Directions should be given after medication has been filled rather than from the prescription pad. Color of the pill as well as its name should be described; use visual aids with teaching.[36]

Errors are increased when the senior does not know the nature of his illness or the purpose of his drugs and when there is inadequate communication between physician and patient. Often the physician is unaware of the total number of drugs that has been ordered or is taken by the person. As a result, unpleasant drug interactions occur.[24] The more drugs the person takes, and the more the pills look alike, the greater the chance for error.[26]

Other factors also influence whether or not a person takes the prescribed medications. The person who lives alone or without much social stimulus or encouragement becomes apathetic about his treatment and omits doses. If the person feels hostile toward his doctor or authority figures generally, feels that taking medication means drug dependence and loss of control, or is suspicious about the doctor or medication, he is less likely to take prescribed medication. He may secure over-the-counter drugs to overcome such feelings. If the person is impulsive or overconscientious, he may take more than the prescribed amounts.[26]

The patient-practitioner relationship is important. Patients are less likely to follow the medication regimen if expectations about care are not met, if they perceive a lack of warmth or interest in the practitioner, or if the practitioner does not explicitly convey that he believes the treatment is worthwhile.[26]

Sometimes the senior does not take drugs in the routine prescribed by the doctor for a good reason. By trial and error he had learned how many and when to take them so that he feels most comfortable. Health professionals should realize that the subjective physical feelings are an important cue and work with the senior in drug adjustment.

Diet teaching is important, as described earlier, since any arthropathy of a weight-bearing joint will be aggravated by increasing weight. Dietary instruction should begin soon after admission. The community health nurse can continue assessment and teaching in the home after discharge. The person with reduced activity and an arthropathy should be discouraged from a diet high in calories—candy, cakes, pies, cookies, snacks such as potato and corn chips, donuts, sugar-coated cereals, jelly, fried foods, or soda. Many individuals living alone and confined secure most of their daily pleasure from eating. Making food that is high in nutritional value interesting and tasty for the person who has little motivation or energy for preparing or eating may be difficult. If the senior is instructed in the reasons for a well-balanced diet, one that includes his cultural, religious, or individual preferences, he is more likely to cooperate.

Help the senior and family recognize the strong relationship that exists between emotional state and onset and exacerbation of arthritic symptoms. The symptoms become worse when the person is emotionally upset, angry, or feeling a sense of loss or deprivation. Emotions related to stress are apparently associated with dysfunction of the immunologic system. Stressful experience affects production of adrenocortical hormones, which may be immunosuppressive. Hypothalamic regulation of immune response may also be adversely affected by stress.[38,41,43,44] Help the person/family consider how they can avoid or minimize stress and cope more effectively with unavoidable stress. Help the person find constructive outlets for anger, such as doing light work in the yard, cleaning house, going for a walk, or expressing problems openly if physical activity cannot be an outlet. Often the arthritis improves considerably when the person accepts the relationship between acute episodes and emotional states and finds more effective coping mechanisms.

Limited Mobility Resulting from Fractures and Orthopedic Surgery: Pathology, Treatment, and Nursing Intervention

Fractures are common in later maturity. Osteoporosis is a physical change in later maturity, especially in women, as described in Chapter 9, that predisposes to fractures. The elderly person with brittle bones, changes in vision, tremor, or intermittent ischemic attacks is more likely to experience accidents and resulting fractures. Metastatic cancer also predisposes to pathological fractures.

Other problems also limit mobility. Arthropathies, such as rheumatoid or osteoarthritis, may result in orthopedic surgery, such as total knee or hip replacements. Diabetes and atherosclerosis predispose to reduced circulation to the lower extremities, ulceration, and infection, sometimes necessitating amputations.

Fractures are commonly treated by internal fixation methods, even in patients who are not ideal surgical risks. Most physicians feel that the elderly patient must be mobilized as soon as possible after a fracture. Also, since most elderly do not tolerate heavy casts, walking casts are rarely used. There is no excuse to let the elderly patient die with a painful fracture of the hip left untreated by a surgeon through mistaken kindness.[14]

Table 15.4 summarizes common surgical and medical interventions for different fractures.[14]

Total joint replacement is indicated for osteoarthritis of the hip and knee when the disease has advanced to the point that it prevents enjoyment of life or has become a disability instead of an inconvenience.[14] The procedures used for hip fractures and the hip replacement differ very little except that the replacement is a planned-for procedure; the fracture is usually an emergency. Choice of prosthesis is usually based on the speed with which the patient can become ambulatory. The technique requiring shorter bedrest is the one of choice.

With hip replacement, the patient gets up with your assistance the day after surgery.[14] With knee replacement, the patient is free to move in bed, but ambulation may be delayed until the sixth day when a plaster cylinder replaces the dressing and provides protection for the new joint.[39]

Anticoagulant therapy is usually utilized; the danger of hemorrhage must be considered. All drugs potentiating anticoagulant effects are eliminated (as-

TABLE 15.4   Fractures and Their Interventions

Type of Fracture	Intervention Method
Femoral neck fracture	Excision of the upper fragment and replacement by a prosthesis.
Trochanteric fracture	Pin and plate inserted into trochanter and femur.
Femoral shaft fracture	Pin and long plate, or intermedullary fixation.
Tibial fracture	Intermedullary nail into tibia.
Ankle-area fracture	Internal fixation of ankle with screws or plate.
Humeral shaft fracture	Intermedullary fixation of humerus.
Elbow shattered	Pressure dressing and sling; patient encouraged to do early movements.
Radius or ulna fracture	Plaster cast, if tolerated, or internal fixation with plate and screws or intermedullary rod.
Colles' fracture (wrist and lower arm)	Plaster cast after closed reduction. Patients are usually encouraged to use the fingers, elbow, and shoulder immediately.
Vertebral fracture	Bedrest with gradually increasing head elevation until sitting is achieved; then up in chair and then walking with a corset.

pirin, antihistamines, indomethacin). Therapy is monitored with tests for prothrombin time; anticoagulant doses are prescribed accordingly.[39]

Postoperative exercises, taught preoperatively and performed prior to surgery to the extent symptoms permit, are started as soon as possible after surgery. Isometric exercises usually begin first, with flexion/extension being delayed in the case of knee replacement until the plaster cylinder is removed (3 to 4 weeks postoperatively).[39] Effectiveness of the replacement should not be assessed on the basis of range of motion achieved in the new joint but rather on the extent that the patient is able to do all the activities of daily living.

Knee replacement is less likely to restore movement that has been absent for a long time than is hip replacement. The stiff, painful knee will usually become painless and useful, but full range of motion will not result.[39]

Amputation is required when circulatory impairment has progressed so far that medical and more conservative surgical procedures are no longer effective. An emergency atmosphere usually pervades since gangrene with its associated toxicity renders the patient very ill. If diabetes is also present, the situation is more serious. The surgical procedure of choice is one that preserves as much of the limb, such as the knee, as possible. The surgeon's main aim will be to obtain primary healing.

Whatever method is used, the important thing is to provide some form of early walking aid that will facilitate ambulation within a few days of surgery. These patients have circulatory problems throughout the body and, if complications are to be prevented, exercise and ambulation must be conscientiously provided. Also, confusion preoperatively, due to the toxicity and ischemia, may not totally disappear postoperatively. Providing a natural appearing walking aid will help the patient to be more secure in using it.

Medical intervention in relation to the diabetic and/or vascular condition will be considered in later sections of this book.

Nursing care of the elderly patient with orthopedic surgery presents a challenge. The risks of surgery are increased by preexisting medical problems, especially those of the cardiorespiratory and genitourinary systems. Lowered resistance to infection because of age changes in the immune mechanism, prolonged healing time resulting from diabetes or atherosclerosis, and lower reserves in the renal, cardiovascular, and pulmonary systems increase surgical risk. Urinary retention, oversedation, overhydration, and poor digitalization may occur. The hazards of immobility previously discussed are to be avoided preoperatively and postoperatively.

All of your basic nursing skills will be used, as well as observational skills and ability, to make nursing diagnoses. The nursing care that the patient receives will determine prognosis: Good nursing care may be the difference between life and death.

Patient care goals include to prevent complications, regain preoperative levels of functioning as rapidly as possible, and prevent unnecessary demands on adaptive capacity. Exact chronological age is less significant than the patient's outlook and physiological status. Optimistic outlook, good nutritional state, and reasonable cardiopulmonary and renal reserves decrease the surgical risk.[4]

The preoperative and postoperative care vital to other age groups undergoing surgery is more vital in the care of the elderly. Because the senior has less reserve, his capacity to maintain and restore homeostasis in the presence of continued strain is less than in earlier life.

Since there is a high incidence of hip fracture among the elderly, and since hip replacements do not differ a great deal from the treatment of a hip fracture with a prosthesis, discussion of nursing intervention will focus on care of the patient with a hip fracture.

Preoperative care of the patient with a fractured hip usually includes use of traction to reduce the fracture; precautions must be taken to maintain traction and prevent complications. The weights must hang free and should not be removed unless specifically ordered; the foot piece must not touch the end of the bed. The patient needs instruction about the purpose of the traction and the amount of movement allowed.

Skin care is of vital importance; the back, coccygeal area, and elbows need careful inspection whenever skin care is given. Dry linens, massage of bony prominences every 2 hours, cleanliness, and good nutrition are required if skin breakdown is to be avoided. Use of sheepskin or an air mattress will be helpful, as well as the side-lying position unless it is contraindicated. Skin on the affected limb must be watched carefully for pressure areas, and circulation should be checked regularly.

Fluid and electrolyte balance is also very important. Intake and output should be measured and recorded. Fluids should be given freely unless contraindicated because of a preexisting condition. Constipation also develops because of reduced activity and having to use a bedpan. A laxative that supplies bulk or lubrication may be ordered. Fruit juices, diet adequate with bulk, and fluid intake will help prevent or alleviate constipation. Glycerine suppositories are also helpful. If a catheter is ordered, it is imperative that strict asepsis be maintained in its insertion and in its care. A closed drainage system, daily change of sterile urine receptacle and tubing, and adequate fluid intake help to prevent infections. This author believes that the catheter should be avoided if at all possible. The problems of its removal after it has been in place for an extended period of time can be great and may predispose the patient to being permanently dependent on it. However, urinary retention is a definite indication for its use; urinary incontinence may or may not be. Conscientious nursing care, including placement of the bedpan or urinal at regular intervals, especially after meals, before retiring, and upon arising, and frequent checking of linens for soilage may be all that are needed to avoid the catheter.

Full range of motion must be maintained in all other joints if the patient is in traction. An overhead trapeze can be helpful for the patient to raise up and strengthen upper extremities. Side rails are helpful in turning from side to side and are usually needed for safety. Physical therapy will probably be ordered for muscle strengthening, joint range of motion, and prevention of contractures prior to surgery. Muscle action and joint function must be maintained for early mobilization. Gait training and use of canes or walkers will be taught postoperatively. Recent studies have shown that crutches are, metabolically speaking, very costly. The energy needed tends to make crutches more hazardous to use.[20]

Teaching deep breathing and coughing to prevent pulmonary complications is essential preoperatively. If treatment to assist respirations, such as intermittent positive pressure breathing (IPPB) is ordered, the patient needs instruction about its purposes. Therapy should begin prior to surgery so that he will know how to breathe with the machine without detailed instructions after surgery.

Anticoagulant therapy for patients requiring bed rest, pressure anti-embolus hose, and active exercises are ordered for patients to prevent venous complications.[18]

Tell the patient what to expect in the preparation for surgery and in the environment of the operating suite. Give him an opportunity to ask questions and explore concerns and feelings. Skin preparation, preoperative medication and anesthesia, dressings, drainage tubing postoperatively, and whether or not he will be in a recovery room and intensive care unit after surgery should be explained. The patient may seem confused, but explanation in simple terms and in a soothing voice should always be given.

Informed consent must be secured from the patient. It is the physician's responsibility to inform the patient of the procedure to be done, expected progress, risks involved, and any alternative therapy. You should contact the physician if this has not been done or if the patient has questions or doubts about the surgery. You can clarify what the physician has told the patient, but you cannot assume primary responsibility for informed consent.

You or some other adult may witness the preoperative permit. Witnesses must be of legal age. It is usually at this time that the patient will voice his concerns; you should be alert for signs of misgivings or confusion. The patient can still withdraw his consent after a permit has been signed. A consent secured when the patient is under the effects of a sedative drug or disoriented is not valid; consents secured by coercion, when the patient is in great pain, or from a family member when the patient is capable of consenting himself are also of questionable validity.

Abnormal laboratory values, vital signs, and symptoms of infection should be called to the physician's attention prior to surgery.

Immediately after surgery vital signs should be checked every 15 minutes until they are stable. Check dressings and drainage devices for signs of hemorrhage. Intravenous infusions must be carefully monitored for rate of administration and infiltration. Urinary output must be monitored; an output of at least 40 ml per hour, relative to intake, should be maintained. Remember that elderly persons tolerate a rapid infusion rate poorly because of reduced compliance of their circulatory system and progressive impairment of cardiac and renal function. Pulmonary edema is a serious complication that can result from too rapid administration of parental fluids. Observe for symptoms of shortness of breath, wheezing, cough, frothy sputum, sense of pressure in the chest, and marked increase in pulse and respirations.[4]

Pain must be treated promptly. Studies have shown that patients who know that they can have a pain-relieving medication require less medication than those who do not know. Failure to relieve severe deep pain may cause weakness, hypotension, pallor, sweating, bradycardia, nausea, vomiting, disorientation, and confusion. More benefit is usually obtained from an analgesic if the pain is not allowed to become too intense. Signs of central nervous system depression should be reported promptly, for example, respiratory rate less than 12 per minute or presence of a stuporous state. Pain control will promote more activity as well as facilitate rest.

Know which surgical procedure was performed and what is allowed: the exact positioning of the extremity, turning, transferring out of bed, and standing or ambulating either with or without weight bearing. Since physicians vary in their preferences, detailed postoperative orders should be secured. The patient with a hip prosthesis or hip replacement will be able to bear weight sooner than the patient with an internal fixation by pinning. Most physicians want the patient ambulatory as soon as possible and will order procedures to promote this goal.

The following chart summarizes some of the differences that may be observed in caring for patients with hip procedures. However, these activities should not be assumed to be the ones to be used with a specific patient. The chart is offered as an example of how care can vary, depending on the surgical procedure performed.[7,23]

Total hip replacement	*Austin-Moore prosthesis*	*Internal fixation*
Adduction and external rotation to be avoided. Partial weight bearing as early as 1 to 2 days postoperative. Full weight bearing in 1 month.	Adduction and internal rotation to be avoided. Partial weight bearing as early as 1 to 2 days postoperative. Full weight bearing in 1 month.	Outward rotation to be avoided. Toeing-in position to be maintained in bed. Full weight bearing delayed until completely healed (3 to 8 months).

Adapt care to metabolic changes that occur after surgery, which are similar to those following an injury. Bedrest causes the problems discussed earlier in the chapter, such as catabolism of protein, nitrogen loss, appetite depression, loss of muscle tone, weakness, decubiti, contractures, urinary tract infections, fecal impaction, and calcium loss from bones.[4] Exercise soon after surgery reduces these complications. Observe for thrombophlebitis; leg exercises, avoidance of pressure on calves of legs, adequate hydration, and prevention of hypotension are preventive measures. Anticoagulant therapy may be prescribed to prevent vascular clotting. Pulmonary complications can be avoided through change of position, coughing, deep breathing, and IPPB treatments.

Prevent wound infections; maintain strict aseptic technique in all dressing changes. Adequate nutrition is vital to prevent infection and promote wound healing. Wound disruption is possible; some potential causes are obesity; undernutrition; deficiency of protein, calcium, or vitamin C; diabetes; uremia; Cushing's Syndrome, or carcinoma.

Withhold food and fluid by mouth until the gastrointestinal tract is functioning normally, which is indicated by presence of bowel sound, absence of distention, and the passage of feces or flatus per rectum. When first starting oral fluids, volume should probably be restricted to 15 to 30 c.c. per hour. Fluids should be discontinued if the patient vomits, becomes distended, or complains of a full feeling.[4] Paralytic-ileus may result following any major surgery under general anesthetic. The symptoms are nausea and vomiting more than 12 to 24 hours postoperatively; abdominal distention ("gas pains"); absence of bowel sounds, failure to pass flatus; and X-ray evidence of obstruction.

Nursing care of the patient pre- and post-amputation is similar to that described above except for the change in body image and the sense of loss and grieving that will be greater for the amputee than for another person undergoing orthopedic surgery. Routine physical care is important, but *emotional support* is invaluable. The amputee in later maturity may give up all hope of ever being independent again. Since he probably does not know many of the advances made with prostheses, his conception of the amputee may be the stereotype of a peg leg, or worse yet, the bedbound cripple. Having him speak with another senior who has an amputation and has regained or maintained his independence will be helpful. The patient who feels that amputation is a fate worse than death must be helped to realize that a happy life is possible after an amputation. However, he must not be given false hope and reassurance. Not every elderly amputee is able to use a prosthesis. Rehabilitation to the greatest degree possible is the goal. The gains made in rehabilitation will only equal the effort the elderly person is able to put into it. His attitude and cooperation are important.

Successful rehabilitation of the amputee depends on several things. His general state of health is crucial. If vascular disease is absent in the unaffected limb, the possibility for successful rehabilitation increases. Visual difficulties, arthritis, and osteoporosis hinder rehabilitation. The depressed or confused patient is less likely to be rehabilitated. Advanced age (over 75) also impedes rehabilitation. Probably the most important factors are the patient's state of mind and his desire to be rehabilitated.

In order to use a prosthesis, certain complications must be prevented. Flexion contractures must be avoided. Traction often is applied to prevent this, and sitting for long periods or propping the stump on pillows must be avoided. The prone position is a good one for preventing flexion contracture at the hip, but the prone position may be impossible for the elderly patient.

The rehabilitation program also depends on the surgical method. Today many physicians immediately fit a temporary prosthesis. A rigid plaster-of-Paris dressing is applied in the operating room and is used as a socket on a temporary prosthesis, which allows ambulation to begin a day or two after surgery. Success with this method requires very skillful surgery and exact application of the postoperative cast. Another method is to wait until wound healing has occurred; then a temporary prosthesis is fitted over a plaster-of-Paris cast. As the stump shrinks, new casts are applied until a permanent prosthesis is fitted. This method is probably the one of choice for the elderly amputee. Delayed fitting with a permanent prosthesis is the third method. After the wound heals, a physical therapy program consisting of wrapping, shaping, toughening, and strengthening of the stump takes place. When the stump is ready, a permanent prosthesis is fitted.[9]

If the patient has been unable to use the temporary prosthesis or cannot be fitted for a permanent prosthesis, he should be taught to be as independent as possible with activities of daily living while using a wheelchair. Use of a wheelchair should not be regarded as a failure, for everyone is an individual and cannot achieve the same level of rehabilitation.

The stump requires special attention; it can be easily injured and is subject to infection. Frequent dressing changes should be avoided, and the stump should be protected from being bumped or otherwise injured during routine care and transfers.

Remind the patient to do exercises to strengthen the upper extremities. Push-ups while sitting up or lying prone can be helpful for crutch walking and parallel bar exercises.

Planning for discharge should begin early in the hospitalization, not the day before discharge. Determine how much the family will be able to assist with care. Assess the physical environment of the home to determine the patient's ability to function comfortably within it. A nurse either from the hospital, home health agency, or health department should inspect the home for hazards and adaptability to the senior's use. Suggest helpful modifications. If the family cannot make modifications, often the agency, the community, the hospital, or the church will have an organization or group that could assist in making them.

Necessary referrals to home health agencies and meals-on-wheels should be made. If it seems impossible for the patient to return home, then other arrangements should be made, for example, living with a relative or admission to a nursing home. These plans should be made with the patient involved if possible. Telling a patient the day of his discharge that he cannot go home but is going to a nursing home instead is very cruel. Exposure to the nursing home, either through literature or a visit from one of the personnel, is helpful. Also, if the patient can choose from several alternative homes, he feels that he is still in control of his own destiny. Use the suggestions given in Chapter 7 to assist the senior and his family in selecting a nursing home.

EVALUATION

Evaluation of nursing intervention should relate to the degree of independence that the senior is able to maintain or regain in the activities of daily living. Range of joint motion should improve or remain the same. Prevention of complications should also be evaluated. Absence of contractures, decubiti, ankylosis, and other complications are positive indicators that the patient care goals and plan of care were appropriate and adequately implemented. If the outcomes are not positive, then the plan of care must be reevaluated after a thorough reassessment of the patient and his situation. Patient care goals should also be reevaluated to see if they are realistic, achievable, and known to all concerned in the plan.

REFERENCES

1. ALFANO, GENROSE, "There Are No Routine Patients," *American Journal of Nursing,* 75: No. 10 (1975), 1804–7.

2. BACKUS, F., and D. DUDLEY, "Observations of Psychosocial Factors and Their Relationship to Organic Disease," *International Journal of Psychiatry and Medicine,* 5: No. 4 (1974), 499–515.

3. BATES, BARBARA, *A Guide to Physical Examination.* Philadelphia: J. B. Lippincott Company, 1974.

4. BELAND, IRENE, and JOYCE PASSOS, *Clinical Nursing: Pathophysiological and Psychosocial Approaches,* 3rd ed. New York: Macmillan Publishing Co., Inc., 1975.

5. BENNAGE, B., and M. CUMMINGS, "Nursing the Patient Undergoing Total Hip Arthroplasty," *Nursing Clinics of North America,* 8: No. 1 (1973), 107–16.

6. BERGERSON, BETTY, *Pharmacology in Nursing,* 13th ed. St. Louis: The C. V. Mosby Company, 1976.

7. BIRCHENALL, JOAN, and MARY STREIGHT, *Care of the Older Adult.* Philadelphia: J. B. Lippincott Company, 1973.

8. BREWERTON, D. A., "Rheumatic Disorders," in *Clinical Geriatrics,* ed. Isadore Rossman. Philadelphia: J. B. Lippincott Company, 1971.

9. BROWER, PHYLLIS, and DOROTHY HICKS, "Maintaining Muscle Function in Patients on Bedrest," *American Journal of Nursing,* 72: No. 7 (1972), 1250–53.

10. CARNEVALI, DORIS, and SUSAN BRUECKNER, "Immobilization: Reassessment of a Concept," *American Journal of Nursing,* 70: No. 7 (1970), 1502–7.

11. CLARK, HELEN, "Osteoarthritis: An Interesting Case?" *Nursing Clinics of North America,* 11: No. 1 (1976), 199–206.

12. COMBS, KAREN, "Preventive Health Care in the Elderly," *American Journal of Nursing,* 78: No. 8 (1978), 1339–41.

13. DEGOWAN, ELMER, and RICHARD DEGOWAN, *Bedside Diagnostic Examination,* 2nd ed. New York: Macmillan Publishing Co., Inc., 1969.

14. DEVAS, MICHAEL, "Orthopedics," in *Cowdry's The Care of the Geriatric Patient,* 5th ed., ed. Franz U. Steinberg. St. Louis: The C. V. Mosby Company, 1976.

15. DRISCOLL, PAMELA, "Rheumatoid Arthritis: Part I—Understanding It More Fully; Part II—Managing It More Successfully," *Nursing '75,* 5: No. 12 (1975), 26–32.

16. FINK, STEPHEN, and FRANKLIN SHONTZ, "Body Image Disturbances in Chronically Ill Individuals," *Journal of Nervous and Mental Diseases,* 131: (1960), 234–40.

17. GORDON, MARJORY, "Assessing Activity Tolerance," *American Journal of Nursing,* 76: No. 1 (1976), 72–75.

18. GRIFFIN, WENNIE, SARA ANDERSON, and JOYCE PASSOS, "Group Exercise for Patients with Limited Motion," *American Journal of Nursing,* 71: No. 9 (1971), 1742–43.

19. GRIGGS, WINONA, "Staying Well While Growing Old: Sex and the Elderly," *American Journal of Nursing,* 78: No. 8 (1978), 1352–54.

20. HABERMANN, EDWARD, "Orthopedic Aspects of the Lower Extremities," in *Clinical Geriatrics,* ed. Isadore Rossman. Philadelphia: J. B. Lippincott Company, 1971.

21. HAHN, BEVRA, "Arthritis, Bursitis, and Bone Disease," in *Cowdry's The Care of the Geriatric Patient,* 5th ed., ed. Franz U. Steinberg. St. Louis: The C. V. Mosby Company, 1976.

22. HALSTEAD, LAURA, "Aiding Arthritic Patients to Adjust Sexually," *Medical Aspects of Human Sexuality,* April, 1977, 85–86.

23. HERSCHBERG, GERALD, LEON LEWIS, and PATRICIA VAUGHAN, *Rehabilitation,* 2nd ed. Philadelphia: J. B. Lippincott Company, 1976.

24. HULKA, BARBARA, JOHN CASSEL, LAWRENCE KUPPER, and JAMES BURDETTE, "Communication and Concordance Between Physicians and Patients with Prescribed Medications," *American Journal of Public Health,* 66: No. 9 (1976), 847–53.

25. JUDGE, RICHARD, and GEORGE ZUIDEMA, *Physical Diagnosis: A Physiologic Approach to the Clinical Examination,* 2nd ed. Boston: Little, Brown & Company, 1968.

26. KOMAROFF, ANTHONY, "The Practitioner and the Compliant Patient," *American Journal of Public Health,* 66: No. 9 (1976), 833–35.

27. KRUPKA, LAWRENCE, and ARTHUR VENER, "Hazards of Drug Use Among the Elderly," *The Gerontologist,* 19: No. 1 (1979), 90–95.

28. LOXLEY, ALICE, "The Emotional Toll of Crippling Deformity," *American Journal of Nursing,* 72: No. 10 (1972), 1839–40.

29. MEYEROWITZ, S., "The Continuing Investigation of Psychological Variables in Rheumatoid Arthritis," *Modern Trends in Rheumatology,* 2: (1971), 92–105.

30. MURRAY, RUTH, and JUDITH ZENTNER, *Nursing Concepts for Health Promotion,* 2nd ed. Englewood Cliffs, N.J.: Prentice-Hall, Inc., 1979.

31. OLSON, EDITH, "The Hazards of Immobility," *American Journal of Nursing,* 67: No. 4 (1967), 779–97.

32. PARKER, WM., "Medication Histories," *American Journal of Nursing,* 76: No. 12 (1976), 1969–71.

33. PITOREK, ELIZABETH, "Rheumatoid Arthritis: Part III—Living with It More Comfortably," *Nursing '75,* 5: No. 12 (1975), 33–35.

34. ROBINSON, CORINNE, *Proudfit-Robinson's Normal and Therapeutic Nutrition,* 13th ed. New York: Macmillan Publishing Co., Inc., 1967.

35. "Safety Checklist for the Aging and the Handicapped and Their Families," National Society for Crippled Children and Adults, 2023 West Ogden Avenue, Chicago, Ill.

36. SCHWARTZ, DORIS, "Safe Self-Medication for Elderly Patients," *American Journal of Nursing,* 75: No. 10 (1975), 1808–10.

37. SNYDER, MARIAH, and REBECCA BAUM, "Assessing Station and Gait," *American Journal of Nursing,* 74: No. 7 (1974), 1256–57.

38. SOLOMAN, G., A. AMKRAUT, and P. KASPER, "Immunity, Emotions, and Stress," *Annals of Clinical Research,* 6: (1974), 313–22.

39. TOWNLEY, CHARLES, and LESLIE HILL, "Total Knee Replacement," *American Journal of Nursing,* 74: No. 9 (1974), 1612–17.

40. U.S. Department of Health, Education and Welfare, *Working with Older People: Vol. IV Clinical Aspects of Aging,* ed. Austin B. Chinn. Rockville, Md.: United States Public Health Service, 1971.

41. WALIKE, BARBARA, "Personality Factors—Rheumatoid Arthritis," *American Journal of Nursing,* 72: No. 12 (1972), 1834–40.

42. WEBB, KENNETH, "Early Assessment of Orthopedic Injuries," *American Journal of Nursing,* 74: No. 6 (1974), 1048–52.

43. WEINER, H., "Are Psychosomatic Diseases Diseases of Regulation?" *Psychosomatic Medicine,* 37: No. 4 (1975), 289–91.

44. ZANDER, W., "Problems of Specific Syndrome Formation in Psychosomatic Disease Situations (Psychodynamics of Rheumatoid Diseases)," *Psychosomatic Medicine and Psychoanalysis,* 22: No. 2 (1976), 150–68.

problems of neuroregulation and sensory perception in later maturity

---

Study of this chapter will enable you to:

1. Describe methods of assessing the elderly person for altered neuroregulation and sensory perception.

2. Assess the senior for cerebral, cerebellar, cranial nerve, and sensory function.

3. Determine appropriate nursing diagnoses after analyzing assessment data.

4. Formulate short-term and long-term goals for the senior with a variety of neuroregulatory and sensory impairments: unconsciousness, paralysis, aphasia, perceptual disorders, incontinence, Parkinsonism, deafness, or blindness.

5. Discuss pathology related to a variety of neuroregulatory problems, including cerebral vascular accident.

6. Describe nursing interventions for the physical, emotional, social, and spiritual care of the senior with impaired neuroregulatory or sensory functions.

7. Describe nursing interventions that can assist the family.

8. Implement appropriate nursing measures for the senior with selected neuroregulatory or sensory alterations and for the family.

9. Work with other health team members to provide continuity of care for this patient and family.

10. Evaluate the effectiveness of care given by considering the patient's potential to achieve stated care goals.

16

In Chapter 15 emphasis was placed on problems of mobility arising from musculoskeletal abnormality. In this chapter problems of mobility are further discussed, since mobility can be inhibited by neurological malfunction as well. Other problems arising from a neurological origin, such as aphasia and those related to the special senses, such as blindness and deafness, are also explored.

Again the nursing process will be used as the framework for the chapter. Assessment of neuroregulation and sensory perception will be reviewed first. Aspects of assessment discussed in Chapter 15 should also be incorporated in any patient examination, since many of the parameters relate to the musculoskeletal system and could be indicative of neurological as well as musculoskeletal problems.

ASSESSMENT

Many neurological functions have been studied and reported to decline with age. Reduced intellectual functioning, failing vision, eye movement and pupil size abnormalities, hearing loss, loss of vibration and touch sensation and two-point discrimination, weakness, gait-posture-coordination abnormalities, and absence of certain reflexes have been considered characteristic of aging.[27,60] However, a recent study with 51 socially active, self-declared neurologically normal subjects between 61 and 84 years revealed *no* consistent pattern of neurological deficit that could be labeled as pathological, and less decline in vibration perception was noted than had been reported by previous researchers. The results obtained from that study indicate that many aspects of neurological function are *little affected* by the aging process. These researchers state that most previous clinical studies of neurological function, although showing a decline with aging, were based on clinical experience with hospitalized or ambulatory patients. They tried, instead, to discriminate normal changes for the elderly from those that are manifestations of diseases particularly prevalent in later maturity.[33]

Objectivity in observation is vitally important for accurate assessment. Approach the senior without preconceived ideas about what might be found because he is elderly.

General Cerebral Function

Assessment of the neurological system includes observation of the entire body from head to toe and a mental status examination.

To observe for neurological problems, note *gait, posture,* and *balance.* This can be done upon first meeting the person and was described in Chapter 15.

Next note *general cerebral function.* Five areas are assessed, beginning with *general behavior.* Look at the person's dress, hygiene, manner of communicating, cooperation, and overall behavior patterns. Is there any bizarre behavior, mannerism, tic, or gesture?

Determine *level of consciousness.* Is the person alert and responding appropriately? Is he *confused, mentally slow, inattentive, incoherent, showing a dull perception of the environment?* Is he *stuporous, having greatly reduced mental and physical activity?* Reflexes are preserved in stupor, but the person responds extremely slowly to commands or stimuli. Is he *comatose, unresponsive to stimuli, with most reflexes absent?* Is he *delirious, confused, agitated, and hallucinating?*[2] Confusion, stupor, and coma often occur on a continuum of severity. Delirium is not usually considered in the continuum.

Describe the specific behavior you observe because labels are not always interpreted the same way by all health team members.

Intellectual performance requires that you know and adapt to the senior's educational level and his cultural and socioeconomic background in order to determine whether or not his level of intellectual functioning is deficient and of recent or protracted origin. Judgment, general information, interpretation of proverbs, serial subtractions, recent and past memory, and orientation to time, place, and person are assessed.

Emotional status is observed for appropriateness. Affect (mood) is noted: Is the patient depressed, hostile, irritable, anxious, manic, euphoric? *Thought content* is also assessed. Is he unduly preoccupied with certain thoughts? Does he express paranoid or phobic ideas? Is the thought content illogical, bizarre, or delusional? Is perception distorted (illusions or hallucinations)? For greater detail on mental status assessment, see Chapter 21 on cognitive impairment.

Specific Cerebral Function

Assess for specific cerebral function as you assess for general cerebral function. Visual or auditory *agnosia, faulty cortical-sensory interpretation resulting in inability to correctly interpret what is seen, heard, or felt,* may be present. *Apraxia, inability to perform some purposeful movement,* tests cortical motor integration. Language ability is tested by having the patient speak, write, and demonstrate understanding of the spoken and written word. *Incorrect use or comprehension of language is called aphasia.*

When testing for agnosia, apraxia, and aphasia, use the assessment method described in Table 16.1.

Cranial Nerve Function

Examination of the cranial nerves can be incorporated into the head-to-toe assessment of the patient. Many of the tests for the senses involve the cra-

TABLE 16.1   Assessment of Agnosia, Apraxia, and Aphasia

Test the Patient's Ability to	By
1. Recognize sound	Identifying familiar sounds with eyes closed.
2. Comprehend speech	Answering questions and carrying out instructions.
3. Recognize body parts and sidedness	Identifying right and left sides and body parts.
4. Perform skilled motor acts	Drinking from a cup or closing a safety pin.
5. Recognize an object visually	Identifying an object held up or pointed to.
6. Comprehend writing	Reading a sentence and explaining its meaning or following written instructions if unable to talk.
7. Use motor speech	Imitating different sounds and phrases. Note abnormal word usage during interview.
8. Use automatic speech	Repeating series of words learned in the past, such as days of week.
9. Use volitional speech	Answering questions relevantly.
10. Write	Writing name, address, simple sentence, or the name of an object held up or pointed to.

nial nerves. Table 16.2 summarizes cranial nerve testing.[2,12,20,28] Understanding the functions of the nerves and their locations simplifies testing and can be reviewed in a basic physiology text.

Cerebellar Function

Balance and coordination are controlled by the cerebellum; thus, gait is assessed. Different types of abnormal gaits and the Romberg test for sensory equilibrium were described in Chapter 15.

Tests for coordination include the following:[12]

1. Finger-to-nose	Person touches nose with index finger with eyes open and then closed. Wide missing of the target is called *past-pointing*.
2. Heel-to-shin	Person runs his heel down his opposite shin from knee to ankle while lying down.
3. Alternating motion	Person pronates and supinates hands or taps floor with toes rapidly.

Assessment of the motor system (determining muscle size, strength, and tone, and involuntary movements) is discussed in Chapter 15.

TABLE 16.2   Tests for Cranial Nerve Function

Cranial Nerve	Test
I. Olfactory	Have patient sniff and identify a familiar scent with eyes closed.
II. Optic	Use Snellen Eye Chart for visual acuity. Test visual fields.* View optic disc with ophthalmoscope.* Check color vision with color chart.
III. Oculomotor IV. Trochlear VI. Abducens	Test III, IV, VI as a group: determine extraocular movements,* and check pupillary response to light. Determine ability to elevate upper eyelid.
V. Trigeminal	Touch to determine sensation on forehead, face, and jaw. Touch cornea lightly with cotton applicator to check corneal reflex. Have patient tighten jaw muscles and move jaw laterally.
VII. Facial	Have patient puff out cheeks, wrinkle forehead, close eyes, frown, smile, and whistle. Determine taste for sugar and salt on each side of anterior tongue.
VIII. Acoustic	Test cochlear branch for hearing by having patient identify watch tick, whisper, sound of tuning fork. Test for conductive, perceptive, and mixed hearing loss by using Weber and Renne tests.* Check conductive and perceptive loss.† (Vestibular branch is usually tested by neurologist doing caloric tests).
IX. Glossopharyngeal X. Vagus	Test for IX and X together. Check phonation, gag reflex, swallowing, and raising of uvula when patient says "ah."
XI. Assessory	Have patient shrug shoulders or turn head against force of your hand.
XII. Hypoglossal	Have patient protrude tongue.

* To perform test accurately, review physical assessment text.

† Note conductive loss if the person speaks softly, hears well on the phone, and hears best in a noisy environment. **Conductive loss** *involves reduced bone conduction of sound through the ear canal, tympanic membrane, middle ear, ossicular chain to the footplate of the stapes.* **Perceptive loss** *is a disturbance in the cochlea, auditory nerve, or hearing center in the cerebral cortex. Both bone and air conduction are reduced. Note perceptive loss when the person speaks loudly, hears better in a quiet situation, and states that he hears but does not understand, which indicates poor discrimination.*

Sensory Function

Tests for the sensory system include those for light touch, temperature, pain, vibration, motion, and position. Testing sensation must be carefully performed and recorded. Sensation should be tested in each dermatome of the body.[2] (See Figures 16.1 and 16.2.) Otherwise, a sensory defect may be over-looked or misdiagnosed.

Light touch is tested by touching the person's skin with a wisp of cotton while the patient has his eyes closed; he reports when he is touched. *Pain* is tested by a paper clip; the straightened pointed end and the rounded end of a paper clip are used alternately. Again, the patient closes his eyes and reports either a sharp or dull sensation. *Temperature* is tested by applying two tubes of water—one warm and one cold—to the skin; the patient identifies accordingly. *Vibration testing* is done by placing a 128-cps tuning fork firmly over a joint of the finger, toe, wrist, or ankle; the patient reports when he feels the vibration cease. *Position* is tested by grasping the patient's fingers or toes on their lateral and medial surfaces and raising or lowering them. The patient identifies up-ward or downward motion. *Discriminative sensation* should be tested in order to determine intactness of the posterior columns and sensory cortex. It involves the following:

1. Stereognosis: Patient identifies a familiar object placed in his hand while his eyes are closed.
2. Number identification: Patient identifies a number traced on his palm while his eyes are closed.
3. Two-point discrimination: Patient identifies the minimal distance that can be perceived as two distinct points when two pins are touched to his skin al-ternately with one pin. Eventually, as the pins are moved closer together the patient will perceive the two points as being one. The distance at which this occurs should be noted.
4. Point localization: Patient identifies the point on his skin where he was touched when his eyes were closed.
5. Extinction: Patient describes where he feels the sensation after similar areas on both sides of the body have been simultaneously stimulated.[2,12]

Reflex testing was discussed in Chapter 15. Several abnormal reflexes will be tested. The Babinski reflex is checked routinely by stroking the sole of the foot with a pointed instrument from the heel, along the lateral edge of the foot, and then across the ball of the foot medially. A *positive Babinski, dorsiflexion of the great toe with fanning of the smaller toes,* is a strong sign of pyramidal disease. Withdrawal of the entire leg and flexion at the ankle, knee, and hip may occur in extensive pyramidal tract disease.[28]

Neurological testing and interpretation of the results require a depth of knowledge and an understanding of neurophysiology and neuroanatomy. Since most nurses do not have this depth of knowledge, neurological testing should probably be left to the neurologist or be validated by the neurologist if done by anyone else.[39] However, your accurate observation and recording of the overall appearance, behavior, and signs and symptoms are essential for nursing diagnoses, patient care goals, nursing interventions, and often, for the

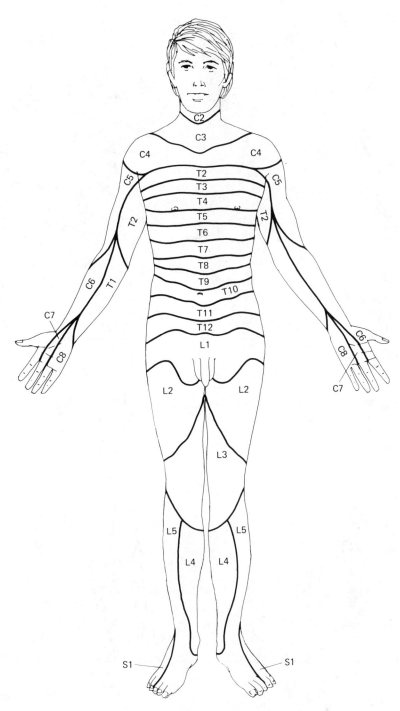

Figure 16.1. Dermatome regions of the anterior body.

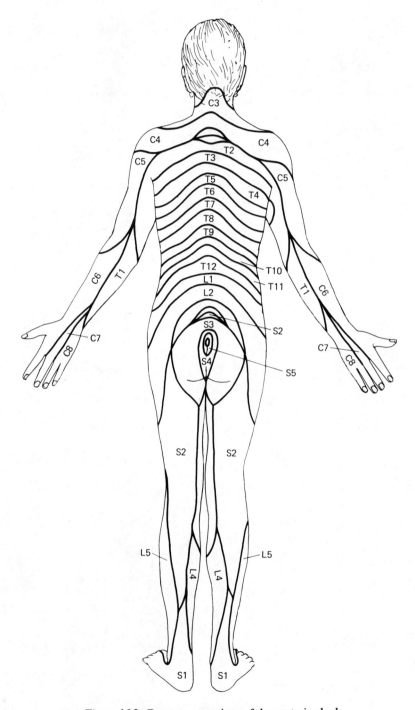

Figure 16.2. Dermatome regions of the posterior body.

medical diagnosis. Further, you are accountable for care given, which means being able to explain why all aspects of care were planned and implemented.

Emotional and social response to altered neuroregulation or sensory impairment is essential to assess. Chronicity, body image changes, sexuality, and interactions with family and others, as discussed in Chapter 15, are also applicable to this patient.

NURSING DIAGNOSIS AND FORMULATION OF PATIENT CARE GOALS

Nursing Diagnoses

Chapter 15 discussed the general aspects of limited mobility and immobility related to musculoskeletal pathology. *Three diagnoses* related to *limited mobility* discussed in this chapter are: (1) limited mobility caused by paralysis (cerebral vascular accident), (2) limited mobility of an extrapyramidal origin (Parkinsonism), and (3) limited mobility of a cerebellar origin. General nursing intervention for limited mobility will not be repeated, but it should be reviewed. Rather, care specific to the above nursing diagnoses will be covered, as will care specific to *other diagnoses* arising from *problems of neuroregulation* and *sensory perception.* These diagnoses are: (1) impaired consciousness, (2) altered communication caused by aphasia or perceptual problems, (3) bowel or bladder incontinence, (4) altered communication caused by impaired hearing, and (5) limited mobility and altered communication caused by impaired sight.

Patient Care Goals

Long-term goals for anyone with limited mobility were outlined in Chapter 15 and would all be applicable here. Additional objectives relative to the diagnoses outlined above are:

1. Paralyzed limbs achieve optimal possible mobility and contracture formation is absent.
2. Communication is reestablished to the degree possible so that needs, feelings, and ideas can be exchanged.
3. Bowel or bladder continence is reestablished.
4. Movement disorders are controlled permitting mobility and a life-style that are as acceptable to the patient and family as possible.

Short-term goals should be written pertinent to the specific needs of the patient.

Because cerebrovascular accident is a medical diagnosis commonly related to the *nursing diagnoses of impaired mobility or paralysis, altered communication caused by aphasia and perceptual disorders,* and *unconsciousness,* the disease will first be discussed. Then nursing intervention for the respective nursing diagnoses will be covered.

Cerebrovascular Accident: Incidence, Pathology, and Manifestations

The term *cerebrovascular accident* (CVA) implies a *vascular occlusion or rupture of a blood vessel.* The occlusion may be the result of thrombus formation or embolism. A gradually developing occlusion will produce a slow onset of symptoms: weakness, slurred speech, tingling sensations, dizziness, and headaches. Intermittent occlusion may cause transient strokes (brief duration, minimal in symptoms and effects). Rapid, sudden occlusion will result in collapse, unconsciousness, hemiplegia, and aphasia.

Approximately 200,000 people die from cerebrovascular accident (stroke) annually; stroke is the third leading cause of death and the main cause of major defects in locomotion. The American Neurological Association estimates that 2.5 million stroke survivors in the United States each year are left with disability requiring special care. Fifteen percent of all stroke patients are so disabled that they require institutionalization. Prevention through recognition and treatment of major risk factors—severe hypertension, obesity, elevated hematocrit, and abnormal electrocardiogram (ECG)—should be the health professional's goal.[56] Other factors identified in increasing risk are: (1) enlarged heart; (2) ECG findings of left ventricular hypertrophy, myocardial infarction or intraventricular block; (3) congestive heart failure, (4) diabetes; (5) evidence on angiograph of cerebrovascular anomaly or vascular stenosis; and (6) familial history of stroke, angina, peripheral vascular disease, and transient ischemic attacks.[38]

Since diagnosis of the cause of stroke is difficult, physicians are beginning to classify strokes according to the length of time involved. This grouping includes:

1. Transient ischemic attacks (TIA): neurologic deficit occurs abruptly and lasts from minutes to 24 hours and then disappears completely.
2. Reversible ischemic neurologic deficit (RIND): lasts from 1 to 3 days before remitting beyond clinical detection.
3. Stroke-in-evolution: begins as a small neurologic deficit and increases in a steplike manner over several hours to days.

4. Completed stroke (CS): the neurologic deficit remains stable over a long period (days to years) and does not completely disappear.[36]

Signs and symptoms of stroke differ, depending on whether the occlusion or hemorrhage has occurred in the carotid or the vertebral-basilar arterial circulation. Carotid circulation defects usually involve one side and include contralateral weakness or numbness. If the dominant hemisphere is involved, the following are observed: dysphasia, apraxia, and confusion; transient monocular blindness and visual field defects; and throbbing headache.

Symptoms of a stroke occurring in the vertebral-basilar arterial circulation tend to be bilateral and generalized. Signs and symptoms include dysarthria and dysphagia; vertigo, tinnitus, and deafness; unilateral or bilateral sensory and motor defects; generalized imbalance; and visual field defects.[57]

Stroke is usually treated medically. However, surgical intervention, endarterectomy, on stenotic neck vessels is useful in increasing blood flow. Surgery is usually performed on low-risk patients with transient ischemic attacks. Surgery may also be indicated in a stroke caused from hemorrhage when an aneurysm is present and the patient is not comatose. Surgery may also prove beneficial in intracerebellar and selected cases of intracerebral hemorrhage.[24]

Treatment of the stroke patient will be symptomatic and supportive. Anticoagulant therapy may be used in nonhemorrhagic stroke. Anticoagulant drugs can be used on a short-term basis to retard the stroke-in-evolution and for transient ischemic attacks on a long-term basis when surgery is not indicated. Much research is currently in progress regarding the use of warfarin and other anticoagulants for transient ischemic attacks.

Often the patient experiencing a stroke will be unconscious, paralyzed, and have impaired communication, perceptual disorders, and incontinence. Nursing care related to these nursing diagnoses will be covered next.

Nursing Intervention for the Unconscious Senior

The patient experiencing a stroke may become unconscious abruptly or gradually. His care during this period of total helplessness is vital if he is to survive. Being unconscious is a high risk to life at any age, but it is even more so for the elderly because he may have several health problems that are taxing his system. Further, the normal changes that accompany age may lessen his ability to withstand the assault of additional pathology.

He should be placed in the intensive care unit of the hospital: ICU care should not be limited only to patients who are young or who have an obviously favorable prognosis. Often the additional care given in the unit or the measures omitted on a general nursing unit will contribute directly to the elderly patient's recovery or death, as well as to his comfort and the peace of mind of his family.

The need for astute observation and committed care is exemplified by the following case study.

Mr. A. L., 76 years old, with chronic congestive heart failure and diabetes, was admitted to the ICU of a major hospital with an acute episode of pulmonary edema. After approximately 24 hours in the intensive care unit, an embolus lodged in his iliac artery. He experienced immediate pain. A surgeon was called to determine what measures to use. The surgeon decided that the occlusion was not complete and that it would be better to take a "wait-and-see" approach. The physician informed Mr. L's daughter that since Mr. L. had experienced one embolus, others would probably occur and an embolus would likely cause a CVA. Apparently, the physician felt that a CVA was inevitable and that Mr. L. would not benefit from the ICU, so they had Mr. L. transferred to a general nursing unit. Approximately 12 hours later, Mr. L. did experience a cerebral embolus, resulting in hemiplegia, aphasia, and gradual onset of coma. Mr. L's daughter stayed with him all night, and when she left in the morning she was told by the house officer that Mr. L. needed frequent position change and suctioning to prevent respiratory complication. When Mr. L's daughter returned in the afternoon, it did not appear to her that Mr. L's position had been changed or the suction apparatus used. Mr. L. died at 7:00 a.m. the next morning.

Mr. L's daughter later questioned why her father could not have remained in the ICU for the additional 2 days or why he was not readmitted to the unit when the stroke occurred. The care he would have received would have been much better. The daughter would have been spared the necessity of going sleepless for 3 days. The patient and his family would have felt much more comfortable knowing that the care he was receiving was the best he could be given.

Maintaining an open airway is the first priority of care with the unconscious patient. After dentures are removed the jaw often sags and the tongue relaxes against the posterior pharynx, which causes obstruction. A side-lying position or an airway can aid in preventing this. Since the unconscious patient cannot cough up secretions, suctioning will be necessary. Intermittent positive pressure breathing will aid in the aeration of the alveoli and prevent atelectasis. Humidified air should be used to prevent drying of respiratory tract tissues and secretions, especially if the patient is a mouth breather. Giving oxygen per nasal cannula to a patient who is mouth breathing is a questionable practice. A mask is best used on patients who breathe through the mouth.

Oral hygiene is also important. Secretions can collect in the posterior pharynx or on the roof of the mouth or posterior tongue. These secretions can obstruct the airway. Tissues in the mouth should be cleansed with gauze squares on a forceps saturated with mouth wash or a hydrogen peroxide and water mixture, especially if secretions have hardened. Glycerine and lemon juice are used to keep tissues moist. Even if the patient has no teeth, he still requires careful and frequent oral hygiene.

Positioning and exercise are essential and will be discussed in the next section.

Elimination, often in the form of incontinence, is a problem for the unconscious patient and will be discussed later in the chapter.

Thoughtful communication is essential with the unconscious patient because hearing is maintained. Never make comments in front of the patient that may be distressing to him. Even though he is comatose, he should be reassured from time to time, told where he is, what has happened, and what is being done. Perhaps your words will prevent him from feeling hopeless; perhaps they will motivate him to live and recover whatever function he can.

Eye care is essential. If the patient's eyes are not totally closed, they must be cared for by using ophthalmic ointments to prevent drying of the cornea. Blinking helps carry tears over the surface of the eye, thus providing moisture. The unconscious patient does not blink his eyelids regularly. Also, the eyes must be protected against trauma, especially corneal scratching. An eye patch may be indicated for this purpose.

Skin care is vital if pressure areas are to be avoided. Cleansing with minimal soap and thorough rinsing should be the rule. Careful attention to genital regions, under the breasts, and any other areas where chafing can occur is required. Light dusting with corn starch can protect these areas. Change of position every hour or two will promote circulation and improve lung expansion. Turning will also reveal any soil that should be cleansed and any reddened areas that require massage. Areas requiring special attention to prevent pressure sores are coccyx, scapula, heels, vertebra, ears, shoulders, and ankles. These areas should be inspected daily. Sheepskin, heel cushions, air mattresses, and any other pressure-reducing devices, plus frequent position change, massage, and cleanliness, should be used to prevent the occurrence of decubiti.

Good nutrition is also important if decubiti are to be prevented. Immediately following the stroke, parenteral fluids will be all that the unconscious patient requires. However, if unconsciousness is prolonged, a means of providing nutritious feeding becomes necessary. Tube feedings per nasal gastric tube or gastrostomy should be suggested to the physician.

Spiritual support by yourself or the patient's clergyman is also important. The patient's family will also benefit from this. You may read a Bible passage or pray aloud so that the patient hears and feels spiritual support. Often the minister, priest, or rabbi can act as a counselor for the family grappling with the pressures of having a seriously ill family member. The clergy may serve as the patient's advocate or as a liaison between the patient and staff. The minister or priest can also be very helpful if the patient's condition deteriorates. The strength, comfort, and support that the spiritual advisor offers should never be discounted.

Care of the unconscious patient is simply good basic nursing. It is far from glamorous and entails much attention to detail. Regrettably, comprehensive, conscientious care involves many of the nursing functions that have been delegated to ancillary personnel. You, the nurse, must remain alert to the necessity of carefully teaching and supervising this care if it is delegated.

Nursing Intervention for the Senior with Paralysis

Emotional and physical care of the person suffering from paralysis would be similar to that for any person with limited mobility and was covered thoroughly in Chapter 15.

However, paralysis does present unique problems related to the prevention of contractures: positioning of joints in functional positions and range-of-motion exercises. Understanding the two types of paralysis and the underlying pathology will help you to be conscientious in joint and muscle care. *Flaccid paralysis* results from lower motor neuron paralysis. The lower motor neuron serves voluntary as well as reflex motor function and is responsible for transmitting a nerve impulse from anterior horn cell to muscle fiber. Flaccid paralysis results in wasting of the muscles and flail limbs. *Spastic paralysis* results from upper motor neuron paralysis. The corticospinal tract is damaged. Reflexes are preserved but voluntary motion is lost or is impaired. Because there is a resistance of muscles to stretch, stiff limbs result. The major causes of upper motor neuron **hemiplegia** (*paralysis of side of the body opposite the cerebral hemisphere containing a lesion*) are cerebral vascular accident, tumor, abscess, injury, and surgical procedure.[26]

The first principle of care is that *both the involved and uninvolved body parts need exercise and positioning* to maintain muscle strength and full range-of-joint motion and to prevent injury to joints, muscles, or skin. The uninvolved side must remain healthy so that rehabilitation is possible.

Exercise should be as strenuous as permitted by the patient's medical condition. If paralysis and immobility have been the result of thrombosis and if his cardiac and mental functionings are adequate, he will be encouraged to turn from side to side and on his abdomen, move up and down in bed, use an overhead trapeze, and participate in his own care. If immobility is the result of hemorrhage or if his cardiac or mental functions do not permit independent exercise, you will be responsible for turning and moving the patient in bed. Range-of-motion exercises also will be determined by the patient's overall condition. Exercise may be active, totally passive, or delayed until danger of further hemorrhage has subsided. Exercise helps to prevent muscle atrophy and joint contractures.

Positioning is essential for paralyzed limbs and general physiological functioning and to prevent the dangers of immobility. Frequent changes of position (using both sides, back, and abdomen) should be performed at least once per hour.

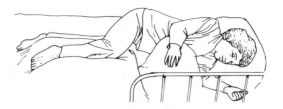

Figure 16.3. Placement for side-lying position.

See Figures 16.3 and 16.4 for side-lying and prone positions. Standing position, if tolerated, is another position that stimulates normal function. The weight bearing produced by the standing position helps to overcome orthostatic hypotension and prevents demineralization of bones with its accompanying urinary tract stones. Frequent changes of position are important in preventing venous thrombosis, decubiti, contractures, and hypostatic pneumonia.

Positioning joints is very important. Physiological functioning of muscles must be considered when doing this. Remember generally that flexor muscles are stronger than extensor muscles. For example, the effect of the flexor arm muscles is to cause adduction of upper arm to the body, flexion of elbow, adduction of forearm to the front of the chest, flexion of the wrist, and curling of fingers. No excuse exists for a situation encountered by this author while caring for a patient who was several months post-CVA. The patient's arm was so tightly contracted that to perform any form of exercise was almost impossible. She had what is called a *frozen shoulder,* a type of contracture that frequently occurs in spastic paralysis. The shoulder joint may also be injured by careless handling of the arm or overstrenuous exercise of the joint. Subluxation may occur from the weight of the arm hanging from the shoulder.

Upper extremity problems can be prevented by careful handling of the arm, use of a sling when sitting or walking, and positioning the arm in functional positions by using pillows and hand rolls. Several arm positions should be utilized, as shown in Figure 16.5. Do not position any portion of the upper extremity beyond the point of resistance or pain.

When applying a sling, always remember that the wrist must be carried in the sling to prevent wrist drop and that the knot must not rest on a vertebra. The weight of the arm should *not* be borne by the neck. The method of sling

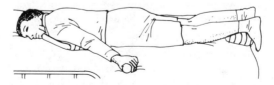

Figure 16.4. Placement for face-lying position.

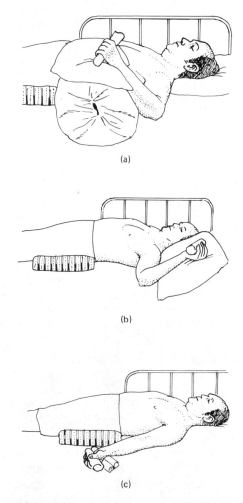

(a)

(b)

(c)

Figure 16.5. Placement for arm and hand positions.

application should place weight bearing on the shoulders (see Figure 16.6). Also, range-of-motion exercises must be performed when the sling is removed.

The lower extremities need attention to prevent foot drop, external rotation of the hip and knee, or hip contracture. Elevation of the head of the bed for any extended period can contribute to hip contracture. Elevation of the knee gatch can result in knee contracture. To prevent external rotation of the hip, support the leg with a sandbag or trochanter roll from above the hip to well below the knee on the outside surface of the leg. Have the feet touch a footboard to prevent foot drop contracture. Pressure on the heels can be relieved by a small block of sponge placed just above the heel to lift it slightly off the bed.[3]

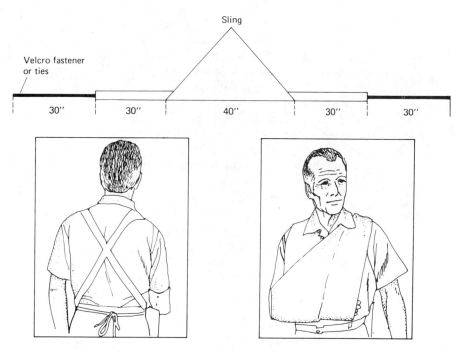

Figure 16.6. Application of sling to arm.

The back-knee deformity should be prevented if possible. Back-knee deformity occurs in patients with return of voluntary functioning when the quadriceps are strong and the hamstrings are weak. It can be avoided by placing a small support under the knees when the patient is supine. However, the support should only be enough to relieve the stretch on the tendons of the extended knee and not enough to cause considerable flexion. The support must not cause pressure in the popliteal space or to the lower leg.[26]

Range-of-joint motion exercises will not be described here. Chapter 15 outlined assessment of normal range-of-joint motion, which would be the degree of movement sought when performing the exercises. Yet, maximum range may not be possible. You should not take range-of-motion exercises beyond the point of pain or resistance before checking with the physical therapist or physician.

Rehabilitative prognosis is dependent to a greater degree on the function of the uninvolved extremities than of the involved extremities. Thus, you must give as much attention to the healthy uninvolved limbs, and the patient must be encouraged to exercise them to maintain their function and strength.

The proprioceptive and superficial sensation changes account for the physiological bases for disturbed body image in paralysis or CVA. Since proprioceptors on the paralyzed side do not give spatial cues to the person, he has no awareness of his paralyzed side. If you ask the senior to do something with the paralyzed limb, he will carry out the activity with the uninvolved limb. Without proprioceptive feedback, he has no idea where his paralyzed limb is unless he is looking at it. Thus, he must be taught to visually check the position and safety of his affected limbs, especially as he transfers or when standing. When you assist the patient in moving, be sure that you do not stand where you obstruct his vision of the affected limbs. Make sure that the room is well lighted and that reference points (doors, mirrors, or furniture) are clearly established as he transfers or tries to walk. Avoid cluttered, dimly lit rooms, wallpapered rooms, a crowd of people, and rapid movement, for all of these confuse the patient's perception of his body. Also approach and talk to him from the unaffected side as you do care, and arrange furniture and belongings on that side of the room.[10, 43]

Body image reintegration is enhanced by having the patient enter into his care as much as possible. Body image changes occur as the person progresses from lying in bed to sitting in a wheelchair. Yet the wheelchair is interposed between the person and his environment, so that the body image remains somewhat distorted because he cannot obtain direct feedback from the environment about body size and position. He misjudges both, and as a result has difficulty getting through doors or narrow spaces. He also has more difficulty if he is visually impaired or is in a dimly lit room.[1]

Body image usually becomes more intact during the year after the paralysis or CVA; apparently it takes about a year to reach major rehabilitative goals. After that the person plateaus physically and he may also feel more vulnerable and less sure of his body boundaries and mental image of self.[45]

Nursing Intervention for the Senior with Impaired Communication Caused by Aphasia or Perceptual Disorders

Aphasia and perceptual disorders have a number of causes, but a common cause for the elderly is cerebral vascular accident. The person who has a CVA may present either a left or right hemiparesis, depending on the side of the brain in which pathology has occurred. The side of the brain that is involved will determine whether aphasia or other perceptual problems are present.

Table 16.3 compares common disorders, their manifestations, and the most likely side of hemiparesis.[3]

Nursing care of the patient with a problem in communicating, perceiving, or with altered inner thinking requires patience, understanding of the problem involved, and careful attention to planning and implementing of nursing approaches appropriate to the diagnosis. Individualizing care is essential. An accurate history is necessary in order to uncover the premorbid personality and determine whether the behavior is the result of pathology or is a lifelong personality pattern. Getting to know the patient and establishing a constructive relationship are necessary if he is to be helped to adjust to the disorder and regain confidence in his abilities. In addition to language or perception problems, the patient may also have visual field alterations and body image problems, and he may be in a state of emotional turmoil because of fear, insecurity, lack of understanding of what has happened to him or where he is, frustration at being unable to communicate or comprehend, and anger at being incapacitated and helpless. *Your thoughtful, kind, understanding, pleasant, and accepting approach* can do much to help the patient overcome these problems and negative feelings.

The patient may have *dysarthria; speech disturbed by muscle paralysis,* as well as *aphasia, loss of language usage.* Either of these conditions causes the person to feel frustrated, out of control, unable to trust himself, and at the

TABLE 16.3   Manifestations of Right and Left Hemiparesis

Type of Disorder	Description	Area of Brain Affected
Expressive aphasia*	Unable to communicate needs and thoughts with language but can understand what is being said.	Right hemiparesis. Left cortex involved.
Receptive aphasia*	Unable to understand what others are saying.	Right hemiparesis. Left cortex involved.
Global aphasia	Unable to use or understand language.	Severe organic brain damage.
Spatial-perceptual difficulties	Fluent speech. Reduced sense of position, body part, or inside/outside. Difficulty integrating movements and objects in the environment.	Left hemiparesis. Right cortex involved.
Agnosia	Unable to comprehend tactile, auditory, or visual sensation.	Left hemiparesis.
Apraxia	Unable to perform acts on command but may be able to do so automatically. May be unable to use speech muscles but is not aphasic.	Left hemiparesis.
Inner-thinking disorders	Alteration in inner language, i.e., language used to talk and think to self.	Both left and right hemiparesis.
Personality disorders	Inappropriate behavior. Rigidity. Unable to adjust to rapid or unfamiliar happenings. Demanding. Agitated. Labile. Withdrawn.	Both left and right hemiparesis.

* Patient may be able to utter sounds, words of endearment or cursing; use automatic speech (repeat verse or prayer without comprehension of meaning); give serial words (days of week, months of year); say ''Yes'' and ''No'' without comprehension.

mercy of others. He fears that he is going crazy, especially when he uses expletives or says something that he does not mean. Talking normally serves many functions: It enhances self-esteem, exchanges ideas and feelings, validates ideas, gains and gives information, modifies opinions or judgment, increases sociability, and maintains contact with reality.

The aphasic's behavior may at times seem inappropriate. He misunderstands what you say, and his behavior is based on his interpretation. Do not label his behavior as uncooperative and stubborn.

Your *nonverbal communication* with the aphasic patient is crucial; he will respond to it more than to your verbal communication. The set of your head, eye and facial expression, body posture, position of hands, and voice tone may tell him more than you realize. Your nonverbal and verbal messages should match.

Always *speak* slowly and in a normal tone of voice; emphasize major ideas. Gestures can help the aphasic patient understand, but they may confuse the patient with perceptual problems. Use simple, short sentences. Do not interrupt and do not belittle attempts at speech. Do not supply words, but it is not advisable to allow the patient to become overly frustrated. All attempts at speech should be encouraged and should not be corrected. Ask direct questions that require a yes/no answer when trying to ascertain needs, but do not bombard him with questions. Be cautious when speaking about the patient's condition to another in his presence. Medical terminology in relation to complications and deterioration can cause apprehension and worry. This caution should be adhered to even for the apparently comatose or nonresponsive patient who may be able to understand even if he is unable to communicate. The patient needs to be treated as an adult. Speaking to him as if he were a child can be very demeaning and demoralizing. He should be encouraged to participate in social activities but should not be expected to communicate to a large group.[3,25,30]

In **receptive aphasia** *the impairment varies from great difficulty in understanding speech to occasional difficulty.* He may hear words, understand them, but not remember them long enough to respond appropriately, or he may remember and respond to only a portion of the request. He may hear correctly but be unable to connect the words with previously learned meanings; thus, he cannot follow verbal directions. The person is not being stubborn; accept his behavior as part of his illness. Ask him to perform simple tasks so that you can determine his level of comprehension. Respond to his gestures; try to understand them by observing their context and his nonverbal messages. Give him one command at a time; if he can follow that, give him two directions together to determine if he is capable of retaining both ideas in his head and responding to them. Work with a speech therapist to learn the exact nature of the patient's aphasia and how the team can be consistent in approach.

In his rehabilitation, teach him by talking slowly, pausing after each sentence to allow him time to interpret and respond. Use gestures with simple, concrete terms, but do not talk down to him. If he cannot respond, rephrase or repeat the directions. Stand near, within his line of vision, so that he can receive your full message. If necessary, demonstrate the task you want him to do in small units and then allow him time to repeat these small units so that he can learn the task. Finally, have him demonstrate the entire task. The patient's ability to understand may vary from day to day, which adds to the frustration level for him and you. Allow enough time in your work with him for the varying impairments you encounter so that his rehabilitative work is not rushed or the cause of a sense of hopelessness or negative self-concept.

In *expressive aphasia, difficulty in speaking,* you should accept whatever speech sounds the patient makes. You should talk to the patient as much as possible because your talking stimulates his desire to reply. Do not demand that he reply. When he cannot reply, carry on an interesting one-way conversation. Give the patient a pad and pencil so that he can write or draw what he wants to tell you. Although the patient cannot talk, assume that he can hear and understand. Give him extra time to answer or interpret your words and respond to them. Since he may not remember from day to day, repeat directions slowly as necessary; say one direction at a time. Avoid distracting noises. Use gestures to help convey your message.

Consider safety. The patient with perceptual problems is prone to accidents and injury because of a tendency to attempt activities that he cannot do. He is unaware of his incapacity. He may be impulsive, use poor judgment, and be unaware of danger because of an inability to perceive himself and his body parts in relation to the environment. This patient will probably not seek assistance when it is needed. He may attempt to go to the bathroom or transfer to a wheelchair without any understanding of how his condition inhibits his activity.[3] Place him close to the nurse's station and anticipate his needs so that you can help cope with the problem. Side rails and a posey belt or jacket may be helpful, but they may also result in a frustrated, angry patient. If they are used, their purpose as a safety measure must be explained and all his requests must be met promptly in order to avoid a negative response.

Adapt your approach to the personality change caused by brain damage that accompanies aphasia. The patient can be easily overwhelmed if the environment is excessively stimulating. A controlled, structured environment and schedule are better than an unstructured, permissive environment. One person, if possible, with as few substitutions as necessary, should be responsible for his daily care. Excessive stimulation and multiple demands should be avoided. Loud noise, too many activities, and frequent, numerous visitors may result in agitation and frustration and may delay adjustment to the new surroundings and rehabilitation. Long-range goals may only be established and achieved once the patient is adjusted to his environment and feels secure with those responsible for his care.

The patient who is withdrawn may require special attention in order to reach him and keep his interest. Stimulation might include showing him something that he is especially fond of and commenting on it, dressing him in his own clothes, giving him something to eat that he especially relishes, or having a special friend or relative visit. A previously enjoyed activity may be initiated, such as watching a sports game on television, going on a jaunt outdoors or to a picnic in a wheelchair, or eating fresh baked goods after watching the preparation. The possibilities are endless and you can use your ingenuity in trying to keep him in touch with his environment. Convey that communication is desirable and possible. Reality orientation, discussed in Chapter 4, is a must for the withdrawn individual. This author has found that the withdrawn patient often responds to a small child or to a cuddly animal. The very regressed often responds to a plush toy. The delight that is often seen in the face of a withdrawn elderly patient when a baby is placed in his lap cannot be adequately described.

Remind personnel and family that mood swings are not an unusual result of the pathology and are not usually related to anything personnel or family members may have said or done.

Encourage and praise the patient who is actively participating in his rehabilitation, for he will become frustrated and anxious if he cannot achieve his goal of expressing a thought or performing a specific task. Frustration can lead to the patient's acting impulsively without good judgment or regard for consequences of the act. Safety measures may have to be used to prevent impulsive behavior. He should continue to attempt the task to his level of frustration, which provides the necessary energy to achieve the task. Beyond this point, however, he may experience an uncontrollable rage-like response called a *catastrophic response.*[13] Since the catastrophic response may result in unconsciousness, overly frustrating activities must be terminated as quickly as possible.

Aphasia and perceptual difficulties can cause feelings of frustration, anger, and helplessness. If you have ever traveled to a foreign country and attempted to communicate with the residents without a knowledge of their language, you will have some understanding of the patient's feelings. In addition to helplessness and frustration, add fear of death or lifelong incapacity, paralysis, and lack of control of daily living activities. Remind yourself of these feelings whenever you care for a patient with aphasia and a CVA. These patients can try your patience, but an understanding of what they are experiencing can make the task easier.

Self-concept, body image, and rehabilitation are affected by loss of the integrative abilities (aphasia, agnosia, apraxia, and perseveration).

The area of the brain that is damaged also affects body image perception. The person with *right hemiplegia* has difficulty in understanding and carrying out verbal orders and in associating words to the body part. Further, he has **right-field hemianopsia**; *he cannot see with the right halves of both eyes.* Thus, he only sees the unaffected portion of himself and half of his environment. The person with *left hemiplegia* has difficulty localizing himself in space because of spatial perceptual impairment. He cannot judge position, distance, rate of movement, form, or where body parts are in relation to other objects. His *left field of vision is cut (left hemianopsia)*, which again interferes with accurate perception of self. The person with left hemiplegia also confuses up and down, right and left, inside and outside. He stays disoriented longer. He misjudges space, often running into door frames. He cannot read because he cannot keep his eyes focused on the page. He may behave as if nothing is wrong; he is overconfident with unfamiliar tasks and is impulsive. He may even be able to describe what he can do but be unable to follow through unless he is given guidance.[45]

Hemianopsia causes one-sided neglect. The person pays no attention to the affected side, even if he suffers injury. He does not recognize a tray of food set on the affected side or food on that half of the tray. Turn the tray around so that he sees the rest of the food and eats it. Because of the limited sensory input, he becomes easily confused. When he walks in one direction, he sees only half of the area. When he returns, he sees the other half and thinks that he is in a different area. He needs help in recognizing the affected side through repeated range-of-motion exercises, your verbal recognition of the affected limbs, or through special stimuli, such as a ribbon or bell attached to the affected limb. While he is prone, turn his head toward the affected side. Have the patient use the unaffected side to exercise the affected side. In the beginning he needs supervision.

Agnosia, decreased ability to recognize the meaning of sensory stimuli (usually visual and auditory), and *anosognosia, denial or unawareness of the disease process and the paralysis,* are behaviors that result from the brain damage associated with CVA and the crisis of his illness. He ignores the logic of time, place, and circumstance in relation to his paralyzed limb. He may believe that the paralyzed limb belongs to someone else and should not be in bed with him. He may see an object or hear a statement but be unable to comprehend the meaning, for example, of a bouquet of flowers or the sound of a siren.

Astereognosis, loss of the ability in the affected hand to differentiate objects by touch, is present. Sense of touch and pain on the affected side is also reduced, which has implications for pressure areas or being burned by hot water bottles or heating pads.

In *apraxia, the ability to direct muscles to act is interfered with.* His hand muscles may be physically able to hold an object, but he cannot direct his hand to do so. He appears clumsy. Or he may not be able to use an object, such as a fork or spoon, because he does not recognize the object or does not recall how to use it. The patient may have to be shown how to use the object.

In *perseveration, the same movement is made repetitiously until stopped by another person.* Since certain movements may be injurious to him, you will have to physically stop a movement that is repeated excessively because the patient cannot stop the movement.

Agnosia, apraxia, and perseveration are difficult to recognize and handle because the patient cannot describe what he is feeling. Further, his behavior may be misinterpreted as stubbornness, disinterest, or lack of motivation. These conditions, along with hemianopsia and aphasia, impair learning: They interfere with memory, attention span, judgment, abstract thought, or transfer of learning from one situation to another. Realistic short-term goals are necessary so that the senior, family, and you can see progress.

Nursing Intervention for the Senior with Urinary or Intestinal Incontinence

Nothing is more demoralizing and injurious to the self-concept than is the loss of control over elimination functions. From earliest childhood we have been rewarded for achieving control of bowel and bladder. Bed-wetting in childhood results in scolding or a trip to the doctor's office to determine the cause and put a stop to it. Thus, the person in later maturity who loses this control may feel guilty, inadequate, regressed, and dirty. The patient will feel embarrassed and exposed when the nurse or family member must clean up the "mess."

Spare the patient embarrassment and protect his feelings of modesty. Careful draping to avoid unnecessary exposure of the body area is essential since the elderly person grew up at a time when covering the body was the norm. Exposure even to family members was considered in poor taste. An accepting, matter-of-fact approach, with neither verbal nor nonverbal negative expressions, is best with the patient. A prompt, quick, thorough clean-up, without undue body exposure, will help the patient.

Urinary incontinence is common in the patient who has had a CVA because of unconsciousness, confusion, and inability to communicate. When he regains consciousness, confusion, aphasia, and paralysis will continue to inhibit him from resuming responsibility for his toileting. Even if he is not confused, he may become so frustrated by attempting to make his need known and not having it met that he will eventually give up and accept his incontinence.

Bowel and bladder continence is possible for the patient with paralysis or a CVA since the nondamaged side of the cortex can control incontinence. The necessity for a schedule of toileting must be emphasized. Offering fluids frequently and achieving an adequate intake (2000 to 3000 ml daily) will contribute to control—a fact that some may find difficult to understand. The bedpan or urinal should be put in place every 2 hours. The more natural the patient's position, the more likely that the effort will be successful. Either a commode or the bathroom is better than a bedpan if either can possibly be used. If the patient is incontinent, note the time and then adjust the schedule of toileting accordingly. Often patients will achieve control if they are toileted on their premorbid schedule. If the patient usually voided upon arising, before retiring, and following meals, the same routine can be attempted. Additional toileting (for example, before meals) may be necessary in the beginning of continence training.

Prevent embarrassment for the patient by providing pads for bed and chairs, rubber sheeting, disposable pads for inserting into underwear, or waterproof panties. Men may be able to use a sheath connected to a leg drainage bag. These aids, however, should not replace the regular schedule of toileting. They should only be used in case of an accident.

An indwelling catheter should not be required in CVA, but if one is inserted, it must be handled aseptically. A closed system of drainage that is changed every 24 hours helps prevent contamination from ascending into the bladder. The following program for reinitiating bladder control should be begun as soon as possible:

1. Indwelling catheter is removed.
2. Toileting is done every 2 hours, increasing to every 4 hours.
3. Catheterize twice daily for residual until it is less than 100 ml.[26]

However, *avoid catheters if at all possible*. According to estimates, within 72 hours a urinary tract infection will develop in 70 percent of catheterized patients.[35]

In upper motor neuron disorders, urination may be fostered by tactile stimulation of the areas innervated by the pudendal nerve.[3] For example, pouring warm water over the perineum may stimulate voiding.

Research has been conducted using a system of rewarding desired behavior and punishing behavior that the nurse is attempting to alter or eliminate. This approach is called *contingency management* and has been attempted with the incontinent elderly patient. A thorough evaluation of the patient's problem and a review of what is rewarding for him are necessary. After a decision is made about what will constitute a reward, the patient is rewarded whenever he is found to be dry on half-hourly checks. If he has been incontinent, no reward is given. Later, this is modified so that rewards are given when the patient is dry for several hours or when he appropriately uses the toilet. Further modifications are made as progress is made, so that eventually rewards are only given when the patient independently uses the toilet at appropriate times.[35]

Infection of the urinary tract can be a serious complication for the paralyzed patient. Normally, the bladder remains sterile because of the constant dilution of the bladder contents by fresh urine and its periodic complete emptying. Residual urine becomes stagnant and is an ideal culture medium. Reflux of residual urine can result in kidney infection. Many organisms that cause urinary tract infections metabolize urea in an alkaline urine. This increased pH contributes to the precipitation of certain minerals out of the urine, resulting in a sediment that can form into stones. If an indwelling catheter is in place, this sediment can collect on the inflated catheter bulb. Later, when the catheter is removed, the sediment may become detached and remain in the bladder, becoming the nucleus for a bladder stone. Or it may make removal of the catheter very difficult; the trauma further contributes to infection.

Be aware of the symptoms of urinary tract infections (chills, elevated temperature, decreased urinary output, hematuria, burning, frequency, urgency) and report them immediately. Fluid intake of 3000 ml daily should maintain dilution and help prevent infection. Juices to achieve an acid urine, such as cranberry and prune, should be offered.

In addition to urinary tract infections, autonomic hyperreflexia may be caused by an extremely overdistended bladder resulting from a blocked indwelling catheter. The symptoms to observe for are anxiety, severe headache, elevated blood pressure, bradycardia, diaphoresis, fever, and pilomotor reflex.[3]

Another complication to observe for in long-term use of an indwelling catheter with a male patient is penial-scrotal fistula. The fistula occurs at the junction of the penis and scrotum and can be observed when the penis is lifted.[3]

Reestablishing urinary control is probably one of the most important factors that will contribute to the total rehabilitation of the patient.

Fecal incontinence need not become a problem following paralysis, even in a severely cognitively impaired patient. *Constipation and impaction can be avoided* by giving a diet that is adequate in bulk and fluids, establishing a regular schedule for evacuation, using stool softeners, and judiciously using suppositories. Remember that patients will have the urge to defecate after a meal, usually breakfast. Check with the patient or his family about the usual time. Then take advantage of this information for planning his care schedule. Place a glycerine suppository at least 2½ inches into the rectum one-half hour before defecation time to soften the stool, provide lubrication, and enhance the normal urge.[26] The normal position for defecation should be assumed.

Paralysis, aphasia, and incontinence are three major problems confronting elderly persons who have experienced a cerebral vascular accident. The nursing care measures just discussed can be applied to seniors who exhibit these problems, regardless of their medical diagnosis.

Nursing Intervention for the Senior with Movement Disorders

Movement disorders caused by either extrapyramidal or cerebellar origin will be discussed together. Paralysis is not present, but the patient experiences difficulty in locomotion and life-style changes because of effects on muscle tone, coordination, and balance. Effects of lesions are compared in Table 16.4.[2]

Parkinson's disease caused by extrapyramidal defects is the most common movement disorder encountered in adults in later maturity. The disease is characterized by progressive rigidity of limb and trunk musculature, decreasing voluntary movement, and posture and gait changes. Neck flexion, elbow and knee flexion, forward leaning, absence of arm swinging, and tiny, shuffling steps characterize the gait and movement of the body as one solid unit. The tremor of Parkinson's increases when resting or walking, occurring rhythmically at the rate of 4 to 6 per second. The tremor of the hands is described as pill-rolling. The tremor may affect hands, feet, head, lips, and tongue. Speech is soft, slowed, and monotonous. Excessive salivation, seborrhea, constipation, and urinary difficulties also occur.

Your nursing care will include measures related to the medical treatment of Parkinson's disease. Levodopa, in a dosage of 3 to 8 gm daily, or 1 to 2 gm when used with carbidopa, relieves the rigidity, slowness, and tremor. You must observe for side effects: nausea, postural hypotension, involuntary movements, blurred vision, confusion, dry mouth, and constipation. Teach the senior to take the medication with meals or an antacid, or use antiemetics to relieve nausea.[24] Instruct him to rise slowly from a reclining position and wait several seconds to minutes before attempting to stand. Remaining close to the bed or couch for a minute or two after rising will help prevent falls from hypotension. A diet high in bulk and adequate fluid intake help overcome constipation. Reducing the dosage will also aid in reducing side effects. Pyridoxine (vitamin B$_6$) will interfere with the drug's effect; patients should be warned against taking vitamin preparations. Anticholinergic drugs such as Artane, Disipal, and Cogentin can be effective in Parkinson's, but the side effects in elderly persons may preclude their use. For example, these drugs are contraindicated in glaucoma, benign prostatic hypertrophy, or tachycardia.

Surgical treatment has not proven as effective in older patients as it has in younger adults with other involuntary movement disorders. Thus, the usual treatment consists of medication, supportive measures, and rehabilitation.[24]

You can assist the senior and his family in adjusting to the problems associated with involuntary movements. Proper balance of rest and exercise is im-

TABLE 16.4.   Comparison of Extrapyramidal and Cerebellar Lesions

Assessment Parameter	Extrapyramidal Lesion	Cerebellar Lesion
Main functions affected	Muscle tone and related movement. No paralysis.	Coordination and balance. No paralysis.
General appearance	Resting tremor noted. Lack of motion otherwise (masklike face).	Appears normal. When asked to perform a task, intention tremor noted.
Strength and voluntary movement	Normal to decreased strength. Slow voluntary movement.	Normal to decreased strength. Uncoordinated voluntary movement.
Movement of extremities by examiner	Increased muscle tone. Rigid, cogwheeling.	Decreased muscle tone.

portant. Exercises prescribed by the physical therapist and speech therapist should be conscientiously performed. Specific exercises of value in helping to counteract the change in tone of muscles controlling speech are: deep diaphragmatic breathing, holding vowel sounds for 15 seconds each, reading aloud, singing, and extending the tongue and then moving it up, down, and sideways. Exercises for other muscle groups include full range of motion for all joints including fingers, toes, back, neck, wrists, elbows, shoulders, hips, knees, and ankles. Marching and bicycle riding movements are good exercises and can be performed in groups or individually.[11] Since symptoms will be exaggerated by fatigue, rest periods must be scheduled several times daily.

The senior should be encouraged and assisted to remain as active as he was prior to the onset of his illness, if possible. He should return to his former employment or hobbies, if possible. If he is retired, occupational and recreational therapy are useful. Or the state or local Department of Vocational Rehabilitation may have a suitable training program. Church groups or various organizations may provide group activities that keep him active.

Family members must become involved in planning for the senior's rehabilitation. They must understand that maintaining activity—physical, social, vocational, or recreational—is important to his adjustment to the illness and gradual incapacity.

Anything that produces or intensifies stress should be avoided because stress intensifies symptoms. Also, if the patient has the inclination to worry, he should be taught to cope with stress in a more direct manner. The patient's family should also be encouraged to avoid increasing stress for the patient.

Consider the patient's intellectual capacity, which is not impaired. Communicate with him on his level; give him reading materials and other forms of intellectual stimulation.

Adapt room temperature as necessary. Heat and cold intolerance may present a problem. Because of the tremor and muscle rigidity, the patient may be uncomfortably warm in what seems to be a comfortable temperature. Frequent changes of wearing apparel may be needed.

Encourage the senior to maintain social contacts and attend social activities as long as possible. Some of the symptoms, such as drooling and tremor, may eventually interfere with attending public social activities. However, he should still be included in all social activities of the family. Celebration of holidays, birthdays, or anniversaries, and family picnics can provide enjoyment and stimulation, even in the severely incapacitated.

Speech therapy can be very helpful in teaching the patient how to maintain control of his tongue and facial muscles. Therapy can be done individually or in groups.

Adapt to his emotional symptoms. The patient's frustration of not being able to control his body is manifested by depression, anger, and crying. The senior's moods should be accepted: he needs to know that the staff and family understand what he is experiencing and do not take his behavior as a personal attack. The patient and family need the support and understanding of a knowledgeable rehabilitation team.

Continuity of care is essential. Drugs have done much to arrest or alleviate symptoms, but a cure has not as yet been developed. Progressive deterioration usually continues over a period of years. The patient needs one person to whom he can relate and with whom he can share his feelings, frustrations, desires, and needs. The private physician is usually the one continuous person with whom the patient has contact. But since the physician cannot usually spare the time required for the patient to express himself, it would be advantageous for another person on the team to be available to provide this continuity of support. The nurse practitioner could provide continuity of care. Organization and payment within the health care delivery system today do not promote continuity of care by the nurse, but they should be goals for the future.

Nursing Intervention for the Senior with Altered Communication Caused by Impaired Hearing

Impaired hearing is one of the most common sensory perception problems encountered by the adult in later maturity. Tinnitus is also a frequent complaint. Together, they can cause communication difficulties, social isolation, severe annoyance, anxiety, and frustration. The person who cannot hear what others are saying often becomes suspicious of others and wonders if others are talking about him, even though they may not be. When the senior must repeatedly ask to have a statement repeated, others become aggravated, angry, fatigued, and rejecting. They are likely to say less. Conversation becomes abbreviated because of the effort it takes to talk to the hearing impaired person. Further, most people prefer not to shout private business or intimate thoughts, whether they are talking about the mortgage, shopping list, or saying "I love you." Others begin to speak less often to the hearing impaired; they talk to each other. Contact with children may become minimal because the person cannot understand them. One senior said, "All I hear is a babble. Unless they talk right to me, I can't get a word of the conversation." He adapted to family gatherings by going into his room and lying on the bed after the initial "hello." No wonder that the hearing impaired thinks suspicious thoughts and feels rejected and isolated.

The type of hearing loss most frequently encountered in the elderly is *presbycusis, a gradual loss of hearing of sensorineural origin.* The cochlea or the auditory nerve, or both, are impaired. Sensitivity for high frequencies diminishes first and gradually progresses to the lower tones as well. Poor speech discrimination also occurs. Loss of hearing is bilateral.

Medical and surgical treatments do not offer much help for this condition. Hearing aids, auditory training, and training in visual recognition of speech (lip reading) offer some hope of improving communication ability.

You can teach the elderly about potential use and limitations of *hearing aids.* A hearing aid is a simple amplifier. Sounds that enter the microphone are amplified at the loudspeaker, which is the earpiece. Hearing aids are designed to deliver enough sound energy so that the person who has some residual hearing can hear speech spoken into the aid. Those who have no residual hearing will be able to feel the vibrations. They will be aware that someone is speaking, be able to follow the rhythm, and with other visual clues from lip reading may be able to understand what is being said.

Hearing aids today are very small and lightweight. Thus, they are more likely to be accepted. However, their small size limits to some degree the quality of sound amplification. Low- and high-frequency sounds are not amplified to the same degree as middle-frequency tones, which along with amplification of other noises, causes additional speech distortion for the senior with presbycusis. Therefore, many elderly reject the hearing aid. Other factors that cause dissatisfaction are the tiny controls that may be difficult to see and manipulate, tiny short-lived batteries, and ill-fitted ear molds that cause sound to escape, be reamplified, and squeal.

The small hole in the ear mold must be kept clear of wax and other debris. If it becomes clogged, the aid loses much of its effectiveness. Daily cleaning and careful drying will prevent clogging and also help prevent earskin irritations.

The cord leading from the earpiece to the microphone needs special attention to avoid tangling and breaking. Rubbing of the microphone against clothing can cause annoyance; therefore, it should be clipped to an area that will receive minimal movement. Hearing aids incorporated into the ear piece of eyeglasses alleviate this problem. However, these glasses will be heavier and may not be tolerated.

All of these care details, plus cost and previous poor experience with aids, causes the older adult to be reluctant to accept an aid. However, the biggest impediment may be his denial of his inability to hear as well as he once did. Denial may arise from a lack of awareness of his problem or its severity and an unwillingness to admit that he has a problem. Hearing aids still carry a stigma that many people feel marks them as old and debilitated.[50]

Teach the family methods of talking with the hearing impaired that are suggested in Chapter 9. The family uses various adaptations, such as speaking more clearly, slowly, and loudly while in face-to-face conversation and eliminating television and other extraneous noise as much as possible. When these adaptations no longer help, the family should be encouraged to have the patient see an otorrhinolaryngologist who will examine him and, if indicated, refer the senior to an audiologist for hearing aid evaluation. The specialist should be seen first, since he is the one to decide whether or not an aid should be recommended, the type, which ear it should be worn in, and the style best suited for the person. The specialist also explains the problem, what can be expected from an aid, and recommends other measures that the family and patient can take to alleviate the problem.[51] The patient and family must be aware of what to expect. If their expectations are unrealistic, both patient and family might be disappointed and reluctant to seek medical help with future problems.

The hearing aid dealer will take the specialist's recommendations and select an aid that best fits the prescription. He will also make the ear mold from an impression of the ear and then fit the hearing aid, adjust it, and demonstrate its operation. He can supply batteries and service as needed.

Auditory training, training in listening to amplified sound, prior to and after purchasing the hearing aid enhances its acceptance and effective use.

Lip reading, or *speech reading, is the process whereby the person derives clues to what another is saying from movement of the eyes, tongue, cheeks, throat, and lips.* Poor vision may preclude the use of lip reading. Also, motivation is probably the most important element in accepting any program to improve hearing. The family's understanding and cooperation with the program and their reassurance and encouragement may make the difference between success and failure. You should be aware of what type of hearing improvement program has been prescribed. If the senior is hospitalized, the nursing staff must be instructed in the care and insertion of the hearing aid, as well as how to communicate with the patient. The elderly person who rapidly becomes disoriented after being hospitalized may be saved this trauma if those responsible for his care keep him reality oriented with use of all possible aids to improve sensory function. Therefore, never let the patient who has been accustomed to using a hearing aid go without it.

Encourage the hearing-impaired senior to remain socially active, and help his family recognize their roles. Often churches and theaters will have special equipment available so that the senior can hear and participate in the activities. Also, special telephone equipment is available for the hearing impaired. Television programs often have subtitles or sign language dubbed in to aid comprehension. Public television stations usually have regular programming scheduled for the hearing impaired. They will make this schedule available if requested. Keeping active mentally and socially is most important to a successful rehabilitation program for hearing loss.

Nursing Intervention for the Senior with Limited Mobility and Altered Communication Caused by Impaired Vision

Vision is important to all aspects of life. Locomotion can be severely limited when sight begins to fail. Activities of daily living become increasingly difficult. Communication is interfered with since the patient no longer can use conventional reading materials and no longer can see expressions on people's faces. The senior can no longer read his mail, pay his bills, watch a movie or television, pursue hobbies that require adequate vision, see the grandchildren grow up, or enjoy the beauty of life as it exists all around us. So much that the sighted take for granted is lost when sight fails.

When the senior no longer has sight for orientation, he becomes more dependent on the other senses. If two or more senses begin to decline, his ties to reality become less secure. The senior who is mentally impaired to a small degree may be thrown into a complete state of confusion by loss of sight and hearing. The nursing staff must never intensify a patient's problems by failing to keep glasses and hearing aids clean, operative, and in place.

Common causes of vision impairment in later years will be discussed. One of the leading causes of blindness is diabetic retinopathy. The best prevention for this condition is careful regulation of the diabetes through close medical supervision. More will be said about this in Chapter 19.

Presbyopia, *increasing failure of the lens to accommodate for close vision,* affects all of us eventually. Although presbyopia does not result in blindness, it can be very annoying and distressing, especially when the adult in his early forties begins to experience this first symptom of the aging process. The person needs to hold near objects farther and farther away from the eyes in order to focus. Presbyopia can be corrected by a biconvex lens for reading. Stronger reading glasses will be needed every few years because the near point (distance from the eye at which near objects can be easily seen) continues to slip farther away. Pride should not keep the patient from securing the correction needed. Bifocals or reading glasses are not half so conspicuous as squinting and holding reading material at arm's length in an attempt to get adequate vision.

Cataract, *an opacity in the lens,* is the most common problem in the aged eye. If the person lives long enough, he will probably develop a cataract. The most common type is senile cataract; the incidence increases with each decade of life. Senile cataracts are of two types. Nuclear cataracts are exaggerations of the ordinary physiologic accumulation of central lens fibers. The nuclear cataract progresses slowly; vision decreases over time. Cortical cataracts are caused by degeneration of the lens fibers, resulting in opacities. Cortical cataracts are mainly in the periphery and may not affect vision until an advanced stage. Until more is known about what causes cataracts, little, if anything, can be done to prevent their formation. Treatment for cataracts is surgical removal of the lens. Newer methods of suturing have eliminated the necessity for long bed rest; the patient is now ambulatory in 24 to 48 hours after surgery. Bilateral eye patches also are no longer necessary so that disorientation and confusion have been almost eliminated.[54] The heavy, thick corrective lenses that did little for peripheral vision also are being replaced by contact lenses and intraocular lens implants. Modern cataract surgery has become very successful and results in restoration of vision in the great majority of patients. It should not be withheld because of age or physical infirmity. Studies have shown that aged persons withstand cataract surgery very well and have good expectancy of recovering functional vision. If the person is up and about, well-oriented, needs and desires the surgery, it should be done.

The idea that a cataract must be ripe or mature is no longer applicable with newer surgical techniques. As soon as the patient is handicapped in his ability to read, write, watch television, or engage in other visual activities, the lens should be surgically removed.

Glaucoma is an increased intraocular pressure resulting from an impaired outflow of aqueous humor from the eye.[8,34,54] Two types that occur in the senior are distinct in their mechanisms, manifestations, and management.

Chronic Simple Glaucoma is the most commonly occurring glaucoma and usually develops slowly. The exact cause of glaucoma is unknown. The eye normally produces aqueous humor, which drains back into the circulatory system through an angle between the iris and cornea. When an obstruction or narrowing of this angle occurs in the anterior chamber of the eye, the fluid cannot escape and pressure builds within the eye. The pathologic change that occurs in chronic simple glaucoma appears to be a degenerative change in the eye's outflow channels. The change inhibits flow of aqueous humor through the outflow channels, causing intraocular pressure to rise. Chronic elevation in pressure and reduced blood supply lead to optic nerve damage. Eventually blindness results if the disease goes untreated. A genetic predisposition to chronic simple glaucoma may exist.

Symptoms are minor until changes in vision occur. The patient may complain of needing a change in his eyeglasses or may clean his lenses frequently to correct the blurred vision. He may experience headache, tearing, halos around lights, difficulty in adjusting to the dark, and reduced side vision. Central vision is not affected until the disease is well advanced. The Schiøtz tonometry reading is elevated. Potential glaucoma is defined as reading from 20 to 25 mm of mercury (Hg). However, some patients with low readings will show optic nerve atrophy, and others with readings up to 30 mm of Hg have no loss of vision, field defect, or flow obstruction. Because of these findings, a wide range of normal exists; the ultimate decision about whether or not one has glaucoma may require prolonged observation.[34]

Since symptoms are not noticed by the patient until visual field loss has occurred, early detection by routine tonometry is a must. Everyone over age 40, any adult with diabetes, or anyone with a family history of glaucoma should have yearly tonometry.

Glaucoma is treated with miotic agents: pilocarpine hydrochloride, physostigmine (Eserine), denecarium bromide (Humorsol), or echothiophate iodide (Phospholine iodide). All of these drugs are applied topically, and the senior must be taught how to administer his eyedrops. A systemic medication sometimes used is acetazolamide (Diamox), a carbonic anhydrase inhibitor, which reduces formation of aqueous humor. Side effects include drowsiness, tingling of extremities, and kidney stone formation. In advanced cases in which medical therapy is not effective in normalizing pressure, surgery may be necessary to prevent further visual loss. The most common type of surgery results in a fistula that drains the aqueous humor externally under the conjunctiva.[54]

Angle Closure Glaucoma, resulting from an anatomic defect in the anterior chamber angle, is much less common than chronic simple glaucoma. The ophthalmologist can study this angle with an instrument called a *gonioscope.* The narrow angle may spontaneously become occluded, and an attack of acute congestive glaucoma results. The symptoms include severe pain, pronounced visual loss, and nausea. The cornea appears cloudy, the pupil is dilated, and markedly elevated intraocular pressure will be present. A subacute attack is characterized by milder pain, headache, and seeing halos around objects. Miotic therapy, acetazolamide (Diamox), or osmotic agents such as Mannitol given intravenously may be utilized.[54] Surgery is indicated for permanent correction. An iridectomy will open the angle and prevent future occurrences.

Nursing intervention may change in a positive direction if you can experience the trauma of visual impairment by assuming the visually handicapped person's situation. Apply a blindfold and then attempt to carry on your usual activities. You will realize the importance of the other senses, the necessity of having things in a specific place known to the individual, and the necessity of always informing the patient before or as you enter the room. Orientation to the environment is crucial to these patients. Knowing how to get help when needed is probably the most important piece of information. Never leave this patient without a means of securing help if needed; always be sure that the call signal is within reach and where the patient expects it to be. Never leave this patient unattended in a strange environment. The feeling of complete helplessness can be very frightening and may cause the patient to panic if he cannot secure help when needed.

The patient fitted with contact lenses after cataract removal should be taught their proper care. Someone in the family should be taught how to remove them in the event of an emergency. The patient should carry a card or wear a Medi-Alert bracelet stating that he has contact lenses. If left in place for extended periods of time, the lenses can cause serious damage. Help the senior and his family realize that visual impairment from cataracts can almost always be corrected. Thus, he can return to normal living.

You should instruct the patient with glaucoma to avoid anything that will increase intraocular pressure. Straining of any kind, such as with defecation, lifting heavy objects, coughing, or sneezing should be avoided. Instruct the person to avoid constipation and upper respiratory infections. Anger, anxiety, and excitement also result in increased intraocular pressure. The senior should take only medications approved by the ophthalmologist. Patent medicines should be avoided, especially cold medications. His medical doctor should be aware of the glaucoma and the medications he is taking. A Medi-Alert bracelet or I.D. card should be carried for all emergencies. Excessive fluid intake over a short period of time may increase pressure and should be avoided. A supply of medication should be kept on hand and not be allowed to run out.

The family's support must be secured so that they can provide the assistance and reassurance the patient needs in coping with his condition. The patient and family must understand that although the glaucoma may not be cured, it can be controlled and further vision damage can be prevented. However, only careful supervision and conscientious following of the physician's orders can result in this controlled state.

If the senior's sight has deteriorated to the point where he would be considered blind (20/200), you must evaluate his environment and suggest aids that will enable him to carry on activities of daily living. Most important is the elimination of dangers in his dwelling, such as open stairways, step-downs, low stools and other low pieces of furniture, or frayed electric cords that he might be unable to see. Everything should have its place and should not be moved. If an article must be moved, the senior should be informed where it has been placed.

If someone prepares his food, food locations on his plate should be described in terms of numbers on the face of a clock.

Mail needs special attention because it usually is something that the senior looks forward to. Someone should make it a point to offer to read the mail to him and write any letters that he might request to have written. Someone will also have to take care of his business, such as paying bills and cashing any checks. Direct deposit to checking or savings accounts is now available for Social Security and other federal government pension checks. This service can save the senior time, worry, and inconvenience, and should be suggested to him.

If he still has some vision, a large magnifying glass can be a valuable tool for both reading and writing. The public library can provide books with large print as well as talking books. Some popular newspapers and magazines (*The New York Times* and *Reader's Digest*) are available in large-print editions and on cassettes. Often public libraries and the Library of Congress can make materials available on records or on cassettes. Braille publications are also available. Often public radio broadcasting stations have special programming for the visually handicapped when news and other general interest materials are read.

The visually impaired senior will need assistance in shopping, not just with transportation but also in selecting items from shelves and in selecting clothing for fit and color coordination. It is also easy for the visually impaired to be cheated when change is returned to him. He should be instructed to carry only one or two denominations of money and keep them separate so that he will know what change to expect. For example, he can carry only five-dollar bills and/or one-dollar bills. He will know how many bills to expect in return from a five easier than he will from a ten because a one can be substituted for a five. Coins can be determined by touch. However, this should be practiced independently before accepting change from someone.

Using a cane can help in discovering sidewalks, curbs, steps, or uneven places. However, use of a cane should also be practiced extensively before venturing outside the home independently.

If the patient never achieves sufficient independence to venture outside alone, someone will have to assume the responsibility for either taking him to the places he must reach or else run the errands for him. A family member, a neighbor, a volunteer from a church, a home health aid, or someone from the local council on aging will usually be this resource. The hospital nurse before discharge, the office nurse, or the visiting nurse should determine his need and then give the intervention needed, implementing referrals as necessary.

The following summary gives general guidelines for intervention with any neurologically impaired senior. Increase his self-esteem by accepting his behavior; being kind, friendly, and matter-of-fact, but setting limits when necessary to protect him. Gradually increase sensory and emotional stimulation to help him respond. Focus on short-term goals; do not try to push the person too fast or he may react with depression, withdrawal, and regression. Help him to achieve tasks within his limits, such as feeding himself, washing face and hands, or wearing his own clothes instead of a hospital gown. Do not tease, goad, shame, or persuade in a condescending manner to get him to do more, which implies that he is not doing well enough. Such an approach only causes hopelessness and more dependency. Treat him like an adult; give an adultlike diet as soon as possible. Pureed foods should be omitted as soon as he demonstrates the ability to chew and swallow. Realize that his impairment may contribute to physical and mental fatigue; do not be overdemanding. The person will feel more motivated if he can finish a small task with a sense of achievement rather than unsuccessfully attempting a larger task. Avoid unrealistic promises for the future; give encouragement and point out his accomplishments to date.

Accept that not all patients progress in rehabilitation. For some, disability is a welcome relief and an acceptable excuse not to face certain responsibilities or problems. Perhaps he now gets more attention than he ever did; therefore, the secondary gratification from being ill may be considerable. Perhaps he is more comfortable in the hospital than in his home. You may have to adjust your goals to his emotional or physical status. You cannot control and you should not try to manipulate another person to meet your own needs. The patient's ability to meet goals should relate to his needs, not your needs.

If the person denies his disability, do not argue with him and do not reject him for his lack of cooperation. If you can help him feel safe and secure and convey to him that he can recover some functions, he may have less need to deny. Then he can begin to face and work with his disability. Directing his attention to the healthy areas of his body, to his strengths and not just his limits, also lowers his anxiety and need to deny. Above all, do not force him to recognize his disability by frequently and repeatedly telling him about his disability. Such an approach would only increase his need to deny because you would heighten his sense of demoralization, frustration, hopelessness, and helplessness.

EVALUATION

Evaluation of care must be based on how goals have been achieved. Have the goals that were outlined earlier in this chapter, such as optimal mobility and prevention of contracture formation, been achieved in the patient with a CVA? Is the patient with Parkinsonism able to maintain his premorbid lifestyle or have one that is acceptable to himself and family? Has the patient with aphasia been able to reestablish a pattern of communication that permits him to lead a happy, productive life? Have corrective measures and devices for sensory impairment been accepted and successful so that the senior is able to cope adequately with his environment? The evaluation of long-term goals is preceded by an ongoing appraisal of progress made in achieving short-term goals.

In order to evaluate the effectiveness of care given to the senior with neurological impairment, determine whether or not the general guidelines for intervention and the specific measures were met.

Consider your feelings and reactions to the neurologically impaired senior. Does his immobility and paralysis threaten your sense of independence, speed, and strength? Does his incontinence repulse you; does it cause you to reject or infantilize him? Do his messy self-feeding practices, the spillage of food on self and in bed, and the drooling caused by one-sided paralysis cause you to feel aggravated, impatient, angry, repulsed, or rejecting? If he uses his fingers instead of eating utensils because he is very hungry—too hungry to try to manipulate the utensils—do you reprimand him? Do you understand that with paralysis a smile may be distorted because the uninvolved side of the face goes up while the paralyzed side sags?

To remain empathic, remember that this person is brain damaged. He is not a child, and he is not trying to act like one. He is a human being in need of physical and emotional nourishment. He relies on you because he can do so little for himself. He feels burdensome and worthless; only your pleasant, courteous, respectful manner can help him to slowly see himself as a person—not a thing.

REFERENCES

1. ARNHOFF, FRANKLYN, and M. MEHL, "Body Image in Paraplegia," *Journal of Nervous and Mental Diseases,* 137: (1963), 88–92.

2. BATES, BARBARA, *A Guide to Physical Examination.* Philadelphia: J. B. Lippincott Company, 1974.

3. BELAND, IRENE, and JOYCE PASSOS, *Clinical Nursing: Pathophysiological and Psychosocial Approaches,* 2nd ed. New York: Macmillan Publishing Co., Inc., 1975.

4. BELLAK, LEOPOLD, *Psychology of Physical Illness.* New York: Grune and Stratton, Inc., 1952.

5. BELT, LINDA, "Working with Dysphagic Patients," *American Journal of Nursing,* 74: No. 7 (1974), 1320–22.

6. BENDER, RUTH, "Communicating with the Deaf," *American Journal of Nursing,* 66: No. 4 (1966), 757–60.

7. BLEDSOE, C., and R. WILLIAMS, "The Vision Needed to Nurse the Blind," *American Journal of Nursing,* 66: No. 11 (1966), 2432–35.

8. BLODI, FREDERICK, "Glaucoma," *American Journal of Nursing,* 63: No. 3 (1963), 78–83.

9. BUCKINGHAM, WILLIAM, MARSHALL SPAIBERG, and MARTIN BRANDFON-BRENER, *A Primer of Clinical Diagnosis.* New York: Harper & Row Publishers, Inc., 1971.

10. BURT, MARGARET, "Perceptual Deficit in Hemiplegia," *American Journal of Nursing,* 70: No. 5 (1960), 1026–29.

11. CARROLL, BETTIE, "Fingers to Toes," *American Journal of Nursing,* 71: No. 3 (1971), 550–51.

12. DeGOWAN, ELMER, and RICHARD DeGOWAN, *Bedside Diagnostic Examination,* 2nd ed. New York: Macmillan Publishing Co., Inc., 1969.

13. EISENSON, JAN, "Therapeutic Problems and Approaches with Aphasic Adults," *Handbook of Speech Pathology,* ed. Lee Travis. New York: Appleton-Century-Crofts, 1957.

14. ELLIS, ROSEMARY, "After Stroke—Sitting Problems," *American Journal of Nursing,* 73: No. 11 (1973), 1898–99.

15. FEUSTEL, DELYCIA, "Autonomic Hyperreflexia," *American Journal of Nursing,* 76: No. 1 (1976), 228–30.

16. FINK, STEPHEN, and FRANKLIN SHONTZ, "Body Image Disturbances in Chronically Ill Individuals," *Journal of Nervous and Mental Diseases,* 131: (1960), 234–40.

17. FOWLER, ROY, and W. FORDYCE, "Adopting Care for the Brain Damaged Patient," *American Journal of Nursing,* 72: No. 10 (1972), 1832–34.

18. ——— and R. Berni, "Operant Conditioning in Chronic Illness," *American Journal of Nursing,* 69: No. 6 (1969), 1226–28.

19. FOX, MADELINE, "Talking with a Patient That Can't Answer," *American Journal of Nursing,* 71: No. 6 (1971), 1146–49.

20. ———, "Patients with Receptive Aphasia: They Don't Really Understand," *American Journal of Nursing,* 76: No. 10 (1976), 1596–98.

21. GARDNER, M., "Responsiveness as a Measure of Consciousness," *American Journal of Nursing,* 68: No. 5 (1968), 1034–38.

22. GODA, SIDNEY, "Communicating with the Aphasic or Dysarthric Patient," *American Journal of Nursing,* 63: No. 7 (1963), 80–83.

23. GUYTON, A., *Basic Human Physiology.* Philadelphia: W. B. Saunders Company, 1971.

24. HARDEN, WILLIAM, "Neurologic Aspects," in *Cowdry's The Care of the Geriatric Patient, 5th ed.,* ed. Franz Steinberg. St. Louis: The C. V. Mosby Company, 1976.

25. HARDIMAN, C., A. HOLBROOK, and D. HEDRICK, "Nonverbal Communication Systems for the Severely Handicapped Geriatric Patients," *The Gerontologist,* 19: No. 1 (1979), 96–101.

26. HIRSCHBERG, GERALD, L. LEWIS, and PATRICIA VAUGHAN, *Rehabilitation,* 2nd ed. Philadelphia: J. B. Lippincott Company, 1976.

27. HURWITZ, L. J., and M. SWALLOW, "An Introduction to the Neurology of Aging," *Gerontologia Clinica,* 13: (1971), 97–113.

28. JUDGE, RICHARD, and GEORGE ZUIDEMA, *Physical Diagnosis: A Physiologic Approach to the Clinical Examination,* 2nd ed. Boston: Little, Brown & Company, 1968.

29. KAY, ELEANOR, and ELIZABETH BOONE, "Stereostatic Surgery for Parkinson's Disease," *American Journal of Nursing,* 72: No. 12 (1972), 2200–2205.

30. KEITH, ROBERT, "Caring for the Aphasic Patient," *Nursing Digest,* 4: No. 3 (1976), 37–38.

31. KERTH, KAYE, "Beyond the Curtain of Silence," *American Journal of Nursing,* 74: No. 6 (1974), 1060–61.

32. KLOTZ, ROBERT, and MILDRED ROBINSON, "Hard-of-Hearing Patients Have Special Problems," *American Journal of Nursing,* 63: No. 5 (1963), 88–89.

33. KOHMEN, E., *et al.,* "Neurological Manifestations of Aging," *Journal of Gerontology,* 32: (1977), 411–19.

34. KORNWEIG, ABRAHAM, "The Eye in Old Age," in *Clinical Geriatrics,* ed. Isadore Rossman. Philadelphia: J. B. Lippincott Company, 1971.

35. MANEY, JANET, "A Behavioral Therapy Approach to Bladder Retraining," *Nursing Clinics of North America,* 11: No. 1 (1976), 179–88.

36. MARSHALL, J., "Recent Advances in Cerebrovascular Disease," in *Some Aspects of Neurology,* ed. R. Robertson. Edinburgh Royal College of Physicians, 1968.

37. MILLER, BARBARA, "Assisting Aphasic Patients with Speech Rehabilitation," *American Journal of Nursing,* 69: No. 5 (1969), 983–85.

38. MILLIKEN, C. H., *The Stroke-Prone Profile, Monograph Vol. IV,* No. 4. New York: American Heart Association, 1969.

39. MORGAN, WM., and GEORGE ENGEL, *The Clinical Approach to the Patient.* Philadelphia: W. B. Saunders Company, 1969.

40. NEU, CARLOS, "Coping with Newly Diagnosed Blindness," *American Journal of Nursing,* 75: No. 12 (1975), 2161–63.

41. OERTHER, BARBARA, "The Blind Patient Need Not Be Helpless," *American Journal of Nursing,* 66: No. 11 (1966), 2436–39.

42. PERRON, DENISE, "Deprived of Sound," *American Journal of Nursing,* 74: No. 6 (1974), 1057–59.

43. PIGOTT, RICHARD, and FLORENCE BRICKETT, "Visual Neglect," *American Journal of Nursing,* 66: No. 1 (1966), 101–5.

44. PILGRIM, MARGARET, and BARBARA SIGLER, "Phaco-Emulsification of Cataracts," *American Journal of Nursing,* 75: No. 6 (1975), 976–77.

45. PULOS, S., *et al.,* "Body Image Alterations in Adults Due to Cerebrovascular Insufficiency," *Journal of Personality and Assessment,* 38: No. 7 (1974), 540–46.

46. *Rehabilitative Nursing Techniques—1: Bed Positioning and Transfer Procedures for the Hemiplegic.* Minnesota: Kenny Rehabilitation Institute, 1962.

47. *Rehabilitative Nursing Techniques—2: Selected Equipment Useful in the Hospital, Home, or Nursing Home.* Minnesota: Kenny Rehabilitation Institute, 1964.

48. ROBERTS, SHARON, *Behavioral Concepts and the Critically Ill Patient.* Englewood Cliffs, N.J.: Prentice-Hall, Inc., 1976.

49. ROBINSON, MARILYN, "Levodopa and Parkinsonism," *American Journal of Nursing,* 74: No. 4 (1974), 656–61.

50. RUBEN, ROBERT, "Aging and Hearing," in *Clinical Geriatrics,* ed. Isadore Rossman. Philadelphia: J. B. Lippincott Company, 1971.

51. SENTURIA, BEN, ROBERT GOLDSTEIN, and WEBB HERSPERGER, "Otorrhinolaryngolic Aspects," in *Cowdry's The Care of the Geriatric Patient, 5th ed.,* ed. Franz Steinberg. St. Louis: The C. V. Mosby Company, 1976.

52. SKELLY, MADGE, "Aphasic Patients Talk Back," *American Journal of Nursing,* 75: No. 7 (1975), 1140–42.

53. SMITH, B., and P. SETHI, "Aging and the Nervous System," *Geriatrics,* 30: (1975), 109–15.

54. SMITH, MORTON, "Ophthalmic Aspects," in *Cowdry's The Care of the Geriatric Patient, 5th ed.,* ed. Franz Steinberg. St. Louis: The C. V. Mosby Company, 1976.

55. SNYDER, MARIAN, and REBECCA BAUM, "Assessing Station and Gait," *American Journal of Nursing,* 74: No. 7 (1974), 1256–57.

56. "Staving Off Stroke," *Medical World News,* 15: (February 8, 1974), 47–53.

57. TOOLE, J., and A. PATEL, *Cerebrovascular Disorders.* New York: McGraw-Hill Book Company, 1967.

58. ULLMAN, MONTAGUE, "Disorders of Body Image After Stroke," *American Journal of Nursing,* 64: No. 10 (1964), 89.

59. WEINSTOCK, FRANK, "Tonometry Screening," *American Journal of Nursing,* 73: No. 4 (1973), 656–57.

60. WOLANIN, MARY, "They Called the Patient Repulsive," *American Journal of Nursing,* 64: No. 6 (1964), 73–75.

problems of transporting and exchanging oxygen and nutrients in later maturity

Study of this chapter will enable you to:

1. Demonstrate ability to assess lungs, heart, and vasculature.

2. Describe the meaning of assessment findings for identifying nursing diagnosis(es).

3. Formulate patient care goals for the individual senior, using information about normal development and pathology.

4. Intervene with the senior who has dyspnea or impaired circulation.

5. Discuss the psychosocial aspects of cardio-respiratory disease for the senior and his family.

6. Work with family members of the patient and other health team members to provide continuity and consistency of care.

7. Evaluate the effectiveness of your care with the senior and his family.

8. Describe the various medical conditions that interfere with transportation and exchange of oxygen and nutrients.

9. Contrast and compare nursing assessments and interventions for elderly patients with obstructive lung diseases, pulmonary tuberculosis, myocardial infarction, and congestive heart failure.

17

Normal cellular metabolism is dependent on a continuous supply of amino acids, glucose, vitamins, hormones, and oxygen. Since the internal environment must be maintained within certain physical and chemical limits, excesses and waste products must be removed. The heart, blood, and vasculature are primarily responsible for delivering and removing these nutrients and waste products.

Levels of oxygen at the tissue level are dependent on air ventilation of lungs, blood perfusion of lungs, cardiac output, tissue demands for oxygen, and the blood hemoglobin level. Tissue hypoxia results if any part of the system is out of balance. The Po_2 (Partial pressure (P) of oxygen (O_2) or oxygen tension) and oxyhemoglobin saturation are measured to determine the lung's ability to provide and maintain adequate oxygen levels in arterial blood. *Below normal arterial Po_2 level is called* **hypoxemia;** **hypoxia** *refers to general or regional lack of tissue oxygen.*[5]

The lungs provide the means for the exchange of oxygen and carbon dioxide and are so intimately associated with the heart that pathology in the heart and blood vessels will affect the lungs, and pulmonary malfunction will adversely affect cardiac function. Therefore, nursing of patients experiencing difficulty with transporting oxygen and materials to and from cells caused by cardiovascular-respiratory pathology will be the focus of this chapter.

Heart disease is the number one killer in the United States; cerebral vascular disease is third. Stroke and the resultant problems were discussed in Chapter 16 and will not be covered here. The major focus will be on emphysematous and atherosclerotic changes; both conditions are prevalent in our aging population.

ASSESSMENT OF PERIPHERAL VASCULATURE, LUNGS, AND HEART

Assessment of the heart, lungs, and peripheral vasculature requires using the skills of inspection, palpation, percussion, and auscultation. It is not the purpose of this text to teach physical assessment skills or differential medical diagnosis, but what a thorough assessment should entail is within the scope of this text. Whether the nurse, nurse practitioner, or physician performs the assessment, the nurse planning care should be aware of the findings of the initial assessment and should continue to monitor these findings for change which may herald improvement or complications. The knowledgeable, observant nurse is in the position to intervene with appropriate care when the patient's condition changes, thus helping to avoid prolonged or unnecessary treatment or increased pain and disability.

Peripheral Vasculature

If oxygenated blood is not being delivered in adequate quantity to the skin, pallor, cyanosis, and cool skin temperature are present. In chronic hypoxia of the extremities, scanty or absent hair growth; thin, shiny skin; skin discoloration and thickened nails; edema; and possibly ulcers are present. Peripheral pulses, such as popliteal, posterior tibial, or dorsalis pedis are faint or absent. Muscles and soft tissues atrophy. In arterial occlusion a dusky, plum-colored rubor develops in dependent extremities and changes to an intense grayish pallor on elevation. Advanced arterial insufficiency causes a bluish-gray mottling which is unchanged by position. Anesthesia (absence of feeling) is also likely to be present.[18,50]

Intermittent claudication, pain in the contracted leg muscle which is brought on by exercise and relieved by rest, may be present. Note the distance the senior can walk before pain occurs and note its frequency.[50]

Any senior who is bedridden is a candidate for thrombophlebitis. Be alert for its symptoms. Superficial venous thrombosis produces redness, induration, tenderness, and a thickened, cordlike vein. Signs of deep thrombophlebitis are: (1) tenderness in the region of the iliac vessels, in the popliteal space, or over the calf; (2) swelling detectable only by measuring and comparing circumferences of both calfs and thighs; (3) low-grade fever; (4) tachycardia; (5) ankle edema; and (6) a positive *Homan's Sign* (*calf pain on sharp dorsiflexion of the foot with the knee slightly flexed*).[16,19,28] Thrombosis of the deep femoral and pelvic veins may by asymptomatic, and a fatal pulmonary embolism may occur without warning.

The Lungs

Observe the senior. Note his physical appearance, color of skin, mucous membranes, and nailbeds. Look for clubbing of the fingers and toes (thickening of the distal end of the phalanges). Note the posture he assumes. Can he lie down without undue distress? Note his respirations: number, depth, regularity, character, and any audible sounds such as wheezes, grunts, or gasps. Are neck veins bulging and venous pulsation visible in them? His face should be carefully observed for indication of pain, apprehension, anxiety, panic. Does he purse his lips on exhaling? Is there a cough? Is it productive? The sputum amount, color, thickness, odor, and any other characteristic should be described. Does he cover his mouth and use cleansing tissues properly? Note breath odor.[3,16,28,52,55]

Only after careful general observation should examination of the chest begin. Examine the chest in a well-lighted room with the patient stripped to the waist. Female patients should be adequately draped to avoid embarrassment. Observe for symmetry, rate, depth, and rhythm of respiratory movements between the two sides of the thorax; location of retraction of intercostal spaces; and retraction of the supraclavicular notch during inspiration or bulging during expiration. Any deformities, such as barrel chest, pectus excavatum, scars, prominences, pigeon chest, kyphoscoliosis, and wounds on the thorax, should be noted.[3,16,28,55]

Palpation is performed to assess symmetry of chest expansion and detect vibration. Placing your hands with fingers spread and thumbs touching on the chest and then having the patient inhale and exhale help in assessing symmetry of chest expansion. *Fremitus* is a *palpable vibration transmitted to the chest wall through the bronchopulmonary system when the patient speaks.* Have the patient repeat a resonant phrase, such as "ninety-nine," which can be detected by using the ulnar surface or ball of the hand. Again, symmetry of vibration is observed. Fremitus is increased over a large bronchus and consolidated tissue. It is decreased when a bronchus is obstructed, pleura is thickened, or pleural space is filled with air or fluid.[3,16]

Percussion is used to detect the density of underlying tissue. The qualities of percussion tones follow:[3,16,28]

Tone	*Detected over*
Tympany	Air filled stomach or bowel
Hyperresonance	Emphysematous lung
Resonance	Normal lung
Dullness	Liver, heart, spleen; replaces resonance over fluid-filled or consolidated lung tissue
Flatness	Thigh muscle

Percussion should be performed over symmetrical areas of the chest at approximately 5-centimeter (cm) intervals down the chest, excluding the area over the scapula, as shown in Figure 17.1.[3] Percussion only penetrates 5 to 7 cm and will not detect deep lung changes.

The level of the diaphragm can also be detected by percussing down the chest wall until dullness replaces resonance. Diaphragmatic excursion is measured by noting the difference of this level on full expiration and then on full inspiration. Normally this is 5 to 6 cm.[3,16,28]

Auscultation provides information on the movement of air in and out of the bronchi. *Vesicular sounds, normal breath sounds, occur over most of the lung and have a soft breezy quality with a longer inspiratory phase and a shorter, almost inaudible, expiratory phase.* *Bronchovesicular sounds are louder, have equal inspiratory and expiratory phases, and are heard over large bronchi and when consolidation is occurring.* *Bronchial sounds are harsh and loud; the expiratory phase is longer than the inspiratory phase.* Bronchial sounds can be simulated

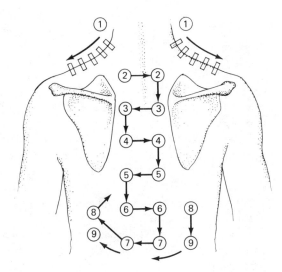

Figure 17.1. Percussion of posterior thorax.

by auscultating over the trachea and are *abnormal* anywhere over the lung because they usually denote consolidation.[3,16,28]

Abnormal sounds are also detected. These include **rales *which occur with inspiration and are caused by fluid in the bronchial tree.*** Fine rales are simulated by rolling hair between the fingers in front of the ear. Coarse rales are louder and are caused by fluid in the larger bronchi or trachea. *Rhonchi and wheezes are continuous and result from obstruction to air flow.* **Wheezes *are high pitched and are caused by obstruction in smaller air passages.*** **Rhonchi *are lower pitched and are indicative of larger airway obstruction.*** **Friction rubs *are grating, rubbing sounds caused by inflamed pleural.*** They occur with inspiration and expiration. While rales, wheezes, and rhonchi can be produced or cleared by coughing, friction rubs will not be so influenced.[3,9,16,28]

If abnormalities of fremitus are detected, then the spoken sound should also be auscultated. Normally, the spoken word is heard very indistinctly through the stethoscope. When consolidation or lung compression caused by pleural effusion is present, bronchophony, egophony, or whispered pectoriloquy may occur. **Bronchophony *is an increased intensity and clarity of the spoken voice.*** **Egophony *is present when the patient says "ee" and it sounds like "a" through the stethoscope.*** **Whispered pectoriloquy *is the clear transmission of whispered words through the stethoscope.***[3,16,28]

The Heart

The pattern of inspection, palpation, percussion, and auscultation is again followed for the heart.

Inspection of the chest should include looking for evidence of cardiac pathology. Note heaves, lifts, prominences, and pulsations in the region of the heart, and note their exact locations. Observe the apical pulse by inspection and palpation if possible. Apical beat is not visible in all patients. A tangential light helps to detect its presence. If the apical beat is seen, measure its location in number of intercostal spaces and in centimeters from the midclavicular or midsternal line.[3,16,28,58] Intercostal spaces are counted by beginning at the angle of Lewis for location of the second rib and counting each space below the rib by the number of the corresponding rib above.

Palpation for heaves, lifts, and thrills should be performed in all areas over the chest. See Figure 17.2.[3,16,28] A *thrill resembles a purring cat and sometimes accompanies loud murmurs.* The aortic and pulmonic areas are in the right and left second intercostal spaces at the sternal border. The tricuspid area is in the left intercostal space at the sternal border. The mitral area is in the fifth intercostal space at the midclavicular line. The epigastric region should also be palpated.[3,16,28]

Percussion of the cardiac outline can be performed to determine enlargement. The left border of cardiac dullness is percussed in the third, fourth, and

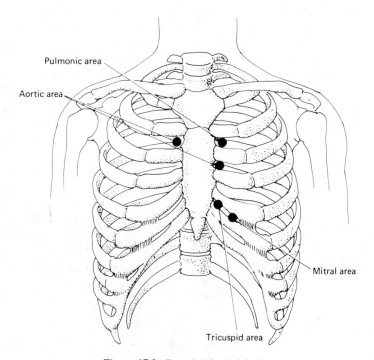

Figure 17.2. Examination of the heart.

fifth intercostal spaces and is then measured in centimeters from the midclavicular or midsternal line. The right border may be percussed in severe enlargement.[3,16,28]

Auscultation of the heart is performed in all valvular areas and along the left sternal margin. The rate and rhythm are noted. Individual heart sounds are then assessed. The first sound (S_1), which coincides with closure of the mitral and tricuspid valves, is louder in the mitral and tricuspid areas. The second sound (S_2), which coincides with closure of the pulmonic and aortic valves, is louder in the pulmonic and aortic areas. A third sound (S_3) may occur during the phase of rapid ventricular filling, and a fourth sound (S_4), which denotes atrical contraction, may occur just prior to S_1. Other sounds that sometimes occur are an ejection click following S_1 which corresponds to the opening of an abnormal aortic valve, and an opening snap immediately following S_2 which marks the opening of a stenosed mitral valve. See Figure 17.3.[3,16,38]

During auscultation the presence of murmurs should also receive attention. Note the following characteristics of the murmur: (1) timing in the cardiac cycle; (2) location according to interspace and centimeters from midsternal, midclavicular, or axillary lines; (3) radiation; (4) intensity graded from 1 through 6, with 1 being the faintest and 6 being audible with stethoscope off the chest; (5) pitch (high, medium, or low); and (6) quality (blowing, rumbling, harsh, or musical).

Other cardiovascular sounds that may be detected are ***pericardial friction rubs,*** *squeaking sounds present in diastole and systole,* and ***venous hums,*** *sounds which can be interrupted by pressing the jugular vein momentarily.* Splitting of sounds may also occur. Wide splitting of S_2 can be caused by right bundle branch block.[3,9,16]

Learning to ausculate the heart effectively takes a great deal of practice,

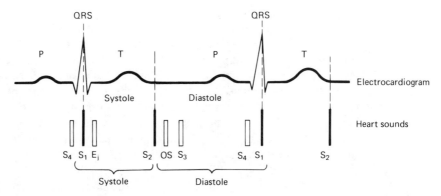

Figure 17.3. Comparison of heart sounds of cardiac cycle to electrocardiogram.

but you should learn to recognize heart sounds and murmurs as well as rate and rhythm changes. Being able to diagnose the underlying pathology is not as important as being able to recognize changes and refer them to the physician for evaluation and treatment.

The nurse visiting an elderly person in his home or the nurse in the nursing home may be called upon to assess a patient's condition before a physician is available. Being able to auscultate the heart and lungs and describe findings can mean the difference in amount of time lost before definitive treatment can be begun. Any nurse in a position where a physician is not immediately available should increase assessment skills as much as possible. Considerable practice with a mentor, however, is a necessity for learning accurate cardiorespiratory assessment.

EMOTIONAL ASSESSMENT

Much feeling can be expressed through the respiratory and cardiovascular systems, because emotions trigger the sympathetic nervous system, causing tachypnea, dyspnea, tachycardia, chest pain, and blood pressure and color changes. It is a vicious cycle. The physical symptoms related to respiratory or cardiovascular disease cause feelings of anxiety, fear, stigma, shame, depression, and anger. In turn, these feelings cause more symptoms. The senior often recognizes the cycle, and he will try to deny or suppress his feelings and avoid excitement. He may isolate himself from others in an attempt to avoid excitement and to suppress his feelings. The feelings that are introjected drain his energy; depression may result, causing other physical symptoms (see Chapter 21). As he withdraws, family, friends, and even health care workers in turn also withdraw.

There is no more frightening nor frustrating experience than being unable to breathe. As his disease progresses, the senior lives with a constant fear of dying from drowning or strangulation. It is not a fear that can be repressed; his fears may cause nightmares or awaken him when he has been able to achieve sleep. Every effort is put into breathing. In his efforts to breathe he becomes frustrated, anxious, and demanding. He fears being alone; he fears neglect. Unfortunately, family, friends, and even health care workers may feel very helpless when they encounter the senior with respiratory or cardiovascular disease, regardless of the cause. To cope with their own fears of death, others may spend less time with the person, which reinforces his fears of neglect and often causes increased demands.

Recognize these emotional reactions and transactions when they occur, for they contribute to other physical symptoms and must be given appropriate intervention.

NURSING DIAGNOSIS AND FORMULATION OF PATIENT CARE GOALS

Nursing Diagnosis

The nursing diagnoses that may be encountered when the senior has a problem of transporting oxygen and materials to and from cells are numerous. Some are described in other chapters: immobility, cognitive impairment, and depression, for example.

Probably one of the most frequently encountered diagnoses is *difficult respiration or dyspnea.* Another nursing diagnosis is *circulatory impairment.* Dyspnea caused by respiratory obstruction, found in most respiratory and cardiac diseases, will be discussed because many of the related nursing measures can be applied to any patient with labored breathing. Common conditions that cause dyspnea in later maturity are: (1) chronic obstructive pulmonary disease; (2) tuberculosis; (3) arteriosclerotic heart disease; and (4) congestive heart failure. The pathology underlying these medical conditions and the *nursing diagnoses* of *dyspnea* and *circulatory impairment* are explored in this chapter.

Patient Care Goals

The *long-range goals* for persons with dyspnea include:

1. Activities of daily living are performed with minimal or no dyspnea.
2. Dyspnea, if it occurs, is reported immediately to the person monitoring the patient's care.
3. Activities that result in dyspnea are not attempted.
4. An activity program is followed that provides adequate exercise and opportunity for socializing without dyspnea resulting.
5. Feelings are expressed verbally instead of through respiratory or cardiovascular symptoms.

Some of these goals may not be possible for a specific senior because of the severity of his condition, his age, or presence of another disability. Therefore, all goals, short- and long-term, must be highly individualized to be achievable.

Write *short-term goals* for a patient you recently cared for who experienced dyspnea.

463

NURSING INTERVENTION APPLICABLE TO PERSONS WITH DYSPNEA CAUSED BY RESPIRATORY OBSTRUCTION

The first action to be taken for the patient with dyspnea is to relieve respiratory obstruction. Care measures depend on the cause and whether it is an upper or lower airway obstruction.

Upper airway obstruction can result from: (1) paralysis of the larynx and pharynx, (2) aspirated foreign body, (3) tumor growth of the upper airway, (4) spasm of the larynx, (5) edema or relaxation of the glottis, and (6) diphtheria. Obstruction is treated by removal manually or through a laryngoscope or by intubation or tracheostomy to bypass the obstruction.[13]

If obstruction is caused by a relaxed jaw in which the glottis occludes the trachea, correction can be accomplished by grasping the mandible at the angle of the jaw and pulling forward. Insertion of an airway will prevent this from occurring when anesthesia or unconsciousness causes jaw relaxation. The absence of teeth also increases the risk of relaxed jaw. Placing the person on his side can help to prevent obstruction since the jaw will be more likely to fall forward simply because of gravitational pull.[13]

Aspirated foreign bodies may be removed by use of the Heimlich maneuver. The patient is grasped around the chest from behind; the person administering the maneuver makes a fist with his two hands and then suddenly and forcefully exerts pressure on the lower sternum. The sudden force is often enough to dislodge the object. However, since aspiration of a foreign object is such an extreme emergency, definitive medical care should be sought. If one or two Heimlich maneuvers are not successful, no further attempts should be made. Medical help should be promptly obtained.

A *lower airway obstruction* may be caused by: (1) chronic airway obstruction as seen in chronic obstructive pulmonary disease (COPD); (2) respiratory restriction from pneumothorax, flail chest, kyphoscoliosis, and decreased diaphragmatic movement; (3) impaired diffusion from pulmonary edema, fibrosis, emboli, pneumonectomy, or tumor; and (4) abnormal ventilation-circulation ratio, which is seen in emphysema, chronic bronchitis, atelectasis, and pneumonia.[40] The alleviation of lower airway pathology includes measures to improve oxygenation, relieve obstruction, and improve ventilation.[25]

Care of the Person with Chronic Obstructive Pulmonary Disease (COPD)

Since all of the therapeutic measures that will be discussed relative to lower airway obstruction are applicable to the patient with chronic obstructive pulmonary disease, a brief description of this pathology precedes the discussion of care. COPD or COLD (Chronic Obstructive Lung Disease) refers to the emphysema and chronic bronchitis complex. Emphysema is the loss of alveolar walls. Incidence of emphysema increases with age. By age 90 nearly everyone has some degree of emphysema. Clinically, emphysema evidences its presence by chronic dyspnea on exertion preceded by cough and progressive disability due to unrelenting dyspnea.[39] Chronic bronchitis may or may not accompany it. Chronic bronchitis refers to chronic cough and expectoration for a period of at least three months. It is almost always found in smokers. Although these two diseases can be described as separate entities, they probably coexist as often as they exist separately.[20,33,39]

Physiologically, ventilatory function tests demonstrate expiratory obstruction in the emphysematous patient. Lung volumes are usually large because of overdistention of alveolae, and residual volume is increased because of expiratory trapping. Gas transport can also be impaired because of reduced alveolar surface. However, hypoxemia and carbon dioxide retention are not observed in emphysema until the disease is advanced unless a complicating illness occurs that places additional demands on the lungs.

Physiologically, chronic bronchitis results in hypoxemia and carbon dioxide retention once the disease is established. Hypoxemia is primarily caused by ventilation and perfusion abnormalities, such as airway plugging and shunting of air through areas of reduced ventilation. Manifestations of chronic bronchitis, such as pulmonary hypertension, cor pulmonale, and congestive heart failure, result from the hypoxemia. Oxygen lack in the myocardium, impaired renal plasma flow resulting in impairment of salt and water clearance, and secondary polycythemia vera contribute to the heart failure.[20,33,39]

Because these two diseases usually occur concurrently, there is no absolute clinical picture of the senior with emphysema or chronic bronchitis. For example, barrel chest deformity, so often described for emphysema, may or may not be present.[20]

COPD consists of two components: the airway component, in which secretions and edema result in obstruction, and a mechanical component in which the collapsing airway increases the work of breathing. The therapy for COPD therefore will be directed toward these two major pathophysiologic entities.

Oxygen therapy is valuable for extremely hypoxemic individuals who demonstrate symptoms of impaired oxygenation in terms of severe disability. Oxygen use should be guided by arterial blood gas analysis. (For example, in chronic obstructive pulmonary disease, only sufficient oxygen to bring the arterial oxygen tension to a range of 55 to 65 mm Hg should be used.) Oxygen therapy is indicated when the Po_2 falls below 50 mm Hg, especially if it is the result of diffusion impairment, ventilation-circulation ratio abnormalities, and the loss of functioning lung tissue. If the hypoxia is caused by airway obstruction or impairment of ventilation, these conditions must be adequately treated. Oxygen is not a substitute for treating the cause. If treatment does not relieve the hypoxia, the addition of oxygen is helpful.[8,39]

There are dangers that you must be aware of when you administer oxygen to persons with chronic carbon dioxide retention. The respiratory center has become insensitive to carbon dioxide as a stimulus for breathing. The carotid and aortic bodies that are stimulated by a decrease in oxygen tension now serve as the primary breathing center. If oxygen is administered in high concentrations, this person's breathing may be suppressed. A second problem also arises when a high percentage of oxygen is administered. A high percentage of oxygen increases the partial pressure of carbon dioxide in the lungs because nitrogen is diluted and carbon dioxide replaces it. This leads to respiratory acidosis, especially if the person is hypoventilated. These dangers can be avoided if a mechanical ventilator is used and is frequently monitored. An oxygen content of less than 40 percent is advisable for patients who are breathing on their own.[8,25]

Table 17.1 summarizes oxygen equipment and the oxygen concentrations achieved.[29]

Removal of accumulation of secretions is the major problem in lower airway obstruction. **Bronchial hygiene** is a term now used to describe *measures to improve airway clearance and to prevent further irritation.* Factors that must be considered in bronchial hygiene are: (1) curtailment of smoking, (2) avoidance of areas with high air pollution, (3) use of electric air filters or air conditioners, and (4) measures to remove secretions.[8,34,40]

Before secretions can be removed, they need to be made fluid and less tenacious. To increase the fluidity of secretions, the person should increase fluid intake, humidify inspired air, and use drugs that have a bronchodilating and mucolytic effect. The bronchodilator aerosol called Bronkosol is one of the most effective. Isoproterenal (Isuprel) or racemic epinephrine (Vaponefrin) are

TABLE 17.1   Oxygen Equipment and Oxygen Concentration Delivered

Method	Flow (liters/min)	Approximate Oxygen Percent Concentration Delivered
Nasal cannula	4–6	30–40
Nasal catheter	4–6	30–40
Mask (with exhalation valve)	6–8	35–45
	8–12	45–65
Mask (with bag)	6–8	40–60
	8–12	60–90
Venturi-mask (Venti-Mask[R])	4–8	24–28–35 (dependent on which of three masks used)
Pressure controlled positive pressure unit		(when driven by oxygen) 40–100
Volume controlled positive pressure unit		21–100

also used. Metaproterenol (Metaprel, Alupint) is a metered dose device. The aerosol is inhaled by the senior and is delivered by means of a hand-bulb nebulizer, a pump-driven nebulizer, or intermittent positive pressure breathing (IPPB) device. Following the bronchodilator therapy, the senior inhales moisture which may be delivered by a heated nebulizer, ultrasonic nebulizer, or a very simple baby bottle warmer with a steam attachment.[39,44]

After treatment to make the secretions more fluid, attempts at their removal are in order. Coughing, postural drainage, clapping and cupping, and tracheobronchial aspiration may be used.

Coughing of the controlled expulsive type should be encouraged. A spasmodic cough usually does not produce sputum and should be discouraged. The patient needs to be taught to cough properly. He should be instructed to inspire deeply, stop, and then forcibly cough. The person with chronic obstructive lung disease may not be able to cough forcibly since collapse of the airway sometimes occurs. He should be instructed to exhale as much as possible. Often this maneuver is enough to move secretions, and this movement will then stimulate a natural cough reflex which on the following deep inhalation generates a spontaneous cough. If a spontaneous cough does not occur, the person should again exhale as much as possible, after which he gives a small cough. This little forceful maneuver compresses the airway and squeezes secretions in front of it. For patients unable to follow instructions, a spontaneous cough can be produced by stroking the neck near the cricoid cartilage. Also, application of force to the abdomen or lower thorax on exhalation may produce a cough. Force must be carefully applied to avoid trauma to underlying bones and tissues.[5]

Mechanical stimulation may be necessary for patients with respiratory paralysis. A Caf-Flater machine, which uses a positive pressure pump to forcibly inflate the lungs and then reverses flow, assists in expiration or cough.[25]

Postural drainage assists bronchopulmonary drainage. However, postural drainage is sometimes difficult to carry out because the senior is unable to assume or maintain the necessary position for any length of time. Then positive pressure assistance prior to and during postural drainage may be helpful.[25] A detailed chart showing the various postural drainage positions is available from the National Cystic Fibrosis Foundation.

Remember that the recumbent position favors the accumulation of secretions in the lungs. Only the prone position slants most of the bronchi in a downward direction that can be acted upon by gravity. An exercise slantboard can be used to promote postural drainage through gravity and is an easier position to assume than the traditional position.

Mechanical measures such as clapping, cupping, and vibrating during postural drainage may be helpful in dislodging secretions. *Cupping is percussion with cupped hands while wrists and arms are very relaxed.* They are *applied rhythmically,* right and left alternately, at 100 to 150 beats per minute for 3 to 5 minutes in each area being drained. Coughing is encouraged during and after.

Vibration *is application of pressure with the flat of the hand along with tremor of the arm.*[25] These measures should not be used over the vertebral column or below the ribs.[5]

Deep airway suctioning may be required if all previously described measures do not maintain patency of the airway and if the patient is comatose. Suctioning carries certain hazards that are not always avoidable: trauma to mucosa, hypoxemia, incomplete clearing of the lungs, and introduction of pathogens.

Reduce trauma to mucosa from the whistle tip catheter by careful insertion and withholding of suction with the use of a Y-connector or a thumb closure device while inserting and removing the catheter. Use as little suction as necessary to remove secretions. Also avoid up-and-down motions. Catheters that reduce the possibility of the catheter's clamping to the mucosal wall are becoming available and will alleviate the problem.

Hypoxemia is produced by extended suctioning. The catheter causes increased obstruction while it also suctions air from the airway. Preoxygenation and short suction periods of no more than 15 to 20 seconds and the reinstitution of oxygen following suctioning can minimize this problem.[8]

With deep suctioning, the catheter is unlikely to enter the left mainstem bronchus without use of a special curved bronchial catheter, knowledge of anatomy, and skill in advancing and turning the catheter. Merely turning the patient's head and hyperextending the neck do not insure entrance of the catheter into the left bronchus. Therefore, it is not likely that adequate clearing of secretions from both lungs will be accomplished.[5]

Another major hazard with deep suctioning is the introduction of pathogenic organisms into the lower airway. Equipment that is used for deep suctioning should be sterile or clean. Catheters should be sterile and should be discarded after each suctioning session. A sterile glove should be worn on the hand that manipulates the catheter. A sterile normal saline solution should be used to lubricate and flush the catheter. A sterile bowl replaced after each use or clean paper cups that are discarded after each suctioning can be used for holding the saline solution. A different catheter should be used for oral and pharyngeal suctioning and deep suctioning through an endotracheal or tracheostomy tube since the mouth and nose are grossly contaminated. Organisms can be introduced into the lower airway if the same catheter is used to suction the oral pharynx and tracheostomy or endotracheal tube. For more detail on suctioning technique, consult a text in Medical-Surgical Nursing.

Patient and family teaching is extremely important in lower airway chronic obstruction. Aggravating or extending the disease should be avoided. Teach the importance of avoiding respiratory infections and areas of heavy air pollution and of seeking medical care immediately when symptoms of a cold occur. Seasonal flu immunizations are helpful for the senior. Cessation of smoking is essential, but it may be difficult for the lifelong smoker. There is a greater susceptibility to upper respiratory infections with chronic pulmonary disease. When infection occurs, edema of the mucous membrane lining of the lung results. This causes increased narrowing and greater difficulty with coughing and removing secretions. When retained, these secretions thicken and become even more difficult to expel. This process results in progression of the disease and should be avoided.[6]

Breathing retraining may also be your teaching responsibility. Slow breathing favors oxygen transport. The patient is taught to relax the abdomen during inspiration and contract it during expiration. This promotes lung emptying, as does exhaling against pursed lips. The maneuver reduces the amount of air that needs to be breathed for a unit of oxygen to be consumed, and gas transport at the alveoli improves.[1,39]

Diet instruction is also important. Suggest adequate fluids to help in liquefying secretions and avoidance of gas-forming foods and overeating that might in turn interfere with abdominal breathing. These patients often are so dyspneic that merely chewing food can be overwhelming. Therefore, easily chewed, well-seasoned, nutritious, small frequent feedings are ideal. If the patient is overweight, a reduction diet will be required. Any excess weight only adds to the problem of dyspnea. However, many times these patients become malnourished because of anorexia and inability to comfortably eat and enjoy a meal. Mouth breathing diminishes the taste of the food; foul secretions to be expectorated can cause anorexia, and medications taken per nebulizer can affect the taste of food. Therefore, frequent oral hygiene is necessary, especially before meals. Swishing the mouth with mouthwash before meals can freshen it so that foods are more palatable. A glass of wine prior to eating can whet the appetite and add interest and enjoyment. Meals should be social occasions; therefore, if meals can be shared with another person, the senior may feel more like eating.

Physical reconditioning may also be necessary. Graded exercises that focus on normal walking improve mobility of the person with chronic obstructive pulmonary disease. Patients are instructed to exercise in appropriate situations around the home and to increase the amount of exercise each day. Morning and afternoon exercises are planned. Exercise tolerance can be increased 100 percent and sustained for 2 years. Increased exercise tolerance can mean increased productivity as well as decreased symptoms.[24]

Emotional support from all members of the health team is essential for caring for a patient with dyspnea and his family. Since emotional state and the ability to breathe are so closely intertwined, your intervention can help to break the vicious circle. Do not avoid the senior. Frequently check on him. Remain calm; be decisive as you give necessary physical care so that he trusts your competency in maintaining his respirations. Help him talk about his feelings; convey understanding of them. Help him explore the changes he must make in life because of his illness, to accept these changes, and to find meaning in his new life-style. The principles of therapeutic communication and emotional care described in other chapters are all useful for this person as well as for the person with other respiratory or cardiovascular problems.

The senior suffers loss of self-image when he realizes that he has a progressively debilitating disease. He feels useless and a burden. What previously brought a feeling of pride, such as employment or physical ability in a particular sport or another hobby, is no longer experienced. If self-esteem can be fostered through some type of achievement, rehabilitation is enhanced. A hobby that can be tolerated, some task not requiring strenuous activity, or development of a meaningful relationship or renewal of a waning one may be what is needed to boost self-esteem. Referral to occupational and recreational therapies and family or group therapy should be suggested.[2,17,32]

Help family members understand what the senior is experiencing. Acknowledge and help them express their feelings of fear, helplessness, frustration, guilt, anger, and depression. Give them guidelines for talking with the senior more effectively. Recognize their coping abilities as they try to care for him. Encourage their continued involvement with their loved one without causing unnecessary dependency. You can be a model for them as you care for the patient. If you can foster a smooth interaction between family and the senior, the patient care goals described earlier are more likely to be met in either the institution or in the home.

You may teach the family how to carry out the physical care measures in the home that were described earlier. Consult a Medical-Surgical Nursing text and booklets from the American Lung Association for effective ways to initiate a rehabilitation program and prepare the home environment for the elderly person with chronic dyspnea.

Acute respiratory failure can occur in chronic obstructive lung disease. This emergency occurs when the oxygen tension rapidly drops to less than 50 mm Hg, the carbon dioxide tension is above 50 mm Hg, or both. If this has been a slowly occurring situation, the patient may be able to tolerate these abnormal blood gas levels.[8,39]

However, the patient who experiences sudden acute respiratory failure is in need of intensive care management. Carefully controlled oxygen therapy at low flow accompanied by bronchial hygiene, inhaled moisture, and other supportive nursing care can realize a 50 to 75 percent of recovery rate. Some patients may require tracheal intubation or tracheostomy with automatic ventilation.[39]

Care of the Person with Pulmonary Tuberculosis

Pulmonary tuberculosis deserves consideration in any discussion of care of the senior because of the predisposition of chronically ill individuals to this infection. It appears that tuberculosis is becoming a disease of the elderly. In the

United States the primary infection occurs any time during life. The tuberculosis bacillus frequently remains dormant after this initial infection and only becomes a clinically overt disease when impaired host response occurs, which may be in old age or during chronic illness.[14]

The cause of tuberculosis is the Mycobacterium tuberculosis which is transmitted by droplet nuclei produced by an infectious person. Close contact is defined as exposure for 10 to 20 or more hours weekly for 3 months. Skin testing for a positive PPD (purified protein derivative) test, chest X-ray, sputum smears, and cultures are used for diagnosis. A positive skin test (induration greater than 8 to 10 mm) evidences a previous contact with the antigen but does not necessarily mean that the person presently has active tuberculosis.[5] The skin test in the elderly population is less reliable because relative degrees of tuberculin anergy are not uncommon in this age group.[39]

Chronically ill persons (incidence highest in older nonwhite males) and very young children (under 3 years) are especially susceptible. Thus, it is essential to screen elderly persons residing in a home with young children. Also, all workers in retirement, convalescent, and nursing homes should receive annual skin tests or chest X-rays. Poor nutrition and crowded living conditions appear to predispose to the infection.

Treatment in most cases requires only chemotherapy. Isoniazid (INH), streptomycin, and para-aminosalicylic acid (PAS) are the traditional drugs used in the treatment of TB. Ethambutal (EMB) has replaced PAS to a large degree since it is better tolerated. Rifampin (Rifadin) is also being used. Rifadin has replaced streptomycin in the three drug regimen because many elderly are especially sensitive to streptomycin toxicity. INH and EMB are usually continued for a 2-year period.[39]

The disease is frequently no longer active after a week of drug therapy, and hospitalization, except in advanced cases, is usually not required. If the senior is hospitalized, isolation procedure for TB should be followed for one to two weeks. Most hospitals keep the patient in a private room that has nonrecirculating air and the door is kept closed. The patient should be taught how to cover his mouth when he coughs and how to dispose of tissues. If he cannot cooperate, he may have to wear a mask that can obstruct the droplet nuclei when they are first expelled. Masks worn by the nurse are of limited value and are probably unnecessary since after evaporation the nuclei are small enough to pass through masks.[39]

Follow-up of close contacts as defined earlier is also required. Prophylactic INH therapy for 1 year is offered to close contacts. Skin tests and chest X-rays are used to determine progress.[5]

The community health nurse should supervise the care of the patient receiving home treatment. Helping the patient understand the importance of following the drug regimen and having regular checkups should be two primary goals. Because the patient's symptoms may be minimal or nonexistent, these goals may have to be regularly evaluated and reinforced.[37]

Care of the Person with Arteriosclerotic
Heart Disease

Arteriosclerotic heart disease is the most frequent type of heart disease in the person over 60 years. Acute myocardial infarction, angina, arrhythmias, and congestive heart failure are the most common manifestations of this pathology. Coronary artery disease increases in prevalence with aging and is present in almost all individuals over 70. Although acute myocardial infarction in the elderly is similar in symptoms and treatment to that in younger patients, mortality increases significantly after age 60. Anterior infarctions, cardiogenic shock, congestive failure, pulmonary edema, and serious arrhythmias also increase in later maturity. Renal failure, sepsis, and embolism are more common complications in the elderly.[29,42]

Atypical and silent myocardial infarctions are more prevalent in the senior. Atypical cases usually do not exhibit the pain pattern of a myocardial infarction. Symptoms more frequently observed are: (1) dyspnea; (2) dizziness, weakness, vertigo, and confusion; (3) mid-abdominal or lower abdominal distress; and (4) syncope. These symptoms are attributable to left-sided heart failure, reduced cerebrovascular perfusion, visceral congestion caused by right-sided heart failure, and complete heart block.[29]

The silent myocardial infarction is usually discovered on the electrocardiogram since there are usually no clinical manifestations or pain, or only the symptoms just listed are felt. Silent myocardial infarctions have not been explained fully, but they may be related to insensitivity to pain, loss of the meaning of pain sensation, memory loss, and a tendency to ignore a new symptom among other preexisting symptoms. Electrocardiograms should be performed routinely on the senior with atypical complaints, unexplained increase in congestive failure, after surgery when incidence of silent myocardial infarctions increases, and as part of periodic exams. Acute myocardial infarction in the elderly is often misdiagnosed as pneumonia or hypertensive heart disease.[46]

The treatment of acute myocardial infarction in the elderly is similar to that of the younger patient. A text in Medical-Surgical Nursing should be consulted and care of the patient with a myocardial infarction should be reviewed at this point. The senior will require special attention in the following areas.

Sensory deprivation of coronary care units plus cerebral hypoxia can result in an agitated depression or acute psychotic response. The best way to avoid this response is to personalize care as much as possible, preserve as normal an environment as possible (lights should not be kept on continuously for 24 hours), provide familiar objects in the environment, and permit family to be present as much as possible. Principles of reality orientation as described in

Chapter 4 should be used to keep the patient in contact with his environment. Excessive sedation should be avoided. Glasses and hearing aid should be kept in place. Calling the patient by name is of vital importance.

Chair treatment, which is reported to place less work on the heart physiologically, a bed-chair regimen with bedside commode, or bathroom privileges and early ambulation will probably be less debilitating to the senior than a long period of bed rest. It is your responsibility to monitor this care and be sure that overexertion does not occur when lifting him in and out of bed, getting him on and off the commode, or ambulating. Being able to feed himself will be very important; but if this is too tiring for him, a staff member or family member must feed him.[5,23,48]

A guide to use in determining whether or not an activity is too strenuous for the patient includes: (1) an increase in pulse of 20 beats per minute over the preactivity pulse, (2) a pulse of 120 beats per minute during the activity, or (3) the pulse does not return to the preactivity rate within 3 minutes after completing the activity.[5] If the patient is being monitored, the development of abnormal beats or rhythms may indicate a need for more restriction on activity.

Nutrition and elimination must be maintained. Foods that are easy to chew and not gas-forming should be taken. Since bowel function is usually of great concern to the senior, special attention should be given to avoiding constipation and straining. Adequate fluids, fruit juices, and stool softeners should be used. If constipation does occur, enemas, if ordered, or suppositories must be administered cautiously to avoid vagal stimulation that can cause cardiac slowing. The patient must also be cautioned not to strain at stool since this causes a Valsalva maneuver. The Valsalva maneuver results in increased pulmonic pressure, decreased cardiac output, and an increased venous return to the heart when the intrathoracic pressure suddenly drops at the end of the maneuver. The Valsalva maneuver may predispose to arrhythmias or ventricular rupture.[29]

Anticoagulant therapy may present special problems in the care of the senior with a myocardial infarction because the aged are susceptible to cerebral and intestinal bleeding. The frequency of hypertension; potential bleeding sites such as duodenal ulcers, diverticula, hemorrhoids, and cystitis; and sensitivity to even small doses of anticoagulants all increase the danger of this type of therapy. You must be alert to any symptom of bleeding when anticoagulants are being used in care of the senior. The loading dose of warfarin is smaller in the aged; 20 mg is usually given initially with as little as 2.5 mg or less per day as a maintenance dose. Anticoagulant therapy is monitored by the prothrombin time which is usually maintained at twice the control (25 seconds). The following drugs lengthen the prothrombin time: aspirin, heparin, phenylbutazone, sulfasoxasole, and quinidine. Other drugs such as phenobarbital, chloral hydrate, glutethimide, and meprobamate shorten the prothrombin time. Warfarin can also potentiate the action of tolbutamide.[46]

Since congestive heart failure is a common complication for the senior who has experienced a myocardial infarction, careful observation is most important when ambulation is begun. Impending failure may become manifest at this time.[51] The treatment of congestive failure will be discussed in the next section.

Drug therapy often produces unexpected results in the senior because of metabolic, circulatory, and excretory changes.

Digitalis toxicity is easily induced because the myocardium in acute infarction is depleted of potassium. Patients who have been on long-term thiazide diuretics may be especially predisposed to this complication. In the senior, abnormal rhythms, ectopic beats, and conduction disturbances may occur with few symptoms. The EKG may reveal a prolonged P-R interval, which should be investigated as a possible indication of digitalis toxicity.[49,54]

After discharge from the hospital the patient should resume activity within the limitations of his disease status. Moderate exertion that does not produce angina, fatigue, or increased congestive failure is desirable in order to promote morale and overall function as well as promote collateral circulation.

Care of the Person with Congestive Heart Failure

Heart failure is a common complication following a myocardial infarction in the elderly. Cardiac output is inadequate to meet the metabolic needs of the body as a result of the heart's failure to pump the blood through the circulation. Research suggests that the myocardial cells lose their ability to contract forcefully because of some physiochemical event related to abnormalities in the heart's cellular metabolism. Although coronary artery disease appears to be the predominant cause of failure in the elderly, multiple other factors may contribute to it, such as: (1) hypertension, (2) cor pulmonale resulting from chronic lung disease, (3) valvular disease, (4) pulmonary embolism, (5) chronic pericarditis, (6) subacute bacterial endocarditis, (7) congenital heart disease, (8) thyrotoxicosis, and (9) myxedema.[46,51]

Right-sided failure is manifested by weakness, fatigue, anorexia, nausea, liver engorgement, ascites, ankle and dependent edema, and generalized body edema (anasarca). Since tissues are being poorly perfused with right-sided failure, decubitus and cellulitis may occur. Malnutrition will also be masked by anasarca.[42,46,51]

Left-sided failure presents symptoms similar to those of pulmonary disease, such as wheezing, coughing, and dyspnea. Insomnia, weakness, fatigue, paroxysmal nocturnal dyspnea, and basal pulmonary rales are other signs. Pulmonary edema is the severest form of left ventricular failure.[42,46,51]

In *pulmonary edema* the fluid transudates from the capillaries to the interstitial spaces surrounding the alveoli and into the alveoli directly. Hypoxia, hypercapnea, intense dyspnea, pink-tinged frothy sputum, cough, cyanosis, diaphoresis, and tachycardia occur, along with intense fear. Chest pain may be present because of the congestion. Respirations are noisy and gurgling.[42,46]

In left-sided failure a ventricular gallop denoted by an S_3, an atrial gallop denoted by an S_4, or a summation gallop which is S_3 and S_4 occurring simultaneously may be detected on cardiac auscultation. The point of maximal intensity is also displaced because of cardiac enlargement.[42,46]

Cerebral dysfunction may result from the hypoxia and hypercapnea of left-sided failure. Thus, the patient cannot be relied on as an accurate informant. His account of symptoms, onset, and other information should always be substantiated by that of a family member or other involved person.

Congestion of the venous system occurring in right-sided failure causes distention of the jugular veins. Assessment of cervical-jugular vein distention is done by observing the pulsations while the patient is in a 45° upright position. The height of these pulsations above the sternal angle is measured in centimeters and gives a rough estimate of central venous pressure.[35,43]

In advanced right-sided failure, pleural and pericardial effusion can result in emergency conditions caused by lung compression and reduction in cardiac contractility. Dyspnea is usually the primary symptom.[46]

Chronic congestive failure involves both right and left sides of the heart and manifestations are a combination of the two. It is an irreversible process; therapy is palliative and is directed toward maintaining circulation and preventing complications that will intensify the failure. Intractable heart failure will eventually occur. It is unresponsive to treatment and terminal in the largest percentage of patients.[5]

Intervention is directed at increasing cardiac efficiency and output, reducing the fluid load, correcting hypoxia and hypercapnea, reducing the oxygen need of the heart and correcting, preventing, or controlling arrhythmias.[5]

Digitalis can be instrumental in accomplishing these goals. Digitalis increases the inotropic force of contraction and slows conduction in the atrioventricular node. Thus, it is beneficial in treating supraventricular arrhythmias such as paroxysmal atrial tachycardia, atrial flutter, and atrial fibrillation. Cardiac output is increased, thus increasing perfusion of the kidneys which results in water and sodium excretion. With reduction in fluid, and increased cardiac output, all tissues of the body are better perfused, improving oxygenation and reducing the carbon dioxide retention.[54]

Digitalis agents, however, carry a small margin of safety because the therapeutic-toxic ratio is extremely low. Toxicity is most frequent when renal function is impaired, in advanced pulmonary disease, in cardiac enlargement, during diuretic therapy, and in the event of pulmonary emboli. These conditions are prevalent in advanced age and make the elderly more susceptible to digitalis toxicity.[29,54]

In addition to these predisposing factors, there is evidence that age itself may be a factor in digitalis toxicity. The noncardiac symptoms of toxicity are subtle and must be carefully observed for. They include gastrointestinal symptoms (anorexia, nausea, vomiting), lethargy, weakness, weight loss, emotional manifestations (depression, stupor, paranoia, delirium), color vision disturbances such as yellow-green, and facial neuralgia. Central nervous system symptoms usually occur later. The cardiac symptoms result from an increase in automaticity and slowing of conduction. Arrhythmias occur; the most common initial one is ventricular extrasystoles, frequently in a bigeminal pattern. These can progress to ventricular tachycardia and fibrillation. Extreme sinus bradycardia caused by sinoatrial block is common in the elderly. Paroxysmal atrial tachycardia with atrioventricular block of some of the impulses is another frequent manifestation of digitalis toxicity.[5,29,54] Consult a pharmacology text for details on specific digitalis preparations.

Be alert to the symptoms of digitalis toxicity. Any significant change in rate or rhythm of the pulse should be reported before administering the next dose of the drug. The drug should be administered at the prescribed time in the prescribed dose and manner. Hypokalemia predisposes to digitalis toxicity and any patient receiving diuretics, particularly thiazides, will be susceptible. Potassium supplement will usually be prescribed. Otherwise, foods high in potassium (see Chapter 15) need to be included in the diet.[49,54]

Reducing the fluid load in the body is accomplished through several measures. Diuretic therapy increases the excretion of sodium and water. A salt restricted diet will usually be prescribed. In acute pulmonary edema the fluid load will be reduced by rotating tourniquets in which the blood flow is temporarily blocked in the extremities, thus reducing the venous return and the load on the heart. Peritoneal and hemodialysis can also be used to reduce the amount of water and salt in the body. Water intake is not usually restricted. In acute situations, a moderate restriction may be used (1200 to 2000 ml per 24 hours), which includes the 700 to 800 ml of hidden fluids in solid foods.[46]

Diuretics such as furosemide (Lasix), ethacrynic acid (Edecrin), and chlorothiazide (Diuril) are those most frequently used today. Lasix and Edecrin can be administered intravenously and are therefore useful in emergency situations, such as pulmonary edema, pleural effusion, and pericardial effusion. These drugs interfere with the tubular reabsorption of sodium. Intravenous potassium therapy often accompanies intravenous diuretic therapy. Potassium overdose can also cause cardiac arrhythmias; therefore, monitor the drip rate carefully.[29]

While the patient is on diuretics the daily weight and intake and output should be recorded. Massive fluid and electrolyte loss after intravenous diuretic therapy can result in dehydration, electrolyte imbalance, shock, uremia, pulmonary infarction, cerebral infarction, as well as digitalis toxicity. Acute urinary retention in elderly males with benign prostatic hypertrophy can also present an acute emergency. Hyponatremia and hyperchloremic acidosis can occur because of rapid excretion of sodium.[46]

Teaching the patient and his family about his drugs is most important. He should be cautioned about the need for taking them as prescribed and about the danger in either increasing or decreasing the amounts taken. Often the elderly shut-in will begin to run out of his prescription and will reduce the dose or stop taking it entirely. Also, if he does not feel well, he frequently will increase the dose. Since this is his "heart" pill, he thinks that a little more will be just that much better. The senior and someone else should be taught to take his pulse and look for signs of toxicity. Any significant rate or rhythm change and any other symptom of toxicity should be reported.

Diet is used to prevent the accumulation of salt. A diet containing 1 to 1.5 gm of sodium daily is usually prescribed. Teach the senior and family not to use salt in cooking and not to put it on the table and to eliminate foods containing high amounts of sodium, such as baking soda and powder and flavor enhancers (MSG). Such measures alone remove much excess salt from the diet. Watching labels for salt and preservative additions containing sodium is also beneficial in reducing sodium intake. The American Heart Association has descriptive pamphlets available about specific sodium restricted diets.

Oxygen therapy, described earlier in this chapter, can be beneficial in an emergency such as pulmonary edema to reduce hypoxia and hypercapnea. In pulmonary edema IPPB will probably be prescribed.

Thoracentesis or paracentesis can be helpful in increasing oxygenation by decreasing the pressure exerted against the lungs, thus increasing lung expansion.

Provide rest and reduce anxiety to decrease oxygen need of the myocardium. During pulmonary edema merperidine (Demerol) should be administered to the elderly in preference to morphine to accomplish this goal.[46] Bedrest or chair rest also is prescribed. The patient in acute pulmonary edema will only accept an upright position. Dependency of the lower extremities will impede venous return to the heart which may be beneficial. However, any pressure behind the knee or on the calves of the legs must be prevented in order to avoid thrombophlebitis.

Both physical and psychological rest are necessary to reduce the oxygen needs of the heart. The family should be cautioned about relating stressful matters. Small doses of tranquilizers may be required. However, in the elderly these may increase confusion and must be evaluated on an individual basis.

Making the patient comfortable while at the same time preventing complications is an important nursing goal. Frequent change of position is important even if the patient is in the Fowler's or semi-Fowler's position. Again, avoidance of the Valsalva maneuver is necessary when the patient is turning. The Valsalva maneuver can intensify the failure already present.

Cardiac arrhythmias can be avoided by careful administration of digitalis and diuretics. Providing rest and decreasing oxygen demand of the myocardium also decrease the possibility of arrhythmias. Drugs such as quinidine may be administered in cardiac arrhythmias. Conversion of an atrial arrhythmia either electrically or medically carries the danger of thromboembolic phenomenon. Some feel that this phenomenon can also occur when anticoagulants are used when mural thrombi are present, such as in long-term preexisting atrial fibrillation. Bedrest also predisposes to thrombi formation. Elastic stockings are worn to prevent the pooling of blood in the patient on bedrest. Leg exercises, such as quadriceps-setting and flexion and extension of the ankle, can foster venous return.

The elderly patient with congestive failure most frequently succumbs to complications rather than to the failure itself. Thus, it is your responsibility to be aware of possible complications and take measures to prevent their occurrence. In one study, bronchopneumonia accounted for one-third and pulmonary embolism accounted for one-seventh of the deaths.[4]

EVALUATION

Since dyspnea is such a common symptom of cardiopulmonary disease, its presence or absence can often be used as a guide to the effectiveness of care. If therapy and nursing care have been beneficial, dyspnea will be reduced or eliminated. If treatment and nursing measures have been ineffective, the dyspnea will be intensified. If the senior remains anxious, fearful, depressed, or demanding, dyspnea and other symptoms of respiratory-cardiac distress related to an intense emotional state will be present, showing that psychological care has been inadequate.

Dyspnea also will determine how other goals are achieved. The patient who is dyspneic will have difficulty with any function or activity. If he is able to eat with enjoyment, resume normal activities, and care for himself, nursing intervention has probably been effective.

When you evaluate your care, determine the patient's compliance to medication and dietary routines, whether or not the patient has been able to follow a rehabilitation regimen, how well the family is managing with home care, how effectively the health team have worked together during the acute stages of the chronic illness, how useful the discharge plan was, and whether the necessary community resources were utilized. Check with the patient and family to learn of their feelings during acute care stages as well as during remissions of the chronic illness.

Finally, consider your feelings as you confronted mortality when the patient had pulmonary or cardiac failure, your sense of helplessness or frustration when the medical condition did not respond quickly to treatment. How did you handle your feelings while you were working with the patient and his family? How well did you help the patient and family to cope with their feelings?

REFERENCES

1. BARACH, A. L., "Diaphragmatic Breathing in Pulmonary Emphysema," *Journal of Chronic Diseases,* 1: (1955), 211.

2. BARSTON, RUTH, "Coping with Emphysema," *Nursing Clinics of North America,* 9: No. 1 (1974), 137–45.

3. BATES, BARBARA, *A Guide to Physical Examination.* Philadelphia: J. B. Lippincott Company, 1974.

4. BEDFORD, P. and F. CAIRD, *Valvular Disease of the Heart in Old Age.* London: Churchill, 1960.

5. BELAND, IRENE, and JOYCE PASSOS, *Clinical Nursing: Pathophysiological and Psychosocial Approaches,* 3rd ed. New York: Macmillan Publishing Co., Inc., 1975.

6. BIRCHENALL, JOAN, and MARY STREIGHT, *Care of the Older Patient.* Philadelphia: J. B. Lippincott Company, 1973.

7. BRAMMEL, H. L., and ARLENE NICCOLI, "A Physiologic Approach to Cardiac Rehabilitation," *Nursing Clinics of North America,* 11: No. 2 (1976), 223–36.

8. BRANNIN, PATRICIA, "Oxygen Therapy and Measures of Bronchial Hygiene," *Nursing Clinics of North America,* 9: No. 1 (1974), 111–21.

9. BUCKINGHAM, WILLIAM, MARSHALL SPAIBERG, and MARTIN BRANDFONBRENER, *A Primer of Clinical Diagnosis.* New York: Harper & Row, Publishers, Inc., 1971.

10. CARNES, G., "Understanding the Cardiac Patient's Behavior," *American Journal of Nursing,* 71: No. 6 (1971), 1187–88.

11. CASSEM, N., and THOMAS HACKETT, "Psychological Rehabilitation of Myocardial Infarction Patients in the Acute Phase," *Heart and Lung,* 2: No. 3 (1973), 382–88.

12. ———, "Stress on the Nurse and Therapist in the Intensive-Care Unit and the Coronary-Care Unit," *Heart and Lung,* 4: No. 2 (1975), 252–59.

13. CHRISMAN, MARILYN, "Dyspnea," *American Journal of Nursing,* 74: No. 4 (1974), 643–46.

14. CLARK, MYRA, "Recent Trends in Tuberculosis Care," *Nursing Clinics of North America,* 9: No. 1 (1974), 157–64.

15. DEBERRY, PAULINE, LENNER JEFFERIES, and MARGARET LIGHT, "Teaching Cardiac Patients to Manage Medications," *American Journal of Nursing,* 75: No. 12 (1975), 2191–93.

16. DEGOWAN, ELMER, and RICHARD DEGOWAN, *Bedside Diagnostic Examination,* 2nd ed. New York: Macmillan Publishing Co., Inc., 1969.

17. DIRSCHEL, KATHLEEN M., "Respiration in Emphysema Patients," *Nursing Clinics of North America,* 8: No. 4 (1973), 617–22.

18. EDDY, MARY, "Teaching Patients with Peripheral Vascular Disease," *Nursing Clinics of North America,* 12: No. 1 (1977), 151–59.

19. FAGAN-DUBIN, LINDA, "Atherosclerosis: A Major Cause of Peripheral Vascular Disease," *Nursing Clinics of North America,* 12: No. 1 (1977), 101–8.

20. FILLEY, G. F., "Emphysema and Chronic Bronchitis: Clinical Manifestations and Their Physiologic Significance," *Medical Clinics of North America,* 51: (1967), 283.

21. FOSTER, SUE, "Pump Failure," *American Journal of Nursing,* 74: No. 10 (1974), 1830–34.

22. FROHLICH, E. D., "Use and Abuse of Diuretics," *American Heart Journal,* 89: No. 1 (1975), 1–3.

23. GOLDSTROM, DEBORAH, "Cardiac Rest: Bed to Chair," *American Journal of Nursing,* 72: No. 10 (1972), 1812–16.

24. GUTHRIE, A., and T. PETTY, "Improved Exercise Tolerance in Patients with Chronic Airway Obstruction," *Physical Therapy,* 50: (1970), 1333.

25. HIRSCHBERG, GERALD, L. LEWIS, and P. VAUGHAN, *Rehabilitation, A Manual for the Care of the Disabled and Elderly,* 2nd ed. Philadelphia: J. B. Lippincott Company, 1976.

26. HURST, J., and R. MYERBURG, "Cardiac Arrhythmias: Evolving Concepts," *Modern Concepts of Cardiovascular Disease,* 37: (1968), 73.

27. JOHNSTON, R., and P. HOPEWELL, "Chemotherapy of Pulmonary Tuberculosis," *Annals of Internal Medicine,* 70: (1969), 359.

28. JUDGE, RICHARD, and GEORGE ZUIDEMA, *Physical Diagnosis: A Physiologic Approach to the Clinical Examination,* 2nd ed. Boston: Little, Brown & Company, 1968.

29. KLEIGER, ROBERT, "Cardiovascular Disorders," in *Cowdry's The Care of the Geriatric Patient,* 5th ed., ed. Franz A. Steinberg. St. Louis: The C. V. Mosby Company, 1976.

30. KRUPP, M., and M. CHATTON, *Current Medical Diagnosis and Treatment.* Los Altos, Calif.: Lange Medical Publications, 1975.

31. LEE, ROBERT, and PATRICIA BALL, "Some Thoughts on the Psychology of the Coronary Care Unit," *American Journal of Nursing,* 75: No. 9 (1975), 1498–1501.

32. MALKUS, BOBBY, "Respiratory Care at Home," *American Journal of Nursing,* 76: No. 11 (1976), 1789–91.

33. MITCHELL, R., T. VINCENT, S. RYAN, and G. FILLEY, "Chronic Obstructive Bronchopulmonary Disease: IV. The Clinical and Physiological Differentiation of Chronic Bronchitis and Emphysema," *American Journal of Medical Science,* 247: (1964), 513.

34. MOODY, LINDA, "Primer for Pulmonary Hygiene," *American Journal of Nursing,* 77: No. 1 (1977), 104–6.

35. MORGAN, WILLIAM, and GEORGE ENGEL, *The Clinical Approach to the Patient.* Philadelphia: W. B. Saunders Company, 1969.

36. NICCOLI, ARLENE, and H. L. BRAMMELL, "A Program for Rehabilitation in Coronary Heart Disease," *Nursing Clinics of North America,* 11: No. 2 (1976), 237–50.

37. PETERSON, LOIS, and JUANITA GREEN, "Nurse Managed Tuberculosis Clinic," *American Journal of Nursing,* 77: No. 3 (1977), 433–35.

38. PETTY, T. L., *Intensive and Rehabilitative Respiratory Care,* 2nd ed. Philadelphia: Lea and Febiger, 1974.

39. ———, "Chronic Respiratory Diseases," in *Cowdry's The Care of the Geriatric Patient,* 5th ed., ed. Franz Steinberg. St. Louis: The C. V. Mosby Company, 1976.

40. ———, and L. NEIL, *For Those Who Live and Breathe with Emphysema and Chronic Bronchitis,* 2nd ed. Springfield, Ill.: Charles C Thomas, Publisher, 1974.

41. POMERANCE, A., "Cardiac Pathology in the Aged," *Geriatrics,* 23: (1968), 101.

42. ———, "Pathology of the Heart with and without Cardiac Failure in the Aged," *British Heart Journal,* 27: (1975), 697.

43. POWELL, ANNE, "Physical Assessment of the Patient with Cardiac Disease," *Nursing Clinics of North America,* 11: No. 2 (1976), 251–57.

44. RAU, JOSEPH, and MARY RAU, "To Breathe or to Be Breathed: Understanding IPPB," *American Journal of Nursing,* 77: No. 4 (1977), 613–17.

45. REICHLE, MARIAN, "Psychologic Aspects of the Acutely Stressed in an Intensive Care Unit," in *Respiratory Intensive Care Nursing,* ed. Sharon Bushwell. Boston: Little, Brown & Company, 1973, pp. 219–29.

46. RODSTEIN, MANUEL, "Heart Disease in the Aged," in *Clinical Geriatrics,* ed. Isadore Rossman. Philadelphia: J. B. Lippincott Company, 1971.

47. RYZEWSKI, JANE, "Factors in the Rehabilitation of Patients with Peripheral Vascular Disease," *Nursing Clinics of North America,* 12: No. 1 (1977), 161–68.

48. SCHMIDT, Y., *et al.,* "Armchair Treatment in the Coronary Care Unit—Effect on Blood Pressure and Pulse," *Nursing Research,* 18: No. 2 (1969), 114.

49. SCHNEIDER, WM., and BARBARA BOYCE, "Complications of Diuretic Therapy," *American Journal of Nursing,* 68: No. 9 (1968), 1903–7.

50. TAGGART, ELEANOR, "The Physical Assessment of the Patient with Arterial Disease," *Nursing Clinics of North America,* 12: No. 1 (1977), 109–17.

51. TANNER, GLORIA, "Heart Failure in the MI Patient," *American Journal of Nursing,* 77: No. 2 (1977), 230–34.

52. TRAVER, GAYLE, "The Nurse's Role in Clinical Testing of Lung Function," *Nursing Clinics of North America,* 9: No. 1 (1974), 101–10.

53. WAXLER, ROSE, "The Patient with Congestive Heart Failure: Teaching Implications," *Nursing Clinics of North America,* 11: No. 2 (1976), 297–308.

54. WINSLOW, ELIZABETH, "Digitalis," *American Journal of Nursing,* 74: No. 6 (1974), 1062–65.

55. ———, "Visual Inspection of the Patient with Cardiopulmonary Disease," *Heart and Lung,* 4: No. 3 (1975), 421–29.

problems of cell proliferation and pain in later maturity

Study of this chapter will enable you to:

1. Teach the senior and his family early signs of cancer and the importance of using preventive measures.

2. Assess presence of cell proliferation through observation, examination, and a history.

3. Assess presence of pain in the senior, including covert signs, and factors that affect pain perception and tolerance.

4. Formulate nursing diagnoses and a care plan related to the type and location of malignancy, degree of pain, and extent of changed body function or structure.

5. Intervene with appropriate physical or emotional nursing care measures.

6. Discuss alternate treatment methods for malignancy with the patient/family.

7. Carry out nursing responsibilities related to surgery, radiation, or chemotherapy.

8. Teach the patient and family how to recognize cancer quackery and give sufficient support so that they do not stop useful medical treatment.

9. Help the senior avoid complications of advancing malignancy.

10. Help the elderly person maintain dignity and quality of life, even as he approaches death.

11. Support the family as it faces the crises of terminal illness and death so that it can in turn remain supportive to the loved one.

12. Evaluate the effectiveness of your care to the terminally ill and dying patient and his family by obtaining their feedback to your care measures.

13. Work with other health team members and consumers to insure provision for quality care for the terminally ill.

18

Cancer is the second leading cause of death in the United States, with a death rate of 163.2 per 100,000 population.[1] More than one-half of these deaths occur in persons over 65 years of age.[2] The leading cancer sites for the age groups 55 to 74 and 75 and over for men and women are given in Table 18.1.[1]

TABLE 18.1   Most Common Sites of Cancer

| | Persons 55–74 years | | Persons 75 years and over | |
	Men	Women	Men	Women
1.	Lungs	Breast	Lungs	Colon and rectum
2.	Colon and rectum	Colon and rectum	Prostate gland	Breast
3.	Prostate gland	Lungs	Colon and rectum	Pancreas
4.	Pancreas	Uterus	Stomach	Uterus
5.	Stomach	Ovary	Pancreas	Stomach

Since cancer of the lung, breast, prostate, colon, and rectum are the more common of the cancer sites in the senior, these will be the ones focused on in this chapter. However, assessment will not be limited to simply evaluating the patient for cancer in these sites but will include all possible sites.

ASSESSMENT

Basic to an assessment for cancer is a thorough history. Each person should also be informed of the following danger signals:

1. Unusual bleeding or discharge.
2. Lump or thickened area in the breast or elsewhere.
3. Sore that does not heal.
4. Change in bowel or bladder habits.
5. Hoarseness or cough.
6. Indigestion or difficulty swallowing.
7. Change in a wart or mole.[4]

These danger signals serve as a concise summary of the major signs and symptoms of most cancer forms. Remember that cancers on the skin, lips, mouth, tongue, vulva, and penis are visible and can be detected by inspection. Cancers of the vagina, anus, rectum, sigmoid, cervix, bladder, larynx, bronchi, stomach, esophagus, and nasopharynx can be observed through instrumentation. Cancers that may be palpated are of the breast, rectum, prostate gland, ovary, bone, lymph nodes, and testes. Other cancers, however, require X-ray and other internal examinations for detection, such as lung, liver, intestine, stomach, pancreas, kidney, brain, and bone.

Systemic Manifestations of Malignancy

Several symptoms may indicate cancer: anemia, fever, weight loss, and urinary or endocrine symptoms.

Cancers that cause chronic blood loss, such as cancer of the stomach and bowel, will be associated with anemia from an early stage of development. Presence of occult blood in the stool may be the first clue to a gastrointestinal cancer and thus should be routinely tested for. Anemia in cancer can also result from depression of hematopoiesis, infection and inflammation, poor nutrition, renal insufficiency, and decreased erythropoietin production.[27]

Fever may be a systemic manifestation of a malignancy, although it is usually the result of infection locally. Resistance to infection may be impaired by reduced neutrophils, deficiency of gamma globulin, and poor antibody reserve.[27] Assessment of body temperature for several days periodically during day and evening hours will help to identify any pattern of fever.

Leukemias will be accompanied by abnormal leukocyte counts. Thus, a white blood count (WBC) and differential should be part of every routine examination.

Weight loss can be a normal manifestation of aging. However, in cancer, diversion of body protein in favor of tumor growth, reduced appetite, depression of normal protein synthesis, caloric expenditure greater than intake, and shrinkage of fatty tissues due to their metabolism for energy can also cause a loss of weight.[27]

Renal insufficiency may occur because of obstruction and pyelonephritis accompanying or resulting from a malignancy. Hypercalcemia in certain bone or parathyroid tumors can result in kidney stone formation. Multiple myeloma is commonly accompanied by proteinuria.[26]

Hormonal overactivity in endocrine tumors can cause typical symptoms associated with hypersecretion of the specific gland. Symptoms that might occur are Cushing's syndrome, hyperparathyroidism, hyperthyroidism, feminization, virilization, and hypoglycemia.

A systematic survey of the body and careful review of systems will assist in detecting any signs or symptoms of cancer.

Head and Neck

The skin of the head and neck is examined by inspection and palpation. Swellings in the area of the salivary glands and enlarged lymph nodes should be noted. The thyroid gland is palpated and inspected for enlargement and nodules. Consult a text on physical assessment for exam procedure.[6]

Figure 18.1 shows the positions of the lymph nodes and salivary glands.

Dentures should be removed so that the buccal mucosa, tongue, roof, and floor of the mouth can be inspected. Areas of leukoplakia, ulceration, and nodules or thickening should be noted. The lips, floor of the mouth, and tongue should be palpated.

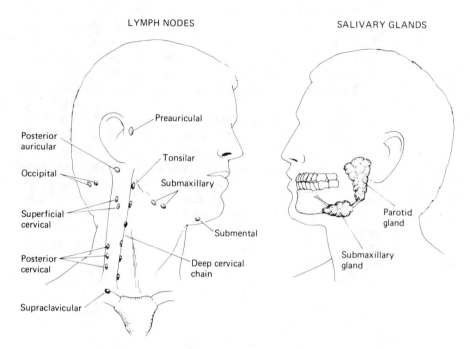

Figure 18.1. Assessment of the lymph nodes and salivary glands.

The nasopharynx and larynx should be inspected with a laryngeal mirror. This procedure requires skill and should only be performed following proper instruction and practice in use of the mirror. A nasal speculum is used to inspect the anterior nares.

Chest and Breasts

Cancer of the lung can be detected through chest X-rays, cytologic smears of sputum, and bronchoscopy. The lung cancer rate rose from 20.6 per 100,000 in 1950 to 52.1 in 1970 in males and from 4.4 to 10.3 in females.[1] Cigarette smoking continues at a high level even though the U.S. Surgeon General's Advisory Committee on Smoking and Health in 1964 stated, "Cigarette smoking is causally related to lung cancer. . . .   The risk of developing lung cancer increases with duration of smoking and number of cigarettes smoked per day, and is diminished by discontinuing smoking." Thus, all adults who smoke should have annual chest X-ray examinations.

Cancer of the esophagus is usually associated with dysphagia, which may be intermittent and related to the texture of the food ingested. X-ray and esophagoscopy are utilized for diagnosis.

Esophagoscopy and bronchoscopy are uncomfortable procedures. You can help the senior before, during, and following the procedure by giving a great deal of support. The senior's response to the procedure must be carefully observed. Topical anesthesia will alleviate much of the discomfort, but the anxiety level should be observed as well as change in vital signs. The gag reflex should be present before food or fluids are permitted.

Cancer of the breast can be detected through regular breast self-examination. However, results of a Gallop Poll conducted for the American Cancer Society show that fewer than one in five women practice breast self-examination. Only 24 percent of the women who were polled received instruction from their physicians on how to examine their breasts. However, among those receiving instruction, 92 percent practiced the examination. This indicates that women of all ages need instruction in the self-breast examination method. The older woman especially needs encouragement to continue breast self-examination. If the physician does not provide instruction, you should assume responsibility for this. Breast cancer is one of the easiest to detect, and yet it remains the number one cancer killer in women. The following procedure should be followed.

The breasts should first be carefully inspected and palpated in a well-lighted area by the woman in the sitting position. Puckering of the skin and change in nipple level should be noted as the arms are raised over the head and the hands are clasped forcibly in front of the chest. The breasts should be compared for symmetry. The nipple and areola are inspected. Any discharge from the nipples should be reported. The axillary and supraclavicular regions are palpated for enlarged lymph nodes. After assuming the supine position each breast is palpated first with the arm over the head and then at the side. A small pillow should be placed under the side being examined. All quadrants of the breast should be systematically examined.[4]

Aspiration and biopsy are of diagnostic value. Biopsy is indicated for solitary tumors and is the only exact means of determining whether or not a mass is malignant.

Abdomen, Colon, and Rectum

Cancer of the stomach has vague early symptoms. However, persistence of any digestive difficulty should be carefully investigated. Upper gastrointestinal series, X-rays, and cytology are frequently used diagnostic measures. A careful history of eating habits, digestive difficulties, and related symptoms is important. Since the senior often has increasing digestive difficulty as enzymes and tone decrease, he may at first dismiss the early symptoms of cancer as part of aging.

Carcinoma of the colon or rectum is frequently diagnosed by a change in bowel habits: either constipation or diarrhea. Blood in the stool should always be investigated. The abdomen should be palpated in all four quadrants; note distention, masses, and organ sizes. Palpate and percuss the liver edge. Attempt to palpate the spleen. Note herniations, femoral pulses, and enlarged lymph nodes in both groins.

Rectal carcinoma may be discovered on digital exam. A bimanual exam may reveal pelvic masses. The anus should also be observed for hemorrhoids.

Proctosigmoidoscopy, visual examination of the rectum and sigmoid colon with a special scope, is a valuable examination for diagnosing cancer of the rectum and colon. A clean bowel is required for the procedure; several enemas and laxatives may be required before examination; often this preparation is taxing for the senior. You will have to carefully observe the senior who receives a bowel prep because he may faint or fall. You can help to allay the person's anxiety during the procedure by telling him what to expect and staying with him. The senior will need a rest period after the examination, and his complaints should be listened to empathetically.

Genitourinary Tract

In the female obtain a history of the earlier menstrual cycle and postmenopausal events. Spotting or bleeding and any watery vaginal discharge should be investigated. A Papanicolaou smear should be performed along with a complete pelvic exam; the Pap smear can detect early cervical cancer. Specimens for the test should be taken from the cervix and the vaginal pool. The cervical specimen should be taken from the squamocolumnar junction where the columnar epithelium that normally lines the endocervical canal meets the squamous epithelium that covers the ectocervix. If this junction is present on the ectocervix, it can be identified by a difference of color and texture. The squamous epithelium is typically pale pink, shiny, and smooth. The columnar epithelium is reddish and has a granular surface. If the two do not appear on the cervical os, then the junction is probably in the endocervical canal. While the speculum is in place the cervix and vagina should be inspected.

The complete pelvic exam should include inspection and palpation. The vulva should be inspected for leukoplakia and ulceration. Digital palpation of the vagina and cervix and bimanual palpation of the uterus and adnexa should be performed.

In the male the prostate gland should be palpated during the rectal examination. Hypertrophy and tumor nodules should be noted.

Men and women both should be questioned about hematuria either in the form of gross bleeding or as a smoky-colored urine, which may indicate microscopic blood. A routine urinalysis with particular attention to the presence of red blood cells is important since cancer can occur in any part of the urinary tract, and bleeding is an important signal.

The Skin

A history should include inquiry about exposure to carcinogenic factors such as sun, radiation, coal tar derivatives, and arsenic ingestion. A change in the color, ulceration, or enlargement of a wart, mole, or sore that has not healed should be questioned and carefully inspected. A biopsy may be necessary to determine presence of cancer.

The skin should be carefully inspected, including the palms, soles, scalp, and genital area. Palpate for thickenings and masses. Sarcomas occur as firm or soft lumps which may or may not be fixed.

Report findings of the assessment accurately and promptly to a physician so that further diagnostic tests, such as biopsy, can be made.

Pain

Pain, although a later symptom of cancer, must be assessed. However, an understanding of the factors influencing pain is necessary before assessment can adequately be done.

Age appears to be an important variable for the degree of pain relief provided by an analgesic. In one study, postoperative patients in the older age group experienced more extensive surgery but reported a lower level of initial pain and a greater degree of pain relief following analgesia.[9] When you assess the elderly, remember that their reports of pain may not be indicative of the extent of pathology and therefore cannot be relied on as any indicator of presence or extent of a neoplasm.

Several theories have been proposed to explain the pain phenomenon. Pain is a complex reaction, and to date no one theory explains it completely. Pain is not a single sensation; it must be recognized as a complex experience involving the total individual.[32] Older theories postulate the anatomy of pain as consisting of specific pain receptors, pain fibers, and pain centers in the central nervous system. The anatomy of the sensory perception of pain has been theorized as consisting of pathways or nerve fibers, one set transmitting rapidly while the other conducts the impulse slowly. In one such theory, A delta fibers, which are large, myelinated, rapid conducting, and passing more or less directly to the thalamus and sensory portion of the cerebrum, alert the person to the pain and its location. C fibers, which are small, unmyelinated, slow conducting, and connecting with the reticular formation, cause the suffering of the pain.[24]

A recent explanation of the pain phenomenon is called the *Gate Control Theory*. This theory proposes a transmission blocking action that closes a gate to impulses entering the spinal cord. The pain mechanism is activated when excitatory pain signals are carried to the spinal cord by small-diameter fibers of the peripheral nerves. If these excitatory pain signals are not blocked, they travel to transmission cells in the dorsal horn and then to the thalamus and cerebral cortex via the anterolateral tract. The substantia gelatinosa, which consists of densely packed cells extending the length of the spinal cord, is theorized to be the site of the transmission blocking action referred to earlier. When the controlling gate is open, it permits excitatory pain signals to reach the transmission cells. When it is closed through some inhibitory mechanism, such as stimulation of large-fiber, afferent, cutaneous nerves by vibration or rubbing, the excitatory pain signals carried by the small fibers do not reach the transmission cells. Pain inhibiting mechanisms also descend from parts of the reticular formation, thalamus, and cerebrum.[14,33]

The pain inhibiting mechanism descending from the thalamus and cerebrum is called the *central control mechanism*. When it is activated, the gate is closed to any further incoming pain signals. The theory suggests that the entire brain is a pain center, since so many areas of the cerebral cortex are responsible for pain perception and response and also because the brainstem appears to act as a central biasing mechanism through its neural connection with various parts of the body. Stimulation of the brainstem produces analgesia in these various connected areas.

Cerebral processes are classified as sensory-discriminatory, motivation-affect, and cognition activities. The interplay of these various functions affect pain perception. The potential ability of the cerebrum to produce an inhibiting mechanism that closes the gate is used to explain the influence of emotional factors on pain perception.[14,33]

This Gate Control Theory should help you better assess and manage the pain phenomenon in patients. This theory demonstrates why a history of the patient's previous experiences with pain is so important. Previous experiences could heighten or reduce the perception of pain. The senior's present state of mind also must be assessed since it influences his perception and reaction to the pain. Awareness of conditions that cause anxiety, fear, and anticipation of pain is also a necessary part of assessment because all have the potential for increasing pain. Observation for signs of tension and fatigue are important since they reduce pain tolerance.[40]

Additionally, assessment must be made of the locations, quality, intensity, duration, origin, radiation, and pattern of the pain experience, including what alleviates and what aggravates or intensifies it. Any associated symptoms accompanying pain, such as nausea, vomiting, diaphoresis, and syncope should be investigated.

Try to determine the meaning of the pain to the senior because this greatly influences the reaction to pain or the psychic component of pain. The meaning of pain to the individual may result in its being greatly reduced or absent. (Studies have compared the pain of seriously injured soldiers admitted to a combat hospital and pain following surgery with similar incisional wounds in civilians. Apparently, soldiers were grateful to have escaped from battle alive and therefore did not report as severe pain as did the civilians, who, rather than being saved from death, feared the possibility of greater injury, pain, or even death.)[16]

Find out whether the senior recognizes the pain as something short-lived and explainable or as something chronic, unexplained, life-threatening, with little hope of significant or long-lasting alleviation. The senior's attitude is important, since overall response to the pain and attempts at its alleviation will be decidedly different.[15]

The senior's outward appearance must also be assessed for pain: Facial grimacing during certain movements or coughing; positions assumed, such as drawing up of legs; writhing; restlessness; walking in a stooped position; carrying a limb in a particularly stiff position; swallowing carefully; holding a part; splinting one side of the chest. Sympathoadrenal activity signifying pain, such as changes in pulse, blood pressure, and respirations; nausea and vomiting; diaphoresis; ashen facies; excitement, irritability, depression, and mood swings should be noted.[32]

NURSING DIAGNOSIS AND FORMULATION OF PATIENT CARE GOALS

Nursing Diagnosis

Following assessment, the following *nursing diagnoses* related to cell proliferation may be made:

1. *Anxiety* related to pain or concern about the family or the unknown.
2. *Acute or chronic presence of pain.*
3. *Body image change* (resulting from change in body function or mutilation of a body part).
4. *Fear of impending death.*

Other nursing diagnoses described in other chapters may coexist with the above diagnoses.

Patient Care Goals

Long-range patient care goals for the senior with a malignancy could include the following:

1. Roles and responsibilities characteristic of his premorbid health status will be resumed.
2. Daily activities of living will be performed and social contacts will be enjoyed to the degree that he maintains a positive self-concept, even if he is unable to resume former roles.
3. Friends and family will demonstrate acceptance of his changed body image if he has undergone disfiguring surgery/treatment; the acceptance is indicated by his willingness to participate in former social activities with them.
4. Acceptance of his changed body structure/function will be demonstrated by the ability to care for himself independently or with minimal assistance.
5. Feelings about terminal illness will be expressed to someone close and preparation for death will be dignified and according to his wishes if at all possible.

6. Chronic, intractable pain will be managed with various treatments and comfort measures so that as much comfort is attained as is possible.

Short-range goals could include the following:

1. Personal hygiene and activities of daily living will be maintained by the person.
2. Pain will be relieved so that activities of daily living can be managed.
3. Self-concept and body image will be reintegrated toward a positive, whole perception.
4. Interest in and activity with hobbies will be maintained.
5. Treatment routines will be followed to obtain maximum effect.

You will think of other short-term and long-term goals appropriate to an individual elderly person who has a malignancy or pain.

NURSING INTERVENTION

Successful treatment of a malignancy depends on early detection. The senior should be routinely examined annually or semiannually, since the incidence of cancer increases with age. Then the carcinoma may be discovered before symptoms become obvious. Local chapters of the American Cancer Society help to sponsor mass screenings where various tests such as breast exams and Pap smears are performed. Health departments often provide free examinations for seniors. You can foster senior citizen participation in these opportunities by informing contacts about their availability and by volunteering to assist with mass screening efforts when assistance is sought. You should also be able to teach the seven warning signals to all seniors whom you contact; women should be taught self-breast examination. If the malignancy is too advanced when it is diagnosed, little definitive treatment is possible. Teach and encourage the practice of good nutrition and other good health habits. Some researchers believe that immunological protection declines when malnutrition is present and that the older person is more likely to develop carcinoma for this reason.[37]

Since certain substances are known to be carcinogenic, the elderly should be warned about their use. Cigarettes are one of these. Pipe smoking appears to predispose to cancer of the lip. The rays of the sun, particularly for fair individuals, may result in skin cancer after prolonged exposure. Overexposure to ionizing radiation is also carcinogenic. The air in industrial and urban areas may contain carcinogenic chemicals. Seniors should be warned about going outside on high smog days, not only for the danger of carcinogens but also for the aggravation that may occur to preexisting lung disease. The Federal Food and Drug Administration attempts to remove most suspected carcinogens from the market. An example of this is cyclamates. Seniors should be informed about the reasons for removal of such substances. It is likely that in the future other substances will be found to be carcinogenic. For example, researchers have found increased incidence of cervical cancer and malignant melanoma in women who have taken oral contraceptives for 4 or more years. It is imperative that you remain informed and in turn inform your clients about carcinogens when additional knowledge becomes available.

Additional information about carcinogens, especially those related to occupations that the senior may have been engaged in, can be found in Chapter 9, *Nursing Concepts for Health Promotion.*[34] Often carcinogenic effects of pollutants, or substances contacted during work, is first apparent many years after the contact—sometimes after retirement.

Cancer can be cured if it is diagnosed early so that surgery, radiation, and drug therapy, alone or in combination, can be effective. If the cancer has metastasized, treatment will usually be palliative, consisting of measures to relieve pain, prevent further spread, and maintain vital functions. Five-year survival rates have continued to increase steadily from the 1940's to the 1970's. For example, the survival rate for cancer of the prostate increased from 37 to 56 percent; survival from breast cancer has only increased from 53 to 60 percent; and survival from cancer of the uterus has increased from 61 to 74 percent. Even though survival rates have not decreased for any cancer site in the past 25 years, they remain very low for too many types of cancer.[1]

Early detection and treatment are the only answers to complete eradication of cancer.

Caring for the Senior with a Suspected Malignancy

The elderly person who suspects that he might have cancer will be under severe emotional stress. Fear of death, pain, disfigurement, helplessness, and being a burden can make him feel trapped or abandoned. He may see death as a better alternative than living a painful, helpless existence for what will seem to be an interminable period.

Seniors often are not aware of advances that have been made in the field of cancer therapy. They often base their fear of cancer on "poor Mom" who died of cancer in agonizing pain back in the 1930's. They may have known someone who had a colostomy that was never regulated or someone who died of metastasis from cancer of the breast. They are, more times than not, only aware of the horrors of cancer and are not aware that early diagnosis and treatment can result in cure or remission.

You must be available to the senior and you must establish a relationship in which he will feel free to express his ideas. You must also be able to dispel some of these fears by informing him about the advances in knowledge and successes in cancer therapy.

The elderly must be considered for the same therapy as a younger patient. The fact that he is older must not be the only basis for discounting his need for a specific therapy. The attitude of medical and nursing personnel should be such that every patient, no matter what his age, is recognized as an individual of innate worth. Avoid the following attitude: "He has cancer but he is old, so we're not going to do too much; we'll just keep him comfortable and let time take its course." Decisions about therapeutic approaches should be based on the individual's total condition (i.e., location, type, and extent of the tumor, and overall state of health).

The patient and his family should be given an opportunity to decide about a particular therapeutic plan. However, decision about treatment can only be made if they have adequate information about the prognosis with or without the therapy and the alternatives available. They must also know what the therapy will involve in terms of pain, disfigurement, risk, length of hospitalization, and possible side effects and complications. They should also be given an idea of the cost of the therapy. It is the physician's responsibility to convey this information, but you must know what the patient has been told so that you can answer questions and reinforce the information he has been given. These are extremely difficult decisions, and the patient and his family will require a great deal of understanding and support not only before but afterward, especially if the results are disappointing or unsuccessful and guilt and blaming occur.

Therapy must be tailored for the individual. It must be accepted by the patient; if he decides not to have the therapy, this also must be accepted by his family and the staff. The decision is his right, and it must be respected.

You should also be aware that the desperation that the senior might experience can lead him to grasp at straws and seek opinions from multiple physicians and even unscrupulous individuals who set themselves up as possessing cures for cancer. You should help patients learn how to distinguish a cancer quack from a bona fide physician. The quack will usually offer to "cure" the patient. He will make unrealistic claims for a specific drug, machine, or treatment. The quack advertises, seeks publicity, and uses testimonials. The "cures" that he promotes are "natural" or are based on a principle previously overlooked by researchers. He usually claims that the medical establishment is persecuting and conspiring against him.[3] Seeing a quack instead of a physician can result in loss of valuable time for diagnosis and in delay in getting treatment that could be beneficial. If the person does not have cancer, it prolongs the worry and financial expense. By educating your patients/clients and the public about quackery, you can help curtail the quack's activities.

When you care for a person with cancer, give support and reassurance that convince him that everything possible is being done. Perhaps as important as a specific treatment is the interest and support given by the physician and nurses. Interest in the patient's response to the therapy and the progress of the disease condition can be a form of protection against the cancer quack. Patients and family need to feel that something is being done that offers hope.[7]

Caring for the Senior Undergoing Cancer Therapy

The therapy will depend on the location, type, and extent of the malignancy, as well as on the patient's overall physical health. The potentialities and limitations of surgery, radiotherapy, and chemotherapy will differ for various forms and presentations of cancer. Often a combination of therapies is decided on.

Care of the senior undergoing surgery was discussed in Chapter 15. A Medical-Surgical Nursing text should be consulted on the care of patients receiving surgery for specific cancer.

Remember that patients of advanced years are greater surgical risks. They do not tolerate complications as well as younger individuals do. Lowered cardiac, lung, and kidney reserves and preexisting diseases often result in or intensify complications. Postoperative mortality doubles for patients with concurrent diseases.[36,45]

Geriatric patients do not withstand blood loss as well as their younger counterparts do, and hypotension for even a very brief period can be fatal. The necessity for careful monitoring of vital signs cannot be stressed too much.

Pulmonary complications, thrombosis, and other hazards of immobility are more prevalent in seniors. Turning, coughing, and deep breathing, plus early ambulation must be instituted immediately postoperatively to prevent such complications. Oral hygiene can help prevent pulmonary complications and parotitis. The patient has to be assessed immediately prior to surgery for any indication of an upper respiratory infection. This must be eradicated before surgery in order to reduce the possibility of atelectasis or pneumonia. If inhalation anesthesia is used during surgery, the likelihood of respiratory complications also increases. These patients require increased surveillance for possible complications.

Fluid and electrolyte imbalances are not tolerated well by the elderly. An output of at least 40 to 50 ml of urine per hour should be maintained. An output below this indicates insufficient fluid replacement. Overloading of the circulation will cause heart failure and pulmonary edema. Transfusions of whole blood seem to increase this risk, especially in patients with heart disease when blood volume is already above normal.

The nutritional status of the senior must be normal. All nutritional deficiencies should be corrected before surgery and oral feedings should be resumed postoperatively just as soon as possible.

Caring for the Senior Receiving Radiotherapy

Radiotherapy must be used very carefully in the elderly. The arteriosclerotic vascular bed present in the elderly patient is further aggravated by the radiation reaction. This reaction consists of an initial damage to the intimal vasculature and arteriolar spasm and a later fibrosis of periarteriolar capillaries and intimal endothelial proliferation. These phenomena together result in a substantial acceleration in the aging process in the areas irradiated. Vascular insufficiency in the elderly reduces the tissues' ability to repair themselves and therefore any secondary infection or inflammation may result in necrosis in the irradiated tissues. Any nutritional deficiency may reduce the body's ability to respond to the stress of radiation. Since the elderly are frequently malnourished, this may present a problem when radiation therapy is attempted.

Radiation damage to the skin is characterized by patchy erythematous areas. If the radiation insult continues, edema and moist desquamation occur, leaving a raw area similar to a second-degree burn. Further damage leaves an area similar to a third-degree burn. This last response should not be seen in radiation therapy.

Care of these areas consists of keeping erythematous areas dry and clean. Patients should be instructed not to wear tight clothing and to avoid strong soaps. Baby powder or corn starch may lessen itching. One percent hydrocortisone ointment may be prescribed for itching. Areas of moist desquamation are treated with lanolin, A & D ointment, and/or antibiotic ointments. Mild antiseptics may be used to cleanse small areas. If areas are particularly painful, 5 percent Nupercaine or Benzocaine in A & D ointment may be prescribed.

The side effects of X-ray therapy depend on the areas irradiated. X-ray to the chest may cause esophagitis, sore throat, cough, and pneumonitis. Abdominal irradiation may result in difficulty with digestion. A generalized feeling of lethargy is present but is transient with any irradiation.[22,31]

Caring for the Senior Receiving Chemotherapy

This is usually used when surgery and/or radiation therapy cannot control the cancer. Chemotherapy can also provide palliation in terminal cases. Since tumors in the elderly generally grow more slowly than they do in younger individuals and because patients over 70 years are less able to tolerate anticancer drugs, they are usually prescribed in a lower dose schedule. Patients in the 50- to 70-year age range can generally tolerate average anticancer dosages. Each patient can only be treated to his tolerance. If toxicity occurs, the drug should be discontinued. Two classes of drugs are being used. Cytotoxic drugs kill or injure cancer cells in dosages that do not kill normal cells. Hormones and some enzymes alter the climate or environment of the cancer cell, thus inhibiting its growth.[7] Cancer drugs used in the elderly and toxic effects are summarized in Table 18.2.

Some of the newer anticancer drugs have not been tried on the elderly cancer patient. Often hormones such as cortisone, estrogen, and progesterone are used. The anticancer drugs are frequently used in combination with other therapy. It is very important that drugs be given according to the prescribed protocol in order to achieve optimum effectiveness.

The symptoms of toxicity must be recognized and treated accordingly.

TABLE 18.2   **Cancer Drugs and Their Major Side Effects**

Methotrexate	Bone marrow depression, nausea, vomiting, mucous membrane ulceration, alopecia, hepatic toxicity.
5-Fluorouracil	Nausea, vomiting, diarrhea, temporary drop in WBC, stomatitis, anorexia, alopecia.
Nitrogen mustard	Nausea, vomiting, bone marrow depression, local phlebitis.
Thio-TEPA	Bone marrow depression, allergic skin reaction.
Chlorambucil (Leukeran)	Bone marrow depression.
Cyclophosphamide (Cytoxan)	Bone marrow depression, alopecia, hemorrhagic cystitis.
Busulfan (Myleran)	Reduction in white blood cell count. Therapy should be discontinued when the level reaches 6000 to 7000 per cubic mm.
Streptonigrin	Bone marrow depression. Nausea, vomiting.
Doxorubicin (Adriamycin)	Myelosuppression, thrombocytopenia, alopecia, stomatitis, cardiotoxicity (EKG changes, hypotension, failure), phlebitis at injection site, local tissue necrosis if extravasated.
Bleomycin (Blenoxane)	Pneumonitis that may progress to a fatal pulmonary fibrosis, alopecia, stomatitis, erythema, nausea and vomiting, weakness, pain in fingertips.
Vinblastine sulfate (Velban)	Bone marrow depression, local burns at injection site if infiltration occurs, neuromuscular disorders.
Vincristine (Oncovin)	Peripheral nerve damage, paresthesias, loss of deep tendon reflexes, permanent paralysis and causalgia, constipation, abdominal pain, cranial nerve paralysis, ptosis, double vision, alopecia.
Procarbazine (Matulane)	Bone marrow depression, gastrointestinal upsets, dermatitis, neuropathies.[7,45]

Bone marrow depression is marked by anemia, thrombocytopenia, and leukopenia. Anemia is treated with drugs or blood transfusions. Bleeding should be observed for and bruising should be prevented. Generally, when white blood cell counts drop to 2000 per cu. mm or platelets decrease to 50,000 per cu. mm, the drug should be discontinued and patients placed in protective isolation. If alopecia occurs, the person should be provided with a wig. Gastrointestinal symptoms such as diarrhea, vomiting and nausea, and mouth ulceration should be treated symptomatically. Giving easily digested, nonirritating, soft, bland foods can be helpful. Warm saline mouthwash can soothe tender mucous membranes.

Give diethylstilbestrol with food to reduce vomiting. Hypercalcemia is a side effect to be observed. Dry mouth, thirst, nausea, weakness, lethargy, thick speech, fluid retention, and convulsions are signs of hypercalcemia. The drug should be discontinued when these symptoms occur. Reestablishment of fluid and electrolyte balance is important. Patients should eat a diet low in calcium while taking this drug.[31]

Perfusion therapy, in which a chemotherapeutic agent is perfused into an artery supplying the area of a tumor removed from the corresponding vein and which can be oxygenated by a pump oxygenator, is now primarily used for tumors of an extremity. *Infusion therapy is the continuous intra-arterial infusion of a chemotherapeutic agent so that tumor cells are exposed to constant drug action.* They are administered on the average of 7 days. Tumors of the liver are treated through the hepatic artery or umbilical vein. Tumors of the head and neck are treated by way of the external carotid. Tumors of the cervix can be treated by way of the external iliac vein. This technique can be used when radiotherapy is impossible. Pharmacologic antagonists are administered systemically. Complications of the technique can include thromboembolism, air embolism, leaks around the catheter, and hemorrhage. The catheter site must be carefully observed.[45]

Caring for the Senior with Advanced Cancer

The most important element of the senior's care with advanced cancer is for you to be convinced that there is still a great deal that can and must be done to help the patient.[7] Maintaining the patient in as independent and productive a life-style as possible, preventing suffering, and maintaining physiologic functions should be your goals in caring for the senior with advanced cancer.

Pain is probably the most distressing problem with which the patient and professional personnel will have to cope. Clinical evidence suggests the conclusion that the elderly are less sensitive to pain, but laboratory data show no decline in pain threshold. Perhaps the senior delays reporting pain because he is reluctant to raise a false alarm.[41] If he has many other concurrent conditions, he may just accept the pain as an unavoidable incident of illness. If he has had a great deal of pain over a long period, he may have conditioned himself to withstand pain for longer periods before requesting relief.

Remember that the senior may be experiencing greater pain than is indicated by his requests for relief, complaints, and other responses. Behavior and systemic reactions discussed previously should be observed for so that the patient is not made to suffer needlessly.

Since anxiety intensifies pain, you should be available when needed to answer questions and dispel fears. Tension contributes to pain intensity and causes fatigue which decreases pain tolerance. Opportunities for rest and promotion of uninterrupted sleep will help the senior cope with the pain. Relaxation exercises, muscle relaxants, and tranquilizers can help.

A system of defense mechanisms is usually developed to cope with chronic pain. If the senior is helped to analyze his situation and make decisions about ways of lessening it, thus redirecting his energy, he will be better able to handle the stress of pain than be immobilized by it. Individual and group therapy can help him to work through feelings and cognitively cope with pain. Hypnosis may also help. Distraction and refocusing of attention on other considerations can help to reduce anxiety and pain awareness. *Waking imagined analgesia* is a method in which the patient is taught to imagine a pleasant situation involving the painful part and then reliving the pleasurable sensation when in pain.[40]

Behavior modification therapy, which uses a system of rewards for non-pain responses, also has been used, but it may teach the person to disregard pain when it is an important signal. Increasing other stimuli such as touching, vibrating, rubbing, and massaging, is helpful. Analgesia through electrical stimulation applied to the skin surface is thought to cause a stimulus that blocks the pain impulse by stimulating the gating mechanism. Percutaneous stimulation is performed by inserting a needle or wire into or near a major peripheral nerve. A ground wire is placed farther down the nerve. The person turns on the current and regulates it to the point that provides the most comfort. Two implantable devices, the peripheral nerve implant and the dorsal column stimulator, are available. Before they are used the patient should be evaluated for emotional stability and the likelihood that the implant will provide relief. Electrical stimulation will not be as successful in patients who have had surgical interruption of nerve pathways such as cordotomy.[19] Persons who receive implanted stimulators require instruction in the instrument's use and care as well as instruction about resulting paresthesias with initial dorsal column stimulation. As the person gains confidence that electrical stimulation can reduce pain, he should be helped to discontinue his reliance on drugs.[21]

Central nervous system depressants and tranquilizers are often given in combination to gain a synergistic action. Specific discomforts should also be treated so that they do not intensify the pain. Relief-giving medications such as antacids, vasodilators, local anesthetics, muscle relaxants, and antispasmodics should be used instead of narcotics for complaints such as indigestion, mouth ulceration, or denuded skin. Nonnarcotic analgesics should be used first for pain, and the dose should be increased no faster than necessary to keep the person comfortable. Then less addicting narcotics should be used for relief of severe pain. Tolerance to the drug can be delayed by accurately controlling the dosage and time intervals between the dosage. Although narcotics should not be administered when other drugs will suffice, do not withhold narcotics and cause the patient to suffer needlessly. Narcotics may not be required or desirable initially for the patient with advanced cancer. However, the euphoria, tranquility, and pain relief that they give are very beneficial later.[17] A pharmacology text should be consulted for a review of analgesic drugs and their effects.

Remember that potent narcotics must be used with extreme caution in the elderly. In patients over 70 years morphine should probably not be used. The undesirable reactions to morphine, including respiratory depression, gastrointestinal effects, and genitourinary difficulties, are potentially more serious in the elderly. However, patients in hospices in England often receive considerable amounts of morphine or heroin during their last days, obtaining pain relief and euphoria without complications.

If psychotherapeutic agents such as the phenothiazines are ordered, they must be used cautiously in the aged. Hypotension occurs more frequently in the older person with atherosclerosis. Extrapyramidal reactions and disturbed liver function also increase when the elderly take phenothiazines.[8]

Cordotomy, interruption of pain-conducting pathways in the spinal cord through cutting of the spinothalamic portion of the anterolateral tract, obliterates pain (but also temperature sensation) below the level that is severed. Other sensation and motor function are left intact. The procedure is performed via a laminectomy or percutaneously. Postoperative urinary retention is common but usually transient. Sexual function in males is impaired.[7]

Rhizotomy is the division of the anterior or posterior nerve root between the ganglion and the cord. Cranial and upper cervical root rhizotomies are used to treat cancer involving the head or neck.[7]

Thalamotomy, thermocoagulation of thalamic nuclei tissue at the site of pain perception, is still experimental and reserved for the terminally ill. Since it can alter the patient's personality, it is contraindicated except in desperate situations.[7]

No matter what therapy is used for pain relief, it is important that you remain with the patient who is suffering acute pain to prevent social isolation and permit the patient to initiate interaction if he wishes. Too often the person in pain is left alone; the nurse may avoid the patient experiencing pain because of feelings of helplessness and guilt for being unable to help. Remaining with the patient is an appropriate response to his anxiety. Apparently the desire to be with someone increases as anxiety increases. Merely being with the senior can imply that you share the experience and are available to help. Physical presence should be coupled with touch. The therapeutic benefits of laying on of hands have not been adequately researched. Touch does convey to the patient that dependency is allowed at stressful times and that he does not have to bear it alone. The type and time of touch must be based on your experience and observation of the patient's response to it.[30]

Nutritional maintenance is a challenge for the senior with advanced cancer. Chemotherapy and radiation usually cause nausea, vomiting, and anorexia. Anorexia may be caused by metastasis to the liver and bowel as well as by mouth ulceration caused by treatment. All of your ingenuity will be called forth in trying to whet the patient's appetite. If antiemetics are ordered for nausea, for optimal effect they should be given 20 minutes before meals if oral or 10 minutes before if intramuscular.[7]

Small, frequent, appetizing, attractive meals should be offered. If the patient needs assistance with eating or with reaching his food for self-feeding, he should be assisted as necessary immediately when the tray is served. Foods at the correct temperature enhance appetite.

Patients with stomatitis should have oral hygiene frequently and especially before meals so that foul tastes can be eliminated. An anesthetic elixir may be prescribed and should be given prior to eating so that the discomfort of chewing can be reduced.

Decubitus ulcers should be prevented if at all possible. The malnourished, emaciated patient is extremely prone to their occurrence. The skin should be inspected by the professional nurse at least once every shift. The patient's position should be changed hourly, the bed must be kept dry, and any reddened areas and all bony prominences should be massaged every 1 or 2 hours. Alternating pressure pads, lambswool, water beds, and other devices may be used to relieve pressure.

If a decubitus does develop, action must be taken immediately to prevent its extension. Keeping it clean and dry, relief of pressure, and exposure to air and light plus adequate hydration and nutrition are necessary to heal the decubitus, regardless of other treatment used. Extensive decubiti require debridement, usually before other treatment can begin. The treatments for decubitis are multiple. Packing with white granulated sugar and covering with gauze has been effective.[5] In a recent study, 1OU of U40 Regular insulin was applied twice daily to the decubitus. It was then exposed to the air to dry. There was an increase in the rate of healing for subjects who received this treatment over a control group. However, the limited sample size detracted from the generalizability of the results.[44]

If *odors* are a problem, assess their source, since odor often signals presence of infection. Cleanliness will usually prevent and eliminate most odors. Changing dressings, bedding, and clothing when they become soiled and removing soiled dressings and excreta from the room immediately will help to reduce odors. Buttermilk or yogurt dressings have been found to be effective in reducing odors caused by foul drainage. Air fresheners may help, but they must be used sparingly since they may contribute to the person's nausea. Opening a window to obtain fresh air when the patient is out of the room helps to eliminate odors.[6]

Complications must be observed for constantly. A common complication with bone metastasis is hypercalcemia. The symptoms to look for were described earlier in this chapter. The metastatic bone destruction causes calcium to increase in the blood and eventually exceed the kidney's capacity to excrete it. Note an elevated calcium blood level and teach the patient to observe for the early signs and symptoms and to get medical care immediately when these appear. Hypercalcemia is treated with hydration of 4 liters of sodium-containing fluid in 24 hours.[6] Patients with urinary insufficiency and cardiac failure cannot tolerate this rate of administration and must be monitored for fluid overload even when lower rates of fluid administration are ordered.

Compression of the spinal cord may result when spinal metastasis causes collapse of a vertebra or when the tumor's increasing size compresses the cord. The patient complains of neck, back, and nerve root pain. Paraplegia or quadriplegia may result. This usually develops gradually, preceded first by motor weakness and then numbness. Sphincter control is lost. If paralysis occurs, immediate relief of the pressure can reverse the paralysis. Surgical intervention must be prompt.[6]

Fractures also occur in metastasis to the bones. These pathologic fractures usually involve the hip. Patients must be cautioned against unsafe conditions that might cause falls. Lifting heavy objects, reaching, and twisting can also result in fractures. Thus, the person's activity must be severely limited at times.

Caring for the patient who is facing death requires that you understand your own feelings toward death. Your presence with the patient, use of touch, meticulous physical care, and support for the family are vital at this time. The senior should be kept as comfortable as possible but not stuporous, unless he requests this. He must know that he is not alone and that he has not been abandoned. Opportunities for taking care of unfinished business should be provided if requested.

All measures should be taken to help the patient maintain a positive self-image. Protecting his privacy, preserving his individuality, respecting his wishes and avoiding any hint of hostility, scolding, punishing, or rejection are vitally important in caring for the patient with cancer. Information from Chapters 3, 7, 10, 11, 12, and 13 may be helpful.

Spiritual support should be available from a religious advisor if desired and from the staff. You can provide comfort by praying with the patient, reading the Bible or religious literature, and helping him maintain religious rituals. Reading Chapter 14 in this book and Chapter 11 in reference 34 may be helpful to you.

Care of the patient facing death is covered in Chapter 13.

EVALUATION

Maintaining the patient at his optimum level of functioning for as long as possible is the primary objective in caring for the senior with a malignancy. If he remains comfortable and maintains his self-esteem, dignity, and sense of pride and satisfaction in himself and his life, you are assured that the goals of care have been met.

An evaluation to which you can honestly answer that everything possible was done for the person that would have been done for someone of any other age is not an easy goal to achieve. A family that feels good about the care of its loved one and feels that it has provided everything to the best of its ability indicates a successful plan of care.

REFERENCES

1. American Cancer Society, "Cancer Statistics, 1975—25-year Cancer Survey," *Ca—A Cancer Journal for Clinicians.* 25: (1975), 2–21.
2. American Cancer Society, *1973 Cancer Facts and Figures.* New York: American Cancer Society, 1972.

3. American Cancer Society, *Combating Cancer Quackery—Cancer News.* 27: No. 1 (1973), n.d.

4. American Cancer Society, *Cancer Detection in the Physician's Office.* New York: American Cancer Society, 1967.

5. BARNES, JAMES, "Sugar Sweetens the Lot of Patients with Bedsores," *Journal of American Medical Association,* 223: (January 8, 1973), 122.

6. BATES, BARBARA, *A Guide to Physical Examination.* Philadelphia: J. B. Lippincott Company, 1974.

7. BELAND, IRENE, and JOYCE PASSOS, *Clinical Nursing: Pathophysiological and Psychosocial Approaches,* 3rd ed. New York: Macmillan Publishing Co., Inc., 1975.

8. BEELEVILLE, J. W., *et al.,* "Influence of Age on Pain Relief," *Journal of the American Medical Association,* 217: (September 27, 1971), 835–41.

9. BENDER, A. DOUGLAS, "Drug Therapy in the Aged," in *Working with Older People, Vol. IV—Clinical Aspects of Aging.* Washington, D.C.: U.S. Department of Health, Education and Welfare, 1971.

10. BIELARS, KAREN, "You Have Pain? I Think This Will Help," *American Journal of Nursing,* 70: No. 10 (1970), 2143–45.

11. BIRCHENALL, JOAN, and MARY EILEEN STREIGHT, *Care of the Older Adult.* Philadelphia: J. B. Lippincott Company, 1973.

12. BUCKINGHAM, WILLIAM, MARSHALL SPARBERG, and MARTIN BRANDFON-BRENER, *A Primer of Clinical Diagnosis.* New York: Harper & Row, Publishers, Inc., 1971.

13. CAPP, LAUREL, "The Spectrum of Suffering," *American Journal of Nursing,* 74: No. 3 (1974), 491–95.

14. CASEY, KENNETH, "Pain: A Current View of Neural Mechanisms," *American Scientist,* 61: (March–April, 1973), 194–200.

15. CASHATT, BARBARA, "Pain: A Patient's View," *American Journal of Nursing,* 72: No. 2 (1972), 281.

16. CROWLEY, DOROTHY, *Pain and Its Alleviation.* Berkeley: University of California Press, 1962.

17. DANKONTIDES, ANNA, "Drugs to Treat Pain," *American Journal of Nursing,* 74: No. 3 (1974), 508–13.

18. EXTON-SMITH, A., and A. WINDSOR, "Principles of Drug Treatment in the Aged," in *Clinical Geriatrics,* ed. Isadore Rossman. Philadelphia: J. B. Lippincott Company, 1971.

19. GAUMER, WILLIAM, "Electrical Stimulation," *American Journal of Nursing,* 74: No. 3 (1974), 504–5.

20. GEORGE, MAUREEN, "Long-Term Care of the Patient with Cancer," *Nursing Clinics of North America,* 8: No. 4 (1973), 623–32.

21. GOLASKOV, JOAN, and PIERRE LEROY, "Use of the Dorsal Column Stimulator," *American Journal of Nursing,* 74: No. 3 (1974), 506–7.

22. GRIBBONS, CAROL, and M. A. ALIAPOULIOS, "Early Carcinoma of the Breast," *American Journal of Nursing,* 69: No. 9 (1969), 1945–50.

23. ———, "Treatment for Advanced Breast Carcinoma," *American Journal of Nursing,* 72: No. 4 (1972), 678–82.

24. HAUGEN, FREDERICK P., "Current Concepts of the Pain Process," *Journal of Chronic Diseases,* 4: (July, 1956), 9.

25. HUBBARD, SUSAN, and VINCENT DEVITA, "Chemotherapy Research Nurse," *American Journal of Nursing,* 74: No. 4 (1976), 560–65.

26. LENHART, DOROTHY, "The Use of Medications in the Elderly Population," *Nursing Clinics of North America,* 11: No. 1 (1976), 135–43.

27. LEWIN, ISSAC, "Neoplasia," in *Internal Medicine,* eds. Peter J. Talso and Alexander Remenchik. St. Louis: The C. V. Mosby Company, 1968.

28. MASTROVITO, RENE, "Psychogenic Pain," *American Journal of Nursing,* 74: No. 3 (1974), 514–19.

29. MCCAFFERY, MARGO, "Nursing Intervention for Bodily Pain," *American Journal of Nursing,* 67: No. 6 (1967), 1224–27.

30. ———, and LINDA HART, "Undertreatment of Acute Pain with Narcotics," *American Journal of Nursing,* 76: No. 10 (1976), 1586–91.

31. MCCORKLE, MARGARET, "Coping with Physical Symptoms in Metastatic Breast Cancer," *American Journal of Nursing,* 73: No. 6 (1973), 1034–38.

32. MCLACHLAN, EILEEN, "Recognizing Pain," *American Journal of Nursing,* 74: No. 3 (1974), 496–97.

33. MELZACK, RONALD, "The Perception of Pain," *Scientific American,* 204: (1961), 49.

34. MURRAY, RUTH, and JUDITH ZENTNER, *Nursing Concepts for Health Promotion,* 2nd ed. Englewood Cliffs, N.J.: Prentice-Hall, Inc., 1979.

35. OWEN, MARGARET, "Special Care for the Patient Who Has a Breast Biopsy or Mastectomy," *Nursing Clinics of North America.* 7: No. 2 (1972), 373–82.

36. SCHEIN, CLARENCE, and HERBERT DARDIK, "A Selective Approach to Surgical Problems in the Aged," in *Clinical Geriatrics,* ed. Isadore Rossman. Philadelphia: J. B. Lippincott Company, 1971.

37. SCHWIND, JUSTIN, "Cancer: Regressive Evaluation," *Nursing Digest,* (1975), 54–56.

38. SHAPIRO, SAM, P. STRAX, and L. VENET, "Periodic Breast Cancer Screening in Reducing Mortality from Breast Cancer," *Journal of the American Medical Association,* 215: (1971), 1777–85.

39. SHEPARDSON, JAN, "Team Approach to the Patient with Cancer," *American Journal of Nursing,* 72: No. 3 (1972), 488–91.

40. SIEGELE, DOROTHY, "The Gate Control Theory," *American Journal of Nursing,* 74: No. 3 (1974), 498–502.

41. STORANDT, MARTHA, "Psychologic Aspects," in *Cowdry's The Care of the Geriatric Patient,* 5th ed., ed. Franz Steinberg. St. Louis: The C. V. Mosby Company, 1976.

42. SUTHERLAND, ARTHUR, and CHARLES ORBACH, "Depressive Reactions Associated with Surgery for Cancer," in *The Psychological Impact of Cancer.* New York: American Cancer Society, 1974.

43. "The New War on Pain," *Newsweek,* April 25, 1977, 48–50.

44. VAN ART, SUZANNE, and ROSE GERBER, "Topical Application of Insulin in the Treatment of Decubitus Ulcers," *Nursing Research,* 25: No. 1 (1976), 9–12.

45. WRIGHT, JANE, *et al.,* "Cancer," in *Cowdry's The Care of the Geriatric Patient,* 5th ed., ed. Franz Steinberg. St. Louis: The C. V. Mosby Company, 1976.

problems of chemical regulatory balance in later maturity

Study of this chapter will enable you to:

1. Consider the interrelationship of metabolism, nutrition, and fluid and electrolyte balance in maintaining chemical regulation in later maturity.

2. Discuss the mechanisms and possible causes of anabolism and catabolism.

3. Describe nutritional needs of the elderly person.

4. Identify causes of fluid and electrolyte imbalances.

5. Assess signs and symptoms of nutritional, fluid, and electrolyte imbalances.

6. Assess general signs and symptoms of endocrine dysfunction.

7. Assess signs and symptoms of diabetes mellitus.

8. State nursing diagnoses and formulate patient care goals, based on your assessment.

9. Adjust the treatment regime and self-care measures to the *unique* needs and abilities of the senior and his family.

10. Teach the senior and his family how to manage the disease and adjust to necessary changes in their life-style involving diet, exercise, recreation, hygiene, and use of medications if prescribed.

11. Intervene with the elderly diabetic by carrying out necessary treatments or care measures when he is unable to do so.

12. Teach the senior and his family how to prevent diabetic complications.

13. Institute prompt treatment when you assess the presence of hypoglycemia or ketoacidosis.

14. Evaluate the effectiveness of your care through diagnostic tests and feedback from the senior and his family.

19

This chapter will attempt to look at those mechanisms within the body that are responsible for chemical regulation. There are many mechanisms that could be included. Those that will be explored are metabolism, fluid and electrolyte balance, and nutrition.

The approach of this chapter will be slightly different since these mechanisms, as they are affected by aging, will be discussed first before applying the steps of the nursing process. The assessment step of the nursing process will include an overview of observations to be made for multiple problems of chemical regulation. Intervention will focus on the care of the elderly with diabetes mellitus.

METABOLISM

Metabolism is all those changes taking place within cells of the internal environment, including building-up, breaking down, and functional activities. *Anabolism is the synthesis of larger molecules from smaller ones. It is a building-up mechanism and involves energy saving. Catabolism is the breaking up of large molecules into smaller ones. It is a breaking down of energy-containing compounds into lower energy compounds or into carbon dioxide and water.*[2]

Anabolism and catabolism occur continuously throughout life and are balanced in the normal adult. When new tissues are being added to the body, anabolism exceeds catabolism. When tissues are being broken down, such as in dieting, starvation, and serious illness, catabolism exceeds anabolism.

In advanced age, an imbalance between anabolism and catabolism exists. Anabolism and synthesis are reduced while catabolic processes increase with a slowing of the building processes, in contrast to youth when the rate of anabolism and synthesis are high.[2]

Mechanisms that control metabolic reactions are not known. Endocrine balance is constantly shifting, and biological assays are not refined enough to accurately reflect glandular function. Some researchers suggest that reduced sex hormones cause not only altered endocrine balance but also altered metabolic processes. Androgen reduction may result in reduced anabolism. The basal metabolic rate also gradually becomes lower. However, reduced oxygen consumption does not appear to be the result of reduced thyroid secretion but may result from decreased skeletal muscle mass. Other researchers feel that the elderly are not able to utilize the thyroid hormone as well as in earlier life, even though thyroid secretion appears to be within normal limits. Regardless of the cause, this reduction in overall body metabolism is a strong influence in bringing about lowered resistance to factors resulting in disease and illness and is an important factor in bringing about the frailty of old age.

Metabolic changes may be mediated by secretion from some endocrine gland other than the thyroid. Gonadal hormone secretion is reduced with a concomitant reduced adrenal corticosteroid production. In combination, these phenomena should theoretically result in increased catabolism, with resultant effects on protein and calcium metabolism.[5]

NUTRITION

The cells in the body carry out functions such as muscle contraction, nerve impulse transmission, glandular secretion, absorption, and excretion. *Homeostasis is defined as the steady state maintained in an organism through the coordination of its complex physiological processes.* Homeostasis is maintained by the continuous regulation of the transport of materials across membranes and of their extracellular fluid environment. Energy is required for the maintenance of homeostasis. Metabolism of energy, glucose, fatty acids, amino acids, and calcium are some of the complex processes involved in homeostasis.

The body maintains a *metabolic pool, which is a supply of nutrients instantly available through absorption from the intestinal tract plus those released by catabolism and the secretory activity of the cell.* This metabolic pool is necessary for the maintenance of homeostasis. Cellular functions depend on an adequate supply of the following: (1) materials that produce energy, such as glucose, fatty acids, and amino acids; (2) materials that are used for tissue building, such as all amino acids, some fatty acids, carbohydrates, calcium, phosphorus, sodium, potassium, magnesium, and others; and (3) materials for the synthesis of regulatory substances, such as hormones and enzymes.[2,3]

The maintenance of metabolic activities depends on the cell's ability to synthesize enzymes and to synthesize or recover the chemicals needed for the metabolic process. Many enzymes require coenzymes. Vitamins largely function as coenzymes.[19] Thiamine is required for carbohydrate metabolism. Riboflavin, niacin, pantothenic acid, biotin, vitamin B_{12}, folacin, and vitamin B_6 are required for energy and amino acid metabolism. A deficiency in any of these coenzymes interferes with the metabolic process so that anabolism or catabolism cannot occur. Enzyme activity also requires mineral elements, such as magnesium, iron, copper, molybdenum, zinc, and manganese.[2]

From this brief review the importance of nutrition is obvious. The quality of the older person's life will be largely dependent on what he eats. Much debate goes on today, however, about the requirements of the aged for calories and other nutrients. A general nutritional prescription for the aging population cannot be made. There are too many individual variations among the aged as a result of the insults of disease, variations in body structure and metabolism, and different levels of physical activity.[2,3,19] We can define *good nutritional status as a physical and mental state of health that cannot be improved by providing or withholding food.* The definition implies that both an inadequate and excessive intake of nutrients can result in a poor nutritional state.[25]

Energy requirements are related to body size, age, activity, climate, and growth needs. The recommended allowance at age 65 for a 70-kg (154-pound) male engaged in light activity is 2200 to 2400 calories; 1600 to 1800 calories is recommended for the 50-kg (110-pound) woman.[19,25] Recommended daily allowances should be based on desirable weight for height, sex, and frame. For example, the desirable weight range for the man who is 6 feet tall is 157 to 174 pounds. The desirable weight range for the woman who is 5 feet, 5 inches tall is 120 to 133 pounds. If the person is malnourished, he will need more calories than the recommended daily allowance. If he is obese, calories may be reduced.[25] You must assess each individual not just nutritionally and medically but also emotionally. The pleasure of eating may be one of the few satisfactions left in late life. Therefore, it may not be wise to restrict the obese person's diet drastically, unless there is a very good reason for doing so. It is very difficult to change the habitual diet of the elderly, and dieting may impose hardships and stress that may be out of proportion to the effects to be achieved. Some of the factors to consider before reducing caloric intake are: (1) emotional health, (2) physical health and effect of the obesity on increasing severity of disease or debility, (3) magnitude and importance of the effects sought by dieting on the total health picture, (4) facilities for food preparation, (5) economic resources and burden to be placed on others, and (6) the person's ability to cope.

FLUID AND ELECTROLYTE BALANCE

With age the total body water diminishes. Extracellular fluid volume remains constant and therefore constitutes a larger percentage of total body water in the senior. The intracellular fluid compartment is reduced because of tissue loss. Plasma, blood, red blood cell volume, and total plasma protein remain unchanged. Serum albumin, however, appears to decrease while serum globulin increases.[14]

Electrolyte levels of sodium, potassium, chloride, and bicarbonate and the blood pH and P_{CO_2} do not significantly change with age, but when challenged by an acid load, the serum bicarbonate takes longer to return to its basal level in the elderly than it does in the younger person. Renal function is directly related to the interval necessary for correcting an acidosis. The capacity of any person to return fluid and electrolyte composition to a normal level diminishes proportionately with a decrease in renal function. The average 80-year-old has about one-half as much renal function as that of a normal 30-year-old as indicated by glomerular filtration rate. Therefore, it takes about twice as long to correct any fluid or electrolyte abnormality.[14]

See Table 19.1 for a summary of the symptoms and causes for common fluid and electrolyte imbalances of the elderly.[14]

ASSESSMENT

General Signs and Symptoms

Since many metabolic processes are controlled by endocrine function, the following signs and symptoms of endocrine dysfunction should be observed:

1. Headache: Frontal or bitemporal in location if caused by a pituitary tumor.
2. Impairment of peripheral vision: Optic chiasm is compressed by a pituitary tumor.
3. Increased perspiration: Excess production of growth, thyroid, or adrenal medullary (epinephrine) hormone.
4. Changes in skin texture: Soft, warm, moist skin associated with hyperthyroidism; rough, thick, dry skin associated with hypothyroidism.
5. Excess dark body hair: Disorders of ovary or adrenal cortex in which there is excessive androgenic activity.
6. Temporal and vertex hair loss: Panhypopituitarism.
7. Changes in hair texture: Thyroid dysfunction.
8. Excess pigmentation (darkening) of skin: Addison's Disease.
9. Fatigue and weakness: Addison's and Cushing's diseases, primary aldosteronism, hyperparathyroidism, hyperthyroidism and hypothyroidism, testicular and pituitary failure.
10. Lightheadedness or faintness, especially upon sudden standing: Addison's disease.
11. Muscle cramps or spasms: Hypoparathyroidism and primary aldosteronism.
12. Intolerance to heat and cold: Hyperthyroidism and hypothyroidism, respectively.
13. Excessive volume of urination: Hyperparathyroidism, primary aldosteronism, and diabetes.
14. Protrusion of the eyes: Hyperparathyroidism and thyrotoxicosis.
15. Excessive hunger and thirst: Diabetes.
16. Change in facial or body configuration: Trunkal obesity, thin extremities, moon face, and buffalo hump seen in Cushing's Syndrome; facial, hand, and foot bone changes seen in acromegaly.

Diabetes Mellitus

In the aged the onset of diabetes is usually gradual and mild. Often signs and symptoms of complications will be what first prompts the patient to obtain medical care. Renal disease, retinopathy, and peripheral vascular disease are the complications frequently seen. Obesity in the elderly and family history of diabetes also are common.

TABLE 19.1   Fluid and Electrolyte Imbalance in Later Maturity

	Causes	Symptoms
Dehydration	Inadequate intake of fluids in neglected or unconscious persons, e.g., CVA, organic brain syndrome, psychosis. Obstructive lesions of upper gastrointestinal tract. Damage to thirst center, e.g., aneurysm of Circle of Willis. High-protein nasogastric feedings without adequate water intake. Abnormal losses from the gastrointestinal tract or kidneys, e.g., diarrhea, vomiting, fistula, loss of concentrating ability of the kidney, or increased urinary solute load as in diabetes mellitus. Diabetes insipidus.	Thirst. Fever, flushing. Dry skin and mucous membranes. Loss of tissue turgor. Tachycardia. Personality change. Severe dehydration: hallucinations, delirium, manic behavior, convulsions, coma.
Overhydration	Salt retention with osmotically obliged water, e.g., congestive heart failure, cirrhosis, nephrotic syndrome, and renal insufficiency.	Edema, ascites, anasarca. Heart failure and pulmonary edema.
Hyponatremia	Low serum sodium with decreased extracellular fluid volume, e.g., loss of body fluids high in sodium and replacement with electrolyte-free solutions; parenchymal renal disease; diaphoresis, vomiting, diarrhea, and gastrointestinal fistulas.	Muscle weakness. Apathy, lassitude, headache. Postural hypotension, tachycardia. Muscle cramps. Severe hyponatremia: confusion, delirium, delusion, coma. Skin turgor and elasticity decrease.
	Low serum sodium with increased extracellular fluid volume, e.g., heart, liver or renal failure and gross edema, causing limited ability to excrete salt and water in the urine; salt restriction without fluid limitation; anti-diuretic hormone syndrome seen with pulmonary and cerebral neoplasms, head trauma, CVA, encephalitis, subarachnoid hemorrhage; and primary water intoxication.	Strange behavior, confusion, delirium, muscle weakness, seizures, and coma.
	Low serum sodium with normal extracellular fluid volume, e.g., chronic pulmonary disease, arteriosclerosis, and malnutrition.	No symptoms. Low serum sodium.

TABLE 19.1 (*Continued*)

	Causes	Symptoms
Hypernatremia	Increased serum sodium with inadequate intake of fluids in neglected or unconscious persons.	Symptoms of dehydration.
Hypokalemia	Inadequate potassium intake. Excessive potassium loss in diuretic therapy; excessive gastrointestinal losses; excessive urinary losses due to adrenal disease (hyperaldosteronism, Cushing's Syndrome) or renal disease (renal tubular acidosis, pyelonephritis, renal artery stenosis). Metabolic alkalosis.	Muscle weakness or tenderness. Apathy. Distention, paralytic ileus. Polyuria and metabolic alkalosis. Electrocardiograph changes—T-wave changes, lengthening of Q-T interval, and arrhythmias. Potentiates effect of digitalis with resulting toxicity.
Hyperkalemia	Increased serum potassium with renal insufficiency. Acidosis. Increased tissue catabolism. Gastrointestinal bleeding. Potassium supplements.	Anxiety, extreme restlessness, apprehension. Stupor. Weakness, hyporeflexia. Electrocardiograph changes— peaking of T-waves, later loss of P-waves, and widening of the QRS complex.
Hypocalcemia	Low serum calcium with inadequate intake or absorption. Excessive gastrointestinal loss from pancreatitis with steatorrhea; excessive urinary loss with renal tubular necrosis. Presence of elevated serum phosphorus, as in uremia.	Tetany. Numbness and tingling of fingers, toes, and perioral region. Muscle cramps. Stridor. Nausea, vomiting, diarrhea. Depression, delirium, psychotic behavior. Convulsions. Papilledema. Long-standing hypocalcemia: skin and nail changes, hair loss, cataracts, dentition abnormalities.
Hypercalcemia	Low serum calcium with excessive absorption of calcium in vitamin D intoxication or in increased reabsorption of bone, e.g., hyperparathyroidism, multiple myeloma, metastatic malignancies, hyperthyroidism, immobilization, and Paget's disease.	Polyuria. Polydipsia. Recurrent stone formation. Nausea, vomiting, constipation, abdominal discomfort. Weakness, lethargy, drowsiness. Mental confusion and toxic psychosis. If uncorrected, azotemia develops

TABLE 19.1 (*Continued*)

	Causes	Symptoms
		and is first reversible but later irreversible.
Metabolic Acidosis	Renal insufficiency. Diabetic keto-acidosis. Loss of bicarbonate with diarrhea and fistula drainage. Shock (lactic acidosis). Starvation. Intoxication with methyl alcohol, ethylene glycol, salicylates, paraldehyde.	Asymptomatic until carbon dioxide content falls below 18 mEq/L. Then symptoms of weakness, malaise, headache, nausea, vomiting, abdominal pain, Kussmaul's respirations. Other symptoms depend on the cause, e.g., in diabetic acidosis, severe dehydration, loss of skin turgor, shock, hyperglycemia, glycosuria, ketonemia, ketonuria.
Metabolic Alkalosis	Excessive intake of alkali, e.g., sodium bicarbonate abuse. Abnormal losses of acid, e.g., excessive vomiting or gastric suction. Potassium depletion.	Shallow respirations. Elevated P_{CO_2}.
Respiratory Acidosis	Pulmonary disease with impaired ventilation or perfusion dynamics, e.g., emphysema, pulmonary edema. Hypoventilation due to respiratory center pathology producing carbon dioxide retention.	Increase in plasma P_{CO_2}. Dyspnea.
Respiratory Alkalosis	Hyperventilation, e.g., emotional disturbance, central nervous system lesions, and cirrhosis.	Decrease in plasma P_{CO_2}. Numbness, tingling. Dyspnea. Smothering sensation, lightheadedness. Chest pain. Severe symptom: tetany.

The fasting blood sugar and the presence of glucosuria are not always accurate determiners of diabetes in the elderly. Nondiabetic older people, as was mentioned in an earlier section of this book, show increased fasting blood sugar, especially in times of stress. Also, since it is frequently a mild disease in the older population, blood sugar levels may be low enough to be interpreted as normal. Fasting blood sugar levels in the following ranges have been established for older people:

110 mg % or below—normal
110 to 130 mg %—further study required
130 mg % and over—highly probable diabetic level[8]

The 2-hour postprandial blood sugar test appears to be of greater diagnostic value than the fasting blood sugar; 2 hours after a 100-gm carbohydrate meal a blood sugar test is done. The following scale has been established for the elderly:

110 mg % or below—normal
110 mg %– 140 mg %—equivocal
140 mg % or above—highly likely diabetic value[8]

The oral glucose tolerance test is performed when equivocal results are obtained. A diet containing at least 150 to 300 gm carbohydrate (for malnourished individuals) is given for 3 days. Commonly accepted results are as follows:[7, 8]

	Standard Value	Maximum Borderline Value	
		Age 55 to 64	Age 65 to 84
Fasting	110 mg %	110–120 mg %	110–120 mg %
1 hour	160 mg % or 170 mg %	160–180 mg %	190–200 mg %
2 hours	120 mg %	120–130 mg %	140–150 mg %
3 hours	110 mg %	110–120 mg %	130–140 mg %

These figures do not take into account the age-related changes in glucose tolerance. There is some evidence that a higher peak and an increased delay in return to the fasting level exist in nondiabetic aged persons.[7] Since an inadequate diet prior to the test can result in a false positive curve, questionable test results in older people with inadequate intake should be followed with a repeated test after the diet has improved.[7]

Often diabetes in the elderly becomes obvious during a hospitalization or treatment for an infection. Physiologic stress appears to be a risk factor in diabetes and is a powerful stimulus to hyperglycemia. Stress stimulates the sympathetic nervous system, which decreases insulin responsiveness to glucose. A diminished carbohydrate tolerance and hyperglycemia result. Diuretics, such as ethacrynic acid (Edecrin) and furosemide (Lasix), and other drugs, such as nicotinic acid and estrogen, lower glucose tolerance.[7] Some risk factors associated with the development of diabetes are: age over 65, obesity, genetic predisposition, infection, severe mental anguish (which many seniors suffer because of the stresses they endure), surgery, diabetogenic drugs (thiazides, cortisone), and prolonged bed rest.[16]

Assessment for complications of diabetes should also be performed. Complications include coronary artery, cerebrovascular, and peripheral vascular disease; hypertension; neuropathy; retinopathy and glaucoma; glomerulosclerosis, arteriolar nephrosclerosis, and pyelonephritis; and coma of diabetic acidosis.

Assessment of the patient suspected of having diabetes must also include psychologic and social factors, especially those that will affect his ability to assume self-management. Declining physical and mental ability may limit his understanding and performance of self-care activities related to the diabetes. The ability to learn and perform manual functions is vital. Loss of memory for recent events, loss of perceptual-motor skill affecting speed and quality of performance, or loss of ability to process information can all interfere with learning ability.

A nutritional assessment is also vital. If a dietitian is not available, you may have to do it yourself. Nutritional assessment should consist of a diet history focusing on the current or recent diet in order to determine the nutritional status and plan for diet changes. Careful questioning of the senior or one who is familiar with his eating habits should reveal patterns of eating, especially a change to new patterns. Ask about ingestion of supplemental vitamins, which is often unrelated to need. Give attention to the amount of bakery and carbohydrate snack foods consumed, since these may be the senior's major source of calories, at the expense of protein. Learn who purchases the food and prepares the meals: If someone other than the senior does this, the person will need as much or more instruction than the senior receives. If the senior buys and cooks for himself, you have to motivate him to follow instructions.

Information about physical activity and amount of sleep is necessary for determining calorie requirements. Changes in behavior, mental state, endurance and activity, and relations with others may be associated with poor nutrition and therefore should be investigated.

Physical assessments that should be made include:

1. Weight, including recent changes.
2. Estimate of adipose tissue, based on thickness of skin folds over the triceps, subscapular area, and lateral abdominal wall.
3. Signs of nutritional deficiency which are seen frequently in the aged:
   (a) Glossitis: Red, painful, fissured tongue (B group deficiency).
   (b) Pale atrophic tongue (related to anemia).
   (c) Fissures in the corners of the mouth with maceration (niacin, riboflavin, or pyridoxine deficiency).
   (d) Dryness and pigmentation of the skin, increased thickness over pressure points, hyperkeratosis and nasolabial seborrhea (indicative of multivitamin deficiencies).
   (e) Thickening and opaqueness of bulbar conjunctiva (vitamin A deficiency).
   (f) Enlargement of liver
   (g) Enlargement of parotid gland
   (h) Tenderness of calf of leg
   (i) Decreased vibratory sense
   (j) Absent tendon reflexes
   (k) Petechiae and ecchymosis

   } Symptoms of medical diseases of multiple origins can be related to nutritional deficiencies.

4. Laboratory tests indicative of undernutrition in the aged include the following:
   (a) Hematocrit below 40 in males and 38 in females.
   (b) Hemoglobin below the usually accepted range of normal.
   (c) Serum albumin level below 3.5 gm per 100 ml.

Assessment for fluid and electrolyte balance should include observation for those symptoms outlined in Table 19.1. Patients experiencing problems with fluid and electrolyte balance should have intake and output measured and recorded daily to aid in assessment. Daily weight for gain or loss of edema fluid may also be necessary and should be done at the same time every day, with the same amount of clothing, and on the same scale.

NURSING DIAGNOSIS AND FORMULATION OF PATIENT CARE GOALS

Nursing Diagnosis

Some of the *nursing diagnoses* that may be made after assessing the senior with a chemical regulatory imbalance are:

1. *Rejection of food and resultant malnutrition.*
2. *Undernutrition caused by unbalanced intake of adequate calories.*
3. *Excessive caloric intake resulting in overweight or obesity.*
4. *Noncompliance to diabetic treatment plan.*
5. *Deficient intake or output of fluid.*
6. *Deficient intake or output of specific electrolytes.*

Patient Care Goals

When the nursing diagnosis has been made, long-term and short-term goals should be identified. *Long-term goals* could include the following:

1. The senior regularly eats each day the nutrients recommended by the National Research Council and ingests sufficient calories to maintain desirable weight.
2. The diabetic senior adheres to his treatment plan as demonstrated by blood glucose and urinary glucose determination and ability to resume or maintain a satisfying and productive level of activity and social interaction.
3. Fluid and electrolyte imbalances do not occur as demonstrated by normal serum electrolyte levels and absence of symptoms.

Short-term goals could include the following:

1. The senior or the person responsible for his food preparation is able to plan a one-day menu including foods from the Basic 4 food groups and approaching the daily allowance of prescribed nutrients.

2. The senior is able to test his urine and accurately assess the results.
3. The senior takes prescribed medication at the prescribed time. If insulin is prescribed, he is able to draw up the correct amount and aseptically administer it to himself.

NURSING INTERVENTION IN DIABETES MELLITUS

Remember that the senior with newly diagnosed diabetes has existing emotional and physical problems apart from his diabetes. The imposition of rigid controls that cause fear and anxiety about possible complications is cruel and unwarranted. He may already be depressed, anorexic, anxious, agitated, and suffering from undernutrition or insufficient physical and recreational activity. Diabetes can add emotional and financial burdens in terms of dietary restrictions and medication. Visual problems, memory defects, and limited mobility all compound the problem.[18]

Diet

In most older people with diabetes, the condition is mild and can be controlled by diet. In spite of great effort directed toward proper diet, control may be difficult to achieve. Changing lifetime eating patterns is difficult because of the energy saved by following habit, personal preferences, and ethnic considerations. The inability to shop for groceries; the cost of recommended foods, especially protein; and the lack of energy, manual skills, or memory needed to prepare a meal all interfere with getting the proper diet for the senior. Lack of or ill-fitting dentures may inhibit his chewing ability and interfere with enjoyment of food. Telling the person to avoid high carbohydrate foods or sweets may fall on deaf ears or may be looked on as a terrible hardship, especially when other foods are more difficult to secure and prepare and when carbohydrate foods are one of the few remaining pleasures. Living and eating alone also may remove any incentive to prepare a meal, much less eat it.

Minimal modification of food intake is essential. Instead of focusing on strict adherence to measuring foods in specific food groups, the goal should be two, three or four balanced meals daily. The three-meal plan typically described in texts may be unrealistic for the senior because it may not fit into his sleep and activity patterns. Elimination of foods high in pure sugar is important, if at all possible. The diet should contain 40 to 50 percent carbohydrate, 15 to 20 percent protein, and 35 to 45 percent fat.[20] People over 65 who are sedentary should receive 25 calories per kilogram of ideal weight. One gram of high-quality protein per kilogram of weight should be supplied.[13,14]

If food exchange or food group lists are required, the senior should be taught how to use them. Copies of *Exchange Lists for Meal Planning* are available from the American Diabetes Association, 600 Fifth Avenue, New York, New York 10020. A diet prescription may also be given in points. In this system, foods are assigned point values. Points allowed in each food group are then prescribed. Copies of this point system are available from the Kansas Wheat Commission, 1021 North Main Street, Hutchinson, Kansas 67501. Simply handing the senior a sample diet may result in his eating only what is on the sample diet and never substituting other foods from the appropriate group. This, needless to say, can be very monotonous and conducive to the development of nutritional deficiencies as well as discontinuance of the diet.

If the senior does not have the facilities for preparing food or the incentive to prepare it, investigate senior citizen centers where meals at minimal cost may be available, meals-on-wheels programs, or restaurants specifically catering to the needs of the elderly. Cost, convenience, style of cooking, feelings of control in the program, and personal preference must all be considered when you explore any program, and any one of these factors can cause the senior not to begin or to discontinue a program's use.

Exercise

Exercise lowers the blood glucose level through promotion of insulin secretion and improved utilization of glucose by skeletal muscles. The senior with diabetes should be informed why exercise is necessary. This can serve as an incentive for him to do his exercise.

The elderly person usually has reduced his activity, especially after retirement from employment. Some other activity should be substituted. If the person has enjoyed physical exercise during his life, he will tend to continue it. However, if he has not, then you should explore with him his level of activity and any activity that he enjoyed in the past but may no longer be participating in. Interests should also be explored. Today physical exercise is the vogue. Health clubs offer programs of activity tailored to one's needs and desires. Senior citizen centers often incorporate a physical fitness program into their activities. The local YMCA or YWCA, local high school, or college may offer programs of physical exercise for senior citizens. The senior should have recommendation from his physician before participating in any such program.

Walking is a form of exercise in which most seniors can participate unless they are severely incapacitated. During inclement weather an indoor exercise program should be encouraged. Range-of-motion exercises and walking within the house may be acceptable substitutes for walking out-of-doors.

Medications

Oral hypoglycemic agents are frequently prescribed for the patient with adult-onset diabetes when the disease is mild. It is questionable how necessary the drugs are in controlling the diabetes. In a recent study when the hypoglycemic drug was discontinued, one-third of the patients were totally unaffected, one-third required more rigid dietary management, and one-third required insulin.[22] These drugs have apparently been overprescribed. There is also evidence of an increased cardiovascular mortality rate associated with their use. Administration of tolbutamide and phenformin (DBI) have been linked to an increase in cardiovascular deaths. Other studies found that patients receiving oral hypoglycemic agents had almost twice as many myocardial infarctions and strokes and twice as high a death rate as those using diet alone or diet plus insulin.[1,10,17] Tolbutamide (Orinase), chlorpropamide (Diabinase), acetohexamide (Dymelor), and tolazamide (Tolinase) are the only oral hypoglycemic agents currently approved for use.[7]

If oral hypoglycemics are prescribed, remember that hypoglycemia can result from their use. Sulfonylurea agents are the main cause of hypoglycemia. Hypoglycemia in the elderly can be a very serious condition. Cardiac arrhythmias may result from release of catecholamines caused by hypoglycemia. The central nervous system symptoms in the elderly may be more severe because of pre-existing atherosclerosis. You should carefully monitor the patient on oral hypoglycemic agents for signs of hypoglycemia, especially if he is taking sulfonylurea agents. The hypoglycemic action of tolbutamide and other sulfonylureas is potentiated by use of salicylates, probenecid, coumarin, phenybutazone, inderal, and sulfonamides. The action of alcohol and barbiturates may also be increased when given to patients receiving sulfonylurea agents.[66] The senior should be instructed about the necessity for eating the prescribed diet and should be told to contact his physician if he is unable to eat. He and someone close by or living with him should be instructed about the signs of hypoglycemia. They include hunger, nervousness, weakness, nausea, diaphoresis, shakiness, irritability, headache, yawning, lethargy, lassitude, confusion, inability to carry on a conversation, convulsions, and coma.[20,21] However, remember that hypoglycemia in the elderly may not be heralded by the same symptoms and signs as in a younger person. The person may become unconscious without warning. Also, episodes of bizarre or psychotic-appearing behavior or disorientation, confusion, or somnolence are often mistaken for signs of cerebral atherosclerosis. Nocturnal headaches, nightmares, sleep disturbances, unusual sleep postures, and inability to arouse the person easily could also be indicative of hypoglycemia.[21]

When a meal is delayed, 5 to 10 gms of glucose should be taken. One-fourth to one-half glass of orange juice or a Life Saver contain enough glucose to prevent hypoglycemia. If insulin reaction occurs, four ounces of orange juice, sugar cubes, a regular (not diet) soft drink, hard candy, or six or seven Life Savers can correct it. Glucagon is given parenterally if the person is unable to take anything by mouth. Someone who is usually available to the patient should be taught how to administer Glucagon. Observation for improvement is important. Either therapy can be repeated if improvement does not occur in 15 minutes. If he does not respond in 30 minutes, emergency medical care should be sought.[20]

Insulin may be required even though most seniors with adult-onset diabetes will be able to be controlled without it. Since the danger of hypoglycemia in the senior carries greater risks than it does in a younger person, hypoglycemia must be vigorously avoided. An intermediate-acting insulin will probably be ordered. If vision is a problem in using an insulin syringe, a magnifying glass and additional lighting may help. Otherwise, preset syringes may be required, or someone other than the senior will have to be taught to administer the insulin. The increasing visual impairment, diabetic neuropathy, and cerebrovascular complications may make self-administration of insulin difficult and hazardous; therefore, continuous surveillance at frequent intervals is a necessity. A family member or a visiting nurse may be able to assume this responsibility. If the person cannot be monitored at frequent intervals, it is probably better that insulin is not prescribed. Medications are prescribed by the physician, but often only the nurse can give the physician information about the senior's living arrangements, his daily habits and the resources available to him.[21]

Hygiene

Learning and maintaining self-care are very important for the senior with diabetes. Measures he should be taught include:

1. Careful inspection of all parts of the body, especially the feet, including the soles. (A mirror is helpful for seeing soles, shoulders, and neck.)
2. Toenails should be cut by a podiatrist. Corns, calluses, athlete's foot, and injury to the feet require prompt medical care.
3. Note any change such as swelling, discoloration, pustule formation, or break in the continuity of the skin. Garters, knee hose, and sitting with legs crossed interfere with circulation and should be avoided. Buerger-Allen exercises should be performed regularly to promote collateral circulation.
4. Note any functional change and presence and location of pain.
5. Use of mild soaps, lukewarm water, gentle cleansing, and careful drying of all body parts, especially between the toes.
6. Avoid use of any medication not prescribed, including local applications such as corn plasters. Toes that overlap should be separated by lambswool.
7. Apply prescribed medications as ordered.
8. Avoid clothing and shoes that cause friction (shoes should be inspected for worn linings and nails through insoles), and shoes should be interchanged at least daily with another pair to relieve pressure. Avoid going barefoot. New shoes should be broken in gradually.
9. Safety hazards in the patient's environment should be eliminated. Heating pads and hot water bottles should not be used on the feet. Extra covering or socks should be used.
10. The person should remain under medical supervision and seek care im-

mediately when infections or injuries occur. The person should also carry identification indicating that he is a diabetic, along with the physician's name and any medications that the person takes.[21,24]

Occurrence of Ketoacidosis

A small proportion of elderly diabetics may develop ketoacidosis as a result of emotional or physical stress or following omission of insulin.

The *pathophysiology* of ketoacidosis is complex. Ketoacidosis occurs when utilization of carbohydrates by the tissues is diminished, allowing an increased breakdown of fats from adipose tissue, with the resultant elevation of free fatty acids in the blood. Stores of glycogen quickly become depleted. Fatty acids undergo partial oxidation to acetyl coenzyme A. Ketone production and synthesis by cholesterol become the major means of acetyl coenzyme A disposal. There is an increased release of glucose despite hyperglycemia. Ketogenesis is accompanied by hydrogen ion release, resulting in metabolic acidosis. Hyperglycemia and ketonemia result in diuresis, with loss of water and electrolytes. Hypovolemia and hypotension develop. Hyponatremia is common. Serum potassium is normal or elevated, though most patients have suffered potassium deficits.

In the senior these events have a greater impact on homeostasis than they do in a younger patient. Long-standing renal disease could have reduced the nephron count and renal reserve so that they do not readily handle an increased hydrogen ion load. Hypotension further reduces the renal blood flow. Cerebral blood flow can be interfered with by the ketoacidosis and shock, producing reduced cerebral function and possible cerebral vascular accident.

Therapy is directed toward correcting losses of water, salt, and potassium and toward administering adequate amounts of insulin. Bicarbonate may be administered to correct the acidosis. When diabetics with severe acidosis are treated with sodium bicarbonate, insulin requirements are reduced.

In the elderly you must constantly watch for cardiac complications during administration of saline. The patient must be observed for overhydration and cardiac failure. The serum potassium must be carefully monitored, especially if the patient is receiving digitalis or if coronary artery disease is present. Blood sugar levels rather than glycosuria should be used to determine therapy. The goal of therapy is to reestablish carbohydrate tolerance, as indicated by the absence of signs of acidosis.   The response of the patient to therapy and his ultimate prognosis depend on the promptness with which therapy is initiated. You may be called on to prepare, administer, and supervise the regime. You may be responsible for observing the patient and his reactions to therapy and for modifying therapy relative to the effects observed.

The patient and those living with him should be taught signs of ketoacidosis. They should be taught how to test the urine. The second voided specimen before meals or at bedtime should be used. Unstable, insulin-dependent diabetics should use a copper-reducing agent, such as Clinitest. When urine sugar is elevated, they should also test for ketonuria with Ketostix or Acetest. Testape or Diastex is satisfactory for more stable diabetics to test for glucose. You must remember that certain drugs affect urine testing results, giving false positives or negatives. Cephalosporins, chloramphenical, levodopa, methyldopa, nalidixic acid, phenazopyridine, probenecid, salicylates, sulfonamides, tetracyclines, vitamin C, and cancer antimetabolites are common offenders.[15,16] During infections, testing before meals and at bedtime is recommended to help prevent acidosis. Signs and symptoms that the senior and family should be taught are: (1) drowsiness and weakness, (2) dry skin and mouth, (3) thirst, (4) abdominal pain and vomiting, (5) fruity odor to breath, (6) acetone in the urine and glucosuria, (7) frequent scant urination, (8) slow, deep inspiration, (9) increased pulse rate, and (10) coma.

Although diabetic coma is not common in the elderly diabetic, it is such an acute emergency in the senior when it does occur that judicious assessment should be undertaken when a senior is admitted in coma or with drowsiness and other suspicious symptoms. Diagnostic tests should include those for ketoacidosis.

Adherence to treatment routines is most likely to occur when the senior and his family feel that the senior has a warm, trusting, supportive, and caring relationship with his nurse and doctor.

EVALUATION

Problems of chemical regulation can be multiple and complex. This chapter has just touched on some of the problems that cause or result in chemical regulatory dysfunction. Evaluation of the effectiveness of care that the senior has received may be measured against laboratory results and the general health status.

Effective care has been given in the following situations:

1. The diabetic senior has been able to resume or continue in a productive, satisfying mode of living.
2. The diabetic senior has been able to avoid complications by following the treatment regime.
3. The undernourished senior has followed a balanced diet and is now approaching his ideal weight.
4. The obese senior has reduced his intake while following a balanced diet and has lost weight so that his health status has improved.
5. The senior has not felt emotionally distressed by the treatment regime or your approach in teaching it.

Evaluating care through an appraisal of goal achievement is an appropriate way to appraise the quality of care given. This should be done routinely during and following the implementation of a care plan.

REFERENCES

1. ABRAMSON, J. H., ed. "World Health News: Apparent Rise in Mortality from Diabetes," *Israel Journal of Medical Science,* 7: (1971), 1209.

2. BELAND, IRENE, and J. PASSOS, *Clinical Nursing: Pathophysiological and Psychosocial Approaches,* 3rd. ed. New York: Macmillan Publishing Co., Inc., 1975.

3. BIRCHENALL, JOAN, and MARY EILEEN STREIGHT, *Care of the Older Adult.* Philadelphia: J. B. Lippincott Company, 1973.

4. BOZIAN, MARGUERITE, "Nutrition for the Aged or Aged Nutrition?" *Nursing Clinics of North America,* 11: No. 1 (1976), 169–77.

5. CHINN, AUSTIN, "Metabolism, Homeostasis, and the Older Patient," *Working with Older People—Vol. IV Clinical Aspects of Aging.* Washington, D.C.: U.S. Department of Health, Education, and Welfare, 1971.

6. DAVIDSON, J. K., Panel on Diabetes in Epidemiologic Studies and Clinical Trials in Chronic Diseases; Symposium, Pan American Health Organization Advisory Committee on Medical Research; *PAHO Science Publication,* No. 257 (1972), 44.

7. ELIOPOULOUS, CHARLOTTE, "Diagnosis and the Management of Diabetes in the Elderly," *American Journal of Nursing,* 78: No. 5 (1978), 884–87.

8. GITMAN, LEO, "Diabetes Mellitus in the Aged," *Working with Older People—Vol. IV Clinical Aspects of Aging.* Washington, D.C.: U.S. Department of Health, Education, and Welfare, 1971.

9. GRANCIO, SUSAN, "Nursing Care of the Adult Diabetic Patient," *Nursing Clinics of North America,* 8: No. 4 (1973), 605–15.

10. HADDEN, D., D. MONTGOMERY, and J. WEAVER, "Myocardial Infarction in Maturity—Onset Diabetes," *Lancet,* 1: (1974), 475.

11. JUDGE, RICHARD, and GEORGE ZUIDEMA, *Physical Diagnosis: A Physiologic Approach to the Clinical Examination,* 2nd. ed. Boston: Little, Brown & Company, 1968.

12. KNUTTERUD, G. L., *et al.,* "Effects of Hypoglycemic Agents on Vascular Complications in Patients with Adult-Onset Diabetes—IV A Preliminary Report on Phenformin Results," *Journal of the American Medical Association,* 217: (1971), 777.

13. LEVIN, MARVIN, "Diabetes Mellitus," in *Cowdry's The Care of the Geriatric Patient,* 5th ed., ed. Franz Steinberg. St. Louis: The C. V. Mosby Company, 1976.

14. LINDEMAN, ROBERT, "Application of Fluid and Electrolyte Balance Principles to the Older Patient," in *Working with Older People—Vol. IV Clinical Aspects of Aging.* Washington D.C.: U.S. Department of Health, Education, and Welfare, 1971.

15. LUNDIN, DOROTHY, "Reporting Urine Test Results: Switch From + to %," *American Journal of Nursing,* 78: No. 5 (1978), 878–79.

16. NICKERSON, DONNA, "Urine Testing," in *Nursing Management of Diabetes Mellitus,* ed. D. W. Guthrie and R. A. Guthrie. St. Louis: The C. V. Mosby Company, 1977.

17. REID, D. D., and J. EVANS, "New Drugs and Changing Mortality from Non-infectious Disease in England and Wales," *British Medical Bulletin,* 26: (1970), 191.

18. RIFKIN, HAROLD, and HERBERT ROSS, "Diabetes in the Elderly," in *Clinical Geriatrics,* ed. Isadore Rossman. Philadelphia: J. B. Lippincott Company, 1971.

19. ROBINSON, CORINNE, *Proudfit-Robinson's Normal and Therapeutic Nutrition,* 13th ed. New York: The Macmillan Publishing Co., Inc., 1967.

20. SLATER, NORMA, "Insulin Reactions vs. Ketoacidosis: Guidelines for Diagnosis and Intervention," *American Journal of Nursing,* 78: No. 5 (1978), 875–77.

21. THOMAS, KATHERINE, "Diabetes Mellitus in Elderly Persons," *Nursing Clinics of North America,* 11: No. 1 (1976), 157–68.

22. TOMKINS, A. M. and A. BLOOM, "Assessment of the Need for Continued Oral Therapy in Diabetes," *British Medical Journal,* 649: (1972), 651.

23. "University Group Diabetes Program: A Study of the Effects of Hypoglycemic Agents on Vascular Complications in Patients with Adult-Onset Diabetes, II: Mortality Results," *Diabetes 19*: Supplement 2 (1970), 747.

24. VENTURA, EMMA, "Foot Care for Diabetes," *American Journal of Nursing,* 78: No. 5 (1978), 886–88.

25. WEIR, DAVID, HAROLD HOUSER, and LEITA DAVY, "Recognition and Management of the Nutrition Problems of the Elderly," in *Working with Older People— Vol. IV Clinical Aspects of Aging,* Washington, D.C.: U.S. Department of Health, Education, and Welfare, 1971.

EMOTIONAL ILLNESS IN LATER MATURITY:
Related Nursing Process

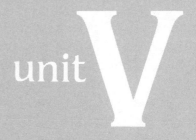

unit **V**

cognitive impairment in later maturity

Study of this chapter will enable you to:

1. Discuss personal feelings about the loss of cognitive functions and the value of the deteriorating person.

2. Describe general etiology and manifestations of cognitive impairment and reversible and nonreversible brain disorders.

3. Contrast abilities and limitations of the person with impaired cognitive function with those of the cognitively unimpaired person.

4. Discuss how to generally differentiate the person with a functional illness from one with organic brain disorder.

5. Use an appropriate assessment tool to determine a nursing diagnosis of cognitive impairment.

6. Formulate patient care objectives and a care plan for an elderly person with reversible brain disorder and one with irreversible brain disorder.

7. Adapt nursing intervention to the needs of the senior with cognitive impairment related to etiology, signs, symptoms, and behavior.

8. Work with other health team members to initiate or continue a reality orientation program.

9. Evaluate the effectiveness of your care by looking at your feelings, approach, and patient's response.

20

Whether you work in an acute, extended care, psychiatric, community, emergency, or home setting, you may encounter the cognitively impaired elderly person. While only 2 or 3 percent of persons over 65 years are institutionalized as a result of cognitive deterioration or psychiatric illness, 3 out of every 10 patients in mental institutions are over 65 years of age, and 94 percent of these elderly have been diagnosed as suffering from chronic brain disease or cerebral arteriosclerosis.[22,48] However, the cognitive impairment may be a result rather than a cause of institutionalization.[9] In the general population from 4 to 6 percent of the people over 65 suffer organic brain diseases.[29] These numbers are significant enough to command attention because the impact upon the elderly and society is tremendous in terms of sorrow and human life. You need to understand as fully as possible what cognitive impairment is and what can be done to improve life for the elderly who are suffering from it.

DEFINITIONS

Cognitive impairment is caused by a variety of conditions associated with brain tissue dysfunction.[4] Many terms are used to explain or classify this impairment, and they can be confusing. First, the terms organic and functional illness are related to causation. The term *organic refers to cognitive impairment resulting from brain tissue changes.* Agents of causation include: (1) intracranial and systemic infections; (2) drugs, poisons, and systemic intoxication; (3) brain trauma; (4) epilepsy; (5) disturbance of metabolism, growth, or nutrition; (6) intracranial neoplasms; and (7) degenerative disease of the central nervous system.[8] The term *functional* is used if *there is no discernible or identifiable cause,* such as in psychosis or neurosis.[16]

In early times dementia was the term used to denote madness; however, later it meant organic loss of intellectual ability. Today it is used much less, and some condemn the usage.[34] As people began living longer and evidencing more cognitive difficulty, senile dementia was separated in the literature from arteriosclerotic disease. Functional problems began to be differentiated according to symptoms, such as depression, delusional thinking, and paranoia. Roth later classified all disorders of later life into affective, senile, and arteriosclerotic psychoses.[41] In the *American Psychiatric Diagnostic and Statistical Manual,* acute and chronic brain disorders were classified into psychotic, neurotic, and behavioral reactions.[3] As if this were not confusing enough, in *Manual II* the classifications were changed to psychotic and nonpsychotic disorders.[4] The *nonpsychotic conditions are those in which the person, though troubled, can test reality and handle basic daily habits of living without presence of gross perceptual distortions,* such as hallucinations and delusions. The *psychotic reactions are those in which the person has impaired reality testing and gross interference in the ability to meet the demands of life because of deficits of language, memory, or perception.*[46]

Most of the literature today speaks of the reversible (acute) and nonreversible (chronic) brain disorders because of their descriptive usefulness. An acute condition may become chronic if damage remains and impairment persists.

ASSESSMENT OF THE PERSON

The Interview

When you first meet the person in the assessment interview, rely upon your observations and listening skills. Although you may observe obvious data about failing cognition as the person walks into the room, you will probably have to look for subtle changes, such as clues in conversation, memory, judgment, affect, and orientation. If the person is interviewed with family members, their perception can be exceedingly important. They may openly state such symptoms as, "Mom wanders around the house at night," or "She laughs and cries all in a matter of minutes." They may say no more than, "Mom is failing." Follow these clues until you have a clear understanding of the symptoms. As the interview begins, you may observe that the person's anxiety is increasing, which in turn increases the confusion. Perhaps you notice that the family discusses the senior as if he were not present, and speaks of him negatively. Determine how to progress with the interview. You may want to talk to the family or the patient alone. You may want to make a first-level assessment of the senior quickly and then continue further assessment later in several short sessions.

The first interview usually produces fear in the elderly person. Even in the best situation, such as his home, he is struggling to think and to hold on to his mental capabilities. With the added stress of new people, ideas, or an unfamiliar setting, he experiences greater difficulty. He feels uneasy, vulnerable, fearful, and confused.[35]

Adjust the interview to the person you are meeting. Patience and gentleness can help to promote a sense of safety in the setting. If you try to create a safe, comfortable setting, you will usually be rewarded with enough information to make an early assessment. Do not feel that you must ask every question on the interview tool. Do not rush the patient. He should be allowed time and space to tell his own story. If he is pushed, he may become more anxious and disorganized, and your purpose may be defeated.[49] While the interview is progressing, carefully notice the level of functioning. You may want to apply more stress by challenging a point he has made or date he has given you in order to observe his reaction. You may want to provide more structure to assess whether or not he can function within a more defined framework. *Never press the patient more than is necessary.* Whenever possible, respond to him in a helpful manner. You can support him with an empathic statement, or you can give a reassuring smile to convey the impression that he is in good hands. At times, you may be able to make a sound assessment in one interview; in other cases, it will take longer. Now is the time to begin the nurse-patient relationship, which may be the most helpful tool in the assessment process.

No typical patient complaining of confusion, suffering cognitive impairment, with either acute or chronic organic brain syndrome, exists. A wide range of behaviors is seen from patient to patient. Behaviors change. Severity changes. Complications are as varied as are the personalities of the individuals concerned. The type and severity of the behavior are not always related to the extent of brain damage. The person with little neuropathology sometimes shows severe behavioral change. Those with profound pathology may have only mild symptoms. In some instances, even normal-behaving people may have brain changes as marked as others with senile or arteriosclerotic disorders.[14,27]

Case Studies

The two following examples are very different people with different problems; yet, both are suffering from cognitive impairment or organic brain syndrome. The first case is typical of reversible (acute) syndrome. The second is typical of nonreversible (chronic) brain syndrome.

Mr. L. V., an 82-year-old farmer, complained of a severe headache for 4 or 5 days. He continued to do morning and evening chores, and, other than an occasional cough, he had no symptoms. He began to lose consciousness, fluctuating from disorientation and garbled speech to stupor. He ate little and became incontinent. On being admitted to the local community hospital, he was diagnosed as having pneumonia. For several weeks the anoxia caused by this systemic infection caused him to continue to exhibit symptoms of impaired intellect—loss of memory, lack of concentration, and confusion. Even after his pneumonia was cured and he was discharged from the hospital, his memory was spotty, and he was less alert than before the illness. However, a month after he was discharged he was again as alert and active as before the illness; he showed no signs of cognitive impairment in managing the farm or in daily living.

Miss M., an elderly spinster who lived alone, was having progressive memory difficulty. She made lists to remind herself of activities and asked friends to call before each meal. With friends she laughed inappropriately; yet, she was careful to discuss experiences of 20 years ago that were familiar and easily recalled. She often dressed in clothes that were not color-coordinated, or she wore several layers of dresses, blouses, and skirts. Heavy make-up and a big, floppy hat finished her attire. At first, friends considered her eccentric—even funny. Later they began to realize that her behavior had progressively deteriorated in the past year. One day she was brought home by the police because she had been causing a disturbance in a nearby city park. Her only living relative, a cousin, was notified. When he arrived to visit, he found that her bookkeeping and bank balancing were disastrous and that her pantry was stocked with boxes of perishable items. He found tea bags, food, and feces in drawers, all of which exuded an unpleasant odor throughout the house. Since she demonstrated an inability to adequately care for herself, arrangements were made to admit her to a local nursing home.

The wide range of symptoms or behaviors manifested by cognitively impaired seniors is caused by a variety of factors: long-term personality patterns; the crisis of loss; death of loved ones; complications of neurotic, psychotic, and behavioral disorders; stressful social and economic environments; lack of religious or family support; or pathology located in different areas of the brain.

Common Symptoms

Regardless of the degree of severity, the basic features of cognitive impairment are found in the acronym, *JOMAC* (Judgment, Orientation, Memory, Affect, Cognition). They include: (1) faulty judgment; (2) sensorium impairment, such as impaired orientation, loss of memory, and disordered intellectual functioning; and (3) lability of affect.[16] As indicated by the following discussion, assessment of these areas aids differential diagnosis between reversible and irreversible cognitive impairment and functional illness.

Judgment is the ability to perceive and distinguish relationships or alternatives with the capacity to make reasonable decisions. When you are assessing the person's ability to make judgments, you will be looking at the form, speed, and content of his expressed thought. You may ask him to explain a fable or old saying. During the interview you may notice little sequence of thought, inability to make and act on a decision, or unrealistic thinking. If you observe illogical thinking, you have reason to question the person's ability to judge and decide. As judgment deteriorates, so does ability to think in the abstract. Perhaps the most difficult problem encountered by the senior struggling with impaired judgment may center around situations in everyday living. The family may tell you about his unwise investments, permissive sexual activity, or family embarrassments from behavioral indiscretions. He may change his will or give away money. Friends may comment about his "change of living" or "going back to childhood." You may observe inappropriate dress, excessive make-up or perfume, or an unkempt, dirty appearance. The patient with severe functional problems, such as schizophrenia or mania, also has difficulty in judgment, which may cause difficulty in diagnosis differentiation.[15]

Orientation is the ability to locate self in one's environment as to person, place, or thing.[19] Loss of orientation is fairly easy to assess. Disorientation for time—day, hour, month, or year—occurs first; it can readily be determined by questioning. Disorientation about location or place seems to occur next. To determine place disorientation, ask the following questions: "Where are you? What city do you live in? What state do you live in? What country do you live in?" Next the senior loses the identity of the people around him; finally, he loses knowledge of himself. Ask the person who he is, what his name is, or whom he sees in the mirror. Disorientation may be first noted at night when sensory stimulation is lower, as the person wanders around, gets lost, or does not answer to his name. Major difficulties in orientation usually accompany advanced brain disease.

In the senior diagnosed with reversible brain syndrome, the disorientation may fluctuate from hour to hour, but a person with nonreversible brain syndrome may have periods of disorientation, become oriented, and then return to disorientation. In comparison, patients with functional illnesses often lose sense of identity first, and then they lose their orientation for time, place, and person.

Secondary symptoms such as hallucinations, illusions, delusions, may also interfere with the elderly person's orientation. He may *hallucinate, have vivid sensory experiences without presence of sensory stimuli.* Some clinicians believe that true hallucinations occur only when there is neurological change or disease. *Illusions, misperception of sensory stimuli,* may occur because of hearing, vision, or tactile impairment. The elderly person may also have *delusions— false beliefs.* A suspicious, frightened patient may refuse food because he believes that it is poisoned. Or he may hide in his room because he thinks that the nurses are going to steal his money. The schizophrenic or manic patient may also have sensory perceptions that promote disorientation, but the hallucinations or illusions are much more bizarre and symbolic. Often the delusions are more autistic and are poorly understood by others because they are responses to personal fears and fantasies.

Memory is the retention of material over a period of time and involves differing forms of response. You may tell the person several items of information at the beginning of the interview and later ask what information he was given in order to check recent memory loss. *Immediate memory, reproduction, recognition, or recall within a period of not more than five seconds,* may be tested by showing a picture, removing it, and asking the person to tell you about the picture. *Recent memory, reproduction, recognition, or recall after 10 seconds or longer,* may be tested by reading a story or showing a list of words and asking him to repeat them to you.[16] This type of assessment must be done carefully and sensitively; you must wait for the person's reaction. In some cases, he may think that it is a game or a fun situation and not respond accurately. He may feel used, especially if the assessment can be done in other ways. If he feels vulnerable and frightened, such assessment might be perceived as exploitation or ridicule.

Assessing memory of the person is not easy. When the person is able to compensate, detection may come only with time or detailed questioning. In the early stages of memory loss, the person may have difficulty recalling names and may use phrases for places and events. He may be *circumstantial, talking around the topic,* or he may *confabulate, filling in gaps of conversation with fantasy.* When the person is trying to hide the loss from others and himself, he may communicate with pleasantries and banter. Some people are consciously aware of the initial loss. The person may show signs of anxiety about his condition without wanting to share it with you. Note these emotional clues; then make further inquiries. For example, during the interview Mr. Black hesitates, searches for words, flushes, and begins to tremble when he is asked, "What day is it?" He states that the day is Tuesday, the 4th, when he was told earlier in the day that it is Monday, the 24th. As the development of memory loss continues, the deficit will be noticed more frequently in situations involving people. The person may forget names of close family members, relatives, or neighbors. He may call out, "Oh Mary, I haven't seen you in years. How I remember the good times we had together." In reality, they are strangers.

The last memory deficit to be noted is that of the self. In the interview the person may also complain of fatigue or exhaustion because of the amount of energy needed to maintain integrity and cope with his failing memory and intellectual ability.

A common belief is that elderly people suffering from advanced brain disorders have well-preserved remote memory. In fact, their remote memory is significantly inferior to that of normal persons of comparable age and education. However, even the person suffering from greater deterioration will retain longer the events that have made an impact and have been repeated many times; the remote memory is better than the recent memory.[34]

Recent memory loss does occur with many elderly people. In cases in which they view it as a feared mental illness, the problem may be exaggerated. Memory loss frequently occurs in conjunction with depression and anxiety; however, usually with a functional illness there will be little difference between recent and remote memory loss.

Affect refers to the emotional expression, reaction, or stability of the person. Though definite emotional changes occur in brain disease, earlier personality characteristics and manner of response normally become more pronounced as age progresses. A common feature is *lability of affect, rapid fluctuation in emotional response.* The senior reacts excessively and inappropriately, laughing one minute and crying the next. He may mimic your emotions; if you appear angry, he may also. He may look sad, cry, and say, "I don't know why I am crying; I don't feel that bad." A later characteristic is the emotional outburst, called *emotional incontinence, in which he is unable to control aggressive or sexual impulses.*[11] The elderly person will be less able to hold back or defend against his unacceptable feelings and loosened inhibitions; he may become more angry, irritable, or depressed. As the disease progresses, a leveling of affect takes place. Spontaneity, range of response, and appropriateness are lost. Response becomes more apathetic, dull, and monotonous.

Throughout the illness the person may suffer from added stress and experience symptoms of psychotic, neurotic, and behavioral disorders. These disorders may in turn present emotional symptoms that will cloud the picture. Depression, for example, may either result from a changing neurological picture or it may be a reaction to severe cognitive impairment.

In the interview try to determine the person's feelings about certain issues. When this is effectively done, you obtain more data, and he feels that you are interested in *him* and what is happening to him, not just in his physical complaints, family life, financial situation, and mental status.

Cognition involves the ability to know, think clearly, concentrate, and function intellectually. This area, as well as the others described, varies in degree of impairment and may be classified from mild to severe. Clinical observation and neuropsychological testing help to determine general intelligence, reasoning, problem solving, speed and flexibility of response, attention and concentration, language performance, and extent of deterioration.[20] Assess level of education, manner of speech, topics of conversation, comprehension, flow of thought progression, and manner of communication. You need information about previous performance in order to make an accurate comparison; consider prior occupation and organizational involvements. (Do not assume that the ditchdigger was less intellectually bright or less complex than the traveling salesman, for example.) Look for impoverishment of ideas, reduced flow of thoughts and ideas, and inability to abstract.[11]

Assessment Tools

Assessing cognitive function is a subjective area. The interview and the use of JOMAC as a guide are essential. The assessment tool in Chapter 2 may be helpful. You may find simple ways to assess cognitive function, such as using pictures or having the person copy simple drawings (a circle or square). Various psychological tests can be used. You may find Goldfarb's 10-point scale helpful for assessing the extent of the impairment. The questions to ask are:

1. Where are we now? (place orientation)
2. Where is this place located? (place orientation)
3. What month is it? (time orientation)
4. What day of the month is it? (time)
5. What year is it? (time)
6. How old are you? (memory)
7. When is your birthday? (memory)
8. Where were you born? (memory)
9. Who is the president of the United States? (general information and memory)
10. Who was the president before him? (general information and memory)[22]

The evaluation is done by counting up the number of incorrect answers:

0–2	No impairment to mild impairment
3–8	Moderately impaired
9–10	Severely impaired[18]

Another scale used to assess deterioration in the spheres of orientation, emotional control, motor ability, and communication was developed by a team at Kingston Psychiatric Hospital in Canada. Content and scoring of the scale are described in detail by the authors.[33]

Remember that test results can be influenced by many factors, including response to the test and the tester. Do not be hasty in your conclusions about the past and present functioning.

COMPARATIVE ASSESSMENT OF REVERSIBLE AND NONREVERSIBLE BRAIN DISORDERS

The previous discussion on assessment relates generally to anyone with cognitive impairment. However, it is useful to know the different manifestations of reversible (acute) and nonreversible (chronic) brain disorder. The following discussion and Table 20.1 help to clarify the differences. Usually cognitive impairment, both reversible and irreversible, have multiple causation.[30,34]

Reversible Brain Disorder

Reversible (acute) brain disorder is a confusional state in a severe, fulminating form and produces symptoms related to functions of the brain area involved. For example, subdural hematoma or epidural bleeding in the temporal lobe might cause olfactory hallucinations; bleeding in the occipital lobe would cause visual hallucinations.

Frequently, however, the total brain reacts in a diffuse manner. You may observe clouding of consciousness, disorientation, fluctuation of confusion, and reduced attention span. Perceptual disturbances usually occur in severe cases. The patient may complain of various perceptions when awake or upon awakening, or he may experience them as nightmares during sleep. Hallucinations are common, vivid, and frightening. Illusions are also common; the patient may misinterpret common objects in the environment to be animals, insects, or frightening people. Often the perceptions produce fear and anxiety. Many patients with acute brain syndrome are also delusional. Frequently the delusions are persecutory in nature, and the patient may feel that he is being trapped or endangered by someone or something.

You should note not only the various physical and behavioral symptoms but also the duration, fluctuations in severity, and possible precipitating causes. Such observations can help determine the diagnosis.

Just as a child may react to an elevated temperature with a seizure, so the elderly adult may react to elevated temperature, immobility, fecal impaction, stress, pain, and the other etiologic factors given in Table 20.1 with confusion or a variety of other symptoms of impaired cognition.[44]

TABLE 20.1 Comparison of Reversible and Nonreversible Cognitive Impairment

Characteristic	Reversible (Acute)	Nonreversible (Chronic)	
Onset	Sudden	Slow, insidious.	
Etiology	Temporary, diffuse disturbance of brain function which results from a toxic process. Examples include cerebral hypoxia; intracranial tumor or abscess; head trauma; infection; altered cellular content; dehydration; electrolyte imbalance; malnutrition; metabolic disorder such as uremia or diabetes; intoxication by poisons, drugs, or alcohol; seizure disorders; sensory deprivation; liver dysfunction; hemorrhage, anemia; psychological abuse.	Permanent, diffuse disturbance of brain function which results from progressive deterioration. Examples include atrophy of neurons and total brain mass; enlargement of ventricles; senile plaques on brain tissues; cerebral vascular insufficiency or arteriosclerosis. Deterioration from vascular insufficiency and arteriosclerosis partly reversible in early stages.	
		Deterioration from Old Age (Senile Dementia)	*Deterioration from Poor Blood Supply (Cerebral Arteriosclerosis)*
Age of onset	Any age, depending on etiology.	Age 65 to 70 years, or later. May not occur.	Age 50 to 65 years. May not occur until later.
Sex	Either	Females more frequently.	Males more frequently.
Physical symptoms	Related to etiology. Any organ system may be affected. Delirium, stupor, coma.	Fatigue, nocturnal restlessness, deterioration of self-care habits, disturbed sexual behavior, incontinence.	Dizziness, headaches, hypertension in 50 percent of cases, fatigue, drowsiness, syncope, marked physical deterioration, stiff and shaky voluntary muscles, ataxia, poor coordination. Often have symptoms of a small stroke.

TABLE 20.1 (*Continued*)

Characteristic	Reversible (Acute)	Nonreversible (Chronic)	
		Deterioration from Old Age (Senile Dementia)	Deterioration from Poor Blood Supply (Cerebral Arteriosclerosis)
Speech pattern	May or may not be abnormal.	Dysphasia—impaired ability to speak and perhaps to comprehend.	Dysphasia. Slurred speech.
Mental symptoms	Rapid impairment of orientation, memory, intellectual function, judgment. Confused.	Disoriented, confused, impaired abstract thinking, memory, judgment.	Poor concentration and judgment, memory loss.
Emotional symptoms	Impaired affect; may have psychotic or neurotic reaction.	Anger and irritability; emotional lability; use of rationalization, denial, or projection; increased dependency; helplessness; possibility of suicide or accidents.	Personality degeneration; may have insight into difficulty up until the last stages, which causes depression and anger; suspicious; delusions.
Clinical course	Brief. Recovery unless there are physical complications that do not respond to treatment.	Intellectual and physical deterioration progressing for years, ending in death.	Death from cerebral vascular accident.

Often, diminished cognition is a presenting sign of other problems, although the person cannot label his symptoms clearly or recognize his abnormalities. Or he may indirectly tell you that he is ill by complaining about food, mobility, and relatives, or by restating past complaints. Emotional lability, confusion, disorientation, or poor judgment frequently precede myocardial infarction, cerebrovascular accident, congestive heart failure, or cardiac arrhythmias.[50]

The acute physical adaptive process itself may cause further difficulty. Toxins from tissue damage are circulated to all body cells, cutting off adequate oxygen supply and, with it, nutrients and fluids, thus upsetting the body chemistry. In the end this causes more confusion.[37]

Many times the well-functioning elderly person temporarily reacts to a change of environment or stress with complaints of not knowing where he is, misinterpreting people around him, or forgetting what he has just been doing. While the younger person who has suffered a toxic state or a head injury may return to normal functioning rapidly, the elderly person is not so likely to do so. Even without a history of degeneration, he has a greater chance of nonreversible cognitive impairment because deterioration is begun or accelerated by the acute assault. It seems that since the elderly person has moved to a more precarious mental position, any one of a number of factors may cause disorganization of mental abilities and brain functioning.

Nonreversible Brain Disorder

Assessment of *nonreversible cognitive impairment* (*chronic brain disorder*) may be easier and more accurate in the home. During visits to a family, you can check the elderly members for beginning signs of mental difficulty: amnesia, misidentification, disorientation, confusion, defective judgment, and poor impulse control. Your assessment in the home will be more accurate than in an institution, since the senior is functioning at the highest level in familiar surroundings. Further, you can also assist the family to understand and deal with behaviors they are noticing for the first time, and to intervene in the early stages. If the senior is diagnosed with chronic brain syndrome, you must also assess for various physical problems. Common problems could be cardiac decompensation, cardiac attacks, cerebral hemorrhage, fractures, decubitus, circulatory problems, anemia, uremia, infection, and pulmonary complications. Further, observe for signs of depression, suicidal ideation, withdrawal, alienation, loneliness, and disengagement. While working with this patient, you must be attuned to many nursing specialties.

The following case studies compare the two types of nonreversible brain disorder: deterioration (senile brain disease) and cerebral arteriosclerotic syndrome.

Miss L. grew up in a large family in a Midwestern city. She was a dedicated accountant in a local business until she retired. She lived alone in a large white house. After 65, she occupied herself with her garden, Golden Age Club, and housecleaning. Later, Miss L. became forgetful, particularly for recent and immediate events. This trend progressed rapidly, and soon it was accompanied by difficulty with speech and comprehension. Apparently unaware of what was happening to her, Miss L. would fill in memory gaps by confabulation or fantasy, or she would blame other people for misplacing or hiding items. Her habits began to deteriorate; she became sloppy in appearance and careless about housework. Interest in activities rapidly diminished. Wandering at night became a problem. She would knock on neighbors' doors, looking for her mother or father. Though neighbors and friends were concerned about her safety, they were unable to talk to Miss L. about her condition. One day when she was trying to cook a meal, she started a fire in the kitchen. She went to her neighbor, who immediately called the fire department. Since the house, though only moderately damaged, was no longer livable, Miss L. was persuaded to move to the Old People's Home in the area. Upon admission, she was confused and helpless.

Miss L. lived 2 more years, and then died from pneumonia and other complications. An examination of her brain revealed atrophied brain substance, layers of shrunken and abnormal cortical cells, and ventricle enlargement.

Miss L.'s behavior and clinical findings are typical of one of the major causes of chronic brain syndrome, Senile Brain Disease, deterioration apparently caused by advanced age.

Mr. B. had always wanted to be a lawyer. He grew up as an only child in a large metropolitan city. His parents sacrificed to send him to Columbia University, where he was studious and industrious. On returning to his home city to set up practice, he had little difficulty getting clients; in time he had a flourishing clientele. Mr. B. married, had five children, and became a stable member of the community. At 55 he began having headaches and dizziness. His usual energy began to wane and, after a blackout spell, he sought help from his physician. Hypertension was found; medication was supplied. At age 60 he suffered a series of little strokes with accompanying slurring of speech and confusion. He began to have periods of disorientation. When he was oriented, his family would take him to the office where he functioned adequately. He continued to deteriorate. His gait became shuffling with small Parkinsonian-like steps; he had more difficulty with concentration. This behavior upset him, and he would weep for long periods. His depression increased; he became more and more difficult to live with. He became crude, explosive, and self-centered. At age 63 Mr. B. died of a cerebral hemorrhage.

On autopsy, the brain of Mr. B. was marked by softening and discoloration of tissue caused by insufficient blood supply. Mr. B. exhibited behavior similar in some ways to Miss L., but he was diagnosed with the second largest type of chronic brain disease, Cerebral Arteriosclerotic Syndrome.

Diagnostic Procedures

Brain disorders are usually discovered by careful observation and interview; the JOMAC assessment by the nurse; a history noting abnormalities in physical, neurological, and psychological examinations; or an electroencephalogram or brain scan. Skull X-rays, lumbar puncture, arteriography, ventriculography, and pneumoencephalography may be done.

Diagnostic measures should be directed toward the whole person. Often, the physician will look for the precipitating cause of the acute state and complications of the physical problem. In the hospital the patient may be diagnosed with diabetes, heart disease, or any number of chronic illnesses, and no one notes the acute brain syndrome the patient is suffering. If the acute brain syndrome is not diagnosed, complications may occur.

A variety of diagnostic studies is more likely to determine if the symptoms result from a temporary condition, age deterioration, or vascular problems. Very specific body chemistry tests and X-rays help to diagnose a physical disease that is causing an acute confusional state. In cerebral arteriosclerosis, symptoms of cerebral hypoxia are caused by the waxy deposit from cholesterol on the vessels, which causes the vessels to thicken and harden.[37] The patient usually has generalized arteriosclerosis; he is having cardiac, kidney, lung, and vascular complications as well. Neurological symptoms are common. In senile dementia, various skull X-rays may show diffuse cerebral atrophy or shrinking with dilatation and enlargement of the ventricles and widening of the cortical sulci.[20] Senile dementia may be positively confirmed at autopsy when a higher than normal density of senile plaques are found on the brain.

Some elderly people who function adequately have been found at autopsy to have advanced brain pathology. Patients diagnosed with either type of disorder may have atrophy, plaques, and softening of the brain. The degree of influence that functional or emotional aspects have upon symptom development is unknown. Many times depression will cause some of the same symptoms as chronic brain syndrome; differential diagnosis is difficult.

NURSING DIAGNOSIS, PATIENT CARE GOALS, AND INTERVENTION

Your nursing diagnosis of impaired cognitive function may include the following assessments of the person:

1. Demonstrates varying degrees of impaired alertness, orientation, and rationality.
2. Demonstrates various amounts of inaccuracy when responding to directions.
3. Is unable in varying degrees to recall data appropriate to the situation.
4. Displays varying inability to think through situations; encounters difficulty in making decisions; judgments are not based on data.
5. Shows pattern of involving self in hazardous situations or in situations that will somehow jeopardize him in varying ways.
6. Responds apathetically or inappropriately to stimuli that might otherwise be expected to elicit interest and curiosity.

Patient Care Goals

The long-term goals listed in Chapter 10 for the cognitively unimpaired senior are goals we also envision for the cognitively impaired person, but the goals must consider limitations. *Long-term care goals* could include the following:

1. Tasks related to all spheres of daily living are accomplished to the fullest degree possible, considering limitations.
2. Information that is essential to daily living is retained or learned to the fullest possible degree, considering limitations.
3. Cognitive impairment is realistically accepted to the degree possible, and adequate feelings of self-esteem and hope are retained.

Short-term goals could include the following:

1. Reality contact is maintained.
2. Problem-solving activities appropriate to daily living are accomplished.
3. Creativity is encouraged through self-expression.
4. Memory is stimulated through doing various activities appropriate to the situation.
5. Information pertinent to health or self-care is learned or maintained.
6. Expression of feelings is encouraged in appropriate situations.

You may formulate other goals for patients for whom you are caring.

General Intervention Approaches

"Begin with hand-holding, shoulder-patting, praise, and human warmth."[43] These were the words of the head nurse on a research unit for brain-diseased patients at a Midwestern Veterans Hospital in answer to the question, "How do you begin your nursing intervention?"

This may not be your recipe for working with the confused patient; however, the important quality is to be sincere, respectful, and responsive to the patient. If you can be with him and for him (empathic), your interventions have meaning for the patient. Recognize the patient as a unique person and feel compassion for his suffering, and he will in turn be touched and respond with as much growth as he is capable. If you believe that this person, who may be unable to remember the time of day or your name, is less than human, you do little for him. In fact, you may be disturbing to him.

Most nurses have real empathy for a patient suffering from malignancy or chronic emphysema, but they may have little understanding of the realness of the experience, the suffering, and the fear that confusion, disorientation, failing memory, and hallucinations produce. The pain of terror is as great as the pain of physical suffering.

The following discussion differentiates intervention for reversible and nonreversible brain disorder. Yet, care is similar in many ways. In either case, the patient needs excellent physical care; a helpful, trusting relationship; empathic communication appropriate for his condition; touch; adequate sensory and emotional stimulation; protection from injury; social interaction from loved ones or a peer group, depending on his condition; and spiritual care based on his beliefs. He is not just a diagnosis. He is not just senile. In fact, striking the word senile from the medical vocabulary would probably do a great deal for many elderly persons. The word clouds our vision and creativity; it causes us to feel hopeless and to consider only custodial care.

Intervention for Reversible Brain Disorder

Immediate treatment and intervention must be related to the stressor, precipitating cause, and degree of impairment of the acute state. For example, if the patient has pneumonia, the immediate care must relate to the bacteria or virus. Antibiotics must be given regularly. Oxygenation must be maintained. Fluid and electrolyte balance, nutrition, and elimination require careful monitoring. Rest is essential. All prescribed treatments must be done. Nursing intervention would also relate to the specific mental and emotional problems the patient is having.

In addition to the specific physical treatments, you would include the following main areas of care, which are necessary for patients of any age but must be modified for the specific needs of the elderly:

1. Communication for sensory stimulation and emotional closeness.
2. Diet and fluid therapy.
3. Protective measures, such as drugs (and restraints as a last resort), and provision for rest.
4. Support to the fearful person.

Communication for sensory stimulation and emotional closeness is essential. Whether he is showing signs of confusion, disorientation, delirium, stupor, or coma, the patient has probably reached an isolated, nonadaptive state. To continue to reach out to him, provide human contact, and maintain a stimulating environment, you must provide a continual verbal and nonverbal line to him. Listen carefully to anything he says, no matter how brief or difficult it is to hear. Speak in a slow, gentle manner to this patient. Familiar face, voice tone, and language are important. Kindly and concisely give directions, for example, "Open your eyes, Mr. Brown," or "Raise your arm." Present orienting conversation, such as "You are in St. Christopher's hospital, Mrs. Baron." Make supportive comments, such as, "You are progressing; your temperature is nearer normal today." Long sentences confuse the patient. Avoid negative, condescending, and joking conversation, or your patient may wonder how interested you are in caring for him and feel frightened. Instead of beginning with a question, you might tell him something of interest. Do not threaten, bribe, or demand. Never assume that he does not understand what you say. Usually patients will have partial amnesia after an acute episode but remember threatening or anxiety-provoking experiences.[16, 35, 44, 49]

Establishing trust is basic because it allows the patient in this very vulnerable position to feel secure and depend on you. The patient who is forced to be dependent for complete care may feel that he will not be cared for properly and become suspicious, guarded, and delusional. This may trigger further problems of agitation and panic. Everything discussed in Chapter 3 about a helping relationship applies to this person, even if he appears stuporous or delirious at the time.

The person may benefit by being in a room with another patient, keeping him close to the nurses' station, or asking family to remain with the patient. Visual and auditory devices are important if the individual is able to wear them. Glasses and hearing aids, as well as dentures, provide environmental contact and maintain a sense of identity and body image.

Communication may be nonreciprocal; that is, you may have to continue without much response from your patient. You may find that without any feedback your communication suffers. You may continue to care for him physically but perceive him as less than human. Watch for your feelings of anxiety, boredom, irritation, hopelessness, and discouragement. Such feelings reinforce the patient's anxieties if he is conscious and cause him to feel more insecure and worthless. Or, the patient may be unconscious, but the family may sense your feelings and be concerned that their loved one will not get good care. Explore your feelings with another person to determine why you feel the way you do. Fully expressing these feelings may neutralize them and free you to respond to your patient more positively through your care, your touch, and your spirit.

Nutrition, fluid and electrolyte balance, and state of mind are closely related in the elderly. The well-adjusted senior living in his home may suffer confusion from an inadequate intake or a slightly elevated temperature. An elderly person in a nursing care unit who is malnourished or dehydrated may begin to show subtle signs of confusion. A newly admitted patient suffering from chronic illness such as arthritis may have a serious electrolyte imbalance and an acute brain syndrome. When the imbalance has been discovered and treated, a rapid return to equilibrium usually occurs.

Adequate nutrition is essential to provide nutrients and energy. Intake and output must be accurately recorded. Daily infusions of intravenous fluids, usually with vitamins and minerals, are given if the patient is unable to take fluids by mouth. Carefully observe the speed and amount of fluids given parenterally; always observe for cardiac overload. Daily intake should usually be about 2 liters (8 glasses) of fluids. Adequate protein in the diet is encouraged with supplementary feedings. Always consider the patient's preferences; serving something the patient will not eat is pointless.

A safe, protected, restful environment is essential for maintenance of abilities and improvement. Treatments and care routines should be organized and timed so that they do not interfere with the patient's rest or sleep. Often sleep deprivation adds to the symptoms of brain disorder.

Measures of protection will depend on the severity of the patient's illness. If treatment such as infusions are necessary, assess the patient's ability to understand and cooperate with the treatment. Some patients can keep their arm relatively immobile for an infusion; others cannot. One patient may be able to tolerate a gastric tube in daylight hours but become agitated by it at night. Treatment measures can be modified, depending on response.

Your calm, understanding approach or the presence of a family member will probably be the best protective measure. Do not underestimate the power of purposeful communication and earlier trust feelings in quieting the patient who is agitated, fearful, or potentially self-destructive.

Perhaps verbal reassurance is enough to orient the patient to reality; however, sedative drugs or physical restraints may be necessary.[21] Yet, these protective measures create other problems. All drugs with depressant effects upon the central nervous system may cause confusion, even if given in small doses. Drowsiness caused by drugs may interfere with perception and reality testing, causing further confusion. Chlorpromazine in medium dosages of 50 to 100 mg four times a day or Perphenazine, 4 to 8 mg, given 5 times a day seem successful frequently.[32] However, since individuals respond differently to drugs, you must observe the reaction in each individual case. A hot drink or glass of wine may do more than a tranquilizer.[52]

You may feel that a waist restraint, posey belt, or full restraints are necessary. Physical restraints should be considered a *last resort;* they threaten self-esteem and add to anger. A patient wandering about may fall and injure himself, but a physically restrained patient may have skin damage, become more confused and distraught, or suffer other complications such as pneumonia, decubitus, constipation, or the problems of immobility discussed in Chapter 15. If restraints are needed, other nursing measures are imperative. Frequently tell the patient the reason for the use of the restraint. This is necessary even if it seems to be useless or to cause further agitation. Examine the skin frequently for tears, cuts, and abrasions. Provide skin care by turning and massage; give range-of-motion exercises to maintain circulation, joint mobility, and muscle tone. Offer fluids frequently. Provide communication and sensory stimulation by frequently stopping at the patient's bedside.

Evaluate which method of restraint works best, such as the presence of people, the use of drugs, or physical restraints, but do not threaten the patient. The immediate result of a quiet patient should never have priority over the long-term loss of the patient's sense of integrity. Be certain that use of drugs or physical restraint is an intervention for the patient's well-being and not just a time-saving measure for you. Also evaluate your approach while you are restraining the patient. Many times a severely agitated patient may be provoking and irritating, and even the most accepting nurse might feel satisfaction in restraining him. The patient is the first to pick up feelings of anger, resentment, and punishment in your nonverbal expressions.

Support to the fearful person is essential. The patient in coma or delirium may not be aware of his mental functioning; however, many patients suffering acute brain syndrome are very aware of confusing feelings and thoughts. For example, Mr. S. B., a 75-year-old single man, was admitted to the hospital suffering with acute hepatitis. After being taken to his room, he asked frequently where he was and appeared to receive no reassurance. The disorientation seemed to be more upsetting than his physical symptoms, for he repeatedly asked, "What is the matter with me? I just don't know what is happening."

Symptoms of cognitive impairment are usually a new and bewildering experience to the patient. His response is influenced by present fears and past experiences with confused people, if those experiences were traumatic. He may fear deterioration, becoming insane, or losing his mind. He may have known a neighbor or grandparent who committed suicide or was admitted to a custodial institution. Whatever the degree of organic impairment, it is usually increased by fear and anxiety. Added to his concern about changed mental functioning are fears of strange surroundings, discomfort of physical illness, loneliness, and boredom. Self-esteem and self-concept may be drastically damaged; he feels overpowered by his vulnerability and weakness. Regression and shame become prominent. He may feel very old, worn out, and hopeless.

As a nurse, you come into touch with the human condition—not only your patient's, but also your own. If you have insight into the frailty of the human being, in a holistic sense, and know how fragile a hold any person has on the reality of life, you can be considerably changed. Such insight can help you accept and care for the patient without fear and with the resolution that "Yes, life is hard, it is momentary, but there is hope, and there can be more life ahead." Your nonverbal support and how you feel about the meaning of life, illness, and death may be the most comforting intervention you bring to the patient. You can encourage him to want to live and to deal with his immediate situation. Give him necessary information repeatedly. Let the patient know that you will be available if he needs you.

Intervention for Nonreversible Brain Disorder

Intervention relating specifically to the patient with chronic brain syndrome presents multiple, complex problems that may be present for a long time. Drug therapy has produced little or no results, although a recent study indicated that Naftidrofuge (Praxilene) improved reaction time and short-term memory in patients with mild nonreversible brain syndrome.[7] Therefore, nursing intervention is the crucial factor for this person. This patient needs communication, support, sensory stimulation, adequate diet, fluids, rest, and protection from injury or other illness, just as the patient with acute brain disorder does. He needs privacy, a place for his possessions, a territory to call his own. His modesty must be respected during routine care or diagnostic and treatment measures. Special preferences, such as in food, drink, an activity, or wearing apparel, should be granted whenever possible so that he can maintain a sense of personal integrity. But management and care should begin with careful observation. Mistakes in interaction, treatment, and use of resources can then be avoided. The diagnostic label of nonreversible or chronic often precludes further observation or planning of care. Early, careful, and continued assessment helps you to assist the patient and family to adjust to many practical problems. Many families might be spared much of the guilt they later carry if they were given early information and counseling.

Assess your feelings concerning the future, value, and progress of your patient. You must deal with feelings of pessimism and discouragement as you face mental deterioration, emotional deprivation, suffering, and multiple physical complications and problems. Since this type of patient often is admitted to an institution, such as a nursing home, your intervention should include insights gained from reading about institutionalization in Chapter 7. Because you fear your own death, you may hold yourself back from your patient. You may not want to become involved with your patient because you know that in the end loss is inevitable. You may find the lack of intellectual ability or dependency repulsive to you and feel no empathy and warmth for your patient. You may want to see progress and feel defeated if you only see degeneration. Many times nurses find it difficult to admit such feelings to themselves, but all of us have them. Certainly, at the same time, there are feelings of concern, desire for excellent nursing care, and compassion for another human being. But the negative feelings should be acknowledged because they prevent aspirations for quality care from being fulfilled.

Methods of support discussed in Chapter 10 will help the person maintain whatever cognitive abilities he has. Further, approaching him as a person with abilities, not just impairments, helps you to avoid a pessimistic outlook and to maintain a philosophy of rehabilitation.

Communication is another avenue of intervention. You need to be as skillful as possible in techniques and methods of communication discussed in Chapter 3. You should know the person you are working with, his style of communication, his manner of response, and any sensory impairments. There are many reasons for inappropriate response from the elderly. Often the cause is not confusion, disorientation, or senility, but rather, hearing impairment. In such a case, the methods for communication described in Chapter 9 are applicable. Even though the patient appears confused, realize that what he is talking about may be based on a real experience, on an event much earlier in his life that you do not know about. Listen carefully and ask related questions to help him clarify his story; show respect; stimulate further rational conversation, and promote life review. Your lack of understanding of his conversation may be your confusion, not his! Pick out his meaningful comments and continue talking with him.

Watch for his emotional and nonverbal cues for evidence of how he perceives your communication. The patient's perception of your communication is far more influential on his behavior than what you actually say. Avoid injuring a relationship by making a careless remark about him or his behavior, even if he acts inappropriately.

A major communication barrier is anxiety, which may come from within the senior, yourself, or the environment. The elderly person, with or without sensory and perceptual disabilities, frequently is suffering from a damaged self-concept and body image. Cultural influences and expectations, family goals, personal ideals and aspirations, and many other influences impinge upon him. He may feel that he is losing his life-style, friends, place in society, and sense of hope. He may feel insecure and not worth the time and effort it takes to care for him. He may feel that he has little to say that you would be interested in knowing or that you have some hidden motive for wanting to talk to him. Some factors in the environment that may increase his anxiety are: threatening or hostile staff members, routines that evoke hopelessness and dependency, little contact with the community, or offensive surroundings. Your level of anxiety also influences his feelings.[31]

Another barrier to communication might be the senior's withdrawal, whether it is the physical withdrawal of lying in bed or staying in his room, or emotional withdrawal with its apathy, isolation, bizarre reactions, or unresponsiveness. The more active, aggressive patient receives more attention from the staff. Frequently staff members respond to the withdrawn patient with a withdrawn response, a distancing behavior to cope with their own anxieties and fears.[21] The soundest approach in treating an apathetic or withdrawn patient is to try to establish some rapport and contact. Get to know him so that trust can develop and he can know and respond to your approach.

Other barriers to communication with confused elderly patients are staff unresponsiveness; stereotyping, joking, demanding, or demeaning statements; and talking over the patient as if he did not exist. Such behaviors do not encourage the patient to express his feelings and ideas or talk about his past life experiences with the listener.

Environmental aids for reality orientation, as discussed in Chapter 4, are helpful to the confused, cognitively impaired patient, and they should be consistently used. Be creative about developing new ways of letting the patient know about his reality. Reinforce his realistic behavior. Adjust the environment to fit his failing senses and decreased motor coordination; use brighter colors, better illumination, well-marked exits, color-coded doors and rooms, clocks, calendars, family pictures, and treasured objects to help him remain oriented. Flowers, a fish tank, a bird, or having a small pet makes the environment more homelike. Set limits for the patient's protection, since he cannot rely on his own reality testing. Convey rules clearly and consistently to increase his sense of security.[6, 12, 17, 18, 25, 26]

Physical care is also important as habits deteriorate. The patient may have to be reminded of such activities as brushing teeth and combing hair. A list of activities may be made and checked off as they are accomplished. Encourage him to write, if he is able, any information he wants to remember. Sometimes this causes anxiety and thus defeats the purpose. You may have to give the patient routine care after a period of time if he is unable to accomplish this himself. As time passes complete physical care becomes inevitable.

Social interaction needs to be considered and can begin with reality orientation groups and then progress to more complex activities or group experiences as described in Chapter 4. Family visits, group activities, parties, trips, and shopping tours are important if the patient is able to participate. Encourage friendships between patients and responsibility one for another. It may be helpful to two patients if one is assigned to take the other for a walk. One benefits from the socialization, and the other benefits from the responsibility given him. Both patients receive satisfaction from the adventure. You might ask several patients to decorate the unit or a living room; you give them assistance and support. Music therapy, listening to records, playing an instrument, singing solo or in a group, can promote reality contact, reminiscing, a release of feelings, renewed interaction with others, and a sense of joy. Working with various handicraft projects in occupational therapy can also promote social interaction and meet personal needs. Physical exercise, activity groups, and any manner of stimulation are important in keeping the patient as active and alert as possible and in helping him maintain a sense of identity.[43]

Socialization may be a problem for the elderly person if he is reluctant to join groups because of such problems as urinary frequency or urgency, poor sphincter tone, poor manual dexterity for eating or various tasks, ataxia, or poor memory. Wearing protective apparel may help him avoid embarrassment about elimination. Use of special forks or spoons may prevent him from spilling or dropping food. Unobtrusive guidance may help him cope with ataxia or poor memory.

EVALUATION

Over the years the authors have had many experiences with elderly patients in the community, acute care setting, and nursing homes. Evaluation of care includes looking at relationships, recalling memories of happy and sad human experiences while working with patients with cognitive impairment. Tears were sometimes shed as relationships ended or as a patient recalled memories of his life and better times. Sometimes the patient's subtle sense of humor brightened the day. There were discouraging times as well, such as when a family forgot to visit or a healed decubitus broke down.

An unforgettable experience involved an elderly man confined to a wheelchair. He was disoriented and apparently recognized only his own name and person. He had snow white hair and a kind smile, and he always wore pajama bottoms, a shirt, and a bow tie. One student nurse had been assigned to him for a long-term experience and to learn basic physical care. She had worked with this man for 4 months, and termination of the relationship had been dealt with. On her last day she reminded him that this would be their last visit together. Just as every other day, there was no response—not a word, not a grunt, not a twinkle in his eye. She had always talked to him and had tried to form a relationship with him, but she received very little feedback. In fact, she had told her instructor that it seemed inappropriate to discuss termination because she was not sure that he even knew she was there. As she said goodbye and turned to leave, he said, "Wait." He then pulled her face to his and kissed her on the cheek. The inferences to be made from this experience are that an impaired senior may perceive more of your feelings and care than he overtly indicates and that working with the cognitively impaired elderly can be rewarding.

Evaluation of care should be in terms of the person's ability to maintain or regain some cognitive functions, accept his limitations, work with his assets, and gain satisfaction from personal and group activities. Recovery from the disease that causes reversible brain disorder can be evaluated by various tests. Evaluation of the person's cognitive function and feelings and your nursing approach is more subjective, but it is just as essential. Sometimes the only time you can evaluate the patient's feelings is when an incident occurs similar to the one the student mentioned above experienced.

Eventually the patient may become totally regressed or unable to respond. You know you are effective if you prevent further complications, if family members or other observers recognize that you maintain the dignity of the person, if the family feels comforted by your information and counsel, and if you do unto the patient as you would want done unto you.

REFERENCES

1. ALFANO, GENROSE, "There Are No Routine Patients," *American Journal of Nursing,* 75: No. 10 (1975), 1804–7.

2. AMBURGEY, PAULINE, "Environmental Aids for the Aged Patient," *American Journal of Nursing,* 66: No. 9 (1966), 2017–18.

3. AMERICAN PSYCHIATRIC ASSOCIATION, *Diagnostic and Statistical Manual of Mental Disorders.* Washington, D.C.: American Psychiatric Association, 1952.

4. ———, *Diagnostic and Statistical Manual of Mental Disorders,* 2nd ed. Washington, D.C.: American Psychiatric Association, 1968.

5. ARMSTRONG, PRISCILLA, "Comment: More Thoughts on Senility," *The Gerontologist,* 18: No. 3 (1978), 315–16.

6. BAINES, J., "Effects of Reality Orientation Classroom on Memory Loss, Confusion, and Disorientation in Geriatric Patients," *The Gerontologist,* 14: (1974), 138–42.

7. BRANCONNIER, R, and J. COLE, "The Impairment Index as a Symptom-Independent Parameter of Drug Efficacy in Geriatric Psychopharmacology," *Journal of Gerontology,* 33: No. 2 (1978), 217–23.

8. BURNSIDE, IRENE, "Clocks and Calendars," *American Journal of Nursing,* 70: No. 1 (1970), 117–19.

9. BUSSE, E., and E. PFEIFFER, eds., *Behavior and Adaptation in Late Life,* 2nd ed. Boston: Little, Brown & Company, 1977.

10. BUTLER, ROBERT, D. DASTUR, and S. PERLIN, "Relationship of Senile Manifestations and Chronic Brain Syndrome to Cerebral Circulation and Metabolism," *Journal of Psychological Research,* 3: (1965), 229–38.

11. BUTLER, ROBERT N., and MYRNA I. LEWIS, *Aging and Mental Health*. St. Louis: The C. V. Mosby Company, 1977.

12. CITRIN, RICHARD, and DAVID DIXON, "Reality Orientation—A Milieu Therapy Used in an Institution for the Aged," *The Gerontologist*, 17: No. 1 (1977), 39–43.

13. COHEN, GENE, "Comment: Organic Brain Syndrome," *The Gerontologist*, 18: No. 3 (1978), 313–14.

14. CORSELLIS, J., *Mental Illness and Aging*. London: Oxford University Press, 1962.

15. DAVIES, PETER, ed., *American Heritage Dictionary*. New York: Dell Publishing Co., Inc., 1973.

16. EATON, MERRILL, MARGARET H. PETERSON, JAMES A. DAVIS, *Psychiatry*, 3rd ed. New York: Medical Examination Publishing Company, Inc., 1976, pp. 253–67.

17. FOLSOM, JAMES, "Reality Orientation for the Elderly Mental Patient," *Geriatric Psychiatry*, Spring, 1968, 291–307.

18. ———, and GENEVA FOLSOM, "Team Method of Treating Senility," *Nursing Care*, 6: (December, 1973), 17–23.

19. FOWLER, ROY, and WILBERT FORDYCE, "Adapting Care for the Brain-Damaged Patient," *American Journal of Nursing*, 72: No. 11 (1972), 2056–59.

20. FRIEDMAN, A. M., I. H. KAPLAN, B. J. SADACK, "Organic Brain Syndrome," *Modern Synopsis of Comprehensive Textbook of Psychiatry*. Baltimore, Md.: Williams and Wilkins, 1972, 268–311.

21. GERDES, LENORE, "The Confused or Delirious Patient," *The American Journal of Nursing*, 68: No. 6 (1968), 1228–33.

22. GOLDFARB, A. I., "Psychiatric Disorders of the Aged: Symptomatology, Diagnosis, and Treatment," *Journal of the American Geriatric Society*, 8: (1960), 680.

23. GURALNIK, DAVID, ed., *Webster's New World Dictionary*, 2nd college ed. New York: The World Publishing Company, 1972.

24. HALL, BEVERLY A., "Mutual Withdrawal: The Non-Participant in a Therapeutic Community," *Perspectives in Psychiatric Care*, 14: No. 2 (1976), 75–77.

25. HARRIS, CLARKE, and PETER IVORY, "An Outcome Evaluation of Reality Orientation Therapy with Geriatric Patients in a State Mental Hospital," *The Gerontologist*, 16: No. 6 (1976), 496–503.

26. HIRCHFIELD, MIRIAM, "The Cognitively Impaired Older Adult," *American Journal of Nursing*, 76: No. 12 (1976), 1981–84.

27. JARVIK, L., C. EISENDORFER, and J. BLUM, eds., *Intellectual Functioning in Adults*. New York: Springer Publishing Company, Inc., 1973.

28. KAHN, R. L., *et al.*, "Brief Objective Measures for the Determination of Mental Status in the Aged," *American Journal of Psychiatry*, 111: (1960), 326–28.

29. KAY, D., "Epidemiological Aspects of Organic Brain Disease in the Aged," in *Aging in the Brain*, ed. C. M. Gaitz. New York: Plenum Press, 1972, pp. 15–26.

30. ———, and ALEXANDER WALK, "Classification and Etiology in Mental Disorders of Old Age: Some Recent Developments," *Recent Development in Psychogeriatrics: A Symposium*. Ashford, Kent: Headley Brothers Ltd., 1971, pp. 1–17.

31. KAZMIARCZAK, FRANCES, DOROTHY H. MOSER, and MARY A. RUSSO, "Communication Problems Encountered When Caring for the Elderly Individual," *Journal of Gerontological Nursing*, 1: No. 2 (1975), 21–27.

32. KRAL, V. A., "Confusional States, Description and Management," *Modern Perspectives in the Psychiatry of Old Age*, ed. John G. Howells. New York: Brunner /Mazel, 1975, pp. 356–62.

33. LAWSON, JAMES, M. RODENBURG, and J. DYKES, "A Dementia Rating Scale for Use with Psychogeriatric Patients," *Journal of Gerontology*, 32: No. 2 (1977), 153–59.

34. LILLIE, DOUGLAS, "Attitudes in Geriatrics," *Nursing Times*, 72: (July 15, 1976), lll ff, Supplement.

35. MacKINNON, ROGER, and ROBERT MICHELS, *The Psychiatric Interview in Clinical Practice*. Philadelphia: W. B. Saunders Company, 1971, pp. 339–360.

36. PATRICK, MAXINE LAMBRECHT, "Care of the Confused Elderly Patient," *American Journal of Nursing*, 67: No. 12 (1967), 2536–39.

37. PITT, BRICE, *Psychogeriatrics*. Edinburgh: Churchill Livingstone Publishers, 1974, pp. 24–45.

38. PRESTON, TONIE, "When Words Fail," *American Journal of Nursing*, 73: No. 12 (1973), 2064–66.

39. ROBERTS, ROSEMARY, "Senile Dementia and Depression," *Nursing Times,* 71: (December 4, 1975). 1931–33.

40. ROBINSON, C. W., "The Toxic Delirious Reactions of Old Age," in *Mental Disorders in Later Life*, ed. I. Kaplan. Stanford: Stanford University Press, 1972.

41. ROTH, M., "The Natural History of Mental Disorders in Old Age,"*Journal of Mental Science,* 101: (1955), 281–301.

42. ———, B. TOMLINSON, and G. GLISTED, "Correlation Between Scores for Dementia and Counts of Senile Plaques in Cerebral Gray Matter of Elderly Patients," *Nature*, 209: (1966), 109–10.

43. SAVAGE, B., "Rethinking Psychogeriatric Nursing," *Nursing Times*, 70: (February, 1974), 282–84.

44. SCHWAB, SISTER MARILYN, "Caring for the Aged," *American Journal of Nursing*, 73: No. 12 (1973), 2049–53.

45. "Senile Psychoses May Be Psychologic, Not Organic," *Geriatric Focus*, 8: No. 9 (1969), 1ff.

46. SOLOMON, PHILIP, and VERNON PATCH, *Handbook of Psychiatry*. Los Altos, Calif.: Lange Medical Publications, 1971, 201–9.

47. STEVEN, CAROLYN, "Breaking Through the Cobwebs of Confusion," *Nursing*, 74: No. 8 (1974), 41–48.

48. STOTSKY, BERNARD A., *The Elderly Patient*. New York: Grune & Stratton, Inc., 1968, pp. 108–12.

49. SZANTO, STEPHEN, "Dementia in the Elderly," *Nursing Mirror*, 140: (June 19, 1975), 64–65.

50. WAHL, PATRICIA, "Psychosocial Implications of Disorientation in the Elderly," *Nursing Clinics of North America*, 11: No. 1 (1976), 145–56.

51. WANG, H., "Organic Brain Syndromes," in *Behavior and Adaptation in Late Life*, eds. Ewald Busse and Eric Pfeiffer. Boston: Little, Brown & Company, 1969, pp. 263–88.

52. WHITEHEAD, J. A., "Helping Old People with Mental Illness," *Nursing Mirror*, 138: (March 22, 1974), 76–77.

PERSONAL INTERVIEW

53. HARPOLE, IDA, R.N., B.S., Head Nurse, Veterans Administration Hospital, Jefferson Barracks Division, St. Louis, Missouri.

depression and suicidal tendencies in later maturity

Study of this chapter will enable you to:

1. Define and classify various types of depression.

2. Explore the meaning and feelings of depression in the senior.

3. Discuss the psychodynamics of depression.

4. Assess a depressed elderly person, using parameters discussed in this chapter.

5. Differentiate behaviors of cognitively impaired and depressed elderly persons.

6. Formulate patient care goals related to assessment and nursing diagnosis.

7. Care for the depressed senior, using guidelines for intervention described in this chapter.

8. Work with the suicidal patient, using an understanding of the dynamics and appropriate care measures.

9. Work with the family and health team members as a part of patient/client care.

10. Evaluate effectiveness of your care.

11. Promote community resources and programs to assist the elderly in coping with loss and depression.

21

While not all elderly people are depressed, depression is the most common functional psychiatric problem in later maturity and is related to the rapid and steady losses that are suffered.[24, 43] Loss associated with decreased strength, status, income, health, friends, independence, finances, and eventually death must be coped with. The grief work described in Chapter 13 becomes a way of life with advancing age.[8] If the reaction becomes excessive in duration and degree, and depending on the dynamics involved, pathological depression exists.[11, 40]

Depression is a major health problem not only because of the numbers affected and the reduced productivity, but also because of the suffering endured by the depressed senior.[32] The elderly often state that they are more aware of blue spells and depressive periods than ever before. In one study, 38 percent of elderly persons admitted for the first time to the hospital had affective disorders.[11]

This chapter will help you to differentiate between normal grief work and pathological depression and to recognize overt and masked symptoms in the elderly. You have a responsibility to recognize the depressed and suicidal senior and to intervene appropriately.

DEFINITIONS

Depression is an emotional reaction, altered mood state, and symptom complex accompanied by negative self-concept and lowered self-esteem and associated with regressive and self-punitive wishes.[4]

Hippocrates first described depression and called it melancholy. Kraepelin's description of the behaviors characteristic of depression are still applicable.[35] Freud, in *Mourning and Melancholia*, described the cause of depression: angry, ambivalent feelings associated with a lost love object that are turned inward on the self.[23] Since that dynamic, psychoanalytic interpretation, many methods of classifying and describing depressive illness have developed. Table 21.1 summarizes the descriptive terms used by various authors in classifying types of depression.

THE MEANING OF DEPRESSION

Loss, separation from a loved object, a person, thing, status, or place to which the senior is attached, is the most common precipitant of depression. Loss may be real, such as loss of health, spouse, or job through retirement. Loss may be fantasized; the person may imagine that he is less attractive to others as he ages. Loss may be symbolic; the person may feel less feminine after hysterectomy or less masculine after prostatectomy.

TABLE 21.1 Classification of Depressive States

Classification by	Types of Depression	
Etiology	*Exogenous* Symptoms from reaction to loss; cause outside of person. Reaction to loss excessive in duration and degree because of meaning of loss.	*Endogenous* Symptoms without overt precipitating cause. Due to multiple factors, including long-time faulty life patterns, hormonal, nutritional, chemical imbalance, other disease status.
Symptom	*Reactive* Symptoms a reaction to bereavement. Person more responsive to psychotherapy.	*Endogenous* Symptoms autonomous, without obvious cause. Research concerning biochemical disturbance being done. More evidence of family history. Person more responsive to somatic treatment (electroshock and drug therapy).
Activity	*Retarded* Reduced motor or cognitive function.	*Agitated* Psychomotor restlessness.
Mood change	*Unipolar* One extreme only of mood, usually depression.	*Bipolar* Circular mood swings of elation (mania) alternating with depression.
Reality testing	*Neurotic* Aware of reality. Inappropriate response in relation to feelings about self. No secondary symptoms.	*Psychotic* Inappropriate or faulty awareness of reality in relation to self, others, and the environment. Secondary symptoms of delusions and hallucinations.
History	*Primary* First episode; no known psychiatric history of depression. Depression major problem.	*Secondary* Previous episodes of psychiatric depression. Depression response to another illness.
Disease entity according to Diagnostic and Statistical Manual of Mental Disorders II	Neurotic: Symptoms reaction to loss but built on neurotic character structure. Psychotic: Symptoms of severe depression with impaired reality testing. Manic–Depressive: Symptoms of severe cyclic depression alternating with mania. Involutional Melancholia: Symptoms of depression beginning in middle age centering around adjustments to age, sexual, and family changes. Senile Depression: Psychotic depression in the elderly, usually accompanied by delusions and hallucinations.	

Differentiation Between Grief and Depression

Grief and depression have been experienced by everyone to some degree. *Grief is the feeling of sadness related to an objective loss or separation, occurs in predictable phases, varies in degree, and is self-limited.* The physical symptoms that accompany grief are not so intense or long in duration as the symptoms of depression. In grief the person does not suffer either a distorted self-concept or damaged self-esteem. The person's mood shifts from sadness to a more normal state within one day when people show interest in him or other stimuli confront him. The person may be able to smile or laugh a little, to respond briefly to something genuinely funny; and he responds to reassurance and warmth. Friends and relatives usually feel interest in and empathy for the grieving person, but may feel irritation with the depressed person because of his lack of response to them and the lack of an apparent reason for his depressed behavior. Depression may be unrelated to a specific loss or to an objective situation. If the patient does not receive help, a long-term perceived defect in self, the low feelings, and related symptoms are intensified as the person ages, and the depression becomes fixed.

Dynamics of Depression

In depression, the person reacts to perceived loss with intense feelings of decreased self-confidence, loss of self-esteem, and negative self-concept. The person feels damaged, diminished, worthless, and ashamed, and he blames himself for the loss or for what was not achieved, apparently because of long-established high ideals and expectations of self. An important part of himself is gone; he feels empty. Concurrently, the senior experiences feelings of rejection, abandonment, and loneliness related not only to this loss but also to past losses, past failures, or past experiences with important people. Further, anger at the lost object for deserting him is intense, although it is repressed because of guilt feelings about the anger. Perception of self becomes increasingly distorted; finally relationships with others and the ability to function in daily living become ineffective.[5]

An example of this cycle was seen in the elderly man who became severely depressed after the death of his wife. He frequently commented, "She left me; she left me." His tone of voice and enunciation conveyed anger. Yet, he felt very guilty and ashamed because his anger was unacceptable to him. The resulting ambivalent, guilty, and angry feelings were turned inward into self-accusation and depression.

When the person perceives himself as failing, when he thinks less of self and is angry, his adaptive abilities in turn are diminished. He resorts to more primitive mechanisms to try to restore a sense of security and adjustment. He may withdraw from others; deny that he is feeling depressed or that anything has changed in his life; or project his anger onto others so that he conveys that others are angry with him. Or he develops physical symptoms (somatization). The elderly person may respond with global anxiety, expressing it openly and to anyone, much as a young child does. Sarcasm, blaming, or criticism may be directed to another, especially when the senior considers crying or other obvious expressions of sadness and anger as inappropriate.[11]

ASSESSMENT

When you first meet the person, he may not appear depressed. He may even wear a smile, but he does not usually look happy. Observe carefully his nonverbal behavior; listen to his manner of speech as well as to what he says; be aware of your own reaction to him. Continue your assessment over time so that you will be accurate.

As you interview him, you may begin to feel depressed yourself; depressive feelings can be sensed as easily as anxiety. Or you may feel apathetic or hopeless. Be alert to your feelings. Sometimes the patient will deny his feelings of depression, but your ability to sense his feelings may help you determine the nursing diagnosis.

Appearance

Notice the person's general appearance. Often clothing and hair appear disheveled, as if they have received little attention from him. Clothing may be ill-fitted or somber in color. Facial makeup is often not apparent or is sloppily applied. Shoes may be scuffed or inappropriate for the other clothing. Posture is stooped; movement is usually heavy and slow. His facial appearance is sad: dull expression, furrowed brow, worried frown, turned-down corners of the mouth, reddened eyes from crying. Often weight loss, poor muscle tone, dry skin, weakness, and general malaise are apparent. He may look 10 years older than he is. He has tears in his eyes as if he is ready to cry or has frequent crying spells.[24]

If the person is agitated, you will see rapid, restless, jerking movements and walk. He may wring his hands, cry without shedding tears, or laugh inappropriately. His skin may be scratched or bruised from picking at it. He may pull at his hair or clothes. He may be unable to sit still as he talks with you.

Verbal Response

Open the conversation with a broad statement; note how the senior responds. Be conscious of the topics he initiates. He may ask, "What is the world coming to?" or "Life isn't what it used to be, is it?"

His pace of conversation will be slow and halting, with long pauses between phrases or sentences. Do not hurry him, for he responds with silence or agitation. He often appears uninterested in you or the interview. He loses the trend of the conversation or looks preoccupied, confused, or angry. He may lack the energy or motivation to talk or to recall events. Ask direct, simple questions, such as, "Where do you live?" or "Where are you now?" to determine his ability to answer. He may give you a one-syllable answer very softly, or he may look at you and shrug his shoulders. Yet, he is capable of answering if given time; he thinks very slowly.

Physical Symptoms

During the interview the senior may have many physical complaints. Some of the physical symptoms are related to the person's depression, since depression is a systemic disease. As emotional processes slow, so do autonomic, neuromuscular, chemical, metabolic, and circulatory processes. Thus, he may be constipated and anorexic (the elderly depressed person is less likely to overeat than is the young one). He may have dry mouth, headache, hypotension, weight loss, sleep disturbances, fatigue, and lowered libido. His vague aches and pains may rotate from one body site to another. Symptoms may fluctuate daily, for they are related to the diurnal rhythm. He may awaken at 3:00 a.m. or 4:00 a.m.; therefore, he does not get the required amount of sleep. He may feel worse in the morning, with symptoms improving during the day. Or the pattern may be reversed; he may be most depressed in the evening. Note the depressed insomniac's response to hypnotics, which is not the same as in other patients who suffer from sleep disturbances. Barbiturates do not help the depressed person sleep; they may increase the depth of depression and even release feelings of suicide and aggression against self.[45] The elderly person is normally depressed physically and emotionally by barbiturates; respiratory depression and confusion may be severe.

Since the slowing process is related to all body processes, the immune body system is also affected. The senior is more susceptible to illness: colds, pneumonia, ulcers, urinary tract infections, viral infections, boils, decubiti, and other infectious illnesses. The implications are grave. His resistance is already lowered by age and changed body functions; his depressed state makes him even more vulnerable to a severe and debilitating physical illness. Thus, frequent infections may be another clue to a depressive state.

Since anxiety is many times a precursor of depression, the person may describe symptoms related to anxiety, such as muscular weakness, vague aches, tightness in the chest, stomach cramps, shaking, dizziness, palpitations, lump in the throat, sweating, and diarrhea. Anxiety tends to increase as the illness progresses and is the underlying force of agitation.

The depressed senior may have hypochondriacal complaints that have no organic basis but mimic a specific illness. Since he is more prone to physical illness, his complaints should be carefully evaluated. Differential diagnosis is important, but often in the depressed patient the more you explore the symptoms, the less differentiated the illness is.[11]

The senior may deny his depressed feelings and attribute his mood to the symptoms he is experiencing. He may say, "Nurse, this pain is sure getting me down." He cannot perceive that his mood is causing his physical symptoms. He thinks that hopeless feelings are related to the lack of symptom improvement.[11]

The senior may have a *hypochondriacal preoccupation, a strong, intense, almost morbid preoccupation with health.* The preoccupation seems to be more concerned with the gastrointestinal tract and cardiovascular system.[10] The complaints may have a bizarre quality; the person says that the organs are not working right, the brain is all upset, or pain is stirring up the bowels. Many times these complaints are the beginning of *nihilistic or somatic delusions, false ideas concerning bodily function or annihilation of himself or his organs.* He may state, "My stomach is turned to stone" or "My heart is eaten away." A common statement today is, "Cancer is eating up my entire body."

Masked Symptoms

Masked or covert symptoms are those experienced by the patient but which appear to be something other than depression. Many elderly people are likely to deny any symptom of depression as unacceptable. They feel that to have an emotional problem is weak or ungodly. However, physical symptoms may be acceptable to the senior, his family, and community. How do you feel about the elderly person who complains of headache and stomach cramps? About the one you hear complaining of "feeling no good," who is crying and condemning himself? A subtle rejection is frequently noted among professionals concerning psychological symptoms, and this attitude may be found even more so among the older generation, among his friends and his family. It is no wonder that at a time when it is normal and acceptable to have physical problems, he tends to express his depression with physical complaints.

Behavior

The person's verbal response indicates level of alertness, interest, and distorted thinking. The depressed senior has little interest in his surroundings; he neglects his usual interests and responsibilities. His poverty of ideas is shown by his limited conversational response. He has difficulty with concentration and is preoccupied with himself and his feelings. At times he may become mildly aggressive or agitated, but he probably will not do anything impulsive unless it is a self-destructive act.

Agitated behavior is very common with the severely depressed elderly patient. The patient may pace, wring his hands, pick himself, beg for support or reassurance, and appear totally miserable. It is not uncommon as you try to assess or understand the symptoms that the agitated patient answers by begging you to help him to feel better. A basic problem is that in his attempts to gain relief from pain, his attention-seeking behavior pushes away the people whom he needs.

Other symptoms, not easily recognized but having their source in the core problem of depression, relate to daily living. The person might be drawn away from his religious beliefs, complain of an uninteresting job, break up relationships that have been meaningful, begin compulsive drinking or gambling, or find himself in frequent fights with friends and family members. He may be less interested in grooming and habits of body care that gave him a great deal of pleasure in the past. Some changes may be caused by the inability to concentrate or make a decision. Sense of responsibility is usually reduced and energy level is low. Usually disinterest in self relates to negative self-concept and angry feelings toward the self.

How depression can be masked by general behavior is shown by the following case:

Mr. J. M., a 70-year-old miner, was hospitalized for severe headaches and dizziness. He was receiving a thorough medical diagnostic work-up. He demanded release after a 2-week hospitalization. Since no positive findings had been discovered, he was scheduled for discharge the following day. He arose; he did not shave, and he did not eat breakfast. He dressed in old, shabby, dark clothes, left the hospital, went home, and killed himself. Other than physical complaints, the only sign of his depression was his change in dress and changed pattern of living. (Awareness of the symbolic meaning of his behavior could have spared his life.)

Feelings

Note the senior's affect. The depressed person's mood is very sad and dejected, as evidenced by his appearance and behavior. He feels irritable, humorless, apathetic, exhausted, disappointed in himself, and ashamed. He lacks self-confidence and self-respect. He states that he is worthless, empty, and a burden to everyone, and he blames himself for anything that goes wrong. He expresses ambivalence, pessimism, and hopelessness in most situations. He may express depression in the following ways:

"I feel sad." (Direct report)
"I feel heavy." (Descriptive report)
"I feel stripped of pleasure." (Action—descriptive report)
"I feel like a dragging chain." (Metaphor—descriptive report)

The depressed person may know intellectually that he loves his family, but he cannot feel love for or attachment to them. He loses caring behaviors for his spouse, relatives, friends, pets, and home. He may say, "I don't care about anything anymore." He feels no joy as he thinks of previous pleasures. He has many fears, especially of being alone. These behaviors over a period of time tend to isolate him from others.

The depressed person expresses in every way his loss of self-esteem and negative self-concept. He may state that he is empty or vacant; he is speaking of his *sense* of self. He looks at himself in the mirror with disgust. He criticizes or condemns himself for insignificant behavior. He may say, "I feel so guilty," when he has done no great misdeeds. He may have made many important contributions, but he *feels* useless. Ask him to tell you about recent events; he will select the saddest news to report. He may say, "Nothing is any good anymore. There's nothing left in life for me." He feels that he has no future and that the world has no future either. He may move beyond the negative self-feeling to self-destructive behavior.[14]

Suicidal Ideation and Behavior

Suicide is a direct, purposeful action taken by a person to end his own life. Suicide is a more significant health problem in the elderly for both sexes than it is in the younger depressives. Depression is present in 80 percent of suicidal attempts in persons over 60 years, and 12 percent of the attempters will try suicide again within 2 years, usually in an identical setting.[9, 26, 58]

Many factors contribute to suicide in the elderly: physical illness, perceived mental decline, intense loneliness, hopelessness, a deprived living situation and economic insecurity, and severe guilt reactions following loss of a loved one. Suicide may be seen as a way to rejoin deceased loved ones. The anniversary date of an important loss is frequently a time for a suicide attempt. In paranoid states the suicide may be an attempt to escape tormenting delusions. The person may attempt suicide as a way of controlling or beating death; suicide does not necessarily mean death to the person. Or the senior may try suicide in order to die while he is still physically and mentally able to be in charge of himself, especially if he faces a debilitating, terminal illness and is alone. Even if early moral and religious training taught him that suicide is wrong, his belief that he has a right to choose when and how to die may overcome his guilt feelings. The person may attempt suicide to gain attention from loved ones who have abandoned him. The most common internal conflicts in a suicidal person are those associated with murderous impulses toward a loved person arising out of actual or imagined rejection or abandonment.[53] The person who has attempted suicide before, is alcoholic or psychotic, has had recent surgery, has a depression that is lifting, is hypochondriacal, or is having sleep problems is likely to attempt suicide.[9, 25, 26, 30] The more hopeless the senior feels in any situation the more likely he is to try suicide.[4] The older white male is especially at risk because he reacts adversely to many situations that accompany aging.[6, 9]

Menninger's theory of suicidal behavior is that people have a wish for revenge, a wish to kill; a wish to be killed, with feelings of hopelessness; and fantasies of death and reunion with a wish to die.[38] A study based upon this theory reported that the first two wishes decrease with age but the third wish increases.[20]

Rarely is suicide a gesture. The senior is more likely to succeed in suicide, especially if plans include a violent method and a note is left. He is more likely to use a truly dangerous method such as taking coma-producing drugs, using cutting or piercing instruments, inhaling gas, jumping from heights, or attempting drowning.[5, 26] However, less severe attempts also occur, including subtle methods of self-destruction, such as self-neglect, refusal to eat, and withdrawal, in which the person resigns self, stoically and undramatically, to die.[54, 55]

Every person has at some time in his life thought about suicide. Some have openly stated this wish. The senior who states his wish to die is certainly high risk. He may say, "I am tired of living; I find no joy in going on; I want to die." He may cry and moan, "I am no good, I am worthless, I want to kill myself." He may state a death wish in a more subtle form, such as, "You shouldn't bother about me; I'm a burden to everyone." Or, "Don't do anything special, nurse; it's over anyway." Encourage the person to talk. After listening to cues, and when he seems less anxious, gently ask him, "Have you ever thought of taking your life?" If he answers, "Yes," ask him if he is thinking of suicide now. You will not put suicidal ideas into the person's head by stating the word death or encouraging the person to describe fully his feelings and plans. Learn of others who care for him. Your invitation to share enhances your assessment and may reduce the chance of a suicide attempt. Respond with an empathic statement so that he can see you as a helping person.

Elderly patients are usually ambivalent about the desire to die, in spite of their overt attempts. In a research study investigating communication with family members of 134 elderly persons who had succeeded in taking their own lives, 60 percent of the entire group had talked about committing suicide. One-fourth of the listeners felt the communication was not serious.[49]

If the person has a sense of ego integrity, as discussed in Chapter 11, he is prepared to defend his life against physical, social, and economic threats. Lack of ego integrity and negative self-concept cause a sense of despair, hopelessness, and depression. Suicide may then seem to be the answer.

Differentiation from Cognitive Impairment

The depressed person may be misdiagnosed as cognitively impaired, since persons with irreversible organic brain disease and depression have similar verbal response patterns and overt behaviors. The person with cognitive impairment suffers greater confusion, becomes lost in words, and is unable to respond appropriately even when given time. Memory for remote or recent events is not intact. You will observe emotional lability instead of the consistently dejected mood. Physical complaints are less prominent. Further, the person is not so self-accusatory and suicidal.[44]

NURSING DIAGNOSIS AND FORMULATION OF PATIENT CARE GOALS

Nursing Diagnosis

Your *nursing diagnosis* of *depression with or without suicidal ideation* may include the following assessments of the person:

1. Demonstrates varying degrees of altered mood state, feelings of dejection, helplessness, hopelessness, emptiness, and anger.
2. Complains of various physical symptoms and demonstrates symptoms related to the slowing process of depression, masked depression, anxiety, or agitation.
3. Demonstrates decreased interest in personal, social, spiritual, interpersonal, financial, and occupational activities.
4. Expresses varying degrees of lowered self-esteem and increased self-accusation.
5. Responds with statements of guilt and self-destructive wishes.
6. Demonstrates fatigue and low energy level in a variety of situations.

Thus, your nursing diagnosis relates to the quality, meaning, and degree of depression, which are expressed by a wide variety of signs and symptoms that are not always easily assessed.[17]

Patient Care Goals

Long-term care goals could include the following:

1. Statements and behavior demonstrate acceptance of self and a positive self-concept.
2. Behavior with others shows appropriate interdependence.
3. Statements and behavior express hope and desire to live.

Short-term goals could include:

1. Personal hygiene is managed without assistance.
2. Anger is expressed overtly toward an object that elicits the anger.
3. Physical symptoms are described less frequently and are less extensive over time.
4. Loss of or separation from loved object is worked through realistically.
5. Strengths and limits are realistically spoken of and accepted.
6. Feelings are expressed verbally to professional staff and their meanings are resolved.

You may think of other short-term goals as you care for the depressed person.

INTERVENTION

Interpersonal care, acceptance, and concern make up a major portion of intervention with the depressed senior. You must genuinely care, but you must remain objective enough so that you are not manipulated or controlled by his emotional pain as you guide him toward healthy patterns of behavior. The depressed person needs to feel that he is the center of your care but not the center of the universe. This is a difficult position to try to attain.

Self-Awareness as a Basis for Promoting the Senior's Self-Awareness

How do you feel about yourself when you are with the depressed person? How do you respond to someone who is obviously blue? How do you respond to someone who complains about many physical problems? How do you react to anger? Are you afraid of someone who is angry? Can *you* deal with anger in such a way that the depressed person will be able to accept his own anger and express it? Are you able to control your expression of elation and pleasure? Do you recognize that your optimism and cheerful statements can increase his depression? Do you attempt to define your goals for each interaction? Do you look forward to helping and listening to him? As you listen to the depressed person talk about his loss, you may feel your own unresolved losses. Or you may feel sad about your own aging or the potential loss of loved ones. Look at yourself first. If you don't, you will have difficulty helping the depressed senior look at himself.

Promote Identification and Resolution of Loss

Listen for negative feelings related to specific events or subjects. The elderly person may have suffered loss or deprivation, covered the feeling related to the loss, and forgotten or repressed the precipitating event.[10] Try to connect the present with past events. If anything significant is uncovered, talk with the patient about the event when the time is appropriate. It is not enough for *you* to be aware of his loss; the senior must also understand.

To learn that your elderly patient has lost a son, a home, or a husband may take little time. It may take much longer to prepare him to deal with the experience. Treat this suffering person tenderly. As you would not apply salt to a reddened infected wound, neither should you confront this wounded psyche with painful information too fast or without a caring attitude. The time for confronting the senior about the meaning of his loss depends on the closeness of your relationship, the nurturing attitude of others in the environment, and his personality strengths. There is probably no perfect time to talk about his feelings, but he must be able to attend. The person will not be shattered by what you say if your statement is gentle and conveys concern. Encourage the person to talk; often he will repeat the same things everytime you meet with him. But resolution of feeling is not possible until he can talk about them. Talking is difficult for this patient but eventually it provides a release.

For example, Mr. L. may know that his wife's death caused his depression, but he needs help in talking about what his wife meant to him, the role she had in his life, and how he feels about himself. He needs help in exploring new patterns of living so that he does not rigidly hold on to the depression.

Promote Expression of Anger

A critical element in the feelings of most depressed elderly people is anger. Anger may be manifested in combative, defiant, teasing, sarcastic, obstructive, passive, withdrawn, agitated, or self-destructive behavior.

Most of us usually try to avoid angry people, but encouraging the senior to talk about his angry feelings rather than act them out behaviorally is a goal in treatment. You may first have to tell the senior that you sense that he feels angry about something and that you would like to hear about it. The senior's response may be to sneer, to make a sarcastic remark denying his anger, to withdraw, or to curse. He may be unable to accept that he does feel anger. If you show acceptance of his anger and of him, wait patiently, remain close, and continue to encourage him to talk, he will probably burst forth with angry statements. Since you invited expression of anger, you must be prepared to hear it out, which can take time. Do not take his anger personally, even if he makes derogatory statements to you. Recognize the underlying influences upon his anger and that he is turning it against someone with whom he feels safe. This is not an easy process, for when the senior was growing up in our culture, he was taught to suppress anger or to express it indirectly. Indirect expression, however, does not provide for self-understanding or a full feeling of release.

After the senior has talked about his angry feelings and what he considers the cause, be calm and supportive. Do not appear critical or distant toward him for what he has said, for if you do, he will probably no longer share with you or perhaps any other professional in the future. Gently encourage him to continue exploring causes for his feelings until he can get back to the initial cause or loss. Tell him that you understand his feelings, even if the senior seems inappropriate in his response. If the person is casting blame or making unrealistic statements, you can gradually clarify them. If mutual feelings of trust, respect, and caring exist between the two of you, he will be able to listen as you present another viewpoint. You may gradually be able to help him understand how his angry behavior has kept loved ones away from him, further adding to his problems. You may suggest ways to help him reestablish relations with loved ones.

The principle of reinforcement of appropriate behavior can work over a period of time in this situation. You reinforce the person's expression of feelings by continuing to seek him out, invite his statements, and listen to him. As his anger lessens, you can suggest other ways in which he can get his needs met. You recognize verbally his attempts to change his behavior, to look at himself and others in a new way. Thus, you reinforce him to continue to grow. But he is also reinforcing himself. As he changes his responses to others, others change their responses to him in a positive direction. He begins to feel better about himself. Feelings of worthlessness and being bad or fears of aloneness diminish because others are showing care and affection. This circular process takes time and is completed to varying degrees, depending on how long and how severely the senior has been depressed. If he has been a pessimistic person with depressive tendencies all of his life, the results may not be as obvious. The senior will also have to feel motivated to change his behavior. Yet, people need people, and the depressed senior is no exception. Your concern and assistance can motivate him to try new behavior, and as he sees results and he feels better about himself, he becomes motivated from within.

Some elderly may be unable to express anger and go through the process just described, either because of personal beliefs forbidding such expression, aphasia, brain damage, or various physical, emotional, and social reasons. Here you can help him express anger through constructive activities that he can physically manage, such as hammering, painting, squeezing play-dough or clay, walking, singing, working on a loom, scrubbing floors or walls, or digging in the garden. Activity provides some release, and your attitude of respect, acceptance, encouragement, and care helps him feel better about himself. In turn, he may respond less angrily toward others.

Sometimes the senior can talk about his feelings but only indirectly. He may express anger by complaining about the food, hospital, staff, relatives, or various world events. Your helpful response will be to follow the process previously described.

Promote Resolution of Guilt

Guilt is influenced by the standards and ideals of the person. Most elderly people were raised in an environment that promoted a strict conscience. Depressed people are notorious for having strict, unrelenting rules for themselves and their lives. Thus, the elderly, depressed person looks at himself in a depreciating, accusatory manner; he blames himself for not living up to his standards of perfection and for his loss or problems. He may feel that he is being punished for being bad or worthless. He may feel that he deserves the feelings surrounding depression because he is weak or not good. It is very difficult to grow old in our society and maintain a perfectionistic attitude toward life or strict standards for the self. The person will ultimately end up feeling like an object, less than unique, and worthless if his feelings about self are dependent on what he can or should *do* instead of on what he *is* or can *be*. The anger that arises when he is unable to live up to his expectations will ultimately result in feelings of guilt.

There are times when talking about feelings of anger and thoughts about his self-expectations will alleviate the guilt. As he says the words, he may realize the futility of his strict standards and realize that lowering expectations about his activity is acceptable. He will begin to see reality in a new perspective and blame himself less for events. Your listening and realistic feedback can help the senior moderate his expectations of self and others. Your acceptance of human weakness and failure may help him to accept his own limits. The following statements will be helpful: "You are awfully hard on yourself." "You deserve better treatment than that." "You seem to be blaming yourself for just being human." Your surprised expression upon hearing the senior blame himself when he cannot do an activity any longer will help him realize that others do not expect as much of him as he does of himself. You may say, "I realize that it is difficult for you, but try not to hurt yourself for something over which you have little control." Never hesitate to give encouragement and praise for his efforts in any activities, even in personal hygiene or feeding of self.

Many times the elderly person feels that God is blaming him for his many sins and errors. Convey empathy. Confront him about his perfectionism. Speak of God's love for him. Attend to his spiritual needs yourself or seek the assistance of a clergyman. The depressed person often turns away from his religious life as his depression increases. He may feel that he is being punished. He may believe that God is a just, kind God, and that such a God would not punish him. He then reasons that since he is depressed, there must not be a God. Or the depressed senior who has always been a faithful churchgoer, who feels that he has led a religious life, may now believe that he is being punished for being good. Therefore, God is not just. He either blames God or says that God does not exist. Many seniors were taught by their religion to believe that man is a sinful creature. The depressed senior frequently feels that he is suffering because this is what he deserves, that he is being punished for the sins he committed. There may be varying degrees of added guilt caused by the recent turning away from a lifetime of religious beliefs. It is not your place to convert the senior or to tell him what to believe, but you can help him to find a comfortable and productive spiritual position. If you have an understanding of the person's religious beliefs, you may counsel him. But you must collaborate with a minister, priest, or rabbi who understands the illness of depression and can convey love rather than judgment.[56]

Increase the Senior's Self-Esteem

One of the most crucial areas is how the senior feels about himself.[37] Usually the depressed person has a damaged self-esteem; he feels that he is of no value. First, this destructive concept of self needs to be recognized by the person, if possible. You may think that the person knows how he feels about himself. He may just *feel* all the depressive feelings and not have the slightest understanding that they do not represent his *self*, what he is. The person in the depths of depression has great difficulty seeing the unreality of his thoughts. Instead, he *feels* ugly, bad, lonely, and hopeless; he feels that he does not deserve food, love, space, or life.

Remind the elderly person that most of these feelings are caused by the depressive illness. Repeatedly state that since the feelings do not represent his *true* self, he can work with you to overcome the illness and to feel better. You may say to your patient, "I understand that it is hard to recognize these feelings as the result of the depression, but try to see that many of your ideas are unfounded."

Your acceptance of the senior also conveys that he is valued. Many times, however, the senior will think that you are just being nice to him because it is your job. Yes, caring for him is your job. However, it is also your job to be honest and genuine and to do what is best for him. You can help him to trust you, accept your humanness, and thus grow to accept himself.

Insight comes when he can appreciate you as a helping, unique person, not as a god or all-knowing supernurse, and appreciate himself as a worthwhile aging person, not a helpless, useless person. Such understanding comes gradually as you listen to his many physical complaints, provide needed physical care, convey your honest feelings to him, and spontaneously share a joke, a sunset, or a holiday. Through experiences of human warmth the person can be helped to accept his own human dignity and worth. In turn, he trusts and respects others.

You do not help the patient gain self-esteem by putting your arms around him and telling him that you love him. If you compliment him too early, he feels overwhelmed and cannot accept your warmth. He feels that you are not being honest. The repeated honest appraisal of his strengths through the recognition of an activity he has done well helps improve his feelings about himself. Watch the senior's reaction when you recognize his strengths. He may blush, frown, look away, or laugh. If he accepts your statement without rebuff, you will know that he is beginning to accept your feedback. Move ahead cautiously, always evaluating the effect of your interactions on him. After a while he will say, "If you think I'm O.K., maybe I am." Eventually he will feel positive about himself even when no one is continually supporting him. At that point he has recovered from his illness.

Attend to Physical Symptoms

Whether or not the depressed senior's physical symptoms are directly related to the depression or are a manifestation of his denial and masked depression, he is frequently very disturbed and preoccupied with them. His pain or physical problem is real to him. Usually, the patient does not understand the relationship between his physical complaint and his depression.

At first, listen to his complaints fully and intently. This may help you establish rapport. Also help the senior to be as comfortable physically as possible. Your attention to his needs conveys understanding and hope. Tell him that the physical symptoms can be a manifestation of depression and that there is a good chance he will feel better again. Tell him that by your both working together, many of his symptoms will leave. Get him to feel that you are his ally, a partner in his care. Then the emotional emphasis related to his symptoms should begin.

A behavior modification approach may be used here because repetitious talking about symptoms does not help the patient. His expression of feelings and interest in activities, people, and living is reinforced with positive responses. Preoccupation with himself and bodily symptoms is given no response or only minimal matter-of-fact attention. Be careful that your responses are not phony or that you do not become mechanized in your reaction to the patient. You will need to give treatment to some of his symptoms, but do not focus on them. Further, do not ask "How are you?" as an opening remark because a question like that only encourages his statements of physical complaints. Instead, try to direct the senior's conversation to his emotional state, to important past experiences, or involvement with present interests.

Your goal of emphasizing the emotional impact upon the person's life does not mean that the physical areas should be ignored. Expert care should be given to all areas of difficulty. The senior may be too depressed or listless to eat or too agitated to take the time to eat, or he may refuse food in a suicidal attempt or gesture. Organic changes may result. Record the amount of intake, and determine the presence of malnutrition. Observe his ability to chew. Offer the senior his favorite foods in an attractive setting and sit with him while he eats. Often as you drink a beverage, he too will begin to eat as if he is imitating you. An elderly woman who has prepared meals throughout her lifetime might find it stimulating to assist in preparing the meal with someone's assistance. If the person is in his own home, a meals-on-wheels program may be acceptable. Emphasize having a certain time each day to eat; ask the elderly person when he has the best appetite. Encourage him to set up a timetable around his eating habits. Small, frequent meals may be helpful, for he may not be able to eat a large quantity at once. Give nutritional supplementary feedings. Encourage a well-balanced diet with plenty of fluids. Evaluate the need for natural laxatives (raw or bulk foods) since constipation is a common complaint. Encourage physical exercise and activity early in the day if possible. Encourage him to do certain chores or activities to increase his appetite. To promote adequate nutrition, you must individualize the care according to the senior's desires, needs, and activity.

Many depressed seniors are preoccupied with defecation and bowel problems. Many experience irregularity and constipation because of the slowed body processes. The lack of activity and minimal fluid intake increase the problem. Regression in some oldsters can cause soiling, incontinence, or retention. The manic or agitated depressive may be too active or preoccupied to take the time for elimination. A record should be kept of urinary and bowel elimination; the senior may be able to keep the record himself. From this record determine the person's normal habits of elimination. Ask how the person handled elimination problems in the past.

Laxatives and enemas should be used only when necessary because of their habit-forming effect. Further, consider the meaning of the enema to the depressed person. He may view the procedure as help from a concerned staff. Or he may feel that the enema is a well-deserved punishment, an invasion, a sexual attack, or a means of control. Enemas may become a part of a delusional system. He may say such things as, "My bowels are stone and closed; that tube will kill me." Feelings of fear and suspicion can be the result of a staff concerned only with the physical problem and the means to solve it. The more the patient is made a partner in solving the problem, the more he will feel in control.

A common symptom of depression is sleep disturbance. The severely depressed person may have difficulty falling asleep or he may wake up early; the agitated person may be too active to rest. Explore usual sleep patterns and sleep difficulties. Ask the patient what sleeping means to him. He may fear falling asleep. Many times he will dream. Ask him what he dreams about. If his dreams are filled with fears and are laden with emotion, perhaps talking about some of his fears will be helpful. Discuss with him ways to help him sleep. He will have to adjust his schedule to meet his needs. He should be sufficiently tired, but not too exhausted to sleep. He may need a rest period during the day. Light, rather than strenuous, activity in the evening may prevent exhaustion. If he is able, he might adjust his own environment to enhance rest and sleep. He may like a quiet room, soft music, or a lighted or darkened room. You may help him with muscle relaxation techniques. Or you might try a warm bath, milk, tea, soup, or whatever the patient has used before. Talk softly to the senior in a relaxing tone. Touch soothingly. A backrub is frequently very effective in promoting rest and sleep.

Sedatives and hypnotics should be used as a last resort. Barbiturates should be avoided in the elderly because of central nervous system depression. Barbiturates depress respirations, which are often already compromised in the depressed elderly person. Barbiturates cause confusion and prolonged drowsiness, often the following morning after a night of restless, dream-filled sleep. Paradoxical stimulation may occur so that the person is awake and agitated all night. Other dangers include: (1) falls or incontinence because of the lethargic, confused state; (2) headache and irritability the following day; (3) fearfulness because of the nightmares that may occur with drugged sleep; (4) tolerance so that an increasing dosage is needed; (5) allergic reactions; and (6) dependency and addiction.

A safe sedative for the elderly is an antihistamine such as Benadryl, which has the normal side effect of drowsiness. Some doctors recommend giving the full day's dosage of a tranquilizer at bedtime so that the person sleeps well, awakens refreshed, and remains tranquil during the following day. Table 21.2 summarizes the commonly used nonbarbiturate sedatives and related nursing responsibilities.

Certainly nursing measures to induce sleep are preferable to the use of drugs.

TABLE 21.2   Nonbarbiturate Sedatives/Hypnotics for the Elderly

Drug	Dose	Side Effects	Nursing Responsibilities
Glutethimide (Doriden)	0.1–0.5 gm per os	Nausea. Nonpruritic skin rash. Headache. Dizziness. Stupor. Peripheral collapse rarely occurs.	Use nursing measures to prepare patient for sleep. May be given late at night because of short action and minimal hangover. Assist patient if he gets up after taking medication. Give judiciously; may be habit-forming. An overdose may cause deep sleep or coma lasting up to 72 hours. May not be suitable for suicidal patients.
Methaqualone (Quaalude)	150–300 mg orally	Mild and transient side effects. Headache. Dizziness. Nausea and epigastric distress. Dry mouth.	Prepare for sleep. Give only at bedtime. Limit activity after medication is taken; assist as necessary. May potentiate suicidal tendencies.
Ethchloroynal (Placidyl)	100–500 mg orally	Mild side effects. Bad dreams. Headaches. Ataxia. Dizziness. Nausea and vomiting. Unpleasant taste in mouth. Confusion.	Prepare for sleep. Store medication in dark, tight container. Give glass of fluids with drug to delay absorption and minimize dizziness or confusion. Discontinue drug slowly to prevent untoward effects.

Encourage General Hygiene

Personal appearance becomes disheveled and hygiene is omitted because of decreased interest in the body, lowered energy level, feelings of worthlessness, less interest in the reactions of others, agitation with hyperactivity, and decreased self-esteem. Although interest in appearance and hygiene will return when the depression lifts, the feelings of self-esteem and worth are related to appearance and cleanliness. To encourage a neat appearance seems to encourage the recovery process. A severely depressed senior will be unable to care for himself and will need you to care for his basic needs and make decisions for him. At first you may have to give oral hygiene, hair care, nail care, the bath, apply lotion to dry skin, and protect pressure areas. You may have to choose and assemble hygiene articles and clothing. Work through your feelings about caring physically for the dependent adult. Your approach must be nonpunitive; encourage self-directive, independent behaviors when the patient is able.

Encourage Activities

Your patient may be so caught up with himself and his own sorrow that there is little energy left to be involved with others in group activities. The relationship with the nurse can stimulate interest in others. Do not become so involved in an activity that you forget that the project is only a means to an end. The activity is the means of establishing a relationship, investing interest in someone other than self, or increasing self-esteem through a job well done. If the ultimate goal is making a doll, playing a game, or taking a walk, then nothing much is being accomplished.

Choose activities that reflect the senior's interest. If he is severely depressed, he has a short attention span and is easily fatigued; thus, the activities should be simple. Many times the person will want to make something for someone else—a granddaughter or son. Some seniors become involved willingly in a menial task because it helps to displace anger and guilt. If the patient is severely agitated, the activity should productively use restless energy, such as tearing rags to make a rug or making a flower garden for later bouquets for the day room. If the patient is restless, the activity should not be stimulating or overwhelming and it should have definite limits. In every activity encourage the senior to contact others in order to counteract the loneliness so prevalent in the depressed elderly person.

Responsibility with Somatic Treatments

Part of your responsibility in care of the depressed senior is to assist with somatic treatments, such as electroshock treatment. Convulsive therapy began in 1927 with the use of Metrazol given intravenously to produce a seizure. It was helpful, but many complications and dangers existed. In 1938 an electric current was found to produce the same results but with far fewer difficulties. Electroshock (EST) or electroconvulsive (ECT) therapy has been a major procedure in treatment of depression ever since.[12] The treatment consists of applying a current of 110 volts, 20 to 30 milliamperes, to the temperofrontal region of the brain until there is evidence of a grand mal seizure. A short-acting barbiturate, such as sodium pentothal or Brevital, and a muscle relaxant, usually Anectine, are given intravenously to reduce the severity of the muscular reaction. The nervous system reacts to the stimulation with both the tonic first stage, and the clonic second stage, of seizure. Usually, the first stage is noted by facial twitching or the curling of the toes. Little more than a tremor follows. The electric stimulus causes unconsciousness; however, the suffocating effect of the curare-like medication, Anectine, creates great fear and anxiety; thus, sodium pentothal or Brevital is given. A physician is usually present during this procedure; however, many times nurses are responsible for administering the treatment. Usually, the nurse is specially prepared and has experience in emergency treatments.

The risks are few; 1 in 25,000 has an untoward reaction. Age is not a contraindication. If the senior is suicidal, severely depressed, or agitated, the physician may order this treatment. Cardiac symptoms, hypertension, phlebitis, aneurysm, multiple sclerosis, and increased intracranial pressure are contraindications.

The person must have a thorough physical examination, an electrocardiogram, and a chest X-ray prior to treatment.

Major complications of ECT in the elderly are fractured bones and strained or sprained muscles. Fractures are usually caused by the strength and weight of the large muscles jerking the bone in the spasm of the seizure or result from the osteoporosis common in the elderly. Cardiac arrhythmias are another major area of difficulty, especially in people with a prior history of cardiac disease. The other complications are memory loss and confusion, depending on the amount and number of treatments. The closer the treatments, the greater the confusion. Confusion and some memory loss are always expected with ECT; reassure the person and family that the confusion is temporary. Memory usually returns in a week or two after treatment; however, sometimes impairments last from 6 to 12 months. Some individuals complain of permanent loss and reduced learning capacity.

You must give supportive care before and after the treatment. The older person may ask many questions about the treatment and why it is necessary. Tell him generally what to expect. However, no one really knows why depression lifts after EST. Listen to his fears and try to alleviate his anxiety. Touch is reassuring to the person, and he may request that you go with him to the area where the treatment is given. Hold his hand and talk to him until he is asleep. The patient sleeps for a short time after treatment. During this 15- to 30-minute period, pulse, respirations, and blood pressure are taken until the patient is responding and breathing regularly. As the patient awakens, he will be hazy and confused; this regressed period is an ideal opportunity for nurturing. Further emotional support is needed until he fully awakens, is relaxed and feels more secure.[10]

Drug Therapy

Amphetamines were widely used in the past as a stimulant for depressed patients. They were habit-forming and temporary in effect. In 1950 reserpine was given to patients with high blood pressure, and they also became more calm. Iproniazid given to patients for tuberculosis was observed to produce euphoria. Research indicated that reserpine depleted the level of neurotransmitters while Iproniazid increased their level. Later, other major classes of drugs were introduced: phenothiazides, monoamine oxidase inhibitors, and tricyclic compounds. Monoamine oxidase inhibitors break down norepinephrine, a neurotransmitter, and inhibit an enzyme called monoamine oxidase. Tricyclic imipramine prevents the breakdown of serotonin, the other major neurotransmitter.[5] The actions of these drugs are still not clearly understood, but many antidepressants are prescribed annually. However, the effects are established; the most popular drugs for the elderly are the tricyclic derivatives Elavil and Tofranil. Antidepressant effects occur after a waiting period of 10 to 14 days. The monoamine oxidase inhibitors are not recommended for use with the elderly because of the side effects. Table 21.3 summarizes the tricyclic derivatives commonly given, side effects, and nursing responsibilities.

Lithium carbonate has been used effectively with elderly people with bipolar depression alternating with hypomanic states. Blood levels should be carefully monitored. Few adverse reactions occur when serum lithium levels are below 1.5 mEq/1 liter of blood.

Prevent Suicidal Behavior

Your supportive, warm relationship to the elderly senior is the greatest deterrent to suicide. The more involved the senior can be with you as a person, the more you convey wanting to save his life, the less the chance that he will take his life.

Listen to him, try to see life as he sees it, hear his anger, and give direct, structured support. Let him know that you understand that he is suffering and that life seems so painful that he wants to end it. Tell him that you do not think that he is a bad person because he is thinking of suicide, and tell him that you recognize these ideas as part of his illness. Convey the thought that you care about him, perceive his strengths, want to help him, and that together the two of you can work to improve his situation. You may need to make yourself available by phone as well as directly.

Consider any statement about suicide from the elderly as a cry for help.

TABLE 21.3   **Antidepressants: Tricyclic Derivatives**

Drug	Dosage*	Side Effects	Nursing Responsibilities
Amitriptyline (Elavil)	25–50 mg orally 2 to 4 times daily	This classification of drugs may cause dry mouth, nausea and vomiting, constipation, weight gain, urinary frequency, confusion, insomnia, dizziness, hypotension, tachycardia, arrhythmias, tremor, bone marrow depression, agranulocytosis, jaundice, and Parkinsonism.	Observe for changes in patient's mood while drug takes effect. Note suicidal ideas during therapeutic lag. Teach patient about side effects. Teach mouth care and use of mints, gum, or ice chips for dry mouth. Check bowel and bladder elimination. Weigh weekly. Record intake and output. Use safety precautions. Take vital signs daily. Observe for early signs of granulocytosis: sore throat, fever, and malaise. Take monthly blood counts. Observe for jaundice of sclera and skin. Check with physician if signs of bone marrow depression, liver damage, or Parkinsonism. Do not administer with monoamine oxidase inhibitors.
Desipramine hydrochloride (Norpramin)	25–300 mg; 150 mg average; onset in 3–5 days		
Doxepin (Sinequan)	25–300 mg; 75 mg average		
Nortriptyline (Aventyl)	25–300 mg; 150 mg average		
Protriptyline (Vivactil)	5–60 mg; 30 mg average		
Imipramine (Tofranil)	25 mg orally 1 to 3 times daily		

* Smaller doses may be indicated for the elderly.

Give any gesture or statement serious consideration. Realize that while the senior is overtly withdrawing from any help, at the same time he is hoping that someone will find the answers to his problems. Getting the senior to say the words that he has kept hidden often helps him feel relieved. And his statements also give you a chance to convey your intention to help and your respect for him as a person. Often you can stimulate others in his environment to show more interest. You may also be able to secure practical help to overcome various economic, social, or health problems.[42]

If the suicidal senior tells you that he will contact you when he feels the impulse to end his life and prior to carrying out any plan, you have a safeguard against any suicidal attempt. A study of 600 persons who indicated to medical professionals that they had decided not to carry through their suicide plans showed no fatalities over a 5-year span.[18]

Certainly safeguards need to be taken to decrease dangers in the senior's environment. At the same time, do not dwell on or be obsessive about these dangers. It is impossible to have the senior's surroundings completely free of objects with which he could commit suicide. Your best safeguard is your relationship with the person. Your next safeguards are your observation and caring. You can also carry out unobtrusive measures. Make your rounds at different times, not just at predictable hours. Keep the senior with someone or in the group whenever possible. Observe carefully that he swallows his medications. Many patients pretend to swallow pills but actually accumulate them in order to have them available for an overdose. Listen carefully for clues to his intentions. Even though you are cautious and take necessary precautions, you must also convey that you trust him. Discuss his feelings and thoughts with him frankly and on a continuing basis.

The elderly people who live alone, are depressed, and have little contact with helping people are the ones who are more likely to commit suicide. A community service program could reduce suicide in the elderly.[14] In an English community a program was begun to give a variety of assistance to the suicide-prone senior. The suicide rate dropped over 60 percent.[57] Some of the community resources discussed in Chapter 7 could be developed in order to help all seniors stay involved in life. Certainly any depressed person who has been hospitalized needs follow-up services after discharge to maintain improvement.

Work with the Family and Health Team

Previous chapters have discussed the importance of working with family members and how to include them in care. Such intervention is equally important for the depressed person. Further, no care plan is successful unless all members of the health team who have contact with the patient, including home health care personnel, can plan and work together. When staff members share their assessments and suggestions for intervention, the patient and each staff member benefits. The patient is not distressed by inconsistency or an inappropriate referral. Staff members also have a better understanding of the person and what they are doing.

EVALUATION

Although you cannot presume to make up for the many losses experienced by the person in later maturity, in a symbolic and practical way you can fill in some of the gaps.

Evidence of your effectiveness with the depressed senior is shown in various behaviors. He is increasingly interested in the relationship; he may ask questions about your life, partly from curiosity and partly from wanting to reach out. Answer his questions briefly and then redirect the conversation to him. He will show renewed interest in his surroundings and community events, his personal appearance, group activity, and family life. He will look less dejected and anxious and make fewer or no comments about physical symptoms. He will be alert and mentally active. He will make fewer self-depreciating remarks. He will smile, laugh, or tell a joke.

Expect change to be gradual. At times he will be less depressed; at other times he will relapse into depression.

Determine your attitude toward him and his progress. You should be able to accept relapse and to avoid giving excessive approval when depression lifts.

REFERENCES

1. AMERICAN PSYCHIATRIC ASSOCIATION, Committee on Nomenclature and Statistics, *Diagnostic and Statistical Manual of Mental Disorders II*. Washington, D.C.: American Psychiatric Association, 1968.

2. ANTHONY, JAMES, and THERESE BENEDEK, eds., *Depression During the Life Cycle*. Boston: Little, Brown & Company, 1975.

3. BANKS, SUSAN, "Agitated Depression," *Nursing Times*, 69: (September 27, 1973), 1250–51.

4. BECK, AARON, *Depression, Causes and Treatment*. Philadelphia: University of Pennsylvania Press, 1967.

5. BECK, A.T., *et al.*, "Hopelessness and Suicidal Behavior," *Journal of American Medical Association*, 234: (December 15, 1975), 1146–49.

6. BENSON, R., and D. BRODIE, "Suicide by Overdoses of Medicine Among the Aged," *Journal of American Geriatric Society*, 23: (July, 1975), 304–8.

7. BISHOP, SUSAN, "Depression," *Nursing Times*, 71: (October 2, 1975), 1567–69.

8. BREARLEY, PAUL, "The Deprivation Syndrome," *Nursing Times*, 71: (November 27, 1975), 1914–15.

9. BRODEN, ALEXANDER, "Reaction to Loss in the Aged," in *Loss and Grief: Psychological Management in Medical Practice*, eds. B. Schoenberg, A. Carr, D. Peretz, and A. Kutscher. New York: Columbia University Press, 1970, pp. 199–217.

10. BURGESS, ANN, and AARON LAZARE, *Psychiatric Nursing in the Hospital and the Community*. Englewood Cliffs, N.J.: Prentice-Hall, Inc., 1976.

11. BUSSE, EWALD, and ERIC PFEIFFER, *Mental Illness in Later Life*. Washington, D.C.: American Psychiatric Association, 1973.

12. BUTLER, ROBERT, and MYRNA LEWIS, *Aging and Mental Health*. St. Louis: The C. V. Mosby Company, 1977.

13. CASSIDY, W., N. FLANAGAN, M. SPELLMAN, and M. COHEN, "Clinical Observations in Manic-Depressive Disease," *Journal of American Medical Association*, 164: (1957), 1535–46.

14. COBAIN, WILLIAM, "Depression in the Elderly—Treat It Actively," *Consultant*, 15: (February, 1975), 77–79.

15. COMMER, LEONARD, *Up From Depression*. New York: Simon & Schuster, 1969.

16. "Coping with Depression," *Newsweek*, January 8, 1973, 51–54.

17. CRARY, WILLIAM, and GERALD CRARY, "Depression," *American Journal of Nursing*, 73: No. 3 (1973), 472–75.

18. DRYE, R., R. GOULDING, and M. GOULDING, "No Suicide Decisions: Patient Monitoring of Suicidal Risk," *American Journal of Psychiatry*, 130: (1973), 171.

19. FANN, WILLIAM, JEANINE WHELESS, and BRUCE RICHMAN, "Treating the Aged with Psychotropic Drugs," *The Gerontologist*, 16: No. 4 (1976), 322–27.

20. FARBEROW, N., and E. SCHNEIDMAN, eds., *The Cry for Help*. New York: McGraw-Hill Book Company, 1965.

21. FLOYD, GLORIA JO, "Nursing Management of the Suicidal Patient," *Journal of Psychiatric Nursing*, 13: No. 2 (1975), 23–26.

22. FLYNN, GERTRUDE, "The Development of the Psychoanalytic Concept of Depression," *Journal of Psychiatric Nursing and Mental Health Services*, 6: No. 3 (1968), 138–49.

23. FREUD, SIGMUND, *Mourning and Melancholia in Collected Papers*, Vol. 4. London: Hogarth Press, Ltd., 1946, 152–70.

24. FROST, MONICA, "Depression—the Mental Cold," *Nursing Mirror*, 137: (1973), 46–47.

25. FULTON, R., and G. GEIS, *Death and Identity*. New York: John Wiley & Sons, Inc., 1965.

26. GAGE, FRANCES, "Suicide in the Aged," *American Journal of Nursing*, 71: No. 11 (1971), 2153–55.

27. GODBER, COLIN, "The Confused Elderly," *Nursing Times*, 72: (July 15, 1976), Supplement VII–X.

28. GRAMLICH, EDWIN, "Recognition and Management of Grief in Elderly Patients," *Geriatrics*, 23: (July, 1968), 87–92.

29. GREENACRE, PHYLLIS, *Affective Disorders*. New York: International Universities Press, Inc., 1953.

30. KAPLAN, OSCAR, ed., *Mental Disorder in Later Life*. Stanford, Calif.: Stanford University Press, 1956.

31. KICEY, CAROLYN, "Catecholamines and Depression: A Physiological Theory of Depression," *American Journal of Nursing*, 74: No. 11 (1974), 2018–20.

32. KLINE, N., "Practical Management of Depression," *Journal of American Medical Association*, 190: (1964), 732–40.

33. KRAEPELIN, EMIL, *Manic-Depressive Insanity and Paranoia*, trans. R. Mary Barclay and George Robertson. Edinburgh: E. & S. Livingstone, 1921, reprint 1976.

34. LEONARD, CALISTA V., "Treating the Suicidal Patient: A Communication Approach," *Journal of Psychiatric Nursing*, 13: No. 2 (1975), 19–22.

35. LEWIS, A., "Melancholia: A Historical Review," *The State of Psychiatry: Essays and Addresses*. New York: Science House, 1967.

36. LYONS, D. C., "Endogenous Depression," *Nursing Mirror*, 139: (October 17, 1974), 93–94.

37. MACKINNON, ROGER, and ROBERT MICHELS, *The Psychiatric Interview in Clinical Practice*. Philadelphia: W. B. Saunders Company, 1971.

38. MENNINGER, KARL, *Psychoanalytic Aspects of Depression*. Springfield, Ill.: Charles C Thomas, Publisher, 1960.

39. MITCHELL, ROSS, "Depression," *Nursing Times*, 20: (July 11, 1974), 1085–87.

40. MYERS, J., D. SHELDON, and S. ROBINSON, "A Study of 138 Elderly First Admissions," *American Journal of Psychiatry*, 120: (1963), 244–49.

41. NEYLAN, MARGARET, "The Depressed Patient," *The American Journal of Nursing*, 61: No. 7 (1971), 77–78.

42. PAYNE, EDMUND, "Depression and Suicide," in *Modern Perspectives in the Psychiatry of Old Age*, ed. John Howells. New York: Brunner/Mazel, 1975, pp. 290–310.

43. PFEIFFER, ERIC, "What to do About Mental Disorders of the Elderly," *Modern Hospitals*, 2: (August, 1974), 57–61.

44. ———, "Psychotherapy with the Elderly Patients," in *Geriatric Psychiatry,* ed. Leopold Bellak and Taksoz Karasu. New York: Grune & Stratton, 1976, pp. 199–220.

45. PITT, BRICE, *Psychogeriatrics, An Introduction to the Psychiatry of Old Age*. Edinburgh: Churchill Livingstone, 1974.

46. *Psychology Encyclopedia*. Guilford, Conn.: The Dushkin Publishing Group, Inc., 1973, p. 80.

47. RESNIK, H., and JOEL M. CANTOR, "Suicide and Aging," *Journal of the American Geriatric Society*, 18: (February, 1970), 152–58.

48. ROBERTS, ROSEMARY, "Senile Dementia and Depression, and Rehabilitation of the Patient," *Nursing Times*, 22: (December 4, 1975), 1931–33.

49. ROBINS, E., *et al.*, "The Communication of Suicide Intent," *American Journal of Psychiatry*, 115: (1959), 724.

50. RODMAN, MORTON, and DOROTHY SMITH, *Clinical Pharmacology in Nursing*. Philadelphia: J. B. Lippincott Company, 1974.

51. SCHAPIRA, KURT, "The Masks of Depression," *Nursing Mirror*, 140: (June 19, 1975), 46–48.

52. SCHWARTZMAN, SYLVIA, "Anxiety and Depression in the Stroke Patient: A Nursing Challenge," *Journal of Psychiatric Nursing*, 14: No. 4 (1976), 13–17.

53. STAFFORD, LINDA, "Depression and Self-destructive Behavior," *Journal of Psychiatric Nursing*, 14: No. 4 (1976), 37–40.

54. STOTSKY, BERNARD, *The Elderly Patient*. New York: Grune & Stratton, 1968.

55. ———, "Psychiatric Aspects of Maintenance Care of Aged Patients," in *Maintenance Therapy for the Geriatric Patient*, eds. Jacob Rudd and Reuben Macgolin. Springfield, Ill.: Charles C Thomas, Publisher, 1968.

56. TRAVELBEE, JOYCE, *Intervention in Psychiatric Nursing*. Philadelphia: F. A. Davis Company, 1969.

57. WALK, D., "Suicide and Community Care," *British Journal of Psychiatry*, 113: (1967), 1381–91.

58. WEISS, J., "Suicide in the Aged," in *Suicidal Behaviors: Diagnosis and Management*, ed. H. Resnik. Boston: Little, Brown & Company, 1968, pp. 255–67.

59. "What You Should Know About Mental Depression," *U.S. News and World Report,* September 9, 1974, 37–40.

60. WOLFF, KURT, *The Emotional Rehabilitation of the Geriatric Patient*. Springfield, Ill.: Charles C Thomas, Publisher, 1970.

61. WOODRUFF, ROBERT A., DONALD GOODWIN, and SAMUEL GUZE, *Psychiatric Diagnosis*. New York: Oxford University Press, 1974.

withdrawal and the schizophrenic syndrome in later maturity

Study of this chapter will enable you to:

1. Discuss the continuum of withdrawn behavior and the many situations in which the elderly person may experience withdrawal.

2. Explore the dynamics of withdrawal behavior.

3. Relate withdrawn behavior to the schizophrenic process.

4. Assess symptoms of extreme withdrawal in a senior.

5. Formulate patient care goals and a care plan for the withdrawn senior and individualize the care plan for his unique level of withdrawal and regression.

6. Adapt the principles of communication and relationship to meet the needs of the schizophrenic elderly person.

7. Intervene, working with the senior individually and as a team member, to change the senior's behavior to a higher developmental level.

8. Compare the effects of a supportive environment versus a nonsupportive environment on the senior.

9. Help the family to understand and work with the withdrawn senior member.

10. Evaluate the effectiveness of your care by noting the change in the senior's behavior.

22

WITHDRAWAL: A CONTINUUM

Withdrawal as a Part of Daily Life

Withdrawal is an adaptive or coping mechanism that involves physically pulling away from or psychologically losing interest in an anxiety-producing situation, person, or stressful environment. Examples of this behavior include the child who consistently plays alone instead of with a friend, the adolescent who becomes absorbed in reading instead of being involved in a party, the young adult who jogs to avoid personal contact with others, or the recluse who shuts windows and locks doors to close his life to the world. Everyone will at times withdraw by going on a vacation or to the beach or by reading a book instead of seeking the company of others. But when this pattern is used to distance or isolate the self from people or stressful situations, the withdrawal behavior becomes unhealthy.

The elderly person may withdraw after a series of losses, pulling back in isolation and apathy with a "who cares" attitude. Initially during the grieving process, a normal period of withdrawal occurs; the individual avoids contacts with others. After working through the loss and grief, the senior is ready to invest in other people and interests. But he may fear another involvement and pull back from the risk of being hurt again.

The senior who has been an active person usually returns to an active life after loss, getting busy with cleaning or chores previously ignored and being interested first in objects, plants, or animals. He moves more cautiously into new friendships with people. He may spend time recalling past experiences and memories, not as a reminiscing or life review process, but as a pleasurable fantasy to avoid the present. But the time comes when the senior has to decide whether he wishes to continue a life of self-absorption or to again reach out to other people. If he chooses to remain isolated and consider only his own needs, as time passes he will become more self-centered, alone, despairing, and withdrawn.

Withdrawal as a Part of Illness

Since human beings need to be involved with other people to gain inner happiness, the isolated person is usually bitter and unhappy. Withdrawn behavior may be found in a variety of unhappy people and is a common behavior in a variety of mental disturbances.

For example, the chronically depressed person discussed in Chapter 21 devalues and depreciates himself, feels that he is not worth others' affections, and withdraws. He may give up so many attachments that his attitude hastens death. He may even choose death by suicide.

The hypochondriacal person withdraws into constant preoccupation with his body and its functions. In his self-absorption he loses self-respect. He regresses into the helpless child position, suffering with a variety of infirmities. He waits to be cared for by others. He blames his many illnesses for his failures and his deteriorating relations with others. His behavior causes others to reciprocally withdraw as they become disinterested in his constant complaining and moaning. Friends and relatives pull back from involvement and allow him to suffer alone.

The narcissistic, extremely self-centered, proud, and selfish senior also uses the withdrawal pattern. He has probably always been self-centered, seeking recognition or approval from the external environment but giving little to it. He has little or no energy left to love or feel affection for anyone. The cool, detached style is a cover-up for being easily hurt.

Neurosis in the senior may be manifested by a variety of symptoms: anxiety and withdrawal are common features. In all probability this withdrawal pattern has been a predominant feature in the individual's life for years. Through the years he uses more and more defensive mechanisms to save his self-esteem and to cope with the stresses of living. Gradually, he retreats into apathy, seclusiveness, or neurotic withdrawal. The neurotic retreats after minimal social contacts and waits for support from others. He is very aware of and uncomfortable from his symptoms and anxiety; he longs for contact with others yet continues to live his life in the same self-defeating manner.

An elderly person suffering from organic and intellectual decline frequently withdraws from others in the face of his frustration, embarrassment, and growing distress. Of course, the premorbid personality and characteristic defensive style determine his coping behaviors, but a common behavior is that of withdrawal. He stays home more, avoids contacts with family members, and lives in secrecy.

At the farthest end of the withdrawal continuum is the isolated, disengaged individual who lives in his own world of fantasy and autism. The person regresses or decompensates to an early phase of development that is comparable to the phase in which the child had difficulty perceiving the self as "me" or the outside environment as "not me." This autistic, daydreaming state can become the decompensated, regressed state of schizophrenia.

THE SCHIZOPHRENIC PROCESS

What Is Schizophrenia?

Schizophrenia is a severe psychotic disorder that affects the mood, regulation of emotion, thought process, and behavior. Schizophrenia affects the total personality integrity.[10] It is a long-term illness, sometimes called *chronic schizophrenia, process schizophrenia, nuclear schizophrenia,* or *nonremitting schizophrenia.* The prognosis is considered poor. Less severe or less chronic forms of the illness are differentiated as schizophreniform and may be identified as *schizoaffective, remitting acute schizophrenia,* or *reactive schizophrenia.*[19,28] Schizophrenia is thought of as a variety of illnesses because of the diversity of symptoms, etiologic factors, and treatment approaches. Schizophrenia may be found to be a number of distinct functional disorders.

Schizophrenia was first systematically described in 1896 by Emil Kraepelin. He called the behaviors and symptoms *dementia praecox,* meaning a deteriorated, hopeless condition with poor prognosis. He divided the behaviors and symptoms into four major disease types: simple, catatonic, hebephrenic, and paranoid.[5]

The term *schizophrenia* was first used by Bleuler in 1911 to emphasize the schism or splitting-off of the mind between the functions of feeling and thinking.[4] Many people falsely think of schizophrenia as the splitting of the personality into two parts; the term actually was meant to describe the disorganization of the thinking and emotional processes.[17]

Bleuler also set up criteria—primary and secondary symptoms—still used today for diagnosis of schizophrenia. The primary symptoms are denoted by the four A's: (1) autism, (2) ambivalence, (3) affective disturbance, and (4) associational disturbance. Secondary symptoms include: (1) illusions, (2) delusions, (3) hallucinations, (4) motor symptoms, (5) withdrawal syndrome, and (6) lack of touch with reality.[4]

Sigmund Freud and Kraepelin believed that schizophrenia had a poor prognosis because the person could not develop a relationship or transference phenomenon. Later therapists challenged their pessimism. After World War II psychoanalytic therapists such as Sullivan, Fromm-Reichmann, Rosen, Lidz, and others worked with schizophrenic patients with commitment, optimism, and greater prognostic success.

Etiology

Almost every conceivable cause has been given for schizophrenia. The psychosocial and organic or biological theorists have all produced material to substantiate their stands. Organic theory includes genetic predisposition and biochemical, endocrine, and neurological factors.[23] Psychodynamic theorists hypothesize the cause to be a psychic conflict, much like the conflict causing neurosis but more severe, or an ego or personality defect caused by organic, neurophysiological, neurobehavioral, or environmental factors. Between these two extremes are many other positions.[27]

West and Flinn integrate the various models of etiology. They feel that people who become schizophrenic are highly vulnerable to stress in the internal and external environments. Causes of stress include ecological, developmental, learning, hereditary, and neurophysiological.[27]

Most authors agree that schizophrenia is a multifactor illness and may have a variety of causes, especially in late life. Throughout this book many of the factors causing the senior to be vulnerable are discussed.

Why Now?

Schizophrenia is normally thought of as a disorder of the adolescent or young adult years, although it can begin at any age. Butler states that in his experience he rarely saw a newly developed schizophrenic disorder in an older person.[7] Most writers consider that the elderly schizophrenic has been a chronic schizophrenic patient who in the past two decades has been maintained on phenothiazines or with close supervision in the community or nursing home. The aging process may have caused a further deterioration in the disease process.

However, some persons become severely withdrawn schizophrenics for the first time in late life. The schizoid personality intensifies as time passes and more stresses are encountered, so that the senior may regress into an autistic state and develop schizophrenia.[25] Yet, the schizoid personality, that aloof, distant person, has a protection during the senior years. Since he has lived uninvolved with people, he is protected from the loss of loved ones in late life. Another possibility is that a progressive decompensation occurs after the middle years if the losses that occur in the middle years and thereafter are not resolved. The person becomes heavy with conflicts, self-absorbed, hypochondriacal, withdrawn, and disengaged. Finally, if regression is severe, the senior may further decompensate into a psychotic schizophrenic state. The person who becomes schizophrenic in late life is probably the person who has adjusted poorly to life all along. Somehow he managed earlier to patch up his life after various difficulties, alternating between stress, regression, and minimal adjustment. Because of his immature personality structure, he learned little from the situations he encountered. With increasing age, he handles even less well the cumulative stresses.[11,12] When complete decompensation occurs, he is either diagnosed as schizophrenic or misdiagnosed as chronic brain syndrome.[25]

Perhaps many new cases of schizophrenia are not diagnosed in late life because the senior who has lived successfully for 65 or more years is adaptive and has a high resistance to mental illness.

ASSESSMENT

Differentiating a patient suffering an organic illness from an acute psychotic schizophrenic state can be difficult. When an older person manifests confusion, disorganized thought, and inappropriate judgment and affect, the most common diagnosis is that of chronic brain syndrome, which is the most common medical diagnosis of the elderly population in the United States. It is an easy diagnosis to make and is expected by medical workers.[7] Perhaps with more careful observation, the diagnosis of an acute psychotic state could be made, which implies a better prognosis. Characteristics of an acute illness include a good premorbid adjustment, a precipitating event and sudden onset, absence of family history of mental illness, an altered state of consciousness, and presence of prominent affective and paranoid symptoms.[10] A complete history helps to differentiate between the functional and organic illness. Clinical symptoms also differentiate the two states. Certainly, the two problems may coexist. The basic withdrawal pattern, the recoiling or the pulling back, is consistently seen in schizophrenia.

The following assessment will pertain to the schizophrenic process and will cover thought, affective, identity, and communication disorders. Compare these symptoms of extreme withdrawal with the symptoms for cognitive impairment described in Chapter 20.

Thought Disorders

Cognitive or thought disorders include illogical thinking processes, inability to perceive a whole pattern, unrealistic thinking, and childlike primitive thinking.

Illogical, scattered, and incoherent pattern of the patient's thoughts is apparent as you talk with him and is a cardinal sign of schizophrenia.[10] Normally when you talk to a person, his ideas have a logical plan that holds the ideas together. Words are associated by a common idea that pulls the sentences toward a goal. When you talk to a schizophrenic, his thought pattern is loose. The words do not hang together; few links connect the ideas to progress toward a logical ending. A 70-year-old chronic schizophrenic man, when asked what difficulties he was having at home, answered: "The gulls flew into the mother and daughter. Why not? Why not? Hm-m hm-m-m hmm-m-. White bread in a chair." The fragmented thoughts in this statement are an extreme example. Sometimes a patient may sound lucid; the only clue is your sense of confusion. As the patient stops talking, you may wonder, "What was that all about?"

Inability to perceive a whole pattern or unity of a situation exists. The average person perceives a gestalt or the whole of anything, whether it be a tree, a bush, or a picture. The healthy person envisions the sum total of the subject or situation. If you show the patient a picture, he may not notice that it is a picture of a baseball game or a park. He will point out one small area and dwell on it, talking about it in detail, for example,

"The cap on the man . . . Looks like red, red flame, red flame."

The senior may talk in detail about a specific topic, yet be vague and unorganized about other aspects of the whole idea or situation. The unity of the personality has been ruptured; in turn, the person has difficulty seeing unity in the environment.

Unrealistic thinking, obvious fantasy, or symbolic thought is a major feature of the disease. Jung termed schizophrenia the waking dream. The person's thinking may sound like a dream. The psychological mechanisms of condensation, symbolism, displacement, and dissociation produce thoughts and mental pictures of people, objects, and places that are understood only by the person. Thus his thinking is autistic. He may use words that he has "coined" or made up; these words have special meaning and significance only to him. The words he uses do not have the same meaning to the listener, and the meaning may change from time to time. Rubbing his nose may represent a danger signal one time, but 2 hours later it may represent sending a message. His thinking is unrealistic. Unless the patient is grossly psychotic, his thinking may constantly fluctuate between fantasy and reality. The senior cannot grasp the reality around him. To him, the world seems confusing.

Childlike, primitive thinking occurs, although the child's thinking is basically logical. The patient thinks in specific, concrete, tangible terms. The schizophrenic is unable to think abstractly or conceptually. An object exists only if it can be seen. A proverb or a joke will not be understood. Primary, childlike thinking is also characterized by absence of a sense of time; the person lives in the present. He is unable to wait, to imagine alternative modes of action, or to make specific decisions.[25] To test the lack of abstraction or conceptualization, ask the patient, "What is the same about a fork, a knife, and a spoon?" The obvious answer is that they are all eating utensils. The person with impaired thinking disorder might tell you that his mother used to insist he eat with a fork, or he might list the different foods that might be eaten with each utensil. Thinking disorders occur in both organic brain disease and schizophrenia. The major difference is the symbolic nature of the thought content in the functional disorder which is best assessed by exploring the person's ideas and thought processes.

Look for the following symptoms to assess thought disorders in the schizophrenic: (1) ideas without logical connections; (2) words that sound alike spoken together; (3) concretization of words denoting specific objects; (4) circumstantial speech (moving indirectly toward a verbal and mental goal); (5) stereotyped or rigid thinking; (6) automatic knowing (feeling that others know his thoughts); (7) unclear referents (assuming that others know the object or person he is speaking of); and (8) splitting phenomenon, in which the thoughts, feelings, and actions are not consistent.[13]

Affective Disorders

Since schizophrenia is considered primarily a thought disorder, emotional changes may be overlooked. Yet, they are of major importance. Disorders of affect or emotion are withdrawal, inability to show emotions or respond appropriately, uncanny sensitivity, extreme anxiety, senile regression, emotional arrest, and accessory symptoms.

Emotional withdrawal is a major and fundamental symptom of schizophrenia in the elderly. The senior fears that he will be hurt emotionally by others; therefore, he pulls back from others to avoid rejection. The environment seems so frightening that he retreats to his own thoughts and fantasies. His fear of the external world, for whatever reason, may be greater than the fear of his own world, even though his world seems chaotic and alien to us.

Emotional withdrawal may be seen in many ways. The family may tell you that the older person no longer sees his friends and that he remains alone in his home. You may observe him staring into space, covering his face, watching television with a blank stare, or being unresponsive. You may feel as you talk to him that you are not in contact with a person. You may feel unresponsive, apathetic, without empathy or understanding for the pain and suffering that the patient is experiencing. Your feelings are an important clue. Isolation of his feeling is a prominent defense, and you may sense that you are relating to little of his real person. As the patient withdraws, his thoughts and energies are directed inward. He makes an inner fantasy life which is usually confused, chaotic, and frightening.

Inability to externalize or show emotion is characteristic. He has a flat, cold, indifferent facies; little feeling or emotion is evident. He may look at you without any warmth or recognition. It may be difficult to differentiate a flat affect from a deeply depressed, retarded affect. Look for other symptoms; never expect one symptom to give you a picture of a total behavior or illness. Many times you will feel a depression yourself when you are talking to a depressed person, while the lack of feeling is present when you interview the schizophrenic.

Inability to respond appropriately with the proper emotion at the proper time is characteristic of the schizophrenic senior. He may tell you that he came to the clinic because he lost his wife and then laugh giddily. Seconds later he may cry when he looks at his hand or is given a piece of gum. This inappropriate response may also carry over into anger. He may submissively follow the rules and regulations of the institution and then defiantly resist an insignificant request.

Uncanny or extreme sensitivity to or ability to perceive any feeling or thought another person is having which might be threatening to him is a feature of schizophrenia and of few other mental illnesses. He has an uncanny, unusual way of appraising anger, fear, and frustration in another, and yet he may have little or no awareness of positive feelings, such as kindness, interest, or concern toward him. You may be aware of his uncanny sensitivity to your feelings and your state of mind at one point; later you may note his complete insensitivity to any feelings or the overall situation. Many times the schizophrenic patient is able to perceive feelings and attitudes of staff which are unspoken and covert and yet which affect the entire attitude of the unit. During the interview listen to the patient's words. He may be speaking of another place or time, but the message may be related to the present situation and directed to you. He may say, "The birds are restless today, restless. Wonder what is trouble?" "Can you believe the world we live in . . . all the bickering, and fighting." "Trouble, trouble, trouble, makes the little people worry." Such statements may pinpoint areas of difficulty in an interview, a one-to-one relationship, staff relationships, the team approach, or the ward atmosphere.

Extreme, overwhelming feelings of anxiety, feelings akin to panic, are experienced by the schizophrenic senior because his weakened ego is unable to handle the internal and external stresses and organic changes. The anxiety may be observed overtly in tremors, perspiration, laughing, pacing, or wringing of hands. The anxiety also leads to regression, secondary symptoms, and sometimes to consumption of alcohol and drugs. It is cruel to suggest that this person should not be given medication for relief from the inner pain.

Senile regression consists of retreating to the behavior of an earlier phase of development.[23] Regression can occur at any age and any time, but the elderly patient who is unable to deal with reality has even more limited reserves. The person under stress takes a backward step to relive past experiences that were safe and more rewarding.[25] Early regressive symptoms may be transient and occasional, such as beginning withdrawal or memory failures. Or the person may lose articles, forget names, and have difficulty placing events in proper order. Later, a second phase of regression is shown by increased withdrawal into his autistic world and fantasy. There may be loss of impulse control, periods of rage, and failure to think logically or recognize familiar people. The environment may be perceived as hostile. The functions of mental life learned last disappear first as the individual continues to regress. If this process continues, symptoms become more severe and more constant, and they tend to be less reversible. During the last stage the chance of return to normal adjustment becomes less optimistic. The person fades into a psychotic fantasy; he is disorganized, isolated, and confused, and he hallucinates. But his regressive thoughts and speech are influenced by his past experiences.[25] The depth of regression can be measured by the developmental age of the person's experiences. If he is talking about his sister when they were adolescents, he is less regressed than if he talks about his mother who died when he was 2 years old.

Regression can be found in any elderly person. During stress, the well-adjusted person may begin to deteriorate for a short period but he readjusts. Regression is a prominent feature in chronic organic illness and in the schizophrenic process, and it causes a decompensation of personality in both illnesses.

Arrested emotional development causes symptoms of emotional immaturity. According to Erikson's stages of development, the schizophrenic senior is still emotionally in the first crisis period. Symptoms of lack of trust of self and others and a fear of being rejected are readily seen upon first meeting the person. The senior is aloof and distant; he creates an emotional barrier so that secondary symptoms are unnoticed. Communication is limited; mutual contact is

10.30
17 Fitzgerald Rd

BRISTOL AND WESTON HEALTH AUTHORITY

From

To

Our Ref. ....

Your Ref. ....

Date ....

minimal. The infantile developmental level is a prominent feature in the schizophrenic process. Other characteristics of emotional immaturity include ambivalence, dependency, and lack of insight. The senior may say that he has no problem, that his children just want to get rid of him or get his money. During the first interview, you usually feel the dependency or note the senior's desire to be cared for or protected. Yet, if you project yourself toward him in an overtly protective manner, he will pull back in fear and anger, demonstrating his ambivalence.

*The major accessory symptoms are **delusions**, false beliefs; **hallucinations**, false sensory perceptions without external stimuli; and **ideas of reference**, thinking that situations around him refer to or are pertinent only to him.*[8] All these symptoms are frequently present in autistic thinking; hallucinations are more common in the withdrawn schizophrenic and occur in about two-thirds of the patients. Delusions and ideas of reference will also be discussed in Chapter 23. The withdrawn patient's delusions are not as systematically organized as are those of the paranoid patient, and the content is more dissociated from or lacking in emotional input. Ideas of reference are related in the schizophrenic to his self-centered thinking in which almost anything in the environment pertains to self. The paranoid's ideas of reference are related to his suspicion and his fear. *Illusions, misperceptions of external stimuli,* may also occur.

Hallucinations result from the projection of inner ideas or thoughts into the environment, which are perceived as real experiences. Signs of hallucinating include the patient's looking into space as if attending to some person or object. He may answer back, cry out, laugh inappropriately, or say that the voices told him to run. He may ask you if you heard a sound or look at you to see how you are responding. The experiences are usually auditory, but they may be visual, tactile, or olfactory. The patient may see frightening animals or people. He may taste or smell something unusual. One patient said, whenever he ate, "The food is horse dung." He actually perceived that everything he ate tasted like animal feces. While you assess the presence of accessory symptoms, also assess the meaning that the thoughts or hallucinations have to the patient. The patient who tasted horse dung was probably relating his feelings of worthlessness and attempting to organize his perception of the world by saying that if he were worthless, he needed to eat horse dung.

Identity Disorder

The schizophrenic patient's sense of identity is very tentative. The sense of self is weak; the body boundary and the sense of "who I am" and "if I am" fluctuate. Many schizophrenics express the fear of not being. As the senior ages, he may begin to lose touch with reality, mainly the reality of self. As a result, the senior does not use personal pronouns (you and I), and he may refer to himself in the third person, such as "he." One patient always referred to himself only as "one." When asking for anything, he would say, "May one have———?" As you talk to the patient, notice how he addresses himself, if he does. Or loss of identity may occur as he feels himself merge with or become another person or object, as shown by the following example. One elderly schizophrenic patient saw a nurse write his name in the chart on rounds one morning. When the nurse had difficulty finding him for medication that afternoon, she was reminded in all seriousness by him, after she did find him, that she should have looked in the chart because he had been put there.

A group of five elderly schizophrenic patients were occupied in painting one day. Each patient had a sheet of paper. Each was busy painting and coloring. After a period of time the group leader took one large piece of paper and asked each member of the group to paint the same picture he had drawn on his own sheet of paper on the large sheet as a mural to decorate the wall. The patients looked frightened. One patient began pacing; one patient became angry; another patient sat down and refused to move, and two patients began to paint. The fourth patient never got anything on the paper, and the last drew a small painting in the far corner of the paper. This is a dramatic yet symbolic example of how many patients fear merging and losing their very identity. Many patients complain of feeling lost or engulfed when they are touched by another person.

The unstable ego state also causes confusion of body image. As you watch a schizophrenic patient walk, you may notice that he moves his body differently from most people. There may be rigidity; the patient may look at his legs to see if they are moving, or he may place his feet down as if they were not connected to the rest of him. His posture conveys his unsureness of his body structure as he moves.

Surgery, an illness, or a temperature may give this patient a feel of body contour that presents him with a feeling of identity. One patient was extremely lucid one day and said to the nurses on the division, "I am whole, I am whole." He was later found to have an elevated temperature, which emphasized awareness of his body. The next day the temperature was gone, and so was the lucidity and perceived, defined body boundaries. This relationship has been observed by nurses for years.

An easy way to get in touch with the patient's sense of identity is to ask him to draw a stick figure of himself. A student nurse was talking with an 80-year-old patient who was diagnosed as a chronic undifferentiated schizophrenic. She continued to question him about his early life. Her probing was nontherapeutic, which was demonstrated by the stick figures he drew. The pictures show that he was becoming progressively disorganized while she was questioning him. This demonstrates how a stressful situation can cause identity loss.

The schizophrenic patient loses his sense of self early in illness, but the person with acute or chronic brain disease loses his sense of self last.

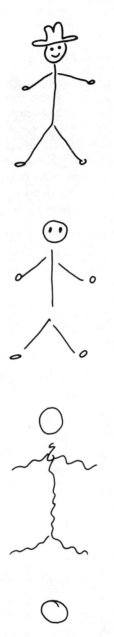

Communication Disorder

The communication process of the schizophrenic patient may be disturbed in several ways. His words may be *autistic, have meaning only to himself,* or they may be jumbled by very personal thoughts or meanings. Words may be incoherent or mixed together incorrectly in a sentence. Some of the lack of communication may be a defensive distancing maneuver to keep people away. If a person can speak only in a monotone or cannot be understood, he will be unable to become involved with other people. The patient with organic brain disease may be unable to state his words or form any thoughts, but the symbolic nature of the content is not present.

NURSING DIAGNOSIS AND FORMULATION OF PATIENT CARE GOALS

Your *nursing diagnosis* of *withdrawn behavior* may include the following assessment of the person:

1. Shows a pattern of pulling back in a variety of ways when encountering anxiety-provoking, threatening situations.
2. Remains alone or engages in purposeless or little activity in order to maintain physical withdrawal.
3. Displays various degrees of emotional withdrawal, such as through daydreaming, fantasizing, or autistic communication.
4. Demonstrates self-centered preoccupation and has little interest in other people or activities.
5. Demonstrates a variety of primitive ego defense mechanisms to cope with anxiety.

Patient Care Goals

Long-term goals may include the following:

1. A feeling of security is developed about the self and environment to the fullest extent possible.
2. Some degree of trust is established, as demonstrated in a satisfying relationship.
3. Interest in other activities is shown and helps him to be more realistic.
4. Appropriate speech and nonverbal behavior express thoughts and feelings to others in an understandable way.
5. Constructive mechanisms to cope with feelings of anxiety are demonstrated to the greatest degree possible.

Short-term goals may include the following:

1. Presence of another person is tolerated.
2. Interest in a brief activity shared with another is stated.
3. Some of his feelings are stated realistically to another person.
4. Sentences are progressively more understandable.
5. Different or more appropriate behaviors to handle anxiety are tried with encouragement.

You will think of other goals as you care for patients.

INTERVENTION

Develop Self-Awareness

While planning for care and intervening with the elderly, extremely withdrawn patient, you must constantly monitor your own feelings. The progress of the patient is usually slow; achievement of your goals should be measured not by time or amount of change but by efforts that are extended. Until you have developed skill and self-knowledge, discouragement and frustration are common feelings as you work with the patient. A cure is usually not within reach, but hopefully the patient has a remission. Increasing ability to relate to others is possible.[14]

Fulfill Responsibility with Medical Treatments

Use of tranquilizers is a humane method to alleviate many of the accessory symptoms associated with the schizophrenic illness. You have an important function in giving the medication, helping the person understand the medication and why he is taking it, and in achieving a dosage with maximum effect and the fewest possible side effects.

Monitoring of any drug given is essential since the elderly patient's tolerance for medication has decreased and his susceptibility to toxic effects has increased.[3] Maintenance dosage is usually smaller in the elderly.

Major tranquilizers for the elderly person include the following phenothiazine derivatives:[3]

Generic Name	Trade Name
Chlorpromazine	Thorazine
Triflupromazine	Vesprin
Trioridazine	Mellaril
Trifluparazine	Stelazine

Generic Name	Trade Name
Perphenazine	Trilafon
Prochlorperazine	Compazine
Thiopropazate	Dartel
Fluphenazine	Prolixin
Acetophenazine	Tindal
Chloroprothixene	Taractin
Thiothimene	Novane
Haloleridol	Haldol

Table 22.1 summarizes the side effects and related nursing measures for the phenothiazines just listed. Acute toxicity is low.[3]

Other somatic treatments, electroconvulsive therapy (ECT), or *psychosurgery, incising the frontal lobe of the cerebrum,* are used infrequently. The ECT is

TABLE 22.1   Summary of Phenothiazine Side Effects and Related Nursing Implications

Side Effects	Nursing Implications
Discomforts Drowiness Dizziness Blurred vision Faulty reflexes and faulty perceptions	Explain the value of the drug in spite of unpleasant effects. Ensure safety precautions. Encourage rising slowly or holding onto furniture. Assist patient initially if necessary. Avoid slippery floors or clutter on floor. Warn that drug may interfere with driving, especially when he begins therapy.
Dry mouth	Encourage sucking on mints or ice chips, chewing gum, holding fluids in mouth. Vaseline may be applied to lips.
Nasal stuffiness	At home, add humidity to room through steam. Use vaporizer.
Weight gain	Encourage low-calorie diet and exercise within limits.
Constipation	Encourage bulk and fluids in diet, exercise, regular times for elimination; may need mild laxative.
Dermatological effects Photosensitivity Pruritis Skin discoloration (grayish-purple)	Warn to avoid exposure to sun because sunburn, rash, and discoloration are intensified in direct sunlight. Lotions relieve itching. Lowering dosage should decrease discoloration.
Blood dyscrasias Agranulocytosis (more common in women and after 40 years of age)	Teach patient to report fever, sore throat, unusual malaise, any infection such as vaginitis, dermatitis, gastritis. Should have periodic complete white blood count and differential. Dosage decreased if dyscrasia occurs.

TABLE 22.1   (*Continued*)

Side Effects	Nursing Implications
Jaundice, liver damage	Prolonged treatment or high dosage may cause decreased liver function. Teach family to observe for yellowish sclera or skin. Should have occasional liver function tests.

Neurological effects
Extrapyramidal reactions (Parkinsonism)
  Rigid limbs and face
  Drooling
  Tremors of hands and limbs
  Skin taut, waxy
  Gait and posture changes
Akinesia
  Weakness, fatigue
  Limbs may become painful
Tardive dyskinesia
  Involuntary movement of face, jaw, tongue
  Convulsions may occur
	Occurs most commonly in people between 15 and 18 years, the elderly, and in women. Reduce dosage. Antiparkinson drugs usually ordered. Promote safety measures. Modify care and activities so that patient maintains self-esteem. May need assistance with eating, hygiene, and grooming.

Acute dystonia
  Increased muscle tone
  Oculogyric crisis
	Teach family to recognize signs: fixed stare, nystagmus, open mouth, protruding tongue, head back, facial expression of pain. Encourage to lie in darkened room with little stimulation.

used carefully with the elderly person because of the chance of complications, although the motor and accessory symptoms and mood may be improved. Psychosurgery is outdated, drastic, and may or may not be effective. Personality is changed; behavior is less spontaneous. Regression may occur.

Maintain a Helpful Environment

Milieu therapy, using the environment as a treatment measure, has proved successful. Both within an institution and in the home setting, the environment should be considered as a means to produce comfort and alleviate anxiety. Today, the emphasis is to keep the withdrawn person from becoming dependent on the institution. Thousands of elderly withdrawn and schizophrenic persons have been placed in nursing homes, apartments, or foster homes. They have been encouraged to participate in community activities. It is far better to have them in the community where they can be more independent and free from the hospital rules and restraints. The paradox is that since so many of these people are unable to feel free in their own minds, they are as isolated in the community as they were in the hospital. Often they receive no treatment in the nursing home and are without the supportive environment in the community that is necessary for healthy functioning. Unless they are in an environment that is secure and promotes trust, the move into the community may encourage more symptom formation instead of lessen it.

In the hospital setting you can maintain a safe, secure environment for the patient. The setting can be attractive. A team approach that provides consistent care and emphasizes gradual involvement with others is important. Continuity of such care into the home environment is more difficult but necessary. The public health nurse, social worker, vocational counselor, and psychiatrist must continue to plan together for the senior's care. Home management goals would include securing support of family or friends, involvement in social activities, and pursuit of hobbies. An excellent opportunity for a psychiatric nursing experience for student nurses would be working in community home-care facilities with elderly withdrawn persons.

Begin Contact with the Senior

Even though this person conveys a desire for closeness and affection, he will maintain distance until the emotional barrier of lack of trust and fear of rejection can be broken. Your first task is to establish some contact with the person. This may be done symbolically by lighting a cigarette, giving a piece of candy, or bringing a book, which represents giving of yourself and being received by the person. Be sensitive to your patient's fears; if you are too enthusiastic and assertive in giving support, warmth, or gifts, the senior may feel so anxious that he breaks off contact by leaving the immediate area or the agency or asking for another nurse. Move slowly and with genuine concern in establishing emotional and physical closeness. His dependency may call for help; yet, he may push you away as you offer guidance. His infantile, unrealistic thinking may demand attention from you to the extent that you may feel overwhelmed and have difficulty maintaining interest. He may be so cold and aloof that you feel that you are not getting anywhere and will want to quit.

Establish a Relationship

Read again Chapter 3 on nurse-client relationship and apply the information with the withdrawn person. Establishing a relationship is difficult because the patient expects you to cause him pain. Thus, after he moves a step closer, he pulls away. Just as you use the four A's in diagnosis of the schizophrenic patient, use the four A's as a guide to forming a relationship. Focus on (1) Acceptance—accept yourself and your shortcomings and the senior's experience; (2) Awareness—listen to verbal, nonverbal, and symbolic communication; (3) Acknowledgment—recognize his fears and communication; and (4) Authenticity—show honest human-to-human contact.[2] The key to helping the patient is to develop trust. With your encouragement he first learns to feel good about being with you; then he can gradually feel secure with others.

If the ability to trust remains underdeveloped, the senior is flooded by disorganizing anxieties. To defend against the anxiety and loneliness, he freezes into "I-It" relations. He tries not only to master the material world, but he also tries to manage others as objects in order to compensate for his loneliness. But neither the highest managerial success nor the solitary perfection can meet the need for trust in others and self, being accepted and understood by another. Trust is a basic human need; it can be rekindled in the senior. Trust promotes personality integration, turns despair to hope, and permits acceptance of the limited freedom and responsibility of his unique existence.[26]

Encourage Involvement

Relatedness is the emotional, perceptual, and cognitive capacity to become involved with another person.[22] The withdrawn individual must slowly but progressively become involved with life and do this through another human being. You must also *slowly* become involved with him. You represent the rejecting, fearful world but offer him another experience with that world that is more comfortable. The senior may have suffered many losses and may have been rejected too often. At first, he is unwilling to risk; therefore, he responds slowly to your presence, conversation, and concern. If the blocks are not too great, his anxiety can be overcome. He may pull back several times and manifest the symptoms discussed previously. You must wait. Give him distance, and then seek him out again. If people have caused him too much hurt and if your own approach is too brusque, too fast, or too pushy, he may never move out at all. If you are perceptive to his feelings as you attempt to form a bond, and if you try over and over, you will be given a chance to succeed. The bond, the involvement, will continue, depending on the time you both have and the ability of both you and the senior to become emotionally close.

The nursing profession and the field of psychiatry may be moving to a more scientific approach to care. This may mean the emphasis upon cognition to solve problems, the emphasis upon organic causes of mental illness which appear exact and defined. Only the future will answer the unresolved questions, but one very basic fact about man is that *caring* and *relatedness* must be in feelings, not just words, to produce growth. Growth and recovery from extreme withdrawal or other emotional disorders do not come about in many instances because the *risk to move close* is not shared by both people, the health worker and the patient. The feeling level must be present as well as the knowledge and skill to have the bond succeed. The mother who is bonding with the newborn child may say all the right words and have the proper sound and method, but if she does not really care for or love the infant, or if fears and anxieties block the feelings of love, the infant will go without the close tie that is so important for the nurturing process to continue. Let us work and desire that nursing, as a *caring profession,* will continue not only to develop knowledge but will also continue to *care.*

Focus on Tangible Issues

The withdrawn senior is hard to live with. When the person is trying to solve a problem, especially in an area ridden with conflicts, he may tend to have more difficulty in thinking. He may become vague, more disorganized, unsure of perceptions, and unable to focus on issues. He says things that make no sense. You have to guide him through the vagueness so that he can gain a sense of past and future. As he feels more secure, as he begins to identify with you, you may be able to help him describe events in daily living which cause him difficulty and determine how to handle these events. Carefully look for causes of the difficulty and reasons for failure, withdrawal, regression, or secondary symptoms. The following case is an example of how a very ill person can work through reasons for behavior when she trusts the nurse. Only then is problem solving possible.

Mrs. K., a 70-year-old widow living alone, was reported by neighbors to be acting strangely. The neighbors told the public health nurse that they were concerned about Mrs. K.'s safety. Since the nurse had made several successful contacts previously, she felt that she could visit Mrs. K. without difficulty. She talked to Mrs. K. over the phone for a short time. Learning nothing, the nurse set a time to visit. When she arrived, she found Mrs. K. untidy; her hair was uncombed; there was food on her chin, and she was obviously regressed. The house was covered with newspapers, filth, and dirty clothes. Mrs. K. covered her nose and mouth with her hand and muttered sounds over and over. Several times she clearly stated, "When I let them in, the hard rail cut the red knob." Then she would begin to mutter incoherently. The nurse contacted the community mental health clinic, and Mrs. K. was admitted to the hospital for observation and treatment. The nurse continued to visit her. As the hospitalization progressed and Mrs. K. became more comfortable with the staff and the public health nurse, she became more clear in her language and more understandable. A certain amount of organic impairment and personality fragility was noted by the attending physician, but they felt that some precipitating event might have caused this severe psychotic regression. The public health nurse began to talk with Mrs. K. about events in the past weeks. The nurse tried to make connections with Mrs. K.'s early comments about the "hard rail." These words had recurred on several other occasions. As Mrs. K. continued to progress, she began talking about a man. On one occasion she said, "hard rail—a man." The nurse who was talking to her asked "What about the man, the hard rail?" Upon further careful inquiry, Mrs. K. described that a man in the neighborhood had entered her house, raped her, and stolen her savings.

Mrs. K. was in time able to express her fears and anger. In discussing this further, the staff was able to explore with Mrs. K. the events that precipitated the senile regression and schizophrenic break, help her to express feelings associated with the attack, and consider future precautions to take.

Hallucinations can also be handled as a tangible issue. The elderly patient can recognize hallucinations, realize that they occur only in certain situations, and that certain events can cause them. This is called the *listening attitude,* for he learns to anticipate and listen or watch for these experiences. He may tell you about his hallucinations, for example, voices he hears and what they are saying to him. Many patients have been told by the hallucinatory voices never to trust anyone with the information the voices give them. Thus, only after some time in a relationship, after a deep trust has been established, will the patient share information about the voices, sounds, people, or other hallucinations. As you discuss these experiences with your patient, explore when he expects to hear the hallucination.[1] Ask, "What happens right before the voice? What brings the voice about?"

A student nurse visited Mrs. R., an elderly patient, in her home. During each visit she took Mrs. R. shopping. Each time they returned home, Mrs. R. would tell the student that the voices were saying Mrs. R. was dumb. As this information was examined, Mrs. R. was able to see that when she expected to hear the words, she would hear them. The words were based on her own feelings that she was a dumb person, on her own feelings of inadequacy and worthlessness. Much later, the voices in the store disappeared because Mrs. R. was able to recognize the precipitating cause and her feelings.

The senior may or may not be able to gain this kind of insight. Such connections may be too anxiety-provoking or too abstract. However, other simple cause-and-effect relationships may be attained in lieu of this deeper insight.

In exploring any hallucinating experience, be aware of the anxiety or other feelings as the cause. Listen to the underlying conflicts, needs, and wishes. Carefully present reality to the patient by telling the patient that you do not hear the voice or see the situation but that you can understand how the experience is real to the patient. Do not go along with the hallucinations or encourage them in any way. Try to decrease the anxiety or underlying feelings. Over time, explore the precipitating feelings, events, or places so that the patient can relinquish the hallucinations and meet his needs in a more realistic way.

Promote Understanding of Dynamics

As you empathize with and get to know your patient and his situation, begin to explore with him the pattern of behavior, defense mechanisms, the background for his feelings and self-concept, the people who are important to him, and how he relates with others and with you. As you begin to make sense of his life and understand the underlying dynamics, help him to clarify his feelings and focus on his difficult life situations. You can help him to make some decisions about his life that will produce some success instead of failure.

Gradually he will learn to understand himself to some degree, the reasons behind his behavior, and its effect on others.

Be a Role Model for the Patient

As much as you can, become a companion to the senior, but maintain objectivity. As you talk with him, you present reality. As you share your ideas and support his efforts, he will learn to deal with life's realities. Gradually he will gain enough strength to return to activity and the community. To experience with the senior may give him courage to become more involved in other relationships, social activities, and former interests, as is shown by the following case.

One elderly patient, Miss J., was discharged from the state hospital to live with another ex-patient in an apartment. The other patient dominated Miss J. so that Miss J. withdrew more and more into herself. She sat by the window and looked out hour after hour—bored, listless, and apathetic. She had always loved to cook but was fearful of doing so in this situation. The visiting nurse spent two visits baking cookies from a cookie mix with her. The next time she baked cookies, the cookies were made from a recipe. Miss J. had gained enough confidence from the mutual experience to bake cookies from a recipe by herself.

Such encounters can lead the way to a fuller life. As you become more involved in a mutually trusting bond, you may cry, laugh, or express anger with the senior, and through this experience teach him how to live.

Strengthen Identity

The confusion of identity can be strengthened by the senior's identification with you, by gaining a greater sense of self-worth through the relationship, by being treated as a unique person, and also by having personal possessions. *Always call the senior by name.* Allow him a certain space. Refer to his possessions, and handle them with care. Support his unique qualities and show respect for him as the worthwhile individual that he is.

Personal hygiene is important for a whole body image and self-respect. Physical activity, such as walking, playing ball, or swimming, may be good. Activities using the five senses and touch may give him more of a sense of self. Think of your patient and some of his symptoms and difficulties; then plan activities for him.

Be careful to touch the patient only if he responds comfortably to being touched. If he does not mind being touched, it can be a helpful contact to reinforce body boundaries. If he freezes or tightens, wait until he is responsive to physical closeness.

Encourage Communication

In the early stages of a schizophrenic break, the major communication is nonverbal. The way to reach the person is by understanding his primitive feeling and thinking level. Gradually, communication may be attempted at a higher, more cognitive level. Try to understand the senior's words when he sounds illogical or incoherent. Look for topics, themes, and symbols. Ask your patient to help you understand. Paraphrase what you think are his thoughts or feelings: verbalize the implied. Say the words that you think he is saying. Help him to say the words coherently if at all possible. Never try to fool this patient by saying you understand when you do not. If trust is a very basic problem, you must be honest: If you do not understand, say so or remain silent until you think you may have an idea. It may be helpful to ask "Are you saying ———?" or "Do I hear you telling that———?" Always let the patient know that you want to understand and that you appreciate how difficult it is for him. Try to be creative by allowing the senior to find alternate ways of communicating. Some patients can draw or make figures while others are expressive in other nonverbal methods: gestures, mime, singing, or dance.[6] The most important method of communication is the unidentifiable energy that moves between people that says, "I care about you."

Activity groups have been found to alter the self-concept of the withdrawn person while increasing interaction. Lancaster chose 12 patients, 6 people from each of two wards, and established two activity groups. Twelve other patients, 6 from each ward, served as control subjects. The group members selected activities—drawing, reading, looking at pictures, baking, and playing the piano. Discussion would sometimes center around activities but sometimes on thoughts and feelings. There was a significant change on Osgood's Semantic Differential Score for Self-Concept within the experimental group but no significant difference within the control group.[12] Review Chapter 4 for ideas on the kinds of groups that can be helpful to the withdrawn senior.

EVALUATION

You will observe an improvement in the senior's behavior as you work with him over time. However, the importance of relationships is not just intuitively understood.

Nursing interventions were evaluated in a study done on the motivation of withdrawn and regressed institutionalized, chronically ill, elderly patients. The nursing intervention consisted of a one-to-one trust relationship in which interactions were held daily, averaging three hours a week for two months. Intervention also included planning rehabilitative, therapeutic, and recreational activities, and mutual reevaluation and modification of nursing plans. The result of the study showed significant behavioral changes; withdrawn and re-gressed behavior was decreased.[9]

Nursing could do much more with therapeutic relationships. Relation-ships take time and effort, but the effort produces results. You may notice signs of renewed interest in surroundings and activities, an increased interest in clothing, food, or, most significantly, in other people. Perhaps the best evalua-tion can be based upon the senior's capacity to respond to you. The senior's testing behavior decreases; he smiles as you approach; he shows excitement about an activity you are planning together. You may first become aware of a setback in the senior's behavior when you miss a day or take a vacation. Grad-ually, you will sense a bond developing between you. Then the senior moves closer to others as well.

REFERENCES

1. ARIETI, SILVANO, "Psychotherapy of Schizophrenia," *Treatment of Schizophre-nia: Progress and Prospects,* eds., Louis West and Don Flinn. New York: Grune & Stratton, 1976.

2. ARNOLD, HELEN, "Working with Schizophrenic Patients—Four A's: A Guide to One-to-One Relationships," *American Journal of Nursing,* 76: No. 6 (1976), 941–43.

3. AYD, FRANK, "The Major Tranquilizers," *American Journal of Nursing,* 65: No. 4 (1965), 70–78.

4. BLEULER, E., *Dementia Praecox of the Group of Schizophrenias.* New York: In-ternational Universities Press, 1911.

5. BURGESS, ANN, and AARON LAZARE, *Psychiatric Nursing in Hospital and Com-munity.* Englewood Cliffs, N.J.: Prentice-Hall, Inc., 1976.

6. BURKETT, ALICE, "A Way to Communicate," *American Journal of Nursing,* 74: No. 12 (1974), 2185–87.

7. BUTLER, ROBERT, and MYRNA LEWIS, *Aging and Mental Health.* St. Louis: The C. V. Mosby Company, 1977.

8. EATON, MERRILL, MARGARET PETERSON, and JAMES DAVIS, *Psychiatry,* 3rd. ed. New York: Medical Examination Publishing Company, 1976.

9. GELPERIN, E., "Psychotherapeutic Intervention by Nurse Clinical Specialist," *Journal of Psychiatric Nursing and Mental Health Services,* 14: No. 2 (1976), 16–18.

10. HOCK, PAUL, "Differential Diagnosis," in *Clinical Psychiatry,* eds. Margaret Strahl and Nolan Lewis. New York: Science House, 1972, pp. 601–48.

11. KAY, D., and M. ROTH, "Environmental and Hereditary Factors in the Schizo-phrenias of Old Age," *Journal of Mental Science,* 107: (1961), 649.

12. LANCASTER, JEANETTE, "Schizophrenic Patients: Activity Groups as Therapy," *American Journal of Nursing,* 76: No. 6 (1976), 947–49.

13. MANSER, JANICE, and ANITA WERNER, *Instruments for Study of Nurse-Patient In-teractions.* New York: Macmillan Publishing Co., Inc., 1964.

14. McARDLE, KAREN, "Dialogue in Thought," *American Journal of Nursing,* 74: No. 6 (1974), 1075–77.

15. MELLOW, JUNE, "The Experiential Order of Nursing Therapy in Acute Schizophrenia," *Perspectives in Psychiatric Care,* 6: No. 6 (1968), 249–55.

16. OSTENDORF, MARY, "Dan Is Schizophrenic: Possible Causes, Probable Course," *American Journal of Nursing,* 76: No. 6 (1976), 944–47.

17. *Psychology Encyclopedia.* Guilford, Conn.: The Dushkin Publishing Group, 1973, 86, 242–43.

18. ROBERTS, SHARON, "Territoriality: Space and the Schizophrenic Patient," *Perspectives in Psychiatric Care,* 7: No. 1 (1969), 28–33.

19. ROBINS, E., and S. B. GUZE, "Establishment of Diagnostic Validity in Psychiatric Illness: Its Application to Schizophrenia," *American Journal of Psychiatry,* 126: (1970), 983–87.

20. ROBINSON, ALICE, "Communicating with Schizophrenic Patients," *American Journal of Nursing,* 60: No. 8 (1960), 1120–23.

21. ROTH, M., "Interaction of Genetic and Environmental Factors in the Causation of Schizophrenia," in *Schizophrenia,* ed. Richter. New York: Pergamon Press, Inc., 1957.

22. ROUSLIN, SHEILA, "Relatedness in Group Psychotherapy," *Perspectives in Psychiatric Care,* 11: No. 4, (1973), 165–71.

23. SOLOMON, PHILIP, *Handbook of Psychiatry.* Los Altos, Calif.: Lange Medical Publications, 1971.

24. STEWART, BARBARA, "Biochemical Aspects of Schizophrenia," *American Journal of Nursing,* 75: No. 12 (1975), 2176–79.

25. VERWOERDT, ADRIAAN, *Clinical Geropsychiatry.* Baltimore: The Williams & Wilkins Company, 1966.

26. WEIGERT, EDITH, *The Courage to Live.* New Haven, Conn.: Yale University Press, 1970.

27. WEST, LOUIS, and DON FLINN, *Treatment of Schizophrenia.* New York: Grune & Stratton, 1976.

28. WOODRUFF, ROBERT, DONALD GOODWIN, and SAMUEL GUZE, *Psychiatric Diagnosis.* New York: Oxford University Press, 1974.

29. ZERBIN, EDITH, and P. RUEDIN, "Genetics," *Modern Perspectives in the Psychiatry of Old Age,* ed. John C. Howells. New York: Brunner/Mazel, 1975.

suspicion and the paranoid process in later maturity

Study of this chapter will enable you to:
---

1. Identify stresses that contribute to suspicious thinking and behavioral patterns.

2. Describe the continuum of suspicion and the dynamics of the paranoid process.

3. Assess the paranoid process in the elderly person, either as the primary mental illness or as part of the symptomatology of another illness.

4. Formulate nursing diagnosis, patient care goals, and a plan of care for the senior who is manifesting the paranoid process.

5. Intervene with the senior in such a manner that he does not have to adhere to the paranoid process.

6. Help family members to adapt their behavior so that they can live more comfortably with the suspicious senior.

7. Work with the health care team to maintain a constant approach to and secure environment for the senior.

8. Evaluate changes in the person's behavior that indicate an effective approach.

9. Accept that the senior may continue part of the paranoid process even after appropriate intervention.

10. Promote reduction of community stresses that contribute to paranoid thinking in the elderly.

23

Societal attitudes described in Chapter 5 create a hostile environment for many of our elderly and cause many of them to feel suspicious of their surroundings.

*The **suspicious** or **paranoid thinking process** is a reaction to anxiety and insecurity, whereby **projection**, attributing personal feelings and thoughts to others, is the basic defense mechanism used. Additionally, the person mistrusts and blames others, rationalizes this behavior, is wary of and feels persecuted by others, and misinterprets others' behavior.*[23]

Many elderly people sound suspicious. However, Butler's statement is worth remembering: "Show me one truly paranoid person and I will show you ten who are truly persecuted."[5]

CONTRIBUTING FACTORS

Old age is a time of many stresses, as discussed in Unit II. Stressful experiences frequently predispose to suspicious thinking. For example, stressors include illness, sensory deprivation, loss, rejection, and loneliness. All of these cause anxiety, insecurity, and decreased adaptability.

In one study the elderly rated illness as their most severe problem, resulting in restricted social contact as well as physical distress.[2] Lowered energy and chronic and debilitating illness seem to evoke suspicious thinking;[20] a high incidence of physical disorders occurs in paranoid seniors.[13]

Sensory deprivation, resulting from loss of sight, hearing, taste, and touch sensations, contributes to paranoid thinking because the person lacks external stimuli to help him evaluate his surroundings. This is especially true with hearing loss, although patients who have their eyes covered after certain eye surgery or treatments also temporarily have acute paranoid reactions. Reduced sensory input often causes frustration, anger, and finally suspicion.[6,7,12,20]

Research shows that the deaf child is usually more suspicious than the normal child is, in spite of all the support and assistance the deaf child is given. Thus, you can understand why the elderly is suspicious of others when he can no longer hear or see; he has few or no supports and must cope with a rejecting, hostile social attitude as well. Others are less sympathetic to the deaf senior than they are to the deaf child because deafness is expected as a part of aging.

Loss, whether financial, social, emotional, physical, or intellectual, causes the senior to lose self-esteem, feel inadequate and anxious, and rely more on internal stimuli and thoughts as social contact is reduced.

Rejection is also a major stressor. Members of the extended family have often moved away or have died, and friends are often fewer or more distant, either because of death, poor health, immobility, or geographical moves. Thus, the senior feels rejected and alone. Solitary living often increases fear and suspicion. Sometimes the senior's suspicions are real; some neighborhoods and communities either reject the senior entirely or do not help him. Sometimes rejection is fantasized, or minor slights are perceived by the senior as rejection.[4]

Most seniors feel more lonely than they did earlier in life. Old relationships are gone, and the senior may find it hard to join social clubs or make new friends. Loneliness may also be a part of other emotional problems: depression, withdrawal, physical preoccupation, and cognitive impairment. The more lonely the person, the more likely he is to respond to his own thoughts, fears, and inadequacies, misinterpret others' behavior, and enter the paranoid thinking process.

DYNAMICS OF PARANOID THINKING

The suspicious person feels insecure, uncertain, unsafe, and vulnerable. He lacks confidence in his own ability to deal with situations. The more threatened he feels, the more self-esteem and sense of personal integrity suffer. Increased anxiety results. The more anxious the person becomes, the more primitive and less integrated are his responses. If the senior has a paranoid personality structure, he responds to anxious feelings with anger and mistrust. The more he responds this way, the harder he is to live with, thus creating difficulty for himself and for those with whom he is associated.[23] It is important not to label the person as a "crabby old man" or "nasty old lady"; instead, see that the person is in emotional distress and understand the reasons for his behavior.

The senior who feels mistreated, inadequate, low self-esteem, and worn out cannot fully acknowledge just how inadequate he does feel. Thus, he *denies* his feelings. Although he feels angry at himself for his predicament, he *blames* others instead of himself. He accuses others as responsible for his own feelings. His feelings become a part of the "not me" portion of his personality as he places them onto others. (This process of externalizing feelings occurs in the young child who blames the chair for his fall or in the young adult who blames the teacher for his failing grade.) The worse the senior feels, and the more unacceptable the feelings, the more he has to attribute his feelings to others (projection).

Projection is supported by *rationalization, a logical sounding, acceptable reason for his response.* The use of rationalization keeps motives and feelings out of the senior's awareness. When he feels inferior to others, he also uses reaction formation by acting superior or being condescending to others.

As the senior encounters more stress and anxiety, the denial, externalization, and projection are inadequate to help him feel secure. He formulates *delusions, false beliefs,* in an attempt to make sense of his world.

The delusion may begin with the *idea of reference, interpreting actions of others as being related to the self.* (Reference implies a relationship between "me here" and "them over there.")[28] For example, the senior may see the mailman talking to a couple of people in front of his house. He assumes that the mailman is saying something about him to the other people. The idea of reference (mental relationship between himself and the other party) may be positive, but it is usually accusing, evil, and hurtful. The senior may also feel that he is actively influencing the other person, or he may feel that he is passively receiving something from the other. Interestingly, a younger person often has ideas of reference and delusions about a group such as the CIA or FBI, but the older person's ideas of reference and delusion usually relate to his family or neighborhood.[19]

There is a basic bit of truth in every delusion, usually the feelings behind the statement, such as rejection or guilt. The initial piece of information is misinterpreted and built upon. The more organized and systematic the delusion becomes, the more logical and realistic it may seem. If the senior has little organic damage and his ability to form connections is intact, he may build upon the basic premise with such logic and precision that the delusion is difficult to detect. But since the basic premise is incorrect, the last deductions are also incorrect. The organically confused person will be unable to organize a logical, complex delusion statement. Often as you listen, you may wonder about the truth of the statement but may be unable to refute it.

At times, delusions are **encapsulated**, *held apart from the rest of the person's life.* One area of his life is dominated by the delusion, but other areas of life are intact, integrated, and little influenced by the delusional idea.

Figure 23.1 diagrams the dynamics of paranoid thinking just discussed.

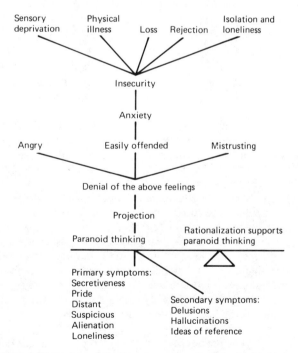

Figure 23.1. A model of the dynamics of paranoid thinking.

Suspicion on a Continuum

Suspicious thinking can be found in people of any age during times of stress. Suspicious thinking is also stimulated by facets of our culture and society.[23] For example, the conflict between labor and management brings out suspicious thinking in both parties. Even when there are no real hostilities, either party may perceive them to be present.

You probably know elderly people who feel that the world is against them, their family has it in for them, and their neighbors hate them. Certainly in many situations these ideas may be true. But the pathologically suspicious or paranoid person uses this attitude of "a bad world" to help him feel more adequate, good, important, or secure.

The Paranoid Personality

The paranoid personality is typically one who has a *pattern* of being suspicious, nontrusting, secretive, rigid, and proud. Such a personality pattern often begins in earlier life and continues until death. The person may be able to live fairly successfully, but probably not as fully as if he had been more open to others. The senior may maintain borderline stability, or his personality traits may cause real difficulty with others. He may be perceived as cantankerous, eccentric, and demanding. He may be easily hurt and unforgiving, and he may hold a grudge for a long time. The more insulted and alone he feels, the more seclusive, angry, alienated, and bitter he becomes.

The paranoid senior is relatively harmless to others; the real suffering is within the person himself as he becomes more isolated and alienated. Others may avoid him to the extent that he sees only delivery men or governmental workers such as tax collectors unless physical illness forces him to seek help.[5] The following case study is an example:

Mr. Brown had been an outgoing, active man all his life. He lived in a small Ohio town and never married. He supported himself as a salesperson in a local real estate office. He was a member of the Catholic Church and active on the board of a local children's home and adoption center. After retiring, he became increasingly more involved in gardening and reading and less involved in any social life as his hearing impairment increased. Later, he developed a cardiac condition, so that gardening activities had to be curtailed. As he became more ill and isolated, he became suspicious of the neighbors; he thought that they were talking about him and were sending X-rays to attack, change, and poison him. His thoughts caused him to become more frightened, and he shut himself in his home. He received no outside visitors. He did occasionally call the police to check up on the neighbors, especially if the neighbors tried to initiate any contact. When he stopped picking up his mail, the neighbors became concerned and finally called the authorities to check. Mr. Brown was found dead, and he had been dead for several weeks.

Often the paranoid person refuses help when it is offered by others, and even when he knows he desperately needs help. If he had an unhappy experience with a health professional, which feeds his delusion of persecution about health workers, he puts *all* health professionals into his delusion and considers them as "out to get him." Even the well-intentioned professional may have a hard time understanding this senior's thinking process and may become resentful and rejecting. When the senior makes accusations about him, the professional may leave the senior alone although he needs help. Yet, the suspicious person may later accept help if the worker has been gentle and patient. If the Protective Services described in Chapter 8 are legally available, both worker and senior benefit because the worker feels that he has the legal protection to take the time and to persist in trying to help a senior in need and to call in other services or workers who may be more successful with the person.

Paranoid States

The elderly person suffering considerable stress may regress to a *paranoid state, a transitory psychotic, delusional state of behavior precipitated by the stress.* Often a major, rapid loss causes this decompensation. The more the loss pertains to an important area, such as the sense of manliness or femininity, or involves separation or rejection from a loved one, the more likely the person will formulate a delusion to offset the loss. Often, after the delusion is formulated, the person appears to adjust to the loss, returning to earlier behavior, especially if familiar activities intervene.

The following case is an example:

John B. was an outgoing, successful businessman and accountant who retired at age 65, at which time he also suffered the death of his mother with whom he had lived. At the mother's funeral, John loudly accused his brother of cheating him out of his inheritance. After the funeral, John quickly sold the mother's house and moved into an apartment. He went to a local lawyer and began to file for damages against his brother. Then, when he was asked by a local accounting firm to do some part-time work, he became involved in his work and settled into his apartment. Shortly thereafter, he dropped the legal proceedings and never mentioned suspicion of his brother again.

Presence of Paranoid Process in Other Conditions

The senior with *reversible or irreversible cognitive impairment* is often suspicious.[20,28] At first he may deny his confusion and disorientation. Then, as he becomes less capable of functioning, he explodes with indignation when someone confronts him about his behavior. He denies or leaves the room. Then he makes excuses for his behavior, attributing his feelings and behavior to others as if others are to blame for his condition. Usually the people who are closest to this senior will get the most blame and will be worked into his delusion. However, his delusion is easily recognized for what it is, since it is poorly organized, may change from day to day, is self-aggrandizing, and is obviously an unrealistic statement.[20] Yet, his mistrusting statements can be difficult for others to cope with.

The *depressed* senior is often suspicious of others; he accuses others of poisoning or persecuting him and maintains these delusional beliefs in spite of reassurance to the contrary. The more worthless the person feels, the more likely he is to say that everyone is out to get him. His mistrust of others prevents him from accepting helpful gestures from others. He feels that he is bad and projects that all of the world is bad.

The *withdrawn* senior may be diagnosed as having ***paraphrenia**, a late life schizophrenia with paranoid ideation.* This person is usually a female who lives alone, is partially deaf, is considered eccentric, and has few close relatives or associates. The person appears to have an intact personality but demonstrates an organized, strongly-adhered-to delusion, with or without hallucinations. When hallucinations do occur, they are vivid, exciting, and threatening.[10,14,18,20,22,24]

Often the person's response to the delusions and hallucinations is to run away, but the thoughts and sensations continue to oppress the senior until he may commit suicide. If this person is treated successfully with phenothiazines, he still lacks insight into his illness. He will say, "The _____ is gone" instead of saying that he was sick and the medicine helped him.[20]

The following case is an example of a paraphrenic senior:

Mary Smith, age 66, became suspicious of her minister. She saw the minister gesturing in the pulpit during a church service and said he was signaling for her to get away. She phoned the minister and told him that she had sent him a dollar and wondered when she would receive the return. He did not understand and asked her what she meant. She yelled at him, calling him a fool and a cheat. Then she became suspicious of her neighbors; she thought they were talking about her when she saw them talking to each other. Soon she began to hallucinate, and the voices, which were loud and rude, called her dirty names. As time progressed, she became more isolated, for she believed a young teen-age neighbor was waiting to rape her. She closed her windows and blinds, locked her door, and had her groceries delivered. Gradually, she believed that the teen-age neighbor had the key to her house and was waiting to come in. When this belief became fixed, she moved from her home where she had lived for 50 years.

Classical Paranoia

Classical paranoia is a relatively rare state in which a person holds to a well-organized rigid delusion that relates to only one area of his life; otherwise, he has a well-integrated, functioning personality. The senior frequently has been successful and relatively well-adjusted in his earlier life, and the length of time he has experienced delusional thinking is unknown. Often someone who has known him well will recall that he had the delusional idea for a long time. Only when the person experiences the difficulties of old age and the related decompensation will other people begin to recognize his beliefs as a delusion. The delusion often becomes more pronounced and the senior is less discreet in talking about it. Yet, the senior with paranoia continues to function adequately in other spheres of life. No one knows how many people go to their death believing a systematized delusion that even their relatives do not know about.

ASSESSMENT

Statements

Assessment of the paranoid thinking process may be difficult, for the illness is often hidden by an extrovertive or aggressive behavior. The senior appears to be in firm control of himself; his personality appears intact because he usually can compensate to hide his mistrust.

If you listen closely, however, you will hear a pattern of denial, rationalization, and projection. He will first deny the obvious. He might say things like: "No, I am not sick." "No, I do not need help." "I came here (to the hospital) for a rest." You hear him deny the effects of aging, for example: "Somebody keeps moving my glasses." "People keep taking my things." "Nobody remembers to tell me things." You might also hear denial of his own defensiveness: "I'm not touchy; they are all prima donnas." "I'm not irritable." "I've always been easy to live with."

Then you become aware of how much the senior blames others for his difficulties. For example, he says that he lacks certain things because: "My family is too busy." "The mail is too slow." "The storekeeper is too greedy anymore." He might say things like: "They let me go at the plant because the bosses are no good." "Did you ever notice how everybody is starting fights these days?" "Nobody has time for an elderly person."

If you regularly hear such statements dispersed throughout the senior's conversation, you can be sure that he is suspicious, even if you do not see any other evidence. Eventually you will see more signs of mistrust, anger, rationalization, and projection. Or you may first notice a number of rationalizations, as if the senior were hiding something. If the delusions and suspicious thoughts are firmly entrenched, and if he is sure of his misgivings about other people, the rationalizations are operating within the paranoid process and may not be openly stated. If the paranoid process is wavering, or if he is cognitively or emotionally struggling to maintain adaptation, he may begin to openly rationalize to help himself feel more adequate. Then you will hear such things as: "Nobody likes to listen to me because they are all jealous of my experience and knowledge." "People keep taking my things because I have collected invaluable items throughout the years." "Nobody likes to listen to me because they know I have the answers." "They won't let me back in the office to straighten things up; they're afraid of me."

Behaviors

You may first be aware of the senior's angry, hostile behavior. He may be openly aggressive, he may berate others for a variety of abuses, he may be controlled so that he expresses his anger about unimportant issues or neutral topics, or he may demand and expect too much from others and attack them for their inadequacies or weaknesses.

Another prominent behavior is the ever-present suspiciousness or mistrust. He walks into the room glancing about, looking for flaws and minor details. He approaches you and others warily. He listens carefully to your words, looking for meanings as if to catch you in an act of harm to him. He listens defensively to protect himself from imagined hurts. His body language may express suspicion; he carefully moves about, sits on the edge of his chair, or perhaps sits with arms folded as if closed to a "hostile world."

Usually he will also be secretive. He seems wary or sensitive about being seen. He may need to hide himself from you in order to feel safe. He may talk to you in a guarded manner, screening his words and protecting his thoughts. He withholds, gives out information carefully, and evaluates your intentions before exposing himself. You may observe this secretive behavior as you watch how he holds his papers, states his history, talks about the money he has in the bank, or clutches the change in the purse.

A third cluster of behaviors consists of the attitudes of superiority, pride, and aloofness. The person may discuss his achievements and emphasize people he has known or places he has been. He may struggle to show you his superior knowledge and experience. He may use words as a filibuster to maintain distance and prove his ability. He may try to control the conversation between the two of you. He may respond to you in a condescending manner. In the hospital he will have difficulty accepting and following the patient role. In his home or apartment he will remain distant or even refuse to open the door rather than trust a health professional to work with him. He may ask for his own room, stating that he fears sleeping with another person. He actually feels that he is better than you, other people, or the other patients in the hospital. He will have difficulty telling you about any problem he is having. He may never be able to say that he has no one to love, no one to care about him, or nothing worthwhile to do.

History

As the senior tells you about his life, listen to his overt and hidden statements, observe the defenses and behaviors he uses, and examine carefully the manner in which he tells you his history. He may be very circumstantial, explaining everything in extreme detail without ever getting to the point. He may hesitate, filling in the conversational spaces with information that seems to fit logically at first, but later seems irrelevant. If you listen carefully to whatever information has relevance and significance for him, that can be a clue to his delusions.

As he tells his history, carefully listen to the content. Listen for ideas that do not seem to fit together or are not in tune with reality. Sometimes he jumbles related ideas together as he expresses a delusion so that you feel confused. For example, as you listen to such a conversation, you would feel uncertain about whether the senior is losing his home to a greedy landlord, losing his money to an unscrupulous caretaker, or being taken advantage of by an unloving daughter. Listen carefully for information that either does not fit together or is of such a bizarre nature that you know that the material is delusional.

Personal Feelings

Be perceptive to your feelings as you contact the suspicious senior. Your own feelings about the person, especially if they validate the overt symptoms, can help you to make a nursing diagnosis. You may feel the distance and notice the lack of emotional contact between you. You may feel "put down" as the senior struggles to feel superior to you. The most diagnostic feeling you will have is that of being attacked, assaulted, belittled, stupid, or dumb, since the suspicious senior projects and blames others for his difficulties. Eventually the helping person—you—becomes the object of his projection, blame, and delusions. His behavior may cause an open confrontation between you and him. When you feel yourself pulling back from the onslaught of his behavior or if you feel a desire to retaliate, you have an important clue that the patient is projecting, and you are the recipient.

NURSING DIAGNOSIS AND FORMULATION OF PATIENT CARE GOALS

Your *nursing diagnosis* of *suspicious or paranoid ideation* may include assessment of the following behaviors:

1. Demonstrates behavior that is aggressive, abusive, angry, or hostile.
2. Demonstrates varying degrees of mistrust and secretiveness.
3. Responds to stress situations with statements that distort and indicate misunderstanding.
4. Blames other individuals or groups when he feels inadequate or uncomfortable.
5. Acts aloof or remains solitary in order to maintain feelings of superiority over others.
6. Makes statements that convey feelings of insecurity, jealousy, possessiveness, fearfulness, or distrust of others.

Patient Care Goals

Long-term goals could include the following:

1. Feelings of trust toward family or close associates who are helpful to him are described.
2. Work or play is engaged in with others as appropriate to the life situation.
3. Stressful situations are handled without excessive or prolonged denial, projection, or blame.
4. Negative societal attitudes are realistically appraised and handled without loss of self-esteem.

Short-term goals could include the following:

1. Tolerates increasing physical and emotional closeness of yourself or other significant persons.
2. Engages in activities of daily living with others as appropriate.
3. States strengths and limits realistically.
4. Enters into activities with others for a limited period of time.

You will think of other goals as you work with suspicious patients.

INTERVENTION

Develop a Satisfying Relationship

Trusting, caring contacts are difficult to establish, but they are essential for the senior to overcome his suspicious thinking.[4,19] Practice of the behaviors described in Chapter 3 and understanding of the dynamics of behavior just described will help you to develop a therapeutic relationship.

Convey to the senior that you are aware that he has feelings that he wishes to express. Give him an opening by saying, "You feel you have not been treated fairly" or "You seem upset about what is happening." Listen carefully to statements that subtly convey his feelings and then validate with him that you heard his feelings.

The suspicious person often has real difficulty in maintaining contacts with others unless he can keep an emotional distance. Allow him to set the pace for closeness and involvement. Listen to his words carefully; he will give you clues when you are moving in too fast and getting too close. For example, he may be talking about the weather or the food, but he will state that he is feeling closed in, attacked, or taken over. Do not move in too fast emotionally or be overly friendly or assertive.

Instead, consistently be reliable; do what you say you plan to, and do not respond defensively to his anger or condescension. Appeal to his healthy behaviors. Let him know that it is acceptable for him to ask for help. If you handle his personality with care, you may become very important to the senior. From you he can learn that people can be trusted, can be dependable, and can help him feel valued. As the relationship with you becomes closer, look for a family member or friend who will add to the senior's life. Help the senior gain social skills so that he can expand his contacts and activities. The person who has mistrusted for a long time will always remain cautious, but he can relearn that people can be friendly.

You, or other important people, cannot always be present when the senior wants to talk about his feelings, fears, or stresses. Have him write what he would say to you or another person. Help him extend himself to others gradually since you have other people to care for and will eventually terminate the relationship. Help him realize that his memories of important relationships, including his relationship with you, can help sustain him when he is alone.

Have a Genuine Attitude

To be effective, be honest in a constructive way. Never be dishonest to the suspicious person. Evaluate your feelings and be genuine with the senior, for he is having a difficult time trying to evaluate what is true and what is not. Being honest and open does not mean that you can take advantage of the senior by being irritable, venting your anger, or telling him that you are bored. There is never any reason or excuse for being hostile toward or for belittling the person. Rather, you must solve your own problems and work through your own feelings before you try to help the senior meet his needs and solve his problems. Yet, an excessive compassion or an overly loving approach can also be based upon anger. Any suspicious patient has a particular facility for finding your weaknesses. You will not fool him. If your caring and affection are not genuine, he will know it.

Increase the Person's Self-Esteem

Your lack of retaliation to the patient's anger and abrasiveness can do more than anything to help him accept himself. Further, as you listen to his feelings, complaints, and opinions and act on them when indicated, you show that you value him as a person. Reinforce his accomplishments and give praise and recognition when he has earned it. Praise him for reliability. Encourage him to make choices. Give opportunities for demonstrating abilities and skills. Assist him in acquiring social skills by including him in activities, games, and social affairs. Have him write his autobiography so that you better understand him. Such an activity also stimulates life review, helping him realize the worth of his life. As his self-esteem rises, so also will his ability to trust himself—one of the major needs of the patient with paranoid thinking.[25]

Explore Reality

When the senior begins to feel safe with you, explore alternatives to his paranoid ideas. When he realizes that the spontaneous expression of his feelings, especially hostility, causes him difficulty with others, he may want to find another way of handling his feelings. Discuss ways for him to check himself before he explodes or to control his irritability. Help him train himself to delay expression of feelings by looking intellectually at the facts before responding. Encourage the senior to put limits on his own behavior, but realize that he will sometimes fail. He will not be able immediately to make major changes, but if he can keep his behavior from getting out of bounds, and at least keep the paranoid process from progressing, the senior is accomplishing a great deal. Although the senior can change, do not expect too much change too fast.

The delusional patient is not realistic; he is misinterpreting his surroundings. Much of the literature says that you should present reality. But first you must listen carefully, understand what he is really saying, and have an established relationship. Otherwise, if you say that something is not true, the senior will turn you off and not talk about his innermost ideas. Asking questions to get further information neither encourages nor agrees with the delusion; asking questions helps you to know what he is thinking. Then you can create doubt about the delusion. The more subtly you do this, the more successful will be the result. Ask the elderly person, "Do you believe that the mailman has it in for you?" or "Is it possible that your daughter is out to get you?" Question with a doubting voice instead of challenging, opposing, or arguing, or the senior might feel that he must defend his delusion. If he asks, "You believe what I am saying, don't you?" respond to his feelings rather than the false belief. Reply, "I realize you *feel* the way you say and that it is hard for you right now to see things another way." Or you may say, "I do not believe your daughter wants to hurt you, but I know you feel that she does. It is important for us to discuss your ideas because I know they cause you much pain." This gives you an opening for further discussion but still you are presenting reality.

The more you encourage the senior to talk about how he felt before, during, and after an incident, the more you can help him recognize the falseness of the delusion and the motive for it. Since the delusion defends him against anxiety, it is important to help the senior to feel safe rather than anxious. You cannot reason the senior out of the delusion, and it will not help to tell him that his idea is crazy.

The delusion has meaning to the senior. The content usually is organized around two main themes: his wishes and his fears. The senior usually fears that he is not going to live up to his own expected standards; he is unable to maintain his level of perfection. When his fears lessen and he either obtains or dismisses his wishes, then he can give up his delusion.[24]

Eventually he can look at himself and the world more realistically as the result of your consistent response and caring.

Reduce Stress

As you increase his self-esteem and develop a close relationship, you will help the senior feel less hopeless and helpless. As he feels more in control of himself, he will feel better able to handle stressful situations.

Certain aids are necessary. Eye glasses or a hearing aid help overcome sensory impairments. Illnesses should be treated so that the person has the energy to cope with other stresses. Safety hazards in his environment should be removed. Community resources should be used to obtain necessities, such as food or shelter, when indicated. Crisis intervention principles described in Chapter 13 can help him work through loss, rejection, or loneliness.

The physician may order phenothiazines, described in Chapter 21, to help alleviate anxiety. Drugs of choice include Thorazine, Mellaril, and Haldol.[3] These drugs are best given in liquid form to the paranoid senior; it has been estimated that 70 percent of the pills given to paranoid patients are not taken.[19] All of the phenothiazines come in liquid form.

Intervene Appropriately in the Patient's Behavior

Response to the patient's *suspicious behavior* should be matter-of-fact and honest. A consistent, secure environment is important. Avoid creating suspicion. Avoid touching unless you have found it successful with this person. Speak clearly and concisely. Avoid laughing in groups near the person. Whenever you make changes, allow for his personal interpretations. He may ask, "Why did you move the chair over there?" "Why are we eating at 4:00?" "Why are you coming to see me at 4:00 instead of 6:00?" Listen to his inquiries. Don't argue. Confront him carefully with the suspicious nature of questioning, but give the reason for change in a calm manner. Because he mistrusts everything and everyone, he may even ask you to taste his food before he eats it. Do so, and state matter-of-factly that it is not poisoned. If he wishes to check out his room, allow him to do so. Tell him in a calm, gentle manner about the reality of the situation and that you have nothing but good in mind for him. Be considerate of his feelings; respond to him with kindness even when he irritates you.

Although the senior's suspicious questioning and behavior may cause you to feel defensive, carry on your activities normally. Somtimes when you have someone checking your every move, you behave differently. But do not be maneuvered by his questions or behavior. When he feels more comfortable with you, he will be less suspicious. You must have patience to wait out his gradually increasing comfort.

The suspicious senior will probably be more fearful in groups of people. He needs experience first with one person whom he trusts before he learns to trust a group. Explain that he will not be harmed by the group. Encourage involvement in group activities; however, he will need to feel in control and set his own pace of involvement. Avoid competitive, aggressive activities and those necessitating close bodily contact. He will need your support; he will need to check out with you the reaction of the group members. Always remember that this person is a lonely, frightened person within the group even if he reacts to them with anger instead of fear.

The suspicious senior is often *angry, hostile, and demanding.* Do not take this behavior personally and do not retaliate with like behavior. Retaliation does not "teach him a lesson"; instead, it increases insecurity and acting-out behavior.

Do not argue to try to give advice to the angry patient. Do not tease him to attempt to humor him out of his feelings. Try to understand what caused his explosive behavior, why he is feeling threatened, rather than to belittle what he believes to be the difficulty. Remain calm, kind, and accepting of him as a person. Let him know that you care about him but that you cannot allow behavior that is harmful to himself or to others. Confront the senior with the results and implications of his behavior so that he can see its results. This cannot be done early in the relationship. At first the senior may not feel safe enough with you to hear the reality of the situation, but eventually he needs to hear in a nonpunitive way that his anger creates problems in living. Explore more acceptable ways of handling feelings. Help him feel more in control of himself and his immediate situation. Timing is crucial.

Activities may be helpful to an overtly angry person. A long walk, working with wood by sanding or hammering, pounding bread, or riding a bike may release energy to cope with angry feelings.

However, the more direct release of angry feelings comes through talking. Sometimes it helps to discuss neutral topics, so that pent-up feelings can be released and anger can be discussed as an emotion that can be handled. Recognize that frequently projection is operating and the angry feelings are in reality related to himself. Encourage the person to talk about himself and his feelings instead of about others and how they are behaving or feeling. Move very cautiously; the elderly person's ego and self-concept are very fragile when he appears the most threatening or hostile. Support positive feelings about himself so that his behavior can become more positive.

Often the senior is demanding of you and your time. Listen to his requests. Be considerate of him. Do not feel that you must meet all of his requests, but if his requests are reasonable, and you can meet them, do so. When you cannot, explain why. Evaluate his requests and try to understand the needs that he is trying to meet. If limits must be set, set them with kindness and consistency. If you can anticipate his needs before he asks, you can reduce some of his demanding behavior. If you do not know what he wants, ask him to help you by explaining as well as he can. Be calm; avoid punitive measures. Try to help him feel that you do want to help.

The senior with more control and personality integration will frequently be more in command of words and information. He may seem intellectual and use this tool to maintain a feeling of superiority over you. He may act very proud, belittle you, act as if he is better than you, and behave in a condescending manner. Often he will refuse to go along with the rules of the agency or· hospital regulations because he does not want to admit that he is ill or in need of help. Gently but firmly state the rules he must follow, and indicate that it is to his advantage not to create a fuss. Recognize that his proud, superior, condescending manner is a defense, and do not try to top his story or be superior to him. Instead, recognize his accomplishments and experience—where he is realistically ahead of you. Give him the opportunity to excel. When he feels accepted and secure, he will be less condescending.

Work with the Family and Other Health Team Members

Often the suspicious senior comes to your attention because the family can no longer handle him. Often his behavior toward the members is so intolerable that they wish to institutionalize him. At times, no long-term institutional care is available. Although your intervention with the senior in the home or hospital may improve his behavior somewhat, you will also have to teach the family to behave toward him in the manner described under Intervention. Often the family members have difficulty carrying out therapeutic responses; the memories of old harangues with him and habitual responses to him keep intruding. Both the senior and the family may be happier if you can arrange for him to live in his own apartment, with the family's help, or to be admitted to a nursing home if he wishes. Whatever arrangement is made will succeed only if the senior can make the decision, or thinks that it is his decision. Regardless of the arrangement, the family needs your support and helpful suggestions.

Anytime you care for a suspicious person, all health team workers who have contact with him must have a similar approach and be consistent in their behavior toward him. Otherwise, the senior will manipulate team members against each other or obtain favors that are not beneficial to him. Frequently confer with the other health workers who are involved in his care.

EVALUATION

Observe the senior closely for changes in behavior toward you and other people. As the suspicious person recovers from his illness, you may also note that you feel differently toward him. You will feel warmth from him and toward him. As he gains security, he will be more comfortable with others, act less angry, and attack others less frequently.

Can you expect changes in the paranoid elderly person? The prognosis is guarded, although the phenothiazine drugs help. Prognosis is most guarded in the case of the severely suspicious, withdrawn person.[15] In the one-year treatment of 93 paranoid patients over 60 years of age, Post found that 6 achieved employment, and 29 began to carry out domestic duties effectively. Yet, he felt that the results were mostly unfavorable because the patients' way of looking at life did not change very much. Results were highly dependent on adequate drug treatment.[20,21] Favorable prognostic signs are an immediate behavioral response to phenothiazines, marital status, a high social status, and good family relationships.[20,21] Prognosis is also better if the paranoid process has not been a long-term behavioral pattern and if organic brain disease or mental illness is not present.[17]

REFERENCES

1. AARONSON, LUREN, "Paranoia as a Behavior of Alienation," *Perspectives of Psychiatric Care,* 15: No. 1 (1977), 27–31.

2. BEVERLY, VIRGINIA, "Beginnings of Wisdom About Aging," *Geriatrics,* 30: (1975), 116–28.

3. BURNSIDE, IRENE, "Recognizing and Reducing Emotional Problems in the Aged," *Nursing 77,* 7: No. 3 (1977), 56–59.

4. BUSSE, EWARD, and ERIC PFEIFFER, *Mental Illness in Later Life.* Washington, D.C.: American Psychiatric Association, 1973.

5. BUTLER, ROBERT, and MYRNA LEWIS, *Aging and Mental Health.* St. Louis: The C. V. Mosby Company, 1977.

6. CAMERON, J., "Paranoid Conditions and Paranoia," in *American Handbook of Psychiatry,* ed. S. Arieti. New York: Basic Books, Inc., 1959, 475–84.

7. EISENDORFER, A., and F. WILKIE, "Auditory Changes in the Aged," *Journal of American Geriatric Society,* 8: (1972), 377–82.

8. FISH, F. J., "Senile Paranoid States," *Gerontology Clinics,* 1: (1959), 127–31.

9. FREUD, S., *The Complete Psychological Works of Sigmund Freud,* Vol. 14. London: Hogarth Press, 1959, pp. 82–91.

10. GOLLICKER, JACQUELINE, "A New Life at 77," *Nursing Mirror,* 137: (July 13, 1973), 34–37.

11. HINTON, JOHN, "Portrait of a Recluse," *Nursing Times,* 71: (October 30, 1975), 1753.

12. HOUSTON, R., and A. ROYSE, "Relationship Between Deafness and Psychotic Illness," *Journal of Mental Science,* 100: (1954), 990–93.

13. KAY, D. W. K., and M. ROTH, "Physical Accompaniments of Mental Disorder in Old Age," *Lancet,* 2: (1955), 740.

14. ———, "Environmental and Hereditary Factors in the Schizophrenics of Old Age and Their Bearing on the General Problem of Causation of Schizophrenia," *Journal of Mental Science,* 107: (1961), 649.

15. LANGLEY, G., "Functional Psychoses," in *Modern Perspectives in the Psychiatry of Old Age,* ed. John Howells. New York: Brunner/Mazel, 1975, pp. 326–55.

16. LIPSCOMB, W., "Acute Paranoia," *Emergency Medicine,* 1: (1969), 17–23.

17. MACKINNON, ROGER, and ROBERT MICHELS, *The Psychiatric Interview in Clinical Practice.* Philadelphia: W. B. Saunders Company, 1971, pp. 259–94.

18. MARTIN, IAN, "The Intruders," *Nursing Times,* 73: (February 17, 1977), 244–45.

19. PFEIFFER, ERIC, "Psychotherapy with Elderly Patients," in *Geriatric Psychiatry,* eds. Leopold Bellak and Taksoz Karasu. New York: Grune & Stratton, 1976, pp. 191–205.

20. PITT, BRICE, *Psychogeriatrics.* London: Churchill Livingstone Publishers, 1974.

21. RELTERSTAL, N., *Prognosis in Paranoid Psychoses.* Springfield, Ill.: Charles C Thomas, Publisher, 1970.

22. ROTH, M., "The Natural History of Mental Disorders in Old Age," *Journal of Mental Science,* 101: (1955), 201–301.

23. SOLOMON, PHILIP, and VERNON PATCH, *Handbook of Psychiatry.* Los Altos, Calif.: Lange Medical Publications, 1971.

24. SPANTON, JOHN, "Paraphrenic," *Nursing Times,* 71: (December 25, 1975), 2053–54.

25. STANKIEWICZ, B., "Guides to Nursing Intervention in the Projection Pattern of Suspicious Patients," *Perspectives of Psychiatric Care,* 2: No. 1 (1964), 39–47.

26. SULLIVAN, HARRY, *Clinical Studies in Psychiatry.* New York: W. W. Norton & Co., Inc., 1956, pp. 78–90.

27. TRAVELBEE, JOYCE, *Intervention in Psychiatric Nursing.* Philadelphia: F. A. Davis Company, 1969, pp. 177–211.

28. VERWOERDT, ADRIAAN, *Clinical Geropsychiatry.* Baltimore: The Williams & Wilkins Company, 1976.

29. WHITEHEAD, J., *Psychiatric Disorders in Old Age.* New York: Springer Publishing Co., Inc., 1974.

30. WICKS, ROBERT, *Counseling Strategies and Intervention Techniques for the Human Services.* Philadelphia: J. B. Lippincott Company, 1977.

index